OXFORD SPECIALTY TRAINING

The Pocketbook for PACES

Edited by

Rupa Bessant

Course Director PassPACES
www.passpaces.co.uk

T0177518

OXFORD
UNIVERSITY PRESS

OXFORD
UNIVERSITY PRESS

Great Clarendon Street, Oxford OX2 6DP,
United Kingdom

Oxford University Press is a department of the University of Oxford.
It furthers the University's objective of excellence in research, scholarship,
and education by publishing worldwide. Oxford is a registered trade mark of
Oxford University Press in the UK and in certain other countries

© Oxford University Press 2012

The moral rights of the authors have been asserted

First Edition published in 2012

British Library Cataloguing in Publication Data

Data available

Library of Congress Cataloging in Publication Data
Library of Congress Control Number: 2012934756

ISBN 978-0-19-957418-6

Printed in Great Britain
on acid-free paper by
Ashford Colour Press Ltd, Gosport, Hampshire

This book is dedicated to
my daughters,
Olivia and Serena,
who are my inspiration.

Foreword by Derek Bell

I am delighted to provide a foreword for *The Pocketbook for PACES*. Medical professional training and clinical practice, in the UK and internationally, is changing rapidly. As such all clinically based medical examinations must keep abreast of these changes if we are to ensure the highest quality of care is provided for all patients. The MRCP(UK) PACES examination is internationally recognized and has evolved to ensure that clinical practice is assessed in a robust and reproducible manner wherever the candidate takes this examination. Candidates sitting this examination must be competent in all clinical scenarios and in the related clinical domains. This textbook is clearly written and provides candidates with a robust framework to support their preparation for this important clinical examination. No individual textbook will provide a candidate with all the information and advice to prepare for PACES but this book offers the potential candidate a strong foundation as they hone their clinical skills. I would like to personally recommend this pocketbook and wish all readers revising for PACES every success.

Professor Derek Bell BSc MB ChB MD FRCP
Professor of Acute Medicine
Imperial College London

Foreword by Gerald Coakley

It is a great honour and pleasure to write a foreword for *The Pocketbook for PACES*. Elegantly produced with a coherent structure followed consistently throughout the book, it is very clearly focused on the current format and content of the PACES examination, as well as having a chapter aimed at the MRCPI. I am impressed by the level of relevant detail concerning the conditions that commonly feature in the exam, as well as useful examination and presentation techniques. The sections on communication and history are full of helpful information, and provide a logical starting point in preparing for stations 2 and 4, for which I know many candidates find it challenging to revise. By reading the book, I have learned a lot about the modern management of conditions outside my own specialty, and even one or two new things about my own. The distinguished authors have clearly put a great deal of thought into their chapters, informed by long experience in teaching MRCP candidates.

I am an admirer of PACES, believing that unlike many other medical examinations, it helps to make the candidate a better doctor. The examination marks a transition from the novice towards the expert diagnostician. As undergraduates, we are taught the time-honoured ritual of taking a full history, and examining every system in the hope of coming to the correct diagnosis. Experts do not work like this, but rather generate hypotheses as they interrogate the patient, and examine and investigate to rule out differentials to come to the correct diagnosis. Experts make the correct diagnosis more rapidly and with sparser information than novices.

The PACES examination helps to assess whether candidates are starting to make this transition, while also assessing communication and professional skills. The examination helps to sort trainable young physicians from 'book doctors' who know 10 causes of renal tubular acidosis and the path of the seventh cranial nerve, but cannot suggest a sensible approach to help Mrs Jones with her painful erythema nodosum or peripheral oedema.

The PACES examination, in essence, assesses whether candidates have mastered the skill of integrating years of theoretical learning with good history-taking and examination skills, to come up with an appropriate differential including the correct diagnosis for the patient in front of them, and communicate that effectively. I believe that the structure of *The Pocketbook for PACES* will help candidates in making this transition from novice to proto-expert, making them both more likely to pass the exam, and also better physicians.

Dr Gerald Coakley PhD FRCP
Consultant Rheumatologist & Physician
Director of Medical Education
South London Healthcare Trust

Preface

This book aims to provide prospective candidates with a comprehensive, yet concise and convenient guide to the MRCP PACES examination, which is portable and can be used as a constant point of reference throughout routine clinical duties.

Whilst this book is primarily intended to help candidates prepare for PACES, many undergraduate medical examinations and other postgraduate examinations have adopted a similar assessment model. Candidates preparing for these examinations may also find this book beneficial.

The PACES examination forms an integral part of Core Medical Training. Preparation for PACES should not be seen simply as time devoted to passing an assessment, but rather as an invaluable and hopefully enjoyable part of a physician's continuing professional development.

The examiners are not expecting a depth of knowledge commensurate with being a consultant in a specialist field, but rather they are looking for a confident, competent and caring doctor to whom they would be happy to entrust the care of their patients. A logical approach based on experience and understanding, combined with an ability to communicate appropriately with both patients and examiners will stand a candidate in good stead when entering the PACES examination.

Careful preparation is essential and this must include both in-depth reading around common examination scenarios, as well as regular practise of clinical examination, communication and history-taking skills.

Familiarity with the format, marking scheme and time constraints of the examination is essential to ensure that a candidate completes the necessary tasks and scores the highest possible marks at each Station.

Our emphasis throughout has been on equipping the candidate with the knowledge required to tailor their routine clinical examination to the many different scenarios that may be encountered, to make diagnoses appropriate to their findings, to formulate a relevant management plan, to predict the direction of the examiner's questions and answer these competently.

Candidates who are well prepared should approach the PACES examination not with trepidation, but with confidence and maintain that confidence throughout the examination.

The editor and chapter authors have combined their extensive clinical knowledge and practical teaching experience to create a book that we believe will help you to maximize your chances of success in PACES. We hope that candidates will both enjoy and benefit from this book and their PACES preparation. Good luck to you all!

Rupa Bessant

Acknowledgements

Firstly I would like to express my gratitude to the many delightful patients I have encountered during almost 20 years of MRCP clinical teaching. These individuals have regularly volunteered their valuable time to enable today's trainee physicians to develop the skills they require to become tomorrow's consultants and professors.

Secondly I wish to thank all those colleagues who have encouraged me to pursue my interest in medical education, those who supported me in my role as Course Director for the University College London Hospitals and Guy's and St. Thomas' Hospitals PACES Courses, and those who continue to assist me during the PassPACES clinical courses.

I am greatly indebted to all the authors who have contributed their expertise and experience to writing the chapters of this book. In addition my thanks go to Dr Christopher Harvey and Dr Robert Thomas for their radiology input throughout the book.

I would like to thank Olivia Bessant for her artwork and design of the cover of this book.

I am most grateful to Dr Gerald Coakley, Dr Charlotte Ford, Dr Refik Gökmen, Dr Elena Nikiphorou and Dr Marlies Ostermann, for their help with the preparation of the manuscript.

I would like to acknowledge the St. John's Institute of Dermatology and Moorfields Eye Hospital for their permission to use clinical photographs, and the publishers and authors who have allowed us to reproduce their illustrations in this book.

I would also like to thank Christopher Reid, Commissioning Editor at the Oxford University Press, and his team for offering me the privilege of editing this Pocketbook.

Finally I would like to thank my family for their love and encouragement throughout my career. In particular, I would like to acknowledge my husband, David, who has supported me wholeheartedly throughout the long gestation of this book.

Rupa Bessant

Acknowledgements

Firstly, I would like to express my gratitude to the many delightful persons it have encountered on my journey to writing this book...

Rupa Besong

Contents

Contributors

**Behdad Afzali MBBS
MRCP(UK) PhD MAcadMEd**
Clinical Lecturer in Renal
Medicine,
MRC Centre for Transplantation,
King's College London,
London, UK

**Owen Anderson MBChB,
BSc, MRCP(UK), MRCOpth**
Specialist Registrar,
Moorfields Eye Hospital,
London, UK

**David Bessant BSc(Hons)
MBChB FRCOphth MD**
Consultant Ophthalmic Surgeon,
Moorfields Eye Hospital,
London, UK

**Rupa Bessant MBChB MSc
MRCP(UK)**
Course Director PassPACES,
www.passpaces.co.uk

**Jonathan Birns BSc(Hons)
MBBS(Hons) MRCP(UK)
PhD**
Consultant in Stroke Medicine,
Geriatrics and General Medicine,
Guy's and St Thomas' NHS
Foundation Trust,
London
Honorary Senior Lecturer,
King's College London,
London, UK

**Danny Cheriyan MBBCh
MRCPI**
Specialist Registrar in
Gastroenterology,
Beaumont Hospital,
Dublin, Republic of Ireland

**Sanjay H. Chotirmall
MBBCh BAO MRCPI
MRCP(UK)**
Respiratory Specialist Registrar,
Department of Respiratory
Medicine,
Beaumont Hospital,
Dublin, Republic of Ireland

**Gerry Christofi BSc(Hons),
BMBCh, MRCP(UK), PhD**
Specialist Registrar in Neurology,
National Hospital for
Neurology and Neurosurgery,
London, UK

**Jennifer M. Crawley
BSc MBChB MRCP(UK)
(Derm)**
Clinical Fellow in Dermatology,
St John's Institute of
Dermatology,
St Thomas' Hospital,
London
Specialty Registrar in
Dermatology,
Royal Victoria Hospital,
Belfast, UK

**Colin M. Dayan
MA FRCP PhD**
Professor of Clinical Diabetes and
Metabolism,
Cardiff University School of
Medicine,
Centre for Endocrine and
Diabetes Science,
Cardiff, UK

Mike Fisher MBChB FRCP(UK) PhD

Consultant in General and Interventional Cardiology, Institute of Cardiovascular and Medical Sciences, Liverpool Heart and Chest Hospital and The Royal Liverpool University Hospital, Liverpool

Honorary Senior Lecturer, Imperial College, London, UK

Chris J. Harvey BSc MBBS MRCP(UK) FRCR

Consultant Radiologist and Senior Lecturer, Department of Imaging, Hammersmith Hospital, London, UK

Robin S. Howard PhD FRCP

Consultant Neurologist Guy's and St Thomas' NHS Foundation Trust, London

National Hospital for Neurology and Neurosurgery, London, UK

Tevfik F. Ismail, BSc (Hons) MBBS MRCP(UK)

Specialist Registrar Cardiology and GIM, North West Thames Rotation, London, UK

Guy Leschziner MA MRCP(UK) PhD

Consultant Neurologist, Guy's and St Thomas' NHS Foundation Trust, London, UK

Myles J. Lewis PhD MRCP(UK)

Consultant Rheumatologist, Guy's and St Thomas' NHS Foundation Trust, London, UK

Helen Liddicoat, BSc(Hons), MBBS, MRCP(UK)

Specialist Registrar in Respiratory and General Internal Medicine, North East Thames Rotation, London, UK

Michael Nandakumar MB ChB MRCP(UK) MRCGP DFSRH DRCOG DCH DPD

General Practitioner and Honorary Clinical Tutor, Department of Medical and Social Care Education, University of Leicester, Leicester, UK

Julian T. Nash BSc MBBCh PhD FRCP

Consultant Rheumatologist, University Hospital of Wales, Cardiff, UK

Rupert P. M. Negus FRCP PhD

Consultant Physician and Gastroenterologist, Clinical Lead for Acute Medicine, Royal Free Hospital, London, UK

William L. G. Oldfield MSc PhD FRCP

Consultant in Respiratory Medicine and Chief of Service for Emergency Medicine, Imperial College Healthcare NHS Trust, London, UK

Stephen Patchett MD FRCPI

Dean of Examinations, Royal College of Physicians of Ireland, Dublin

Consultant Physician and Gastroenterologist, Beaumont Hospital, Dublin, Republic of Ireland

Andrew E. Pink BMedSci (Hons) BMBS MRCP(UK)
Academic Clinical Fellow,
MRC Clinical Research Training Fellow,
St. John's Institute of Dermatology,
Guy's and St Thomas' NHS Foundation Trust,
London
King's College London,
London, UK

Peter Taylor BSc MBChB MRCP(UK) SCE (Diab/endo)
Welsh Clinical Academic Trainee,
Cardiff University School of Medicine,
Centre for Endocrine and Diabetes Science,
Cardiff, UK

Robert H. Thomas MBBS BSc(Hons) MRCP(UK) FRCR
Specialist Registrar in Radiology,
Guy's and St Thomas' Hospitals NHS Foundation Trust,
London, UK

Jonathan White BSc (Hons) MBChB MRCP(UK)
Consultant Dermatologist and Honorary Senior Lecturer,
St John's Institute of Dermatology,
St Thomas' Hospital, London
King's College London,
London, UK

Symbols and abbreviations

❶	Top Tips
❢	Common Pitfalls
♫	Useful websites
📖	Further reading
⊃	Cross reference
~	approximately
±	plus/minus
↑	increased
↓	decreased
→	leading to
≥	greater than or equal to
≤	less than or equal to
A&E	Accident and Emergency
AAA	abdominal aortic aneurysm
ABG	arterial blood gas
ABV	alcohol by volume
ACE	angiotensin-converting enzyme
AChR	acetylcholine receptor
ACTH	adrenocorticotropic hormone
ADH	anti-diuretic hormone
ADL	activity of daily living
ADPKD	autosomal dominant polycystic kidney disease
AFB	acid-fast bacillus
AFO	ankle–foot orthosis
ALP	alkaline phosphatase
AMA	anti-mitochondrial antibody
ANA	antinuclear antibody
ANCA	antineutrophil cytoplasmic antigen antibody
APB	abductor pollicis brevis
APCKD	adult polycystic kidney disease
APLS	antiphospholipid syndrome
AR	aortic regurgitation
ARDS	acute respiratory distress syndrome
ASD	atrial septal defect
AV	atrioventricular
AVM	arteriovenous malformation

AVN	avascular necrosis
BAL	bronchoalveolar lavage
BCG	bacillus Calmette–Guérin
BD	twice daily
BiPAP	bi-level positive airway pressure
BMI	body mass index
bpm	beats per minute
BSR	British Society for Rheumatology
BTS	British Thoracic Society
CADASIL	cerebral autosomal dominant arteriopathy with subcortical infarcts and leucoencephalopathy
CCF	congestive cardiac failure
CD	Crohn's disease
CF	cystic fibrosis
CIDP	chronic inflammatory demyelinating polyradiculoneuropathy
CIS	clinically isolated syndrome
CK	creatine kinase
CKD	chronic kidney disease
CLD	chronic liver disease
CLL	chronic lymphocytic leukaemia
CML	chronic myeloid leukaemia
CMV	cytomegalovirus
CNS	central nervous system
CO	carbon monoxide
CO_2	carbon dioxide
COPD	chronic obstructive pulmonary disease
CPAP	continuous positive airway pressure
Cr	creatinine
CRH	corticotropin-releasing hormone
CRP	C-reactive protein
CSF	cerebrospinal fluid
CT	computed tomography
CTA	computed tomography angiogram
CTD	connective tissue disease
CTPA	computed tomography pulmonary angiogram
CTS	carpal tunnel syndrome
CVA	cerebrovascular accident
CVD	cardiovascular disease
CXR	chest x-ray
DDA	Disability Discrimination Act

DHx	drug history
DIP	desquamative interstitial pneumonia
DIP	distal interphalangeal
DLCO	diffusion capacity
DMARD	disease-modifying antirheumatic drug
DMT	disease-modifying therapy
DSM-IV	*Diagnostic and Statistical Manual of Mental Disorders,* version IV
DVLA	Driver and Vehicle Licensing Agency
DVT	deep vein thrombosis
DWI	diffusion-weighted imaging
Dx	diagnosis
ECG	electrocardiogram
EDM	early diastolic murmur
EF	ejection fraction
EMG	electromyography
ENA	extractable nuclear antigen
ESM	ejection systolic murmur
ESR	erythrocyte sedimentation rate
ESRD	end-stage renal disease
EtOH	alcohol
EUS	endobronchial ultrasound
F/U	follow-up
FBC	full blood count
FEV_1	forced expiratory volume in 1 second
FHx	family history
FSH	follicle-stimulating hormone
FVC	forced vital capacity
FY1	1st year doctor
g	gram/s
G&S	group and save
GCA	giant cell arteritis
GGT	gamma glutamyl transpeptidase
GH	growth hormone
GI	gastrointestinal
GMC	General Medical Council
GP	general practitioner
hCG	human chorionic gonadotropin
HD	Huntington's disease
HHT	hereditary haemorrhagic telangiectasia
HIV	human immunodeficiency virus

HMG-CoA	3-hydroxy-3-methylglutaryl-coenzyme A
HOCM	hypertrophic obstructive cardiomyopathy
HPC	history of presenting complaint
HRCT	high-resolution computed tomography
IBD	inflammatory bowel disease
ICD	implantable cardioverter-defibrillator
ICU	intensive care unit
IE	infective endocarditis
IgG	immunoglobulin G
IHD	ischaemic heart disease
IHF	Irish Heart Foundation
IL	interleukin
ILD	interstitial lung disease
IM	intramuscular
INO	internuclear ophthalmoplegia
INR	international normalized ratio of prothrombin time
IP	interphalangeal
IPAH	idiopathic pulmonary arterial hypertension
IPF	idiopathic pulmonary fibrosis
ITU	intensive care unit
IV	intravenous
JVP	jugular venous pressure
LA	left atrium/atrial
LDH	lactate dehydrogenase
LDL	low density lipoprotein
LEMS	Lambert–Eaton myasthenic syndrome
LFT	liver function test
LH	luteinizing hormone
LIF	left iliac fossa
LMN	lower motor neuron
LMWH	low-molecular-weight heparin
LTOT	long-term oxygen therapy
LV	left ventricle/ventricular
LVEDD	left ventricular end-diastolic diameter
LVH	left ventricular hypertrophy
LVOT	left ventricular outflow tract
mané	in the morning
MCP	metacarpophalangeal
MCS	microscopy, culture and sensitivity
MCTD	mixed connective tissue disease
MCV	mean corpuscular volume

MDI	metered dose inhaler
MDM	mid-diastolic murmur
MELAS	mitochondrial encephalomyopathy, lactic acidosis and stroke
MERRF	myoclonic epilepsy with ragged red fibres
mg	milligram/s
MHA	Mental Health Act
MI	myocardial infarction
mL	millilitre/s
MMNCB	multifocal motor neuropathy with conduction block
MND	motor neuron disease
MR	mitral regurgitation *or* magnetic resonance
MRC	Medical Research Council
MRCP	Membership of the Royal College of Physicians
MRCPI	Membership of the Royal College of Physicians of Ireland
MRSA	meticillin-resistant *Staphylococcus aureus*
MS	mitral stenosis *or* multiple sclerosis
MSA	multisystem atrophy
MV	mitral valve
MVA	mitral valve area
NHL	non-Hodgkin's lymphoma
NHS	National Health Service
NICE	National Institute for Health and Clinical Excellence
NIV	non-invasive ventilation
NKDA	no known drug allergy
NMJ	neuromuscular junction
nocté	at night
NSAID	non-steroidal anti-inflammatory drug
NSCLC	non-small-cell lung cancer
NSIP	non-specific interstitial pneumonia
NYHA	New York Heart Association
OD	once daily
OGD	oesophagogastroduodenoscopy
OGTT	oral glucose tolerance test
OPMD	oculopharyngeal muscular dystrophy
OS	opening snap
OSA	obstructive sleep apnoea
PACES	Practical Assessment of Clinical Examination Skills
PAF	paroxysmal atrial fibrillation
PAN	polyarteritis nodosa
p-ANCA	perinuclear anti-neutrophil cytoplasmic antibody

PaO$_2$	partial pressure of oxygen in arterial blood
PASP	pulmonary artery systolic pressure
PAWP	pulmonary artery wedge pressure
PBC	primary biliary cirrhosis
PBMV	percutaneous balloon mitral valvuloplasty
PCOS	polycystic ovarian syndrome
PCR	polymerase chain reaction
PDA	patent ductus arteriosus
PE	pulmonary embolism
PEFR	peak expiratory flow rate
PEG	percutaneous endoscopic gastrostomy
PEP	positive expiratory pressure
PET	positron emission tomography
PI	protease inhibitor
PIP	proximal interphalangeal
PJS	Peutz–Jeghers syndrome
PMHx	personal medical history
PML	progressive multifocal leucoencephalopathy
PMR	polymyalgia rheumatica
PNS	peripheral nervous system
PR	pulmonary regurgitation
PRN	as required
PS	pulmonary stenosis
PsA	psoriatic arthritis
PSM	pan-systolic murmur
PTH	parathyroid hormone
PTLD	post-transplant lymphoproliferative disorder
PV	pulmonary valve
PVD	peripheral vascular disease
PVE	prosthetic valve endocarditis
PVNS	pigmented villonodular synovitis
QID	four times a day
RA	rheumatoid arthritis
RAPD	relative afferent pupillary defect
RCT	randomized controlled trial
RF	rheumatoid factor
RIF	right iliac fossa
ROS	systems review
RRT	renal replacement therapy
RV	right ventricle/ventricular
RVOT	right ventricular outflow tract

SAH	subarachnoid haemorrhage
SaO_2	oxygen saturation in haemoglobin
SBP	spontaneous bacterial peritonitis
SCLC	small-cell lung cancer
SHO	senior house officer
SHx	social history
SIADH	syndrome of inappropriate anti-diuretic hormone
SLE	systemic lupus erythematosus
SSc	systemic sclerosis
STI	sexually transmitted disease
SVC	superior vena cava
SVCO	superior vena cava obstruction
T_3	triiodothyronine
T_4	thyroxine
TB	tuberculosis
TBNA	transbronchial needle aspiration
TED	thyroid eye disease
TFT	thyroid function test
TIA	transient ischaemic attack
TIPS	transjugular intrahepatic portosystemic shunt
TLC	total lung capacity
TLCO	total lung carbon monoxide
TNF	tumour necrosis factor
TOE	transoesophageal echocardiography
TR	tricuspid regurgitation
TSH	thyroid-stimulating hormone
TST	tuberculin skin testing
TTE	transthoracic echocardiography
TV	tricuspid valve
U&E	urea and electrolytes
UC	ulcerative colitis
UIP	usual interstitial pneumonia
µL	microlitre/s
UMN	upper motor neuron
UV	ultraviolet
VATS	video assisted thoracoscopic surgery
VSD	ventricular septal defect
VT	ventricular tachycardia
vWF	von Willebrand factor
WCC	white cell count
WHO	World Health Organization

Introduction

Rupa Bessant

Royal College of Physicians

The Royal College of Physicians was founded by royal charter of King Henry VIII in 1518. For nearly 500 years it has engaged in a wide range of activities dedicated to its overall aim of upholding and improving standards of medical practice.

The examination for the Membership of the Royal College of Physicians (MRCP) (London) was first set in 1859. The Royal College of Physicians (Edinburgh) and the Faculty of Physicians and Surgeons of Glasgow introduced their own professional examinations in 1881 and 1886 respectively.

A need to have a unified membership examination throughout the United Kingdom (UK) was identified in the late 1960s, following which the first joint examination took place in October 1968. The MRCP(UK) subsequently developed into the current internationally recognized three-part examination.

The PACES examination

From 2001, the five-station PACES (Practical Assessment of Clinical Examination Skills) examination was introduced, replacing the traditional long case, short cases and viva format. The rationale for this change was to standardize the candidate experience, to permit direct observation of candidate–patient interaction throughout the examination, and to place added emphasis on the assessment of communication skills.

The MRCP(UK) format evolved further in 2009. In response to the development of competency-based training and assessment, the key components of the examination were redefined as seven 'core clinical skills':

A) Physical examination
B) Identifying physical signs
C) Clinical communication skills
D) Differential diagnosis
E) Clinical judgement
F) Managing patients' concerns
G) Maintaining patient welfare.

Each 'core clinical skill' is assessed at several different stations of the PACES examination and the marks for each 'skill' are integrated. A minimum pass mark for each 'core clinical skill' was introduced to ensure that candidates who scored poorly in one 'core clinical skill' area could not pass the examination by scoring highly in another skill (a compensatory marking system had existed prior to 2009). Furthermore, the requirement to obtain a minimum overall test score has been maintained. At the time of writing this book, a score of 130/172 was required to pass (Table 1.1).

The second major change in 2009 was to replace the four short (5-minute) cases in Station 5 (Skin, Locomotor, Endocrine, Eyes) with two 'Brief clinical consultations' (each lasting 10 minutes). This format attempts to accurately reflect the real-life clinical practice of trainees. Since there is no longer any restriction on the type of cases that can be encountered, this permits medical specialities that were previously excluded, such as acute and elderly medicine, to be examined. Nevertheless, cases which previously appeared in the old format Station 5 are still frequently encountered.

Between October 2009 and July 2010 over 4500 candidates sat the MRCP(UK) examination in over 100 centres in the UK and nine international centres in the Middle East and Asia. The mean pass rate during this period was 44.4%.[1]

Whilst this book is primarily intended to help candidates prepare for the MRCP PACES examination, many undergraduate medical examinations and other postgraduate examinations have adopted a similar assessment model. Undergraduate students preparing for medical finals may also find this book beneficial. The cases examined for finals and MRCP are often identical, with the principal difference being in the depth of knowledge required.

Table 1.1 Core clinical skills assessed at each PACES station

Core clinical skill	A	B	C	D	E	F	G	Total
Respiratory	4	4		4	4		4	20
Abdomen	4	4		4	4		4	20
History taking			4	4	4	4	4	20
Cardiology	4	4		4	4		4	20
Neurology	4	4		4	4		4	20
Communication			4		4	4	4	16
Brief consultations	8	8	8	8	8	8	8	56
Total	24	24	16	28	32	16	32	172

Numbers represent maximum mark in each core clinical skill at each station. Individual examiners award a satisfactory (2 marks), borderline (1 mark) or unsatisfactory (0 marks) judgement for each skill. A minimum score of 130 out of 172 is required to pass

Format of the PACES examination

The PACES examination consists of five clinical stations.

In order to ensure that the examination is fair, candidates are assessed at each station by two independent examiners, who are non-specialists in the systems that they are examining. As a result, every candidate will be assessed by ten different examiners. Examiners are not permitted to confer when awarding marks. Therefore, a candidate's performance at one station will not influence their marks at subsequent stations.

Candidates may start their examination at any one of the five stations, and then rotate around the carousel, until they have completed all five stations (Fig. 1.1, page 5). Each station lasts for 20 minutes, with a 5-minute interval between each station.

Stations 1 and 3: Physical examination

Four of the major systems, Abdominal and Respiratory (Station 1), Cardiology and Neurology (Station 3) are assessed individually for a total of 10 minutes each.

The Royal College of Physicians' website states that: 'The emphasis in these stations is on the demonstration of comprehensive and correct physical examination technique, the ability to detect physical signs, the ability to construct a differential diagnosis, the ability to suggest sensible and appropriate treatment and investigation plans, and the ability to treat a patient with dignity and respect'.

The candidate has 6 minutes to perform the physical examination and 4 minutes to answer the examiners' questions.

Station 2: History taking

The history-taking station aims to determine whether the candidate can gather from a patient the requisite information, form a differential diagnosis, construct a management plan and explain this plan clearly to the patient whilst dealing with any concerns he or she may have.

14 minutes are allotted for the history taking, and after a minute of reflection there follows 5 minutes of discussion with the examiners.

Station 4: Communication skills

The communication skills station is designed to assess the candidate's ability to conduct an interview with a subject (who is frequently an actor, but may be a patient, relative, or healthcare worker), to explain clinical information in a manner that the subject can understand, to apply clinical knowledge, including knowledge of ethics, to the management of the case or situation, and to provide emotional support to the subject.

Once again, 14 minutes are given for the interview, followed by a minute of reflection and 5 minutes of discussion with the examiners.

Station 5: Brief clinical consultations

This station consists of two 'integrated clinical assessments' and is designed to assess the way in which a candidate approaches a clinical problem in an integrated manner, using history taking, communication and physical examination skills.

For each of the two cases the candidate has 8 minutes with the patient to elicit the history, examine the patient and respond to their concerns. There follows 2 minutes to discuss the diagnosis and management plan with the examiners.

Candidates should familiarize themselves with the marking scheme for each station

The marking scheme indicates which of the seven 'core clinical skills' are assessed at each station and outlines how a candidate is expected to perform in order to score marks in each category. The current mark sheets can be downloaded from the MRCP(UK) website.

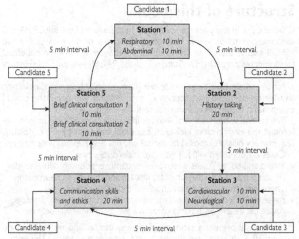

Fig. 1.1 PACES carousel.

Structure of this book

Chapters 2–8 in this pocketbook appear in the order of the MRCP PACES examination stations. The final chapter focuses on long cases for the MRCPI examination. The scenarios in this chapter will also be beneficial to candidates preparing for Station 2 of the PACES examination (History taking).

For the physical examination stations (Respiratory, Abdomen, Cardiology, and Neurology), the first section of each chapter will detail the clinical examination technique appropriate to that system.

The second section will deal with the individual cases likely to be encountered in the examination. Individual cases will focus on specific conditions (e.g. primary biliary cirrhosis) or clinical findings (e.g. hepatosplenomegaly).

Cases encountered will fall into two main categories:

- 'Bread and butter' cases which are frequently encountered in everyday clinical practice e.g. valvular heart disease and peripheral neuropathy. These require a slick presentation and thorough knowledge.
- Rarer and/or complex cases (e.g. with multiple pathologies). Strategic advice for dealing with these cases in a logical manner will be given.

Each case will present a synopsis of the key clinical findings to elicit and present, the relevant investigations and management plan. The topics likely to emerge during questioning of the candidate by the examiners are highlighted and referred to as **Viva questions**.

Whilst general advice relevant to all clinical examination stations is discussed in this introductory chapter, examination techniques that are unique to a particular specialty will be included in the appropriate section (e.g. the ophthalmology section describes the use of an ophthalmoscope).

For those wishing to explore a topic further, many cases include 📖 **Further reading** and 🕸 **Useful websites**.

❶ **Top Tips** and ☞ **Common Pitfalls** will be used throughout the text to highlight some of the most important points.

❶ **Top Tips**
- Talk to senior trainees who have sat the PACES examination recently and learn from their experiences.

☞ **Common Pitfalls**
- Do not delay your preparation until the time of submitting your application to sit the PACES examination, or worse still, the time at which the Royal College sends your exam date to you!
- Many candidates do not appreciate the extent of the preparation required until they begin their revision (having lived in ignorant bliss until that time!).

History taking (⊕ Chapter 4)
The introduction to this chapter offers a structured approach to history taking and includes a template which can be applied to any scenario encountered in the examination.

Communication skills (⊃ Chapter 7)

This chapter provides a strategic approach to enable candidates to handle the sensitive issues and ethical dilemmas encountered. All of the main ethical and legal frameworks are discussed where appropriate in each scenario. The scenarios are grouped according to the main themes that are represented in the examination:

- Breaking bad news
- Explaining a new diagnosis
- Counselling
- Chronic disease management
- Speaking to relatives and colleagues.

Brief clinical consultation (⊃ Chapter 8)

The introduction to this chapter describes how to integrate history taking, physical examination and communication skills within the 8 minutes allocated to each Station 5 consultation. The remainder of the chapter outlines relevant clinical cases, selected on the basis of a survey of previous PACES candidates. These cases demonstrate the strategic approach to the Integrated Clinical Assessment and are divided into:

- Acute medicine
- Rheumatology
- Endocrinology
- Ophthalmology
- Dermatology.

Preparation for PACES

Thorough preparation for the PACES examination is essential to maximize the chance of success. Beyond the examination itself the knowledge and clinical expertise gained will serve as an invaluable supplement to a physician's core medical training, regardless of their eventual specialty.

Revision plan

Early planning is advisable, so that a revision timetable can be incorporated into the busy working weeks leading up to the PACES examination. Starting your revision early will give you the opportunity to address any weaknesses you identify. Once you have decided when to sit the examination, sit down with your diary and calculate the number of weeks that are available for your preparation. Remember to allow for weeks during which you may be changing jobs, on holiday or on nights/long shifts.

Choosing the right PACES books

Most of the theoretical clinical knowledge required will already have been learned during your preparation for MRCP Part I and Part II Written.

In addition to this pocketbook, you should consider buying a larger textbook. Spend some time in a bookshop with a good medical section and select a book that is suitable for your learning style. A good tip is to select a few clinical conditions and compare how these are approached in two or three books – this will quickly identify the text written in the format best suited to you.

Divide the reading up into sections to be covered each week. Remember, when required, you can always supplement the books chosen with further information from Internet-based resources. Many of the cases included in this book have suggested references and weblinks for further reading.

It is recommended that you read through this pocketbook systematically, but also carry it with you when you examine patients, both during your routine clinical work and when you review patients in preparation for PACES. This pocketbook highlights the key points of each case and suggests ways in which you may extend your examination for a particular patient. If you have omitted any part of the examination, you will be able to return to your patient immediately to see if these clinical signs can be elicited. Reading relevant exam-oriented information shortly after reviewing patients will reinforce the key facts for each scenario and help you to recall them during the PACES examination. This process will also help to make the essential techniques of clinical examination second nature.

> **❶ Top Tips**
> - Carrying *The Pocketbook for PACES* with you will facilitate your revision greatly.
> - Reading the main points immediately after reviewing a patient will help you remember these key facts during your examination.

Examining patients

Gather together a group of colleagues who are also sitting the PACES examination at your hospital. Look through your rotas and timetable slots during which you can review patients together – aim to review patients two or three times each week, more frequently as the examination approaches.

Always inform patients that you are going to examine them as part of your PACES preparation, i.e. explain the purpose of your examination. If you are already aware of the diagnosis, be the examiner for one of your colleagues – it is good to practice being on the other side of the fence too!

It is also important to draw on the experience of senior colleagues during your teaching sessions wherever possible. Most hospitals in the UK will have at least a handful of consultants who are willing to teach PACES at the bedside, but you will probably need to ask unless they are very pro-active. Registrars who have recently sat the PACES examination can provide important insights into the examination and act as simulated examiners.

Although examination is part of routine medical assessment, each aspect of the PACES examination is assessed formally and under strict time constraints. Always time each other when practising for PACES. Candidates who have repeatedly practised formal clinical examination of each system will perform this task much better under the stress of examination conditions.

Stations 1 and 3: Physical examination. Aim to complete the basic examination of each patient with a minute to spare, so that the examination can be appropriately extended and your opening statement formulated.

Station 2: History taking. Ask your colleague to introduce a patient to you by describing their presenting complaint. Take a history under timed conditions, followed by 5 minutes of viva questioning.

Station 4: Communication skills. Communication skills preparation is best undertaken in a group of three, with each candidate taking it in turns in the role of the patient/relative, candidate and examiner. Discussion around the case will involve all three candidates.

We would advise candidates to use the 16 scenarios presented in Chapter 7 for this purpose. The 'examiner' and the 'subject' should prepare the scenario, whilst the 'candidate' should not read the scenario in advance.

Station 5: Brief clinical consultations. This station involves focused history, examination and communication with the patient. Whilst this simulates real-life consultations, candidates must be aware that the time available (8 minutes) is very limited. It is therefore essential to focus on the specific clinical issue presented in the scenario. It is crucial to practise for Station 5 by carrying out timed consultations with patients prior to the actual PACES examination.

Remember to get plenty of sleep in the weeks running up to your PACES examination. Tiredness will have an adverse effect on both preparation and also performance on the day of the examination.

❶ Top Tips

- Examining patients and simulating scenarios is the most essential part of your revision, which cannot be undertaken with as much flexibility as the bookwork. Schedule this first and then fit the reading around the practical preparation.
- It is very apparent to an examiner how many times a candidate has carried out a physical examination by the fluency of their technique, so a rapid, reproducible order should be practised for each system.
- The onus of organizing the revision schedule lies with each candidate.

❖ Common Pitfalls

- Do not omit preparation for Stations 2, 4 and 5, which carry a large component of the marks.
- Timing is frequently an issue with the clinical stations, so practise keeping to time!
- If you finish prior to 'the bell' consider how you can extend your examination appropriately – remember that standing in silence will not score any marks and may lead to a feeling of unease for the candidate.

Attend a PACES revision course

Whilst reading and reviewing patients in your own hospital are both essential parts of preparation for PACES, a lot can be gained by attending a PACES revision course.

During a well-organized course you would expect to see most of the common PACES cases and a substantial number of patients with rarer disorders that you are much less likely to encounter during your routine clinical work in the short time available before the examination.

In addition, you can expect to benefit from experienced lecturers who teach and examine in different ways. Examiners are also individuals and have different styles of questioning. It is therefore important that you expose yourself to varied approaches to being examined before your PACES examination.

Finally, your course will prepare you best if it includes a mock examination.

The ideal course balances time devoted to delivering excellent bedside teaching with a wide spectrum of clinical cases and communication/history scenarios. In order to meet these requirements and cover the PACES examination comprehensively, a well-structured course requires 4 full days.

Shorter courses devoted to specific parts of the PACES examination, such as Neurology and Ophthalmology or Communication skills may also be very valuable, particularly if you perceive these to be your weak points.

❶ Top Tips

- Attending a comprehensive PACES course should be viewed as being at a 'finishing school,' completing your preparation, but not as a substitute for the regular review of patients.

The examination day

Dress code

Think about what you plan to wear to the examination beforehand. We would advise you to wear smart conservative clothes. NHS hospitals in the UK currently have a 'bare below the elbows' policy, and you would be advised to enter the examination without a wrist watch, and either role up your sleeves or wear a smart short-sleeved shirt/blouse, and for males, ties should be pinned or tucked in to your shirt.

Many patients have a certain expectation of what their doctor should wear. You need to be able to satisfy this requirement for all patients, and in doing so, will meet the expectations of the examiners.

The examiners should remember you for your clinical acumen, and not the flamboyance of your attire!

Clothes with suitable pockets may enable you to carry your stethoscope and other small items without resorting to a bag.

Ensure that your fingernails are cut short and long hair is tied back neatly.

Presentation on the day

All patients should be treated with the utmost care and respect throughout your career. Despite this ideal, under the pressure of the PACES examination, candidates may respond differently to how they would in normal everyday practice, thereby forgetting that there is a real person in front of them.

Patients accept that a clinical examination may cause a degree of pain because they understand that this is an inevitable part of healthcare and their doctors are trying to help them to recover from their illness. In the PACES examination, however, patients volunteer to be examined by you to help you pass your examination, and they derive no benefit from so doing. It is much more difficult to find patients with the necessary time, motivation and clinical signs, than it is to find examination candidates, and for this reason, examiners are always extremely concerned about the comfort, dignity and respect candidates accord to the patient.

Whilst the advice applicable to each individual system will be discussed in the context of the relevant chapter, the general principles to approaching each patient and their subsequent discussion are addressed here.

❶ Top Tips

- There are 4 people at each station of the PACES examination.
  The ranking order of importance should be:
  1. Your patient comes first and foremost.
  2/3. Examiners rank two and three.
  4. The candidate should place themselves in fourth position!

How to approach the people in the examination: your patient

- **The patient's name** When introduced to a patient, greet them by using their name, 'Good morning/Good afternoon Mrs Davidson . . . Thank you very much for allowing me to examine your . . .' Try and remember their name. Using their name during the consultation shows a more personal approach to the patient and will ensure you appear both respectful and professional.

- **Hand gel** Apply hand gel both at the start and at the end of each examination.

- **Always ask if the patient is in any pain or discomfort** 'Are you in any pain or do you have any discomfort anywhere?' This shows consideration, gains the patient's confidence and avoids the embarrassment of inflicting pain during the examination. If the patient does describe discomfort, adapt your examination accordingly e.g. if a patient informs you that they have tenderness in their knee joint, on examining the lower limbs neurologically, inform the patient (and thereby also the examiners) that you will miss out the assessment of power of knee flexion and knee extension, due to the patient's discomfort. The examiners will understandably disapprove of a candidate who shows no regard for a patient's comfort or dignity, leading to a loss of marks in the Core Skill 'Maintaining patient welfare'.

- **Explain each step of the examination to your patient** Giving a patient clear instructions will also highlight to your examiners that you have a systematic approach to the examination. For example, 'I am going to feel the tone in your arms – do let them go floppy' and 'I would now like to check the power in your arms . . .'

- **Communicate effectively with patients:**
  - Using simple everyday language, avoiding medical terminology. For example, inform them that you are going to 'feel their tummy' rather than 'palpate their abdomen' or ask them to 'straighten their arm' rather than to 'extend their elbow'.
  - Where necessary, demonstrate to the patient what you would like them to do e.g. when asking a patient to invert or evert their feet, use your hands to mimic this action.
  - Ensure that the patient understands the instruction that you have given to them.

- **Maintain the patient's dignity** To preserve the patient's modesty, always attempt to cover them up after you have completed each element of the examination. For example, at the start of a cardiovascular examination, it is important to expose your patient adequately to look for scars. Once this observation is completed, cover up your patient's chest before examining the pulse and continuing up the arm to the head and neck. Expose your patient again for palpation of the praecordium and auscultation. This is even more important with female patients. Cover your patient up again at the end of the examination.

- **Do not keep trying to elicit abnormal signs** If a patient has a loss of the temporal field of vision of the left eye, examine the right eye to determine whether there is a nasal or temporal loss indicating a left homonymous hemianopia or bitemporal hemianopia respectively. Repeating the visual field in the left eye again will demonstrate to the examiner that a candidate lacks confidence in their own clinical findings! It should be apparent at an early stage whether a patient is able to follow an instruction.

- *Thank your patient* To conclude the examination neatly, shake hands with your patient whilst thanking them, after which you should turn and face your examiners.
- *Apply hand gel before moving on to the next station*.

Once again, routine practice of the basic principles described above, on each occasion that you review patients, will help these to become systematically performed and second nature.

Always remember that each patient who you encounter in your career as a doctor, including in the forthcoming examination and its preparation, should be treated in exactly the same manner that you would expect your close relative or yourself to be treated. Be friendly and confident towards your patient at all times. The patients who appear in the PACES examination are there for your benefit, and not their own!

> ❶ **Top Tips**
> - It is vital to make a good impression at both the start and the end of the examination (the parts that examiners most remember!) To begin, apply hand gel, ask for permission and about pain, ensure correct position, exposure and patient comfort before you commence your examination. On completion, thank the patient, help them dress/cover them up and apply hand gel.
> - Remember to behave like a doctor and not an examination candidate!

> ❖ **Common Pitfalls**
> - Avoid starting your presentation by referring to your patient as 'He', 'She', or even worse, 'The patient'! Use the patient's correct title and surname during your initial sentence.
> - In the situation where you have forgotten the name at the time of presenting, refer to them as 'This lady' or 'This gentleman had signs consistent with . . .'
> - Do not ask a patient to repeat an action when their functional limitation does not allow them to carry out an instruction. This will show the examiner that the candidate is unsure of their own findings and may make the patient feel inadequate e.g. on examining hip flexion, a patient who is unable to raise their leg is likely to have weakness of hip flexion rather than not cooperating with the candidate.

How to approach the people in the examination: the examiners

Remember that you will not receive any feedback, either positive or negative, from your examiners. A 'poker-faced' examiner may be awarding you 'satisfactory' marks. Equally an examiner may be encouraging to a candidate if they are not performing as well.

Do not try to evaluate your performance during the examination. A candidate may well be successful at a station in which they thought they had performed poorly. In addition, the examiners in each station are unaware of a candidate's score at a previous station.

How to project yourself

- *Turn and face your examiners* Having thanked your patient, turn and face your examiners.
- *Speak clearly* Talk at a steady pace and in a clear manner. Your voice should be at an adequate level, as the examiners should not need to strain to hear what you are trying to state (but at the same time, not so loud that you appear to be shouting!).
- *Use appropriate medical terminology* when conversing with the examiners e.g. 'Diplopia was present on left downward gaze' rather than 'There was double vision on looking to the bottom left corner'.
- *Maintain eye contact* Eye contact is a key aspect of any professional communication. Remember that whilst one examiner will take the lead role of questioning, the other examiner has an equal share of marks to allocate to the candidate. It is therefore important to look at the two examiners in turn, thereby including them both in the discussion which ensues.
- *Posture* Stand straight and present the key points of your case to your examiners. Do not point to areas of your own body when referring to the elicited signs of your patient. If when nervous, you fidget or point to yourself, keep your hands behind your back.

❶ Top Tips

- Always remember that there are two examiners in the examination.
- If needed, hold your hands together behind your back – this will prevent you from pointing to areas of your own body to indicate where the elicited clinical signs were found.
- Remember to be bilingual in the examination:
  - Use straightforward English to converse with your patients and medical terminology during discussions with your examiners.

❧ Common Pitfalls

- Candidates often only turn their heads to face their examiners, when they begin their presentation. This invariably results in turning back to face the patient again and losing eye contact with the examiners. Always turn your whole body so that you face both the examiners, thus permitting optimal eye contact.
- Lack of eye contact may project an appearance of insecurity.
- Avoid any posturing that may give the appearance of casual conversation e.g. slouching, hands in pockets.
- Remember that you are participating in a professional and formal discussion.

Inspection

Whilst the temptation may be to rush in and examine the patient close-up, always take a few seconds to read the instructions properly and observe the patient as a whole person, not just in relation to the system you are about to examine:

- Look around the patient's bedside carefully for any clues which may guide you in the right direction. For example, when asked to examine a patient's arms neurologically, the presence of a foot drop splint may suggest peripheral weakness in the legs and a more widespread problem involving both the upper the lower limbs.

- Always observe the patient's age group (young, middle aged, elderly), gender and ethnicity. Tailor the differential diagnosis accordingly.
- The patient may themselves have vital clues, for example, to the treatment received (seborrhoeic dermatitis of immunosuppressive therapies or tattoo mark of radiation therapy). They may even be wearing a medic alert or charity bracelet, which will reveal their underlying diagnosis!
- Always look for scars.
- Ask yourself if the patient appears cushingoid (indicating steroid therapy – a treatment used in all specialties).

❶ Top Tips
- Always consider medication by a patient's bedside to have the generic label 'Read me' which may even reveal the underlying diagnosis! The examiners will almost certainly have asked the patient to bring their tablets with them so that they can be placed at a patient's bedside.

Presentation of your case

- *Gather your thoughts continually BEFORE presenting the case* The elicited signs should be continually processed and updated, taking into consideration any new clinical features in a contemporaneous manner. This will enable you to look out for signs which will help to categorize the condition further e.g. establishing whether a patient with a peripheral weakness has myotonia suggesting myotonic dystrophy, or an associated sensory loss suggesting a peripheral sensorimotor neuropathy.
- *Adapt further examination according to the signs elicited* Omit aspects of the further routine examination which transpire to be inappropriate. For example, do not ask a patient about diplopia if they are blind in one eye.
- *Consider the potential questions whilst completing the examination* These should include the positive and *important* negative findings, the most likely diagnosis, the differential diagnosis, investigations related to the case and management of the condition.
- *Comment on observations not related to the system examined first* For example, 'On examining Mr. Banerjee, I noted that he has a left above-knee amputation. Examination of his cardiovascular system revealed signs consistent with mixed aortic valve disease . . .' This will avoid forgetting to mention the amputation once engrossed in a discussion related to the cardiac condition. Failure to comment on findings made on observation may leave an unfavourable impression with the examiners.
- *Opening sentence* This important sentence should convey to the examiners that you have correctly elicited and interpreted the presence of the key physical findings. Follow this sentence through with additional information to back up your case. For example, 'Miss Roberts is a young lady with focal, left-sided cerebellar signs, as

evidenced by hypotonia and past pointing in the left arm. I note that she also has nystagmus on looking to the left . . .'

- **Emphasize the positive and important negative findings** Impart the salient points of the case without deviating attention to irrelevant facts such as listing a series of negative findings. Avoid presenting a long list of signs in a haphazard order, with no interpretation of their clinical significance. Imagine the examination scenario as a post-take ward round, with the consultant having a limited time for each patient. Utilize each second of valuable time to capture and maintain the examiners attention.
- **Extension of examination should be mentioned at this stage** For example, suggest performing fundoscopy in a patient with peripheral neuropathy or a renal transplant.
- **Suggest appropriate investigations** to establish the diagnosis and also the severity of the condition. Always volunteer the expected investigatory findings e.g. in a patient with a renal transplant ask to dipstick the urine, specifying that you are looking for proteinuria and glycosuria.

❶ Top Tips

Capture and maintain the attention of the examiners:
   The opening sentence should inform the examiners that the physical findings related to a particular patient have been elicited and interpreted. Furthermore, it should capture their attention and make them want to continue to listen and engage in further discussion related to a case.

❧ Common Pitfalls

- Do not list any irrelevant negative findings, such as 'this man is comfortable at rest'.

- **Order the differential diagnosis and interpret the signs** in the context of the individual patient you have examined. When formulating the differential diagnosis, always ensure that this is consistent with your clinical findings. Take into consideration:
   - The patient's age, gender and ethnic origin e.g. proximal myopathy is more likely to be secondary to osteomalacia in an elderly Asian lady than in a young Caucasian lady.
   - Specific signs which may also help to subdivide a clinical condition e.g. a young Caucasian lady with focal cerebellar signs is more likely to have demyelinating disease, whereas an elderly patient with global cerebellar disease is more likely to have multiple cerebellar strokes or a paraneoplastic syndrome.
- **Comment on the severity of the condition where possible** e.g. a slow rising pulse and absent 2nd heart sound indicates that the aortic stenosis is more severe.
- **Comment on the complications of the disease or treatment** e.g. pulmonary hypertension in a patient with lung fibrosis or the skin pigmentation of amiodarone therapy.
- **Consider other differential diagnoses** which can be provided if needed.

- *Volunteer the pertinent positive and negative findings in a systematic manner*, particularly if you have not reached a diagnosis or a suitable differential diagnosis. Whilst presenting your case, reconsider the signs elicited and formulate the likely diagnosis, as the examiners will expect a sensible discussion relating to the possible differential diagnoses, with evidence to justify your thoughts.
- *Never highlight your omissions to the examiners* e.g. 'I should have auscultated for radiation of the aortic murmur' or 'I forgot to check for peripheral oedema'. If the examiners ask you about the radiation of the murmur or the presence of oedema, be humble and accept gracefully that you should have looked for these signs, remembering that the examiners have observed your performance.
- *Be forthcoming with discussion* and do not make the examiner drag the information out of you. For example, if you are asked how you would like to investigate a particular patient, mention the tests you would like to carry out and volunteer the expected findings e.g. for interstitial lung disease, 'I would carry our lung function tests, which are likely to show a restrictive pattern with a reduced FEV_1 and FVC, increased FEV_1/FVC ratio (>80%), and a reduced transfer factor'. This will also fully utilize the questioning time by informing the examiner what you *do* know.
- *Respond to the examiners questions directly* If you do not know the answer, do not deviate from the question, but inform the examiners that you are unable to answer that question. This will allow them to move on to another question, where you may be able to demonstrate your knowledge.

Remember that your examiners are trying to find out what you know – thorough questioning does not mean that they are 'against' you!

❶ Top Tips
- Offer a few relevant differential diagnoses in the likely order, structured according to the patient's specific clinical findings, age, gender and ethnic origin, rather than simply reciting a long list. Justify your statements with the key findings.
- Communication is made up of multiple elements including speech, body gesture and eye contact.
- Practise in front of a mirror – it may prove to be an eye opener!
- Ask your colleagues to comment on the manner of your presentation, asking them to highlight any tics or body-language issues that you may be unaware of.
- Anticipate the questions the examiners are likely to ask whilst examining your patient – they are often predictable!

✦ Common Pitfalls

- A list of all examination findings to preface the diagnosis is not necessary and may, in fact, waste valuable time, particularly in the event of an incorrect diagnosis.
- If you are confident of the diagnosis, it is far more impressive to state the diagnosis first and justify it by presentation of the relevant positive and negative physical signs.
- Never highlight your omissions to the examiners – they may have gone unnoticed!
- Answer the question you are being asked; not the one you would like to answer.

Candidates with disability

If you have a disability, seek advice from the consultant who sponsors your application to take the examination. They may well be able to write to the Royal College on your behalf so that any requirements can be accommodated as necessary.

Reference

1. Elder A et al. Changing PACES: developments to the examination in 2009. *Clin Med* 2011; **11**:231–4.

◈ Useful websites

MRCP (UK) PACES website: http://www.mrcpuk.org/PACES/Pages/_Home.aspx.
MRCP (UK) PACES website: http://www.mrcpuk.org/PACES/Pages/PacesMarkSheets.aspx
MRCP (UK) PACES website: http://www.mrcpuk.org/PACES/Pages/PassMarks.aspx.

Respiratory

Sanjay H. Chotirmall*
Helen Liddicoat*
William L.G. Oldfield*

* Joint first authors

Introduction

The MRCP PACES respiratory station offers an opportunity to demonstrate a slick examination technique that is performed on practically all patients. Respiratory diseases, after cardiovascular and musculoskeletal complaints, are the third most common cause for presentation to either the Emergency Department or the general practitioner (GP) and remains proof of the concept that 'common things are common'.

Respiratory disease can be generally divided into 3 major categories: airways, parenchymal and pleural disease. We have aimed to structure the following chapter to reflect this. Certain 'high-yield' or 'favourites' that recur in the PACES examination are covered in this section.

During PACES, examiners assess your ability to *both* **elicit** and then correctly **interpret** physical signs. A general sense exists that a decision to pass or fail a candidate rests on an aura of competence (or incompetence!) during the clinical performance. In essence, the examiners are looking for you to demonstrate correct techniques whilst eliciting the signs and logical thinking when interpreting them. Therefore, eliciting the physical signs is only the first step; the interpretation and presentation are equally, if not more, important.

With this in mind, the following useful general points should be considered:

- The respiratory examination does not need to be a lengthy one. Start at the peripheries with the hands and then move to the back (unless specifically advised otherwise by your examiners). Traditionally the physical examination starts with the anterior chest but it is perfectly acceptable to do the back first then return to the front (most signs and clues to the diagnosis e.g. scars, will be detected by examining the posterior chest).
- A 6-minute period is allowed for the examination portion of the station and it is our advice to spend the *first* 2 minutes examining the patient from a general perspective (including full inspection, hands and face) then the *second* 2 minutes on the posterior chest and the *final* 2 minutes on the anterior chest. As time is limited, palpate for features of pulmonary hypertension or right-sided heart failure at the anterior chest, before moving to the respiratory signs. (The anterior chest signs are likely to be similar to those elicited on the posterior chest.)
- Most cases at the respiratory station involve 'chronic' conditions – the majority of which can be identified well before auscultation. Never underestimate the power of observation, both of the patient and of the surrounding environment!
- The chest is physiologically symmetrical and therefore careful observation may immediately suggest the side of pathology – unilateral pathology includes collapse, consolidation, pleural effusion and pneumonectomy. However, if chest symmetry is preserved, consider airways disease, pulmonary fibrosis or bronchiectasis.
- As with any other system's examination, at the start and the end of the physical examination wash your hands or use hand gel. Having introduced yourself and obtained permission to examine your patient, *ensure* correct *position*, *exposure* and patient *comfort* before commencing. On completion, *ask* yourself whether you have checked

for the following: *evidence of complications* (pulmonary hypertension), *treatment (at bedside)* or *underlying cause* and ensure to *complete your presentation* stating: 'To complete my examination, I would check the peak flow rate, sputum pot and temperature chart'. Remember to *thank* the patient and help them *dress*.

Examination

The key to the examination is practice. Try to collate your examination findings and ensure the signs you elicit fit together (see Table 2.1). Key findings in the respiratory examination are explained in more detail in Table 2.2. A systematic approach to examination of the respiratory system is summarized in Figure 2.2 (p.26).

Inspection

Ensure the patient is comfortably positioned at 45° and is exposed from the waist up. Take time to inspect the patient for important clues from the end of the bed. Stand directly opposite the patient in order to correctly assess any differences in each hemithorax. Remember to cover the patient up after completing each element of the examination in order to maintain dignity.

General appearance

- Consider the patient's age.
- Note the body habitus. Short stature is suggestive of a disease in childhood e.g. cystic fibrosis. Also note their BMI.
- Is the patient short of breath at rest?
- Look for use of accessory muscles (tracheal tug, in-drawing of intercostal muscles, use of abdominal muscles).
- Is there pursed lip breathing (patient providing own positive end-expiratory pressure)?
- Are any audible noises from the end of the bed e.g. wheeze, stridor (suggestive of large airway obstruction), a hoarse voice or cough (note whether this is productive or dry)?
- Note any deformities of the chest wall:
  • pectus excavatum – depression of the sternum.
  • pectus carinatum – outward bowing of the sternum due to chronic respiratory infection or rickets.
  • kyphoscoliosis.
  • barrel-shaped chest, indicating increased anteroposterior diameter and hyperexpansion.
- Is the chest expansion equal?
- Carefully observe for any visible scars on the patient's chest. These are useful to locate at the beginning of the examination (see Fig. 2.1).
- Look for radiotherapy tattoos and radiation-induced skin changes.
- Bedside clues including:
  • oxygen therapy.
  • inhalers or a nebulizer. Ensure that you are familiar with the commonly used inhalers so that you can be specific during your presentation.

- sputum pot.
- walking aids which may suggest the patient has a reduced exercise tolerance.
- Look for complications of disease or treatment e.g. evidence of steroid use (rounded face, central obesity, intrascapular fat pad, thin skin, bruising, hirsuitism, proximal muscle weakness).

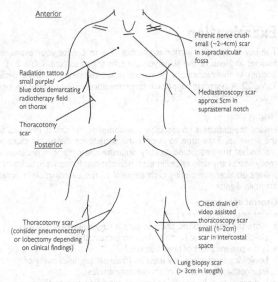

Anterior

Phrenic nerve crush small (~2–4cm) scar in supraclavicular fossa

Radiation tattoo small purple/ blue dots demarcating radiotherapy field on thorax

Mediastinoscopy scar approx 5cm in suprasternal notch

Thoracotomy scar

Posterior

Chest drain or video assisted thoracoscopy scar small (1–2cm) scar in intercostal space

Thoracotomy scar (consider pneumonectomy or lobectomy depending on clinical findings)

Lung biopsy scar (> 3cm in length)

Fig. 2.1 Scars in the respiratory exam.

Hands

- Inspect the hands for:
  - palmar erythema (CO_2 retention).
  - wasting of the small muscles of the hand (Pancoast tumour).
  - changes of rheumatological conditions associated with respiratory disease e.g. rheumatoid arthritis, scleroderma.
- Inspect the nails for:
  - clubbing with the patient's fingers directly in line with your vision so that the nail is observed at 90°. Schamroth's sign (directly opposing distal phalanges of corresponding fingers and looking for the obliteration of the usual diamond-shaped window between the nailbeds) can be performed to assess clubbing.
  - peripheral cyanosis.
  - tar staining and yellow nails (yellow nail syndrome).
- Ask the patient to straighten out their arms and hold out their hands looking for:
  - a fine tremor associated with beta 2 agonist use.
  - a course flapping tremor of CO_2 retention by asking the patient to cock their wrists back as if they were about to stop traffic. Asterixis is more likely to be present in an acutely unwell patient rather than a patient selected for the PACES exam.
- Feel the patient's radial pulse. A bounding pulse is a characteristic sign of CO_2 retention.
- Calculate their respiratory rate by counting the number of respirations over 15 seconds whilst feeling the pulse.
- Pain and/or swelling of hands/wrists suggesting possible hypertrophic pulmonary osteoarthropathy.

Face

Look closely at the patients face for:
- A cushingoid appearance suggesting steroid therapy.
- Stigmata of underlying pathology e.g.:
  - connective tissue disease e.g. telangiectasia and microstomia in scleroderma patients; butterfly rash in patients with systemic lupus erythematosus (SLE); heliotrope rash of dermatomyositis.
  - lupus pernio (sarcoidosis) and lupus vulgaris (tuberculosis) which are most commonly visible on the nose.
- Facial plethora consistent with secondary polycythaemia – evidence of SVC obstruction (facial and upper body swelling).

Eyes

- Suffused conjunctivae present in secondary polycythaemia.
- Horner's syndrome (meiosis, partial ptosis, enophthalmous, anhydrosis).
- Ask the patient to look up and warn them that you are going to pull down gently on their lower eyelid. Look for:
  - anaemia present in chronic disease e.g. cystic fibrosis.
  - jaundice which may indicate malignancy.

Mouth

- Look for evidence of central cyanosis in the lips and the undersurface of the tongue.
- Evidence of oral candidiasis – consistent with steroid use.

Neck

- Look at the patient's neck size (larger collar size increases risk of obstructive sleep apnoea).
- Assess the patient's jugular venous pressure (JVP) at 45° (➔ p.221):
  - A raised JVP may suggest cor pulmonale.
  - Fixed in superior vena cava obstruction (SVCO).
  - JVP waveform: is the a wave prominent (right atrial hypertrophy) or are there large v waves (tricuspid regurgitation)?

Thorax

- **Trachea** Warn the patient that you are going to feel their windpipe and that this may feel slightly uncomfortable. Place your middle finger in the centre of the trachea with your index and ring finger on either side. Look for evidence of deviation or tracheal tug. Check the cricosternal distance (the distance between the suprasternal notch to the cricoid cartilage). This is normally 3 finger breaths and is reduced in hyperinflation.
- **Apex beat** Feel for the patient's apex beat which may be displaced due to mediastinal shift or poorly palpable due to hyperexpansion of the chest.
- **Pulmonary hypertension** Palpate for a right ventricular heave by placing the palm of your hand over the left sternal border and feel for a palpable pulmonary 2nd heart sound.
- **Lymphadenopathy** Ask the patient to sit forward and cross their arms over their chest. Palpate for cervical and supraclavicular lymphadenopathy – ensure you feel all areas (submandibular, pre- and post-auricular, anterior and posterior cervical triangle, occipital and supraclavicular regions). If you find lymphadenopathy offer to examine the axillae.

Expansion

Expansion is a high yield sign but is often performed incorrectly. Place the palm of your hands with fingers in the intercostal spaces on either side of the patient's chest and pull in the subcutaneous tissues slightly. Lift your thumbs off the chest wall so that they meet opposite each other in the middle of the chest. Ask the patient to take a deep breath in and out of their mouth and observe for any asymmetry or reduction in expansion of the chest wall movement. This manoeuvre should be performed in the upper and lower zones of the chest.

Tactile vocal fremitus

Place the ulnar border of your hands obliquely in the intercostal spaces on either side of the patient's chest and ask them to say 'ninety-nine'.

Observe for any difference as the sound resonates through the lungs and chest wall. Repeat this in the upper, middle and lower zones of the chest.

Percussion

You should percuss with your middle finger in a firm connection with the patient's skin. Move the percussing hand from the wrist in order to generate a good sound. Compare each side of the chest in turn and moving down from the apex to the lung bases, not forgetting the axillae. Is the percussion note resonant, dull or stony dull? Absence of hepatic and cardiac dullness may signify hyperexpansion.

Auscultation

Ask the patient to take deep breaths in and out of their mouth and ensure your stethoscope is in contact with their chest wall throughout inspiration and expiration. Consider the following in each area of the chest:

- Is the air entry normal or reduced?
- Are the breath sounds vesicular or is there bronchial breathing?
- Is the inspiratory: expiratory ratio of respiration normal (usually 1:2) or is there a prolonged expiratory phase (airflow obstruction)?
- Are there any added sounds such as wheeze, crepitations or a pleural rub?

Ensure you describe these sounds detailing where they occur in the respiratory cycle as well as their quality, for example, are they fine late inspiratory crepitations or early and course?

Vocal resonance

- Ask the patient to say 'ninety-nine' each time you place your stethoscope on their chest and compare each hemithorax.
- If the vocal resonance is increased, examine for whispering pectoriloquy by asking the patient to whisper 'ninety-nine' and determine if this sound is increased (e.g. over areas of fibrosis). Assess for aegophony (Greek for 'goat voice') which occurs when the lung transmits higher frequencies, giving the speech a 'bleating' quality. If aegophony is present, the patient saying 'a' will sound like 'e' through the stethoscope.

Having examined the posterior of the thorax move onto the anterior of the chest, by which point a good idea of the possible diagnosis should already have been made. Use the rest of the examination to confirm or dispute your findings. Do not forget to examine for signs of pulmonary hypertension if appropriate.

Prior to completing the examination look at the patient's ankles for any evidence of peripheral oedema (cor pulmonale).

Ensure your patient is covered up, thank them and wash your hands.

To complete the examination offer to look at the patient's observation chart and sputum pot (if one is available), to perform a peak flow/bedside spirometry and to look at the patient's chest radiograph (CXR).

❶ Top Tips

- If you are confident of the diagnosis it is better to give the diagnosis first (otherwise present the case in a systematic manner, mentioning the pertinent positive and negative findings).
- Make sure you do not miss out descriptors e.g. specific features of crepitations.
- Attempt to give a possible cause for the patient's underlying respiratory condition e.g. pulmonary fibrosis most likely secondary to rheumatoid arthritis.
- Comment on any complications of the disease or of the treatment e.g. cor pulmonale or Cushing's syndrome secondary to steroid use.
- Make an assessment of severity of disease.

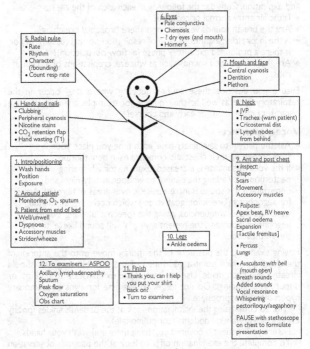

5. Radial pulse
- Rate
- Rhythm
- Character (?bounding)
- Count resp rate

4. Hands and nails
- Clubbing
- Peripheral cyanosis
- Nicotine stains
- CO_2 retention flap
- Hand wasting (T1)

1. Intro/positioning
- Wash hands
- Position
- Exposure

2. Around patient
- Monitoring, O_2, sputum

3. Patient from end of bed
- Well/unwell
- Dyspnoea
- Accessory muscles
- Stridor/wheeze

6. Eyes
- Pale conjunctiva
- Chemosis
- ? dry eyes (and mouth)
- Horner's

7. Mouth and face
- Central cyanosis
- Dentition
- Plethora

8. Neck
- JVP
- Trachea (warn patient)
- Cricosternal dist
- Lymph nodes from behind

9. Ant and post chest
- *Inspect:*
  Shape
  Scars
  Movement
  Accessory muscles
- *Palpate:*
  Apex beat, RV heave
  Sacral oedema
  Expansion
  [Tactile fremitus]
- *Percuss*
  Lungs
- *Auscultate with bell (mouth open)*
  Breath sounds
  Added sounds
  Vocal resonance
  Whispering pectoriloquy/aegaphony

  PAUSE with stethoscope on chest to formulate presentation

10. Legs
- Ankle oedema

12. To examiners – ASPOO
- Axillary lymphadenopathy
- Sputum
- Peak flow
- Oxygen saturations
- Obs chart

11. Finish
- Thank you, can I help you put your shirt back on?
- Turn to examiners

Fig. 2.2 Systematic approach to examination of the respiratory system.

Table 2.1 Summary of key findings in the respiratory examination

Sign	Description	Causes	Pitfalls
Clubbing	1) Loss of the angle at the nail bed (Schamroth's sign) 2) Bogginess of the nail bed 3) ↑ curvature of the nail 4) Drumstick appearance	Chronic suppurative lung disease (empyema, abscess, bronchiectasis, TB), some interstitial lung diseases, lung cancer (non-small cell), mesothelioma Consider other systems (cardiac, abdomen, thyroid etc.)	Beware of diagnosing 'early clubbing'. It is best to describe the features present if clubbing is debatable. The 1st sign seen in clubbing is loss of the angle at the nail bed. It is *not* found in COPD/chronic bronchitis
Crepitations	Short, interrupted, non-musical sounds due to sudden opening of collapsed airways		Timing of crepitations may be helpful in diagnosis but should not be used in isolation Check if they clear on coughing – more indicative of infection/secretions
	Fine: occurring in late inspiration	Fibrosis Pulmonary oedema	
	Coarse: occurring in early-mid inspiration	Infection COPD Bronchiectasis Pulmonary oedema	

(Continued)

Table 2.1 (Contd.)

Sign	Description	Causes	Pitfalls
Wheeze	High-pitched whistling noise due to airway narrowing		
	Monophonic (can be inspiratory ± expiratory)	Localized large airway narrowing due to a fixed obstruction e.g. malignancy or foreign body	Ensure you differentiate this from stridor
	Polyphonic (expiratory)	Noise generated from variable constriction of multiple, different sized airways e.g. asthma, COPD, pulmonary oedema, infection	
Stridor	High-pitched sound with each inspiration	Acute: laryngeal oedema, epiglottitis, croup, foreign body obstruction, smoke inhalation	
		Chronic: malignancy, tracheal stenosis	
Pleural rub	Creaking leathery sound caused by inflamed or abnormal pleura moving against each other and creating friction	Pleurisy	
		Pleural effusion	
		Mesothelioma	

Table 2.2 Patterns of clinical disease

	Collapse pneumonectomy	Pneumothorax	Consolidation	Pleural effusion	COPD	Bilateral fibrosis
Mediastinal shift (trachea/apex)	Towards	No (simple) Away (tension)	No	No or away	No	No
Chest wall expansion	↓	↓ or normal	↓ or normal	↓ or normal	Hyperexpanded at baseline	↓ or normal
Percussion	Dull	Resonant	Dull	Stony dull	No change	↓ or no change
Breath sounds	↓	↓	Bronchial	↓	Variable/↓	No change
Added sounds	No	No	Crepitations	Pleural rub Bronchial breathing at upper border	Wheeze Crepitations	Fine end inspiratory crepitations
Tactile vocal fremitus/vocal resonance	↓	↓	↑	↓	No change	↑ or no change

Interpreting pulmonary function tests

Pulmonary function tests (PFTs) are key to understanding and diagnosing respiratory disease and are frequently asked about during the viva component of the exam.

Flow volume loops (Fig. 2.3)

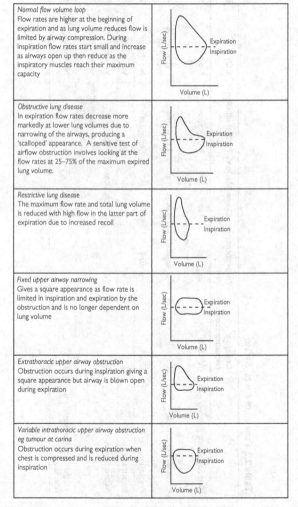

Normal flow volume loop
Flow rates are higher at the beginning of expiration and as lung volume reduces flow is limited by airway compression. During inspiration flow rates start small and increase as airways open up then reduce as the inspiratory muscles reach their maximum capacity

Obstructive lung disease
In expiration flow rates decrease more markedly at lower lung volumes due to narrowing of the airways, producing a 'scalloped' appearance. A sensitive test of airflow obstruction involves looking at the flow rates at 25–75% of the maximum expired lung volume.

Restrictive lung disease
The maximum flow rate and total lung volume is reduced with high flow in the latter part of expiration due to increased recoil

Fixed upper airway narrowing
Gives a square appearance as flow rate is limited in inspiration and expiration by the obstruction and is no longer dependent on lung volume

Extrathoracic upper airway obstruction
Obstruction occurs during inspiration giving a square appearance but airway is blown open during expiration

Variable intrathoracic upper airway obstruction eg tumour at carina
Obstruction occurs during expiration when chest is compressed and is reduced during inspiration

Fig. 2.3 Inspiratory and expiratory flow plotted against lung volume.

Spirometry (Fig. 2.4)

- Forced vital capacity (FVC): from full inspiration patient exhales as long and as forcefully as possible.
- Forced expiratory volume in 1 second (FEV_1): amount of air forcibly exhaled in 1 second
- FEV_1/FVC ratio:
  - Obstructive lung disease indicated if FEV_1/FVC <0.70.
  - Restrictive lung disease (or normality) indicated if FEV_1/FVC >0.70.
- Diffusion capacity:
  - Calculated by inhaling a mixture of carbon monoxide (CO) (which crosses the alveolar membrane) and helium (which does not). The amount of CO transferred across the alveolar capillary membrane into the blood is calculated and adjusted for haemoglobin levels (TLCO, total lung CO).
  - The total lung volume is calculated using helium concentration which would be diluted by gas already present in the lung on inspiration.
  - This allows the kCO (gas transfer per unit volume) to be calculated.
  - kCO is reduced in emphysema and interstitial lung disease.
  - kCO is increased with pulmonary haemorrhage e.g. SLE, Wegener's, Goodpasture's syndrome.
- Total lung capacity (TLC):
  - Measured using helium dilution or body plethysmography.
  - TLC increases in obstructive lung disease with air trapping and hyperinflation.
  - TLC decreases in restrictive lung disease.

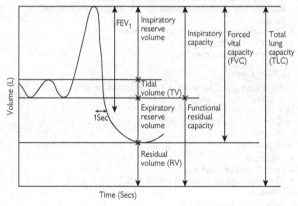

Fig. 2.4 Lung volumes and capacities.

Chronic obstructive pulmonary disease

COPD is characterized by progressive airflow obstruction which shows limited reversibility. It is associated with an abnormal inflammatory response in the lungs due to cigarette smoke or other inhaled particles. Early definitions distinguished between two types of COPD:

- Chronic bronchitis: defined clinically as chronic cough with sputum production for >3 months in 2 successive years.
- Emphysema: defined histologically as alveolar wall destruction, leading to abnormal and permanent enlargement of airspaces distal to the terminal bronchioles.

Clinical signs

- Inhaler devices, nebulizers, sputum pot, oxygen by the bedside
- Cachexia
- Tachypnoea
- Pursed lip breathing
- Barrel-shaped chest
- Use of accessory muscles of ventilation – indrawing of intercostal muscles, tracheal tug
- Peripheral and/or central cyanosis
- Tar-stained fingers
- Bounding pulse (sign of CO_2 retention), asterixis (secondary to CO_2 retention; may be palpable only)
- Reduced cricosternal distance (<3 fingers)
- Hyperinflated chest (vertical >horizontal expansion)
- Hyper-resonance to percussion with reduced hepatic and cardiac dullness (latter due to lingular lobe hypertrophy)
- Reduced breath sounds (especially over areas of emphysematous bullae)
- Prolonged expiratory phase of respiration
- Expiratory wheeze
- Coarse inspiratory crepitations.

❶ Top Tips
- Look for signs of steroid use e.g. cushingoid appearance, thin skin, bruising.
- Look for signs of cor pulmonale.
- COPD is not a cause of clubbing.

Symptoms

- Dyspnoea
- Exertional breathlessness
- Chronic cough with sputum production
- Wheeze
- Recurrent chest infections.

Severity

Can be defined in terms of:
- Symptoms using Medical Research Council (MRC) Dyspnoea Scale (Table 2.3):

Table 2.3 MRC Dyspnoea Scale

1	Not troubled by breathlessness except on strenuous exercise
2	Short of breath when hurrying or walking up a slight hill
3	Walks slower than contemporaries on level ground because of breathlessness or has to stop for breath when walking at own pace
4	Stops for breath after walking about 100m or after a few minutes on level ground
5	Too breathless to leave house or breathless when dressing

- Airflow obstruction using GOLD staging (Global initiative for Chronic Obstructive Lung Disease (GOLD) staging (Table 2.4):

Table 2.4 Gold staging of airflow obstruction

Stage	Severity	FEV_1 (FEV_1/FVC <0.70)
I	Mild	>80% predicted
II	Moderate	50–80% predicted
III	Severe	30–50% predicted
IV	Very severe	<30% predicted or FEV_1 <50% plus chronic respiratory failure

- Both pulmonary and extrapulmonary manifestations of COPD using the BODE index. This calculates severity based on FEV_1, 6-minute walk distance, MRC Dyspnoea Scale and BMI and has been shown to be a better predictor of outcome (in terms of hospital admissions and mortality) than FEV_1 alone.[1,2]

Investigations

Laboratory

- Blood tests:
  - anaemia of chronic disease/polycythaemia.
  - raised inflammatory markers if co-existent infection.
  - low albumin (due to chronic disease).
- Arterial blood gases: hypoxaemia. As disease progresses hypercapnia may develop with evidence of chronic compensation.
- Sputum culture.
- Alpha 1 antitrypsin levels – indicated in patients with early-onset disease, minimal smoking history or family history.

❶ Top Tips

Differentiating COPD and chronic asthma

Airflow obstruction caused by COPD and chronic asthma can be difficult to distinguish.

Clinical findings

- COPD is more likely in smokers with chronic cough and breathlessness which is persistent and progressive.
- Asthma should be considered in patients with variable symptoms and nocturnal awakening with breathlessness and wheeze. Often history of atopic disease.

Lung function

Asthmatic patients can be identified by the following:

- Response to bronchodilators (traditionally a 10–20% or 200mL improvement in FEV_1 is significant; however, due to fluctuations in reversibility testing, guidelines now suggest a change of >400mL).
- Serial peak flow measurements showing >20% diurnal or day-to-day variability.

Functional

- Lung function studies:
  - Airflow obstruction with FEV_1/FVC <0.70.
  - FEV_1 <80% predicted.
  - Minimal reversibility with bronchodilator.
  - ↑ TLC, functional residual capacity and residual volume.
  - Reduced diffusion capacity.

Radiological

- CXR:
  - Low sensitivity.
  - Increased radiolucency of lungs.
  - Flattened hemidiaphragms (≤1.5cm between diaphragm and line connecting the costo- and cardiophrenic angles) or diaphragm at or below the anterior end of the 7th rib.
  - Horizontal ribs.
  - Bullae.
  - Retrosternal air space of >2.5cm.
  - Tubular heart or cardiac enlargement if associated cor pulmonale
  - Enlarged pulmonary arteries with attenuation of peripheral vasculature (peripheral pruning in outer 1/3 of lung) in pulmonary hypertension.
- Computed tomography:
  - Highly sensitive and specific.
  - High-resolution CT (HRCT) used to grade and classify emphysema. Centrilobular emphysema occurs preferentially in upper lobes. Panlobular emphysema involves lung bases. Paraseptal emphysema may be seen anywhere in the lungs and occurs adjacent to visceral pleura and septa.
  - Useful in the evaluation of bullous disease.

Other
- BMI (➜ p.96).
- ECG.
- Echocardiogram (to evaluate possible pulmonary hypertension).

Viva questions

What treatments are available to help patients stop smoking?

Smoking cessation improves symptoms, improves lung function (there is a significantly reduced rate of decline in FEV_1 with a return to near normal age-related decline over time) and is the only treatment shown to alter disease course.

Behavioural treatment
- '5 A' approach endorsed by the BTS: **A**sk about smoking status, **A**ssess readiness to quit, **A**dvise to quit, **A**ssist in efforts to quit, **A**rrange follow-up.
- Patients should be encouraged to identify a quit day.
- Informing patients of abnormal lung function tests increases their likelihood of quitting.
- Group counselling – includes lectures, habit recognition, coping skills and suggestions for relapse prevention.

Nicotine replacement therapy (NRT)
- Insufficient evidence to conclude one form of NRT is more effective than another.
- Nicotine patches, gum, inhalers (can cause bronchospasm), nasal sprays (result in a more rapid rise in plasma nicotine levels mimicking smoking; can cause nasal irritation).

Buproprion
- Antidepressant which enhances CNS noradrenergic and dopaminergic function.

Varenicline
- Partial agonist of nicotinic acetylcholine receptors. Side effects include abnormal dreams, nausea and neuropsychiatric symptoms.

Some evidence of increased efficacy with combination treatment. No evidence for the effectiveness of acupuncture or hypnosis.

Describe the treatment options available for COPD

Non-pharmacological treatment
- Pulmonary rehabilitation:
  - Multidisciplinary programme of care incorporating disease education, physical training, nutritional, psychological and behavioural interventions.
  - Leads to statistically significant improvements in exercise capacity and quality of life and reduces dyspnoea with conflicting evidence regarding effect in reducing hospital admissions.
  - Consider in patients with MRC dyspnoea grade 3+.
- Optimize nutrition:
  - Poor nutritional state associated with increased mortality, impaired respiratory muscle function and reduced immune function.

- Vaccination:
  - Influenza vaccination should be offered to all patients.
  - Pneumococcal vaccination in patient >65 years or <65 years if FEV_1 <40% predicted.

Pharmacological treatment
- Treatment aims to reduce symptoms, decrease frequency and severity of exacerbations, improve quality of life and increase exercise capacity.
- Medication can be delivered by pressurized metered dose inhaler (MDI), dry-powder inhaler (DPI) with or without spacer or nebulizer.
- Inhalers can achieve responses equivalent to nebulizers if used correctly. Inhaler technique should be checked regularly.
- Short-acting bronchodilators:
  - Short-acting beta 2 agonists: act directly on bronchial smooth muscle to cause bronchodilation e.g. salbutamol, terbutaline.
  - Short-acting anticholinergics: inhibit resting bronchomotor tone and affect mucus secretion e.g. ipratropium bromide.
  - Combination treatment has additive effect.
  - Does not alter frequency of exacerbations.
- Long-acting bronchodilators: recommended in patients who remain symptomatic on above or experience >2 exacerbations per year.
  - Long-acting beta 2 agonists: TORCH study[3] (TOwards a Revolution in COPD Health) – salmeterol reduced exacerbation rates, improved lung function and health-related quality of life compared to placebo.
  - Long-acting anticholinergics: UPLIFT study[4] (Understanding the Potential Long-term Impact on Function with Tiotropium) – treatment with tiotropium therapy (versus placebo in patients permitted to use other respiratory medications except anticholinergics) shown to improve lung function, reduce exacerbations and improve health-related quality of life over a four year period.
- Inhaled corticosteroids:
  - Reduce airway and systemic inflammation.
  - Indicated for patients with an FEV_1 <50% predicted who are having >2 exacerbations a year.
  - 12 randomized controlled trials (RCTs) demonstrated reduction in risk of exacerbations versus placebo with no significant effect on mortality.
  - TORCH study: fluticasone propionate reduced rate of moderate-severe exacerbations, improved quality of life and improved lung function versus placebo. Frequency of pneumonia increased in patients using inhaled corticosteroids; however this did not have a significant effect on mortality.
  - Risk of osteoporosis in patients on high-dose corticosteroids in presence of other risk factors.
- Oral corticosteroids:
  - Associated with increased morbidity and mortality and therefore use of oral corticosteroids not recommended for maintenance treatment.
  - Trial of oral corticosteroids does not predict response from inhaled treatment.

- Combined treatment with inhaled bronchodilator and corticosteroid:
  - TORCH study – salmeterol and fluticasone combined improved lung function, health status and reduced frequency of exacerbations compared to salmeterol alone, fluticasone alone and placebo. Mortality reduced compared to placebo but this had borderline statistical significance. Further analysis of study data showed that pharmacotherapy slowed rate of lung function decline, with the greatest benefit seen with salmeterol and fluticasone combined.
- Theophylline:
  - Unclear mechanism of action. Relaxes airway smooth muscle. May improve diaphragm strength and affect mucociliary clearance.
  - Given potential toxicity, drug interactions and need to monitor plasma levels, it is not recommended for initial treatment.

Oxygen
- Long-term oxygen therapy (LTOT):
  - Indicated in patients with PaO_2 <7.3kPa or paO_2 <8.0kPa in presence of secondary polycythaemia, nocturnal hypoxaemia, cor pulmonale or pulmonary hypertension.
  - Need to use >15 hours a day.
  - Improves survival and quality of life.
- Ambulatory oxygen: consider in patients who desaturate on exercise or show improvement in exercise capacity with oxygen.
- Short-burst oxygen: consider in patients with episodes of severe breathlessness not relieved by alternative treatments.

Non-invasive ventilation
- Considered in patients with chronic type II respiratory failure despite adequate treatment.
- May rest fatigued respiratory muscles, improve sleep quality and, by reducing nocturnal hypoventilation, may reset respiratory centre leading to improvements in daytime hypercapnia.

Describe the role of surgery in patients with COPD
Lung volume reduction surgery
- Removing areas of poorly functioning lung (and thus allowing expansion of more physiologically useful lung) can improve exercise capacity, quality of life and mortality in a select group of patients.
- Patients who remain symptomatic despite maximal medical therapy and pulmonary rehabilitation and have FEV_1 >20% predicted, $PaCO_2$ <7.3kPa, TLCO >20% predicted and predominantly upper lobe emphysema should be referred for consideration.

Bullectomy
- Bullectomy improves symptoms and lung function by reducing airway resistance and functional residual capacity, improving elastic recoil, restoring the mechanical linkage between the chest wall and normal lung and moving the diaphragm into a more efficient position.
- Should be considered in patients with progressive dyspnoea despite maximal medical treatment, FEV_1 <50% predicted and bullae >1/3 hemithorax with preserved function in the surrounding lung.

Lung transplant
- Can improve functional capacity.
- The International Society for Heart and Lung Transplant Registry report an overall 1-year survival of 78% and 5-year survival of 51%. However, the true increase in survival over the natural history of COPD is less clear.
- Guidelines for referral include: BODE index >5, post bronchodilator FEV_1 <25 %, resting hypoxaemia and hypercapnia, secondary pulmonary hypertension and accelerated decline in FEV_1.

What causes an acute exacerbation of COPD?
- Infection (60%):
  - Viruses: rhinovirus>influenza, parainfluenza, cornavirus, adenovirus.
  - Bacteria: *Haemophillus influenza*, *Moraxella catarrhalis*, streptococcal pneumonia >*Pseudomonas*, enterobacteria. Incidence of atypical bacteria low.
- Environmental pollution (10%).
- Unknown aetiology (30%).

How are infective exacerbations of COPD treated?
- Controlled oxygen therapy to achieve arterial oxygen saturations of 88–92%.
- Nebulized beta 2-agonists.
- Nebulized anticholinergics.
- Oral corticosteroids: improve lung function and reduce hospital length of stay.
- Antibiotics: initial empirical treatment with aminopenicillin, macrolides or tetracycline.
- Aminophylline:
  - Not recommended as first line treatment.
  - RCTs have failed to show benefit compared to effect of bronchodilators and steroids.
  - Significant side effects including nausea, tremor and arrhythmia.
- Discharge planning should involve a community COPD treatment team.

Describe the use of non-invasive ventilation (NIV) in the treatment of acute exacerbations of COPD
Bi-level positive airway pressure (BiPAP) provides pressure support via a facemask with higher inspiratory positive airway pressure (IPAP) than expiratory positive airway pressure (EPAP).
- Ventilators differ in delivering either a selected volume or pressure and can be timed or patient-triggered, with back-up rates if the patient fails to breathe.
- NIV improves oxygenation, increases the removal of CO_2, increases functional residual capacity, increases tidal volume, improves lung and chest wall mechanics and decreases respiratory effort.

Compared to conventional medical care NIV has been shown to:
- Decrease the need for endotracheal intubation.
- Improve pH and respiratory rate.
- Result in fewer complications (principally ventilator associated pneumonias).
- Result in shorter lengths of hospital stay.
- Reduce mortality.

Indications
- NIV should be considered in patients who despite maximal medical treatment and controlled oxygen therapy have a respiratory acidosis (pH <7.35).
- Patients should be able to consent to treatment and have potential for recovery to a quality of life that is acceptable to the patient.
- Relative exclusion criteria include: life-threatening hypoxaemia, severe comorbidity, confusion, facial injuries, vomiting, fixed upper airway obstruction, inability to protect airway, undrained pneumothorax, haemodynamic instability, bowel obstruction or upper gastrointestinal surgery.
- In patients in whom endotracheal intubation is inappropriate there is flexibility within these guidelines, for example in an unconscious patient secondary to COPD induced hypercapnia.

NB Long-term NIV can be used for patients with end-stage COPD and neuromuscular disorders.

Commencing NIV
- At time of commencing NIV a decision regarding the most appropriate ceiling of care for the patient should be documented (e.g. should they be intubated and mechanically ventilated if NIV fails) and a resuscitation decision should be made.
- Initial pressures recommended are IPAP 12–16cmH$_2$O and EPAP 4–5cmH$_2$O with oxygen adjusted to reach target saturations of 88–92%. Pressures are adjusted depending on patient tolerability and clinical response. Patients should be closely monitored with repeat blood gases 1 hour after commencement of NIV or following change in settings.

How does CPAP (continuous positive airway pressure) differ from non-invasive ventilation?
- CPAP maintains the same pressure support throughout the breathing cycle, splinting open the upper airways, recruiting collapsed alveoli (thus improving lung compliance) and reducing ventilation/perfusion mismatching.
- It is used in the treatment of acute pulmonary oedema, obstructive sleep apnoea and Type 1 respiratory failure.

References
1. Celli BR et al. The body-mass index, airflow obstruction, dyspnea and exercise capacity index in chronic obstructive pulmonary disease. *NEJM* 2004; **350**:1005–12.
2. Ong KC et al. A multidimensional grading system (BODE index) as predictor of hospitalization for COPD. *Chest* 2005; **128**(6):3810–16.
3. Calverley PM et al. Salmeterol and fluticasone propionate and survival in chronic obstructive pulmonary disease. *NEJM* 2007; **356**(8)775–89.
4. Tashin DP et al. A 4-year trial of tiotropium in chronic obstructive pulmonary disease. *NEJM* 2008; **359**(15):1543–54.

ॐ Useful websites
British Lung Foundation: http://www.lunguk.org.
British Thoracic Society: http://www.brit-thoracic.org.uk/ (click on Clinical Information page. Information available on COPD, home treatment teams, NIV and home oxygen).
COPD guidelines: http://guidance.nice.org.uk/CG12.
NIV in acute COPD guidelines: http://www.rcplondon.ac.uk/publications/.

Pneumonia

Clinical signs

- Oxygen/sputum pot at bedside
- Tachypnoea
- Tachycardia

Over area of consolidation:

- Reduced expansion
- Increased tactile vocal fremitus
- Dullness to percussion
- Coarse crepitations
- Bronchial breathing
- Increased vocal resonance/whispering pectoriloquy
- Pleural rub

> **❶ Top Tips**
> - Look for rash:
>   - Erythema multiforme (target lesions) is associated with mycoplasma pneumonia.
>   - Erythema nodosum (red tender nodular eruption on extensor aspects of lower limbs) is associated with streptococcal infections, tuberculosis (TB) and mycoplasma.
> - Look for signs of parapneumonic effusion (stony dull to percussion, reduced breath sounds).
> - Consider whether the patient is at risk of aspiration pneumonia:
>   - Evidence of stroke, motor neuron disease (MND), neuromuscular disorder.

Symptoms

- Cough productive of purulent sputum
- Fever
- Dyspnoea
- Pleuritic chest pain

> **❶ Top Tips**
> *Consider differential diagnoses*
> - Lung cancer:
>   - Look for tar-stained fingers, clubbing, cachexia, signs of COPD.
> - Bronchiectasis:
>   - May be a clue in the history e.g. examine the patient who produces copious amounts of purulent sputum, look for clubbing, early inspiratory crepitations will be heard in multiple areas (unless localized bronchiectasis).

Severity

BTS guidelines recommend using the CURB-65 score to assess the severity of community-acquired pneumonia and guide appropriate treatment and location (Table 2.5). 1 point is given to each of the following parameters:

- **C**onfusion: new confusion defined as an Abbreviated Mental Test Score of ≤8
- **U**rea: raised >7mmol/L
- **R**espiratory rate: raised >30/min
- **B**lood pressure: reduced with systolic <90mmHg and/or diastolic ≤60mmHg
- Age >**65** years

This scoring system has been shown to correlate with 30-day mortality.[1]

Table 2.5 CURB-65 score

CURB-65 score	30-day mortality	BTS guidelines
0	0.7%	Low risk. Consider home treatment
1	3.2%	
2	3%	Increased risk
3	17%	High risk. Treat as severe pneumonia and consider referral to ITU
4	41.5%	
5	57%	

Investigations

- Arterial blood gas if oxygen saturation <92% or features of severe pneumonia (type I respiratory failure).
- FBC, U&E, LFT, CRP.
- CXR – consolidation (with air bronchogram), interstitial infiltrates, lobar collapse, pleural effusion.

Microbiology

- Blood cultures – prior to commencing antibiotic treatment.
- Sputum culture for MCS (and AFB if TB suspected).
- Urine for *Legionella* and pneumococcal antigen in those with severe pneumonia or when suspected on clinical or epidemiological grounds.
- Paired atypical serology: 1st sample sent within 7 days of onset. Repeated after 10 days. Performed in all patients with severe pneumonia and those who are unresponsive to β-lactam antibiotics.
- Serological assays with complement fixation tests for diagnosis of atypical and common respiratory viral pathogens.

Further investigations
- Bronchoscopy: can be of value to exclude endobronchial abnormality, obtain samples for MCS and remove retained secretions.
- CT Chest: consider if poor response to treatment to exclude abscess, empyema and malignancy.

Viva questions

Name the common causes of community-acquired pneumonia
The prevalence of individual pathogens varies depending on whether patients are managed in the community, hospital or ITU setting.

Bacteria
- Streptococcal pneumonia: most frequently identified pathogen (36–39%). Occurs most commonly in the winter.
- *Haemophilus* influenza: more common in COPD patients.
- *Mycoplasma* pneumonia: epidemics spanning 3 winters; occur every 4 years in UK.
- *Chlamydophilia* pneumonia (Q fever).
- *Legionella*: most common in September and October. Over 50% cases related to travel e.g. Mediterranean countries. Epidemics occur in relation to water containing systems in buildings.
- *Staphylococcus aureus*: most common in winter months. Associated with influenza virus infection.
- *Moxarella catarrhalis*: more common in COPD patients.
- Less commonly: Gram-negative enteric bacilli (increased in aspiration pneumonia), *C. psittaci* (mostly acquired from birds and animals), *C. burnetti* (common from April–June in relation to lambing and calving season).

Atypical pathogens (*Mycoplasma pnuemoniae*, *Chlamydia pneumoniae* and *Legionella* species) are identified less frequently in the elderly.

The term 'atypical pneumonia' incorrectly implies there is a characteristic presentation for infections caused by 'atypical pathogens' and hence the BTS recommends this term be abandoned.

Viruses
- Most commonly influenzae A and B.

How can we assess the severity of community acquired pneumonia?
- CURB-65 score – see Table 2.5.
- Other adverse prognostic factors include: presence of coexisting disease, hypoxaemia (SaO_2 ≤92% or PaO_2 ≤ 8kPa), bilateral or multilobar involvement on CXR, albumin <35g/L, WCC >20 or <4 x 10^9 and positive blood cultures.

Describe the treatment of community-acquired pneumonia
General measures
- Oxygen – aim to maintain PaO_2 ≥8kPa and oxygen saturations ≥92%
- Intravenous fluids if evidence of volume depletion
- Nutritional support
- Physiotherapy

Pharmocological treatment

Treatment should be guided by local antibiotic guidelines which take into account local pathogen rates, resistance profiles and side effects such as risk of *Clostridium difficile* infection.

- For non-severe pneumonia (CURB-65 score 0–2) the BTS recommend a penicillin and macrolide (erythromycin or clarithromycin) antibiotic. For those with penicillin intolerance or hypersensitivity a fluroquinolone with enhanced pneumococcal activity (moxifloxacin or levofloxacin) is recommended.
- For severe pneumonia (CURB-65 score >3) BTS recommends either co-amoxiclav or a cephalosporin combined with a macrolide with floroquinolones as an alternative regimen.
- Antibiotics should be administered as early as possible.

Follow-up

Patients should be reviewed 6 weeks post discharge with repeat CXR to ensure resolution of consolidation if there are persistent symptoms or there is a high risk of underlying malignancy.

Prevention

- Influenza vaccination (annually): recommended for patients with chronic lung, heart, renal and liver disease, diabetes, immunosuppression due to disease or medication and age >65 years. Contraindicated in those with hypersensitivity to hens' eggs.
- Pneumococcal vaccination (one-off vaccination with re-immunization after 5 years if required): recommended for patients over the age of 2 years in whom pneumococcal infection is likely to be more common or severe.

Define hospital-acquired pneumonia. What different pathogens are involved?

Hospital-acquired or hospital-associated pneumonia occurs >72 hours after admission to hospital. It is most commonly caused by Gram-negative bacilli, *Pseudomonas* and anaerobes.

Reference

1. Lim WS *et al.* Defining community acquired pneumonia severity on presentation to hospital: an international derivation and validation study. *Thorax* 2003; **58**: 377–82.

♬ Useful website

British Thoracic Society: http://www.brit-thoracic.org.uk (follow link to clinical information then pneumonia).

Bronchiectasis

Bronchiectasis is the abnormal permanent dilatation and destruction of the bronchi caused by a combination of infection, impaired drainage, airway obstruction ± defective host response (Table 2.6). The definitive aetiology may be difficult to identify.

Clinical signs

- (Copious) purulent sputum in cup at bedside
- Cachexia
- Tachypnoea
- Finger clubbing (not always present)
- Central cyanosis
- Hyperexpanded chest
- Inspiratory clicks
- Crepitations – coarse, late, inspiratory (over bronchiectatic areas)
- Wheeze

❶ Top Tips

Look for clues as to the cause of bronchiectasis while examining. For example, in the young Caucasian patient with short stature consider CF (for other causes see Table 2.6).

Respiratory causes of clubbing

- **A**bscess (lung) and **A**sbestosis
- **B**ronchiectasis
- **C**ystic fibrosis
- **D**irty tumours (bronchogenic carcinoma, mesothelioma)
- **E**mpyema
- **F**ibrosing alveolitis (interstitial pulmonary fibrosis).

---

❶ Top Tips

Causes of clubbing and crackles: – 'FAB' you know this:
- **F**ibrosing alveolitis
- **A**sbestosis
- **B**ronchiectasis, **B**ronchogenic carcinoma.

Symptoms

- Dyspnoea
- Cough with daily (copious) purulent sputum
- Haemoptysis
- Recurrent infection
- Pleuritic chest pain
- Weight loss
- History of sinusitis, childhood infection, TB, subfertility, failure to thrive.

Severity

Determined by the following:
- Symptoms: dyspnoea assessed using MRC Dyspnoea Scale
  (❸ Table 2.3, p.33).

- Number of bronchopulmonary segments involved (assessed by imaging).
- Lung function assessment (FEV_1, FVC).

Investigations

Laboratory

- Sputum MCS, AFB and cytology.
- FBC:
  - anaemia of chronic disease, ↑ WCC with neutrophilia. Less commonly polycythaemia secondary to hypoxia.
- Serum immunoglobulins: IgG subclasses, IgM and IgA (hypogammaglobulinaemia).
- Alpha-1 antitrypsin levels (alpha-1 antitrypsin deficiency).
- *Aspergillus* precipitins and serum IgE (ABPA).
- Autoantibodies (if connective tissue disease suspected).

Imaging

- CXR:
  - Dilated and thickened airways (tramlines and ring shadows which may contain air fluid levels).
  - Mucus plugging (bronchoceles – 'gloved finger' appearance).
  - Hyperinflation.
  - Honeycomb patterns seen in severe cases.
  - Normal CXR – 7%.
- HRCT – *the definitive test*:
  - High sensitivity and specificity.
  - Reid classification – cyclindrical (most advanced), varicose and saccular (cystic).
  - Bronchial thickening and dilatation seen as 'tram tracking' in parallel or ring shadows end on.
  - 'Signet ring sign' – thickened dilated bronchi >1.5 times larger than adjacent pulmonary artery.
  - Pus/fluid levels in dilated bronchiectatic segments.
  - Mucus plugging (bronchoceles).
  - Lack of normal tapering with bronchi seen within 1cm of pleura.
  - Associated with obliterative bronchiolitis ('tree in bud' appearance seen as Y- and V-shaped peripheral opacities).

Functional assessment

- Lung function testing: commonly obstructive impairment (FVC ↓ or normal, FEV_1 ↓, ↓ FEV_1/FVC).

Other

- Flexible bronchoscopy (rarely needed. May be necessary to obtain further microbiological samples or exclude other conditions).

Specific tests determined by underlying aetiology

- Cystic fibrosis:
  - Sweat test (chloride >60mmol/L)
  - Genotyping
- Kartagener's syndrome: nasal brushings and electron microscopy.
- Tuberculosis: tuberculin skin test, interferon gamma release assay.

Table 2.6 Causes of bronchiectasis

	Condition	Clues to diagnosis
Congenital	Cystic fibrosis (CF)	Young, Caucasian, short stature, thin, pale
		Clubbing often present
		PEG feeding, long-term vascular access (upper anterior chest wall/antecubital fossa)
		Ask about other systems e.g. diarrhoea, diabetes
	Young's syndrome	Clinical features similar to CF i.e. bronchiectasis, sinusitis, azoospermia but no CF mutation, abnormal sweat or pancreatic insufficiency. Often middle-aged men
	Kartagener's syndrome	Ciliary dyskinesia + dextrocardia, situs inversus, subfertility, sinusitis, otitis media
	Yellow nail syndrome	Yellow nails, pleural effusion and lymphoedema due to abnormal lymphatics
	Abnormal anatomy e.g. sequestrated lung segments, bronchial atresia	
Mechanical	Bronchial obstruction:	Localized/segmental bronchiectasis
	Foreign body	More common in right lung if caused by foreign body
	Carcinoma	
	Granuloma (sarcoid/TB)	
	Compression by enlarged lymph nodes (TB)	
Childhood infection	Whooping cough (pertussis), measles, TB	Look for signs of old TB, stunted growth, ethnic background

Overactive immune response	Allergic bronchopulmonary aspergillosis	Central airway bronchiectasis
		Always consider in patient with 'asthma' resistant to bronchodilators and cough
Underactive immune response	Congenital: hypogammaglobulinaemia	
	Acquired : HIV, leukaemia	
Chemical injury	Recurrent aspiration	Signs of stroke, bulbar neurological disease, chronic alcohol disease
Associated with other respiratory disease	Fibrosis 'traction bronchiectasis'	May also have bronchiectasis
	COPD	30% also have bronchiectasis
		Ask about sputum volume in COPD patient

Treatment

General measures
- Education of patient and family.
- Optimize nutrition:
  - Calorie supplementation.
  - CF patients may need pancreatic enzyme replacement and fat-soluble vitamin supplementation.
- Smoking cessation.
- Vaccinations e.g. Pneumovax, Hib.
- Sputum clearance/physiotherapy:
  - Involves postural drainage, chest percussion, controlled breathing exercises, forced expiration.
  - A variety of devices can be used to provide PEP (positive expiratory pressure) or oscillating PEP.
  - CF patients may use hypertonic saline nebs twice daily prior to physiotherapy.

Medical treatment
- Antibiotics to treat infective exacerbations. These often need to cover pseudomonal species and prolonged courses may be required.
- Prophylactic antibiotics (less evidence based) e.g. azithromycin orally and/or tobramycin nebulized to cover *Pseudomonas* species.
- Bronchodilators (if any component of reversibility).
- Steroids – regular inhaled to decrease chronic inflammation and oral in infective exacerbations.
- Mucolytics e.g. carbocysteine, RhDNAase in CF patients.

Surgical treatment
- Lobectomy/bullectomy (note very specific indications – localized disease with good lung function).
- Transplantation in CF.

Treatment of underlying cause (e.g. immunoglobulins for hypogammaglobulinaemia)

Viva questions

What is the pathogenesis of CF?
- Autosomal recessive disease due to defect in *CFTR* gene (cystic fibrosis transmembrane conductance regulator protein) located on chromosome 7. Over 1250 mutations, most common is ΔF508. Frequency of mutation in Caucasians 1 in 2000–3000 live births.
- CFTR protein located in all exocrine tissues.
- Defective CFTR protein prevents chloride moving out of cells → Na^+ hyperabsorption occuring to keep intracellular electrochemical balance → osmotic pull of water into the cells → dehydration of extracellular surfaces → thick viscous secretions easily amenable to colonization and infection.

What other systems are affected in CF patients?
CF is a multisystem disease with lung disease being the major cause of morbidity and mortality.
- Gastrointestinal:

- Pancreatic enzyme insufficiency with malabsorption of fat and protein.
- Diabetes (cystic fibrosis-related diabetes – CFRD).
- Meconium ileus (in newborns) and distal intestinal obstruction syndrome (DIOS).
- Focal biliary cirrhosis leading to or with portal hypertension.
- Cholelithiasis.
- Reproductive: male subfertility (>95%) due to defective sperm transport. Spermatogenesis is normal.
- Musculoskeletal: osteoporosis.
- ENT: sinus disease and nasal polyposis.

What organisms commonly colonize the respiratory tract in CF patients?

- *Haemophilus influenza* (early childhood).
- *Staphylococcus aureus* (early childhood).
- *Pseudomonas* species (late childhood).
- *Burkholderia cepacia* 'complex' (less common but important):
  - Associated with accelerated decline in pulmonary function and decreased survival.
  - May be a contraindication to transplantation in some centres.

What is the prognosis for CF patients?
Median survival 32 years and increasing, many patients live into their 40s and lead active lives.

Give the main complications of bronchiectasis
Pulmonary complications
- Recurrent infection
- Haemoptysis (can be massive, i.e. >400mL)
- Empyema/abscess
- Cor pulmonale (↑ JVP, right ventricular heave, peripheral oedema).

Extrapulmonary complications
- Anaemia
- Metastatic infection e.g. cerebral abscess
- Secondary amyloidosis.

What other conditions are known to be associated with bronchiectasis?
- Connective tissue diseases (e.g. rheumatoid arthritis)
- Chronic sinusitis
- Inflammatory bowel disease
- Marfan's syndrome.

What are the major pathogens associated with bronchiectasis?
- *Pseudomonas aeruginosa*
- *Haemophilus influenza*
- *Streptococcus* (less commonly).

📖 Further reading
Barker AF. Bronchiectasis. *NEJM* 2002; **346**: 1383–93.
ten Hacken NH et al. Treatment of bronchiectasis in adults. *BMJ* 2007; **335**:1089–93.
O'Donnell AE et al. Treatment of idiopathic bronchiectasis with aerosolized recombinant human DNase I. *Chest* 1998; **113**(5):1329–34.

🔊 **Useful websites**

Cystic Fibrosis Foundation: http://www.cff.org.
British Lung Foundation: http://www.lunguk.org.
British Thoracic Society: http://www.brit-thoracic.org.uk (follow link to clinical information then cystic fibrosis).

Old tuberculosis

Clinical findings of old pulmonary tuberculosis relate both to complications of disease and complications of treatment.

Complications of disease

- Apical fibrosis.
- Bronchiectasis – due to lymph node obstruction causing distal bronchial dilatation, bronchial stenosis and secondary to lung fibrosis (traction bronchiectasis).
- Aspergilloma in old TB cavity.
- Pleural effusion or thickening.

Complications of treatment

Prior to the introduction of effective antibiotics to treat *Mycobacterium tuberculosis* in the 1950s, a number of surgical techniques were used to treat TB. These were based on the theory that inducing lobar collapse would starve the organism of oxygen; however it is now known that *Mycobacterium tuberculosis* can survive in anaerobic conditions.

Techniques included:

- Plombage: derived from the French word for lead 'plomb'. An inert substance, for example wax, plastic balls or gauze, was inserted into the pleural space, thus compressing the adjacent lung.
- Thoracoplasty: ribs were resected thus reducing the intrathoracic volume.
- Phrenic nerve crush: the nerve was crushed or cut to paralyse the diaphragm on the affected side.

Clinical signs

- Chest deformity
- Scars:
  - Thoracotomy scar
  - Phrenic nerve crush in supraclavicular fossa
- Tracheal deviation towards side of old TB in upper lobe
- Reduced expansion
- Dullness to percussion
- Crepitations – either fine end-inspiratory crepitations over area of fibrosis or coarse inspiratory crepitations over area of bronchiectasis
- Bronchial breathing

> ❶ **Top Tips**
>
> Look for kyphosis – may be sign of spinal TB (Pott's disease). This is termed a Gibbus deformity.

Symptoms of active pulmonary TB infection

TB should be considered in any patient presenting with pneumonia, particularly in those with ongoing symptoms:

- Fever
- Night sweats
- Cough productive of sputum
- Haemoptysis
- Dyspnoea
- Pleuritic chest pain
- Fatigue
- Weight loss

Investigations

For initial investigations please refer to ⟶ Pneumonia, p.41. If TB is suspected clinically the following should be considered:

- Sputum for Ziehl–Neelsen/auramine staining and culture: 3 sputum samples. If cough is non-productive sputum can be induced with hypertonic normal saline (requires isolation) or samples obtained at bronchoscopy.
- Early morning urine for AFB (3 consecutive samples, especially if sterile pyuria is present).
- Mantoux testing (tuberculin skin testing – TST):
  - 2 tuberculin units (in 0.1mL of solution) are injected intradermally into forearm.
  - Induces a delayed type hypersensitivity reaction (type IV).
  - Results are read 48–72 hours later and graded. In patients without prior BCG vaccination <5mm reaction is negative, 5–14mm positive, >15mm strongly positive. In patients with previous BCG vaccination <15mm is negative, >15mm is positive.
- Patients who are immunosuppressed, for example with HIV, may have a falsely negative TST due to anergy. Sarcoidosis can also cause a negative reaction due to impaired cell mediated and humoral immunity.
- Interferon gamma release assay (IGRA) e.g. T-SPOT® or QuantiFERON® test:
  - Measures interferon gamma released by antigen-specific T cells in response to peptides derived from (and specific to) *Mycobacterium tuberculosis* e.g. ESAT-6 and CFP10.
  - More sensitive than TST so less likely to produce false negative results, especially in immunosuppressed individuals.
  - More specific than TST. Less likely to produce false positive results, for example in response to prior BCG vaccination.
- HIV testing.
- CXR: hilar or paratracheal adenopathy, pulmonary infiltrates, pulmonary nodules and consolidation, cavitation (classically in upper lobes) and pleural effusion.
- CT scan:
  - More sensitive than CXR.
  - May see consolidation, cavitation, centrilobular nodules connected to multiple branching linear structures originating from a single stalk ('tree in bud' pattern), ground glass opacification, miliary nodules,

> pericardial and/or pleural effusion or thickening, low attenuation lymph nodes, thickening and irregularity of trachea and bronchi.
> • Changes of old TB include fibrosis (predominantly in upper lobes), traction bronchiectasis and pleural scarring.

- Bronchoscopy: to obtain bronchoalveolar lavage (BAL) samples and assess for endobronchial abnormalities.
- Biopsy of extrapulmonary sites e.g. lymph node.

Viva questions

What are the risk factors for active pulmonary TB infection?

- Place of birth – increased incidence in immigrants from sub-Saharan Africa and Asia
- Age – increasing prevalence with age in Caucasian population
- HIV/AIDS
- Homeless
- Previous prison stays
- Sex-workers
- Comorbidities e.g. diabetes, renal disease, malignancy
- Patients on immunosuppressant medication e.g. steroids, chemotherapy, TNFα antagonists

How do you treat pulmonary TB? Name some common side effects of treatment

- TB is a notifiable disease and contact tracing should be initiated.
- Treatment should commence with rifampicin, isoniazid, ethambutol and pyrazinamide whilst microbiological sensitivities are awaited. For fully sensitive disease ethambutol and pyrazinamide can be stopped after 2 months and rifampicin and isoniazid continued for a further 4 months. Dosages are weight related.
- Prior to treatment patients should have their liver function checked, visual acuity documented with a Snellen chart and colour vision assessed using Ishihara plates. Patients should be advised of the common side effects of treatment and given advice to contact doctor if they develop vomiting or jaundice.
- Directly observed treatment (DOT) should be considered in patients with no fixed abode or who have poor compliance with treatment.

Some common side effects of medication include:

- *Isoniazid:* hepatitis, peripheral neuropathy.
- *Rifampicin:* increases activity of hepatic microsomal enzymes with reduced efficacy of medications such as the contraceptive pill and anti-epileptics, red discoloration of secretions and urine (can be used to assess compliance), gastrointestinal disturbance.
- *Pyrazinamide:* gastrointestinal disturbance, hepatic toxicity, peripheral neuropathy, gout.
- *Ethambutol:* optic neuritis.

What are the complications of pulmonary TB?

See → p.50:
- Pneumothorax
- Empyema
- Abscess

What are the extrapulmonary manifestations of TB?

- CNS: TB meningitis, tuberculoma.
- Pericardial TB.
- Spinal TB – most commonly affects thoracic spine, however any joint or bone can be affected.
- Genitourinary: prostatitis, epididymitis.
- Peripheral cold abscess.
- Miliary TB – haematogenous spread, can affect any organ.

New developments

Vitamin D

Recent research has suggested that vitamin D plays an important role in the host defence response to TB. Vitamin D deficiency has been associated with TB disease in a number of case–control studies and there is now a growing body of work demonstrating that vitamin D is metabolized to its active form in TB-infected macrophages, and that this is involved in the production of antimicrobial peptides which defend against TB. Studies are underway to assess the effect of vitamin D supplementation in patients with active TB.

⚲ Useful websites

British Thoracic Society: http://www.brit-thoracic.org.uk (follow link to Clinical Information, then Tuberculosis).

NICE clinical guidelines: http://guidance.nice.org.uk/CG33.

Pulmonary fibrosis

Pulmonary fibrosis is characterized by the development of diffuse paren-chymal lung disease. Whilst there are a variety of causes sharing many clinico-pathological features, there are enough individual distinguishing features to justify labelling them as separate diseases (Table 2.7).

Clinical signs

- Tachypnoea (advanced disease; may see patient on oxygen or portable oxygen at bedside).
- Clubbing (common in idiopathic pulmonary fibrosis [IPF], chronic hypersensitivity pneumonitis; rare in sarcoidosis, collagen vascular disease related-interstitial lung disease, organizing pneumonia).
- Central cyanosis.
- Tracheal deviation to affected side in upper zone fibrosis.
- Flattened chest (affected side, more prominent if upper zone fibrosis).
- Scars from lung biopsy, mastectomy, radiotherapy, phrenic nerve crush (supraclavicular area).
- Reduced chest expansion.
- Increased tactile vocal fremitus and resonance (difficult to appreciate).
- Dullness to percussion (affected zones).
- Auscultatory findings include fine end-inspiratory crepitations (affected zones) or 'squeaks' (hypersensitivity pneumonitis).
- Crepitations of pulmonary fibrosis show distinct features:
  - May disappear or soften significantly when the patient is asked to lean forward so ensure patient is sitting up straight when auscultating the posterior chest or you may miss them completely!
  - Unaffected by coughing thus differentiating them from those caused by pulmonary oedema.
  - Fine quality differentiates them from the coarse crepitations of bronchiectasis or infection (NB as fibrosis progresses, crepitations become coarser therefore 'timing' the crepitations may be more discriminating – 'early inspiratory' in bronchiectasis and 'late inspiratory' in pulmonary fibrosis).
  - Sound like the noise made by rubbing the hair behind the ears with the thumb and index finger; the coarse crepitations of bronciectasis are like Velcro being pulled apart.
- Evidence of pulmonary hypertension (parasternal heave, palpable P2, raised JVP, hepatomegaly and peripheral oedema).
- Evidence of treatment including:
  - Steroid purpura.
  - Oxygen supplementation.
- Features of associated causes (if these have not already been detected):
  - Hands: rheumatoid changes, sclerodactyly (tightening of the skin of the fingers), nicotine staining.
  - Face/eyes: butterfly rash of SLE, heliotrope rash of dermatomyositis, telangiectasia or microstomia of systemic sclerosis, dry eyes (conjunctival injection) or dry mouth in Sjögren's syndrome, lupus pernio of sarcoidosis.

❶ Top Tips

'Zones' of pulmonary fibrosis

Areas affected by pulmonary fibrosis are better thought of as 'zones' (upper and lower) rather than 'lobes' – these will be easier to present when under stressful exam conditions!

Symptoms

- Exertional dyspnoea (in severe cases can progress to occur at rest).
- Chronic dry cough.
- Symptoms of associated conditions (e.g. arthralgia, butterfly rash or photosensitivity associated with SLE).
- The patient may have a history of TB, radiation, metal/dust/drug exposures.

Distribution of the fibrosis

- Fibrosis can affect any lobe or zone but predominant patterns do exist.
- Causes may be symmetrical or asymmetrical:

Symmetrical causes

Upper zone fibrosis ('charts'):

- **C**oal worker's pneumoconioses
- **H**istoplasmosis
- **H**ypersensitivity pneumonitis (fibrotic EAA)
- **H**istiocytosis X
- **A**nkylosing spondylitis
- **A**BPA (allergic bronchopulmonary aspergillosis)
- **R**adiation
- **T**uberculosis
- **S**arcoidosis/**S**ilicosis

Lower zone fibrosis ('ratio'):

- **R**heumatoid arthritis
- **A**sbestosis
- Connective **T**issue disease (scleroderma, PM, DM, Sjögren's syndrome, SLE, MCTD)
- **I**diopathic pulmonary fibrosis (UIP, fibrotic NSIP – see Table 2.7)
- **O**ther causes – bronchiectasis, chemical or drug exposures (❺ Table 2.7).

Asymmetrical causes – usually upper zones, two main causes:

Treated TB (thoracotomy scar and/or phrenic nerve crush).

Malignant disease (radiotherapy marks, lymphadenopathy, small muscle wasting of hands in Pancoast's lesion).

❶ Top Tips

The differential diagnosis of pulmonary fibrosis should be tailored according to the clinical findings in the individual patient, for example if bibasal (lower zone) fibrosis is detected then proceed to give the differential list for lower zone fibrosis first and then state 'other' causes which would include upper zone and asymmetrical causes (explaining that the distribution found on examination make these less likely).

Table 2.7 What causes pulmonary fibrosis?

Group	Causes	Additional information
Rheumatological	Rheumatoid arthritis (RA)	Majority cause lower zone fibrosis; ankylosing spondylitis is the exception causing upper zone fibrosis
	Systemic lupus erythematosus (SLE)	
	Polymyositis (PM)	
	Dermatomyositis (DM)	
	Systemic sclerosis (limited and diffuse)	
	Sjögren's syndrome	
	Ankylosing spondylitis	
	Mixed connective tissue disease (MCTD)	
Pneumoconioses	Silicosis	Upper zone disease associated with eggshell hilar calcification that predisposes to TB
'Group of chronic respiratory diseases caused by inhalation of metal or mineral particles'	Berylliosis	Granulomatous lesions similar to sarcoidosis
	Asbestosis	Lower zone disease associated with pleural plaques and mesothelioma

	Coal workers	3 forms: • Simple (without fibrosis) • Complicated (with fibrosis) • Progressive massive fibrosis
Granulomatous disease	TB	Caseating granulomas
	Sarcoidosis	Non-caseating granulomas, may see hilar lymphadenopathy
Extrinsic allergic alveolitis/ hypersensitivity pneumonitis	Farmer's lung	Mouldy hay
'Acute pulmonary/systemic symptoms occurring 6hrs after exposure to allergen → cough, pyrexia and malaise. If exposure is chronic → dyspnoea and non-caseating granulomatous disease. Treatment: steroids in acute disease and long-term avoidance of precipitating factors in chronic disease'	Bird-fancier's lung	Pigeons
	Byssinosis	Cotton dust
	Mushroom worker's lung	Mushroom spores
	Malt worker's lung	Mouldy barley
Chemical causes	Metals	Steel, brass, lead, mercury, beryllium
	Chemicals	Vinylchlorides (dry-cleaning fluids)
	Poisons	Paraquat

(Continued)

Table 2.7 (Contd.)

Group	Causes	Additional information
Iatrogenic causes or medication 'BBC sport is every MANS Gold'	**B**leomycin	Usually affects lower zones
	Busulphan	
	Cyclophosphamide	
	Methotrexate	
	Amiodarone	
	Nitrofurantoin	
	Sulphasalazine	
	Gold	
Idiopathic interstitial pneumonias (IIPs) These are histological subtypes which are important in determining prognosis and responsiveness to steroid treatment'	Usual interstitial pneumonia (UIP)	• Defines IPF • Also seen in asbestosis, chronic hypersensitivity pneumonitis, collagen vascular disease and chronic drug toxicity • 12% steroid responsive • Mean survival 2.5–5.5 years
	Desquamative interstitial pneumonia (DIP)	• Associated with smoking • 62% steroid responsive • Mean survival 12–14 years
	Non-specific interstitial pneumonia (NSIP)	• Better prognosis than UIP • Similar steroid response and survival to DIP

	Cryptogenic organizing pneumonia (COP)	• Also known as bronchiolitis obliterans organizing pneumonia (BOOP) • Associated with pre-existing chronic inflammatory disease (RA) or medications (amiodarone) • Clinically resembles infectious pneumonia, however suspected following negative cultures and no response to antibiotics • Treated with corticosteroids over 6–12 months (may be longer dependant on response to antibiotics)
	Respiratory bronchiolitis-associated interstitial lung disease (RBILD)	Exaggerated bronchiole response to cigarette smoke
	Acute interstitial pneumonia (AIP)	Hamman–Rich syndrome
Other causes	Chronic pulmonary oedema	
	Radiotherapy	
	Lymphangitis carcinomatosis	

Investigations

Laboratory

- Arterial blood gas (hypoxaemia and hypocapnia):
  - Improves on recumbency and worsens when upright.
  - Desaturation on exercise may be seen in pulmonary fibrosis.
- Specific serum testing dictated by suspected underlying cause:
  - FBC (eosinophilia) and precipitins (EAA).
  - Anti-nuclear factor, rheumatoid factor (RA), anti-centromere antibody (limited systemic sclerosis), anti-Scl 70 (diffuse systemic sclerosis), anti-Jo 1 (DM).
  - Serum immunoglobulins (bronchiectasis, IgE for ABPA) and serum ACE activity (sarcoidosis).
  - CK (associated myositis).

Functional

- Pulmonary function testing with diffusion capacity (DLCO):
  - May be normal in early disease.
  - Generally restrictive defect (FEV_1/FVC >70%) with reduced diffusion capacity (DLCO) indicating functional loss of alveolar function (has prognostic value).
  - Coexisting smoking related lung disease may give a mixed obstructive-restrictive picture.
- 6-minute walk test (6MWT):
  - Involves patient walking for a 6-minute period; total distance walked (in metres), oxygen saturation/heart rate and symptoms are noted; drawback: effort dependant and lacks reproducibility.
  - Different to the 'shuttle walking test' which is a paced test, less effort dependant and more reproducible. Both tests determine the need for portable oxygen.

Radiological

- CXR:
  - Reticulonodular shadowing in affected areas which advances with disease progression.
  - In advanced disease parenchymal destruction with decreased lung volumes occurs (only in UIP, DIP, *not* non-fibrotic NSIP).
  - Some patients may have normal CXR.
- HRCT (1–1.5mSv):
  - Assesses extent, pattern (reticular or nodular) and distribution (upper or lower zones) of disease.
  - Very sensitive (can detect disease in presence of normal CXR).
  - Reticular pattern (frequent finding and due to thickening of intralobular structures).
  - Ensuing fibrosis causes 'honeycomb' appearance when extensive (due to subpleural cyst formation).
  - Evaluate concomitant smoking-related disease.

Others

- Echocardiogram (to assess pulmonary artery pressure).
- Bronchoscopy (with BAL ± lung biopsy – transbronchial, open or video assisted thoracoscopic surgery [VATS]):
  - Cell content from BAL and histological pattern from biopsy can dictate potential treatment responses (➔ 'Viva questions', p.61).

Viva questions

What is Hamman–Rich syndrome?

It is an acute, rapidly progressive lung fibrosis also known as acute interstitial pneumonia (AIP). It may respond to steroids but has a poor overall outcome (6-month survival 22%).

What different types of computed tomography (CT) imaging do you know about and when should each be used?

There are 3 main types of CT scanning:

- High-resolution computed tomography (HRCT: 1–1.5mSv)
  - Involves taking very thin sections (1mm) with high spatial frequency re-constructions with 'skipped' areas between the thin sections (1mm slices every 10mm therefore produces sampling of the lung but not continuous imaging).
  - Images obtained during inspiration and expiration and additionally whilst supine and prone (to exclude dependant change seen on scans which can be mistaken for pathology/disease).
  - Most useful for assessment of interstitial processes such as fibrosis or emphysema and endobronchial changes with 'tree in bud' appearances.
- Dynamic (standard CT: 8mSv):
  - Involves taking thicker sections (10mm) which are then used for reconstruction (provides continuous images in contrast to HRCT).
  - Intravenous contrast may be used as it clarifies anatomy and boundaries of the great vessels and improves assessment of the mediastinum and hilar regions for lymphadenopathy.
  - Most useful for assessment of airspace disease (pneumonia or malignancy) and mediastinal pathology (lymph nodes in staging).
- Computed tomography pulmonary angiogram (CTPA: 8mSv):
  - Involves very thin sections (can be variable e.g. 0.5–0.625mm) in a continuous fashion to obtain images of the pulmonary arteries using multi-detector CT scanning (MDCT).
  - Main diagnostic investigation to detect pulmonary embolism.

NB Protocols for CT slice thickness vary between different hospitals, detector number and re-construction software but general principles remain the same.

What are the main treatments available for 'pulmonary fibrosis'?

Treatment options include the following:

- Corticosteroids (factors contributing to *lack of response* include male sex, severity of symptoms or worse lung function on presentation, neutrophilia on BAL or predominant honeycombing on CT).
- Immunosuppressives (cyclophosphamide, azathioprine, methotrexate and cyclosporine).
- Anti-oxidant (N-acetylcysteine in conjunction with corticosteroids and azathioprine).
- Supplemental oxygen (PaO_2 <7.3kPa or <8.0kPa with cor pulmonale).
- Lung transplantation (60% 1-year survival).

In addition to glucocorticoids and immunosuppressives, are you aware of any other potential treatments?

Agents acting as anti-fibrotics have been suggested for use in the management of pulmonary fibrosis. Evidence for their use is limited and therefore they are rarely used in clinical practice e.g. pirfenidone. Other drugs that may be of use include bosentan and warfarin due to their role in pulmonary hypertension.

Comment on prognosis and list favourable prognostic factors in idiopathic pulmonary fibrosis (IPF)

The median survival is 2.8 years. 5-year survival 50% (65% in steroid responders and 25% in non-responders). Favourable prognostic factors include the NSIP subtype.

Which disorders typically have a high lymphocyte count on BAL?

- Hypersensitivity pneumonitis
- Sarcoidosis
- Organizing pneumonia
- Lymphocytic interstitial pneumonia (LIP).

Describe the possible respiratory manifestations in rheumatoid arthritis ('the rheumatoid lung')

There are 5 main respiratory manifestations of rheumatoid arthritis. It is however important to note that nowadays rheumatoid arthritis-related lung disease is seen much less frequently due to earlier and more aggressive treatment regimens.

- Pleural effusions/pleurisy:
  - Males >females.
  - Usually asymptomatic; respiratory symptoms will only occur if effusion large enough.
  - Characteristically low glucose and rheumatoid factor-positive effusions.
- Pulmonary nodules:
  - May be seen on radiography and precede arthritis onset.
  - Usually asymptomatic but can become infected, cavitate or cause haemoptysis.
  - Predilection for upper lobe location.
- Fibrotic lung disease:
  - 2% of all cases become symptomatic, however subclinical disease is common with a reduced DLCO on PFTs and UIP pattern on HRCT.
  - Can result directly from disease or secondary to treatment (methotrexate, gold). If secondary to treatment, changes may regress on discontinuation of offending drug.
- Caplan syndrome: coal worker pneumoconioses and rheumatoid arthritis.
- Obliterative bronchiolitis:
  - Rare manifestation involving small airways obstruction which progress to necrotizing bronchiolitis.
  - Previously occurred in those treated with gold or penicillamine.

📖 Further reading

Bradley B et al. Interstitial lung disease guideline: the British Thoracic Society in collaboration with the Thoracic Society of Australia and New Zealand and the Irish Thoracic Society. *Thorax* 2008; **63**:v1–v58.

Gross TJ, Hunninghake GW. Idiopathic pulmonary fibrosis. *NEJM* 2001; **345**(7):517–25.

🔊 Useful website

Coalition for Pulmonary Fibrosis: http://www.coalitionforpf.org/index.php.

Pleural disease 1: pleural effusion

'A collection of fluid within the pleural space between the parietal and visceral pleura.'

Symptoms

- Shortness of breath
- Cough (pneumonia, TB)
- Pyrexia (infection)
- Haemoptysis (bronchogenic carcinoma, TB)
- Pleuritic chest pain
- Other features based on underlying cause (e.g. nephrotic syndrome, orthopnoea, rashes etc.)
- History of asbestos exposure (mesothelioma)

Clinical signs *(in affected areas; detectable when >500mL present)*

- Tachypnoea (more frequent in large effusions; patients with mild/moderate congestive cardiac failure may get tachypnoeic with smaller effusion).
- Decreased chest movement on the side of the lesion (may be seen from end of bed).
- Tracheal shift (away from effusion – only seen in large effusions >1000mL).
- Reduced chest expansion.
- Decreased tactile vocal fremitus.
- Stony dull percussion note.
- Diminished breath sounds (bronchial breathing and aegophony at upper border of effusion; ensure that you determine how far the effusion extends).
- Reduced tactile vocal resonance.
- Scars from chest tubes and/or any aspiration marks. (The marks of a plaster removed by the examiner before the exam may be seen!)
- Evidence of underlying cause (if these have not already been detected):
  - Clubbing, tar staining, radiation burns, lymphadenopathy, mastectomy (malignancy)
  - Alopecia, mucositis (evidence of chemotherapy)
  - Fluid overload, raised JVP (right-sided cardiac failure)
  - Hypothyroidism (goitre, dry skin, characteristic facies)
  - Rheumatoid hands (RA)
  - Butterfly rash (SLE).

Types of pleural effusion

- 6 main types of effusions occur:
  - Transudates
  - Exudates
  - Haemothorax (blood)
  - Chylothorax (lymph)
  - Empyema (pus)
  - Drug induced effusions

- Transudates and exudates are defined by Light's criteria – ➔ 'Viva questions', p.69.
- In general, transudates are caused by 'systemic' factors whereas exudates are caused by 'local' factors that alter the homeostasis of the formation and absorption of pleural fluid.

Main causes of pleural effusions
- Transudates ('CHAM'):
  - **C**ongestive cardiac failure (CCF)
  - **H**ypoalbuminaemia (e.g. nephrotic syndrome)/**H**ypothyroidism
  - **A**ll failures (cardiac, renal, hepatic)
  - **M**eig's syndrome (benign ovarian fibromas and transudative pleural effusions; mainly right-sided)
- Exudates ('PINTS'):
  - **P**neumonia
  - **I**nfarction (pulmonary embolism)
  - **N**eoplastic (bronchogenic carcinoma, mesothelioma or metastasis – breast, ovary and pancreas)
  - **T**uberculosis/**T**rauma
  - **S**arcoidosis/**S**cleroderma and other connective tissue diseases (e.g. RA)
- Drugs (exudates >transudates):
  - Associated with drug-induced lupus (quinidine, procainamide, hydralazine)
  - Dopamine agonist (bromocriptine)
  - Disease modifying anti-rheumatics (methotrexate)
  - Anti-migraine (methysergide)
  - Antibiotics (nitrofurantoin)
  - Chemotherapy (procarbazine).

Differential diagnosis of other causes of dullness at the lung base
- Pleural thickening: trachea central, audible breath sounds.
- Consolidation: increased tactile vocal resonance, bronchial breath sounds with associated inspiratory coarse crepitations.
- Collapse: trachea toward affected side, absent breath sounds.
- Fibrosis: trachea central unless upper lobe affected, decreased breath sounds with fine end-inspiratory crepitations.
- Raised hemidiaphragm: phrenic nerve palsy or hepatomegaly: differentiated by 'tidal percussion' where percussion note moves with respiration in the latter.

Investigations
Laboratory
- Pleural fluid analysis (diagnostic thoracocentesis):
  - Often performed under ultrasound guidance.
  - Complications:
    – Pneumothorax.
    – Haemothorax.
    – Intravascular collapse or re-expansion pulmonary oedema (following rapid drainage).

- Serum levels (albumin, LDH) must be sent simultaneously to apply Light's criteria (➔ 'Viva questions', p.69).
- Serum inflammatory markers (CRP/ESR).
- Blood tests (FBC, U&E, LFT, TFT, coagulation).
- Blood cultures (if empyema suspected).
- Tests as appropriate to suspected underlying cause.

Functional
- Echocardiography (ventricular function, valvular lesions).

Radiological
- CXR:
  - Effusion must be at least 300mL to be detected on PA film and 25mL on lateral decubitus view.
  - Dense opacity with associated meniscus sign ('fluid level').
  - Blunting of costophrenic/cardiophrenic angles (earliest sign).
  - Mediastinal/tracheal shift (only if effusion >1000mL).
  - Possible atelectasis of underlying lobe or loculations.
  - Evidence of underlying cause (e.g. bony lesions in metastatic malignancy).
- Pleural ultrasonography:
  - Loculated/small pleural effusions
  - Guided thoracocentesis
  - Closed pleural biopsy
  - Chest drain insertion
  - Differentiates pleural effusions from pleural thickening
- CT thorax:
  - More accurate than CXR in identifying aetiology and guiding interventional procedures.
  - Detects small effusions missed by CXR.
  - 'Pleural enhancement' on CT suggests empyema requiring chest tube insertion.

Others
- Sputum culture (including AFB stain).
- Mantoux/interferon gamma releasing assay test (TB).
- Bronchoscopy ± CT-guided biopsy (when tissue diagnosis required in suspected malignancy).
- Pleural biopsy (performed by 'Abram's biopsy needle' to obtain histological specimen – useful in suspected malignancy/TB).

Viva questions

Outline 5 major processes that lead to pleural effusions
- Increased hydrostatic pressure or decreased oncotic pressure (transudates).
- Increased capillary permeability (exudates).
- Disruption of lymphatic duct (chylothorax).
- Infection within the pleural space (empyema).
- Bleeding into the pleural space (haemothorax).

What important parameters are measured in pleural fluid? How does this help to indicate a diagnosis? (Table 2.8)

Table 2.8 Pleural fluid analysis – what to measure and what is indicated?

Pleural fluid parameter	Interpretation of result	Diagnosis
Albumin & LDH (require concurrent serum levels)	**Protein concentration** >30g/dL exudates <30g/dL transudate **OR Light's criteria:** Exudates demonstrate: • Pleural albumin/serum albumin >0.5 • Pleural LDH/serum LDH >0.6 • pleural LDH >2/3rds upper normal limit of serum LDH	Distinguishes transudates from exudates which can help identify cause (⏵ Main causes of pleural effusion, p.64)
Glucose	Normal >2mmol/L: Low glucose effusion <2mmol/L	Low glucose effusions (<2mmol/L) are remembered as: 'MEAT' effusions: • Malignancy • Empyema • Arthritis (rheumatoid) and • Tuberculosis Chest drain insertion is required with urgency in cases of empyema that show low pleural pH (<7.2) and/ or glucose (<2mmol/L).
pH	Normal 7.4–7.6; abnormal <7.2	<7.2 indicates potential for empyema formation
Microbiology	Gram stain, C+S, AFB staining	• Parapneumonic effusion • Empyema

Adenosine deaminase	↑ levels indicate excessive purine metabolism and/or T-lymphocyte driven process	• TB • Empyema • Malignancy (lymphoma) • CTDs (SLE, RA)
Cytology	Malignant cells	Malignancy
Differential cell content	Red blood cells (RBCs); • Hct effusion/Hct serum >0.5 indicates haemothorax	• Malignancy • TB • Pulmonary embolism • Traumatic tap
	Neutrophils	Parapneumonic effusion
	Eosinophils: • >10% indicates ↑ levels • Does not exclude malignancy	• Benign asbestos related disease • Post haemothorax • Post pneumothorax
	Lymphocytes • ↑ in 1/3 of transudates	• Malignancy (lymphoma) • TB • Collagen vascular disease • Sarcoidosis
Amylase	Not usually increased	• Oesophageal rupture • Pancreatitis • Malignancy (adenocarcinoma) • Pneumonia

(Continued)

Table 2.8 (Contd.)

Pleural fluid parameter	Interpretation of result	Diagnosis
Lipids	Cholesterol & triglycerides: • If TGs >1.3mmol/L: 'chylothorax'	• Lymphomas • Solid tumours • Nephrotic syndrome • Cirrhosis • Occasionally RA
Creatinine	Pleural Cr >serum Cr in 'urinothorax'	Obstructive uropathy
Anti-nuclear factor, RF	Not usually present	Autoimmune/rheumatoid effusions

Are there weaknesses of Light's criteria in differentiating transudates from exudates?

25% of patients with transudates are mistakenly identified as having exudates by Light's criteria. If a transudative effusion is suspected clinically, the pleural albumin should be subtracted from serum albumin giving the serum → pleural albumin gradient. If this value is <1.2g/dL (12g/L), it indicates an exudate with 95% sensitivity and 100% specificity. NB This gradient *is a value not a ratio* as is the case with Light's criteria.

What are para-pneumonic effusions?

These are exudative effusions that accompany approximately 40% of bacterial pneumonias. These can be divided into subtypes;

- Simple/uncomplicated: sterile and resolves with treatment of pneumonia.
- Complicated: occupies >½ of hemithorax or an empyema (requires pleural drainage via chest tube insertion).

Outline the management of a pleural effusion. What additional management is required in cases of recurrent effusions?

Directed at the underlying cause but a few common principles exist:

- Supportive measures:
  - Oxygen.
  - IV hydration.
  - Chest physiotherapy (where applicable).
- Diagnostic ± therapeutic thoracocentesis or chest tube insertion (avoided if possible in mesothelioma due to high risk of seeding).
- Effusions should be drained slowly to avoid haemodynamic compromise, rapid re-accumulation and re-expansion pulmonary oedema.
- Treatment of underlying cause:
  - Antibiotics (empyema).
  - Diuretics (CCF).
- If effusions are recurrent, additional options for therapy do exist:
  - Continuous tube thoracostomy.
  - Pleurodesis (most commonly done in recurrent malignant effusions; can be performed medically with talc or surgically via video assisted thoracoscopic surgery [VATS]). Agents are instilled into pleural cavity to induce an inflammatory response that resolves by fibrosing visceral and parietal pleura together thereby preventing further fluid accumulation. Effective analgesia is essential as the pleura are *very* pain sensitive.
  - Placement of pleuro-peritoneal shunt (rarely used).

Differentiate between a thoracoscopy and mediastinoscopy

A thoracoscopy (VATS) is a surgical technique that involves visualization of the pleural cavity for both diagnostic (e.g. biopsies) and therapeutic (e.g. pleurodesis) purposes. This is different to mediastinoscopy that visualizes the medistinum.

Clinically, a thoracoscopy scar is observed laterally whilst a scar indicating mediastinoscopy is anteriorly located over the mediastinum.

What is 'yellow nail syndrome'?

It is a rare cause of exudative pleural effusions and is a condition of yellow curved nails associated with lymphoedema, bronchitis, bronchiectasis, sinusitis, nephrotic syndrome and hypothyroidism.

📖 Further reading

Heffner JE, Klein JS. Recent advances in the diagnosis and management of malignant pleural effusions. *Mayo Clin Proc* 2008; **83**(2):235–50.

Pleural disease 2: pneumothorax

This clinically important condition is an uncommon case in the PACES exam (but do keep an open mind!)

Types of pneumothorax:

- Traumatic
- Spontaneous:
  - Primary (no lung disease)
  - Secondary (underlying lung disease)
- 'Tension pneumothorax' (life-threatening emergency)

Clinical signs

- Reduced chest movement (affected side).
- Trachea:
  - Central (small pneumothorax).
  - Deviated towards affected side (large pneumothorax).
  - Deviated away from affected side (tension pneumothorax).
  - In the acute setting, the trachea may be deviated away from the affected side but in the context of the PACES exam you are very unlikely to encounter this. For PACES, the trachea is more likely to be pulled toward the affected side secondary to underlying atelectasis.
- Reduced tactile vocal fremitus.
- Hyper-resonant percussion note.
- Decreased/absent breath sounds (affected area).
- Reduced vocal resonance.
- Evidence of pleural aspiration site/prior chest drain insertion.
- Signs of underlying cause:
  - Recent central venous catheter.
  - Thin/marfanoid habitus.
  - Inhalers by the bedside (asthma, COPD).

Symptoms

- Asymptomatic (small pneumothorax)
- Sudden onset or rapidly progressive dyspnoea
- Pleuritic chest pain.

> **❶ Top Tips**
>
> Tell the examiner: 'I would suspect a tension pneumothorax in an unstable patient demonstrating dyspnoea, tachycardia and hypotension requiring urgent intervention'.

Risk factors

- Recent intervention:
  - Pleural aspiration
  - Central line insertion
  - Surgery.

- Relevant medical history:
  - Asthma
  - COPD
  - Chest trauma
  - Marfan's syndrome
  - HIV infection
  - Positive pressure ventilation

Investigations

- CXR
- CT thorax (loculated pneumothorax, underlying lung disease)
- ABG (if patient dyspnoeic)

Management

Depends on size of pneumothorax and patient's symptoms:

- <2cm rim: supportive management.
- >2cm rim or symptomatic: pleural aspiration attempted.
- If failed aspiration: chest drain insertion with underwater seal (may need suction).
- If no resolution/recurrent: surgical pleurodesis or pleurectomy considered.

❶ Top Tips

Traumatic and secondary pneumothoraces almost always require intervention.

Obesity-related lung disease and the Pickwickian syndrome

The Pickwickian syndrome, also known as the obesity hypoventilation syndrome, consists of three components: obstructive sleep apnoea (OSA), hypercapnia and a restrictive defect on PFTs.

Definitions and associations
- OSA is one component of the Pickwickian syndrome:
  - OSA is defined as the 'presence of an increased number of breathing cessations (apnoeas) and/or reduction in tidal volume (hypopnoeas)'.
  - A widely accepted definition of apnoea in adults requires ventilation to be absent for 10 seconds or longer.
  - A hypopnoea is defined as reduction of ventilation to <50% below baseline accompanied by desaturation or sleep arousal.
- OSA remains a separate entity to the Pickwickian syndrome – patients can have OSA alone without having the Pickwickian syndrome.
- More than half of all patients with OSA are *not* obese; consequently this condition remains grossly under-recognized.

Clinical signs
- Obese habitus
- Dyspnoeic or sleepy at rest
- Shallow breathing pattern
- Facial plethora (secondary polycythaemia)
- Central cyanosis (best seen on tongue)
- Maxillary or mandibular hypoplasia
- 'Crowded' oropharynx or enlarged uvula or tonsils
- Increased neck circumference (>16–17 inches/40–43cm)
- Assess for complications:
  - Systemic hypertension (offer to measure the blood pressure)
  - Pulmonary hypertension (left parasternal heave, palpable P2, raised JVP, hepatomegaly, peripheral oedema)
  - Congestive cardiac failure (cardiomegaly, bibasal crepitations, peripheral oedema)
- Assess for evidence of treatment:
  - Domiciliary ventilation – CPAP machine or non-invasive (e.g. BiPAP) ventilator at bedside
  - Oxygen therapy

Symptoms
- Obstructive sleep apnoea:
  - Snoring
  - Witnessed apnoea (collateral from partner)
  - Nocturnal wakenings
  - Early morning headaches (due to hypercapnia)
  - Daytime sleepiness (unrefreshing sleep or falling asleep inappropriately e.g. whilst in conversation or driving, can be assessed by validated scoring systems e.g. Epworth Sleepiness scale)
  - Nocturia

- Shortness of breath
- Large collar size (>17.5 inches)
- Peripheral oedema
- Nocturnal angina
- Heartburn
- History of hypertension
- Family history of obesity

Investigations

- Overnight polysomnography ('sleep study') – gold standard:
  - Performed overnight in a sleep laboratory while patient sleeps.
  - Physiological measurements made include:
    1. Electroencephalogram (EEG), electromyogram (EMG) and electro-oculogram (EOG) which determine stage of sleep (I–V and rapid eye movement [REM]).
    2. Respiratory effort (reflection of chest and abdominal movements) and ventilation (measured as airflow at the nose or mouth) which detect apnoeas or hypopnoeas with classification as central or obstructive (➔ 'Viva questions', p.73)
    3. Microphone to detect snoring may be included.
    4. Oxyhaemoglobin saturation by pulse oximetry.
    5. ECG for assessment of cardiac rhythm.
    6. Body position (detected automatically or recorded manually by technologist).
- Diagnosis of OSA is made by a measurement of severity of sleep disordered breathing. This is assessed in terms of the 'Respiratory Disturbance Index (RDI)' or 'apnoea-hypopnoea index' calculated as the number of each event (apnoea, hypopnoea) occurring per hour of actual sleep (*not* time in bed):
  - RDI >5 (abnormal).
  - RDI 5–15 (mild OSA).
  - RDI 15–30 (moderate OSA).
  - RDI >30 (severe OSA).
- Traditionally, patients undergo diagnostic testing lasting a full night, then a second study for CPAP pressure titration if diagnosis is confirmed. However, to increase efficiency of resources many centres combine diagnostic test with CPAP titration, each lasting approximately ½ of the night, or provide 'autoset' CPAP generators which constantly vary the pressure delivered as appropriate.
- FBC (polycythaemia secondary to hypoxia).
- Thyroid function testing (hypothyroidism is associated with OSA).
- Morning ABG (useful if Pickwickian syndrome suspected): hypoxia ± hypercapnia.
- CXR, ECG and echocardiogram (if pulmonary hypertension or cor pulmonale suspected).

Viva questions

How many types of 'abnormal' respiratory events are described during sleep?

3 types of apnoea or hypopnoea have been recognized:
- Central:

- Results from a cessation of ventilatory drive from the 'respiratory centres' of the brain.
- Breathing can cease for 10–30 seconds.
- No thoraco-abdominal movements are detected.
- It is unknown as to why obese patients are prone to this type of apnoea.
- This form of sleep apnoea is more difficult to treat adequately.
- Obstructive:
  - Results from a collapse of the upper pharyngeal airway consequent to the negative intrathoracic pressure (exacerbated by a short neck, adiposity, large tonsils and micrognathia).
  - Thoraco-abdominal movements are detected but no airflow at the mouth.
  - Consequences are hypoventilation (witnessed apnoea) and hypoxia which trigger multiple awakenings leading to poor quality sleep.
  - Easily and effectively treated with weight loss, removal of obstruction and CPAP (● see viva question below on treatment options).
- Mixed:
  - Starts as one type of event (usually central) and concludes with the other.
  - Most consider that 'mixed' and 'obstructive' apnoeas are clinically the same disorder.

What causes the 'obstruction' in OSA?

At least 2 of the following contributing factors are thought to lead to the obstruction:
- Upper airway narrowing from variety of causes:
  - Obesity
  - Adenotonsillar hypertrophy (children)
  - Macroglossia (hypothyroidism, Down's syndrome)
  - Mandibular deficiency (micro- or retrognathia)
  - Macrognathia (acromegaly)
  - Upper airway tumours
- Upper airway collapse if excess pressure is generated during inhalation (from force required to overcome any nasal obstruction – allergic rhinitis or septal deviation).
- Abnormality in the control of upper airway muscle tone (cause unknown but OSA complicates many neurological disorders).

Outline treatment options available for the management of obstructive sleep apnoea and the Pickwickian syndrome

- Weight loss.
- Reduce or stop smoking and/or alcohol consumption.
- CPAP therapy delivered by nasal/facial mask ± humidification:
  - 1st-line treatment.
  - Prevents apnoeas and hypopnoeas by maintaining upper airway patency through positive airway pressure maintained throughout the respiratory cycle (inspiration and expiration).
  - Main issues are compliance due to dry mouth, discomfort, noise or mask leaks.

- This contrasts with NIV e.g. BiPAP where the inspiratory and expiratory phases of respiration have differing pressures applied (pressure is higher in inspiration to improve ventilation (and hence hypercapnia) and lower in expiration to prevent airways collapse.
  - NIV may be used instead of CPAP in Pickwickian cases (severe hypercapnia).
- LTOT (where indicated).
- Oral appliances: these advance the mandible, hold the tongue anteriorly or lift the palate e.g. mandibular advancement devices, tongue retaining devices.
- Surgery (rarely necessary)
  - Uvulopalatopharyngoplasty (UPPP) (most common procedure used).
  - Genioglossus advancement.
  - Maxillary-mandibular advancement.
  - Radiofrequency ablation (RFA) most commonly directed to the soft palate; least invasive technique available for OSA.
- Drugs:
  - Modafinil (stimulates wakefulness).
  - Fluoxetine (non-sedating antidepressants which suppress REM sleep, the stage associated with the most severe apnoea).
  - Orlistat (anti-obesity agent).

What are the complications associated with obstructive sleep apnoea?

- Cardiac arrhythmias
- Systemic hypertension
- Myocardial infarction
- Stroke
- Obesity-hypoventilation (Pickwickian) syndrome
- Pulmonary hypertension
- Increased mortality

List (i) respiratory problems and (ii) other clinical consequences associated with obesity

Respiratory problems can be summarized as:

- Chronic hypoxia with hypercapnia and cyanosis
- Obstructive sleep apnoea
- Pulmonary hypertension and CCF
- Pickwickian (obesity-hypoventilation) syndrome.

Other clinical consequences include:

- Insulin resistance and diabetes mellitus
- Hypertension
- Cardiovascular disease and lipid abnormalities
- Venous disease (varicose veins, venous stasis, thromboembolism)
- Cancer (mainly endometrial, postmenopausal breast, gallbladder and biliary system)
- Gastrointestinal disease (gallstones, cholestasis and fatty liver)
- Arthritis (osteoarthritis and increased uric acid levels)
- Skin (intertrigo, fungal/yeast infections and acanthosis nigracans)
- Increased mortality (independent of other factors listed).

How can one estimate body fat at the bedside?
Measuring skinfold thickness at the biceps, triceps, subscapular and suprailiac regions. Also see BMI measurement, ➔ p.96.

Differentiate between 'android' and 'gynaecoid' fatness
'Android' fatness occurs when fat is distributed mainly in the upper body (above waist level) where as 'gynaecoid' fatness involves fat distribution in the lower body (mainly lower abdomen, buttocks, hips and thighs). 'Android' fatness carries higher risks for hypertension and cardiovascular consequences including mortality than 'gynaecoid' fatness.

Name some diseases where obesity is a manifestation
● Endocrine disease:
  • Hypothyroidism
  • Polycystic ovarian syndrome (PCOS)
  • Hypothalamic disease (damage by surgery, trauma, inflammation or tumours leading to hyperphagia)
  • Cushing's syndrome
● Genetic disease:
  • Prader–Willi syndrome (almond eyes, acromicria, mental retardation, diabetes, hypogonadism)
  • Laurence–Moon–Bardet–Biedl syndrome (retinitis pigmentosa, hypogonadism, dwarfism, mental retardation, polydactyly).

📖 **Further reading**

Basner RC. Continuous positive airway pressure for obstructive sleep apnea. *NEJM* 2007; **356**(17):1751–8.

🖑 **Useful website**

http://www.sign.ac.uk/guidelines/fulltext/73/index.html (Guidelines for management of obstructive sleep apnoea/hypopnoea in adults).

Lung cancer

Lung cancer is the most common cause of cancer-related death in men and the second most common in women with 1.3 million deaths world-wide annually.

Symptoms
- Cough
- Haemoptysis
- Dyspnoea
- Chest pain (variable in character – dull or pleuritic)
- Hoarseness of voice
- Weight loss
- Bronchorrhoea (production of large volumes of thin, mucoid sputum associated with bronchoalveolar cell carcinoma)
- Symptoms associated with metastases and paraneoplastic syndromes.

Clinical signs
These are variable depending on the associated complications of the tumour.
- Cachexia
- Clubbing
- Tar-stained fingers
- Lymphadenopathy in supraclavicular and cervical regions
- Tracheal deviation:
  - Towards area of collapse or radiation induced fibrosis
  - Away from pleural effusion
- Reduced chest expansion
- Reduced tactile vocal fremitus and/or vocal resonance
- Dullness to percussion over area of collapse, stony dull at base if pleural effusion
- Reduced breath sounds
- Coarse crepitations
- Bronchial breathing
- Wheeze (usually monophonic due to fixed airway obstruction).

Evidence of investigation or treatment (➔ Figure 2.1 [scars in the respiratory exam, p.22])
- Mediastinoscopy scar (small horizontal scar in suprasternal notch)
- Chest drain or VATS scars (small scars in between ribs)
- Radiation tattoos (small purple/blue dots) and radiation skin changes (erythematous areas over chest wall)
- Lobectomy/pneumonectomy scar.

Complications of direct tumour extension
- Hoarse voice (left recurrent laryngeal nerve palsy).
- Stridor.
- Horner's syndrome – suggestive of Pancoast tumour:
  - Ipsilateral partial ptosis, miosis, enophthalmous and anhydrosis due to involvement of paravertebral sympathetic chain.
  - Weakness and atrophy of intrinsic muscles of the hand (T1), pain and paraesthesia in 4th and 5th digits (C8) and medial aspect of forearm (T1) due to invasion of the brachial plexus.
- Superior vena cava obstruction.

Complications of metastatic disease

- Bony deformity or tenderness (Are there walking aids at the bedside?)
- Hepatomegaly, jaundice
- Focal neurology from brain metastases or spinal cord compression.

Evidence of paraneoplastic syndromes

Musculoskeletal

- Hypertrophic pulmonary osteoarthropathy:
  - Clubbing plus pain and swelling at wrists and ankles due to subperiosteal new bone formation.
  - Occurs with any cell type, most commonly squamous cell and adenocarcinoma.
- Polymyositis.

Neurological

- Lambert–Eaton myasthenic syndrome (LEMS; also known as reversed myasthenia ➲ p.381):
  - Slowly progressive proximal muscle weakness, autonomic dysfunction and cranial nerve involvement e.g. resulting in ptosis, diplopia.
  - Muscle strength and deep tendon reflexes can improve after exercise.
  - Disorder of acetylcholine release from presynaptic nerve terminals with presence of antibodies directed against voltage-gated calcium channels.
  - Present in small cell lung cancer (up to 3%).
  - Can predate diagnosis of malignancy by months to years.
- Proximal myopathy.
- Peripheral neuropathy.
- Cerebellar syndrome.

Endocrine

- Hypercalcaemia:
  - Presents with confusion, bone pain, changes in mood and dehydration/constipation.
  - Tumour secretion of parathyroid hormone (PTH)-related peptide, calcitriol and other cytokines.
  - Most commonly caused by squamous cell carcinoma.
  - Treated with rehydration and bisphosphonates.
- Syndrome of inappropriate anti-diuretic hormone (SIADH):
  - Presents with confusion.
  - Results in hyponatraemia, raised urine osmolality, low serum osmolality, raised urinary sodium.
  - 10% patients with small-cell lung cancer (SCLC).
  - Treatment includes treatment of SCLC, fluid restriction (if euvolaemic) and demeclocycline.
- Ectopic adrenocorticotropic hormone (ACTH) secretion:
  - Cushing's syndrome and pigmentation.
  - Common in SCLC.
- HCG secreting tumour: gynaecomastia.

Dermatological

- Thromboplebitis migrans
- Acanthosis nigrans

- Eythema gyratum repens (irregular wavy lines with desquamation on trunk, neck and extremities)
- Dermatomyositis.

Investigations

Performed to obtain histological diagnosis of lung cancer and stage disease.

Laboratory

- Bloods: FBC (anaemia), LFTs (may be elevated with metastatic disease in the liver; NB raised alkaline phosphatase (ALP) often secondary to bony metastases), U&Es (SIADH), bone profile (raised calcium may be secondary to bone metastases or tumour secretion of PTH-related peptide).
- Sputum cytology: positive in 20–25% patients with lung cancer.
- Pleural aspiration: 50–100mL detects 65% malignant effusions, further 30% of samples positive on second aspiration.

Radiological

- CXR:
  - Vast array of appearances depending on histology and stage.
  - Spiculated, non-calcified lesions, collapse, consolidation, pleural effusion, rib destruction, intrathoracic metastases, mediastinal or paratracheal enlargement due to lymphadenopathy.
- CT chest and abdomen with contrast:
  - To evaluate size and stage of tumour, lymph node involvement and metastatic disease.
  - The sensitivity and specificity of CT and magnetic resonance (MR) for the detection of mediastinal nodal disease is approximately 65%.
  - Although CT and MR are accurate in predicting non-involvement of the chest wall and mediastinum, both techniques are less accurate in positively diagnosing invasion of these structures.
- Positron emission tomography (PET)-CT scan:
  - Metabolically active tissue detected by increased uptake of 18-fluorodeoxyglucose. PET-CT provides fusion of functional (metabolically active) and anatomical information.
  - Useful in evaluating regional and mediastinal lymph node involvement and metastases.
  - PET is more accurate than CT/MR in detecting mediastinal disease.
  - PET-CT is the most sensitive technique for detecting extracranial metastatic disease. However, further investigation of isolated tracer uptake (e.g. unilateral parotid) is required to ensure accurate staging and avoid denying patients potentially curable surgery.
- Technetium-labelled bone scan: consider if symptoms, signs or laboratory evidence of bony metastases.
- MR imaging (MRI):
  - MRI is the optimum modality for staging superior sulcus tumours.
  - More effective at evaluating spine and brain metastases.
- Endoscopic ultrasound: role in predicting the resectability of a tumour and identifying and sampling nodal disease.

Lung function testing

- To assess suitability for surgical resection and radical radiotherapy. Post resection lung function and gas transfer can be predicted to ensure adequate postoperative reserve.

Histological sampling

- Percutaneous CT-guided biopsy – for peripherally located lung lesions and bony metastases.
- Ultrasound-guided biopsy/aspiration – of peripheral lymph nodes, liver metastases.
- Flexible bronchoscopy:
  - To assess position within bronchial tree (see Tables 2.9 and 2.10, p. 81 and 82).
  - BAL for cytology.
  - Endobronchial biopsy or brushings.
  - Transbronchial needle aspiration (TBNA) to sample mediastinal lymph nodes.
  - Endobronchial ultrasound (EBUS) with TBNA – superior sensitivity and specificity compared to blind TBNA.
- Transoesophageal endoscopic ultrasound fine needle aspiration for mediastinal node sampling.
- Mediastinoscopy.
- Video-assisted thoracoscopy and pleural biopsy.

Viva questions

Describe the risk factors for developing lung cancer

- Smoking:
  - Estimated 90% of all lung cancers caused by smoking – adenocarcinoma is the only subtype not associated with smoking.
  - Relative risk increases with number smoked per day and duration of smoking.
  - Current smoker of 40 pack-year history has 20 × risk of lifelong non-smoker.
- Radiation therapy.
- Environmental exposure to passive smoke, asbestos, radon, metals (arsenic, chromium, nickel).
- Pulmonary fibrosis.
- COPD.
- Alpha1 antitrypsin deficiency.
- Genetic factors – increased risk in patients with familial history.

Describe the histological classification of lung cancer

Non-small-cell lung cancer (NSCLC)

- 75–80% of lung cancer.
- Squamous cell >adenocarcinoma>alveolar cell >large cell.

Small-cell lung cancer (SCLC)

- 20–25% of lung cancer.
- Rapidly proliferating tumour with early dissemination.

Name the common sites of lung cancer metastases

- Liver
- Adrenal glands
- Bone – osteolytic appearance, most commonly in vertebral bodies
- Brain.

What are the most common paraneoplastic syndromes that affect lung cancer patients?
- Hypercalcaemia
- Syndrome of inappropriate anti-diuretic hormone (SIADH).

Describe the staging classification of NSCLC

Clinically staging disease is important in order to plan best management for patients and assess prognosis. NB Clinical staging may differ from pathological staging following surgery. See Tables 2.9 and 2.10.

Table 2.9 TNM classification of NSCLC

Primary tumour	
T1	Tumour <3cm diameter without evidence of invasion more proximal than the lobar bronchus
T2	Tumour with any of the following features:
	>3cm in diameter
	Involves the main bronchus
	>2cm distal to the carina
	Invading visceral pleura
T3	Tumour of any size which invades any of the following: chest wall (including superior sulcus/Pancoast tumours), diaphragm, mediastinal pleura, parietal pericardium
	Or tumour in main bronchus <2cm distal to the carina but without involvement of the carina or associated atelectasis or obstructive pnuemonitis of the entire lung

Primary tumour	
T4	Tumour of any size which invades any of the following: mediastinum, heart, great vessels, trachea, oesophagus, vertebral body, carina
	Or tumour with malignant pleural effusion or pericardial effusion
	Or with satellite tumour nodules within the same lobe as the primary

Regional lymph nodes (N)	
No	No regional lymph nodes
N1	Metastasis to ipsilateral peribronchial and/or ipsilateral hilar lymph nodes and intrapulmonary nodes
N2	Metastasis to ipsilateral mediastinal and/or subcarinal nodes
N3	Metastasis to contralateral mediastinal, contralateral hilar, ipsilateral or contralateral scalene or supraclavicular lymph nodes

Distant metastasis (M)	
Mo	No distant metastasis
M1	Distant metastasis present (including metastatic nodules in other lung lobes)

Table 2.10 Staging of NSCLC

Stage	T	N	M	Prognosis (approximate 5-year survival)
IA	T1	N0	M0	73%
IB	T2	N0	M0	
IIA	T1	N1	M0	36–46%
IIB	T2	N1	M0	
	T3	N0	M0	
IIIA	T3	N1	M0	9–24%
	T1–3	N2	M0	
IIIB	Any T	N3	M0	
	T4	Any N	M0	
IV	Any T	Any N	M1	2% (median survival 6 months)

Describe the staging classification of SCLC
- Limited disease:
  - Disease confined to ipsilateral hemithorax.
  - Median range of survival 15–20 months.
- Extensive disease:
  - Metastatic disease outside ipsilateral hemithorax.
  - Median range of survival 8–13 months.

What other prognostic factors help guide treatment in lung cancer?
- World Health Organization (WHO) Performance Score:
  - 0: asymptomatic
  - 1: symptomatic but ambulatory and able to carry out light work
  - 2: in bed <50% of day
  - 3: in bed >50% of day and unable to care for self
  - 4: bedridden
- Weight loss.

Describe the management of patients with NSCLC
Patients should be discussed at a lung cancer multidisciplinary team meeting and given information regarding their diagnosis and treatment. Lung cancer nurse specialists are essential to provide continuing support for the patient and coordinate their care.
- Surgery:
  - Surgical resection in the form of lobectomy or pneumonectomy offers the best long-term survival for patients with lung cancer.
  - Considered in patients with stage I and II disease and considered on an individual basis in patients with stage III A disease.
  - Patients need to be carefully selected based on adequate lung function and comorbidities.

- Classically patients with an FEV_1 >2L (or >80% predicted) can tolerate pneumonectomy and FEV_1 >1.5L can tolerate lobectomy. Patients with a DLCO >80% predicted have a low postoperative risk.
- Patients who do not clearly fit a low-risk category can have further testing to assess their predicted postoperative lung function, taking into account preoperative lung function, amount of tissue to be resected and preoperative contribution of tissue to be resected to overall lung function. A predicted postoperative FEV_1 of >40% normal predicted is required for surgery.
- Cardiopulmonary exercise testing is performed to assess the level of work a patient can achieve, measured by maximal oxygen consumption or VO_2 max. VO_2 max<10mL/kg/min is associated with increased risk whereas VO_2 max >15mL/kg/min is deemed acceptable.
- Postoperative adjuvant chemotherapy has been shown to improve survival for patients with stage II disease.
- Radical radiotherapy: CHART (continuous hyperfractionated accelerated radiotherapy) is considered in patients with stage I, II or III disease who are inoperable with a good performance status.
- Chemotherapy:
  - Offered to patients with stage III or IV cancer with a good performance status (WHO score 0–1)
  - Usually a platinum-based drug (carboplatin, cisplatin) combined with a 3rd-generation drug (docetaxel, gemcitabine, paclitaxel or vinorelbine).
  - Combination of chemotherapy and radiotherapy provides a survival advantage in patients with stage III disease.
- Palliative treatment:
  - Stage IV disease.
  - Radiotherapy to control thoracic symptoms.
  - Chemotherapy in patients with good performance status can prolong survival without significant impairment of quality of life.
  - Symptom control with analgesics, anti-emetics, steroids (may improve appetite and performance status).
  - Planning end of life care with the support of the palliative care team.

Describe the management of small cell lung cancer
- Combination treatment with radiotherapy and platinum-based chemotherapy.
- Prophylactic cranial irradiation considered in patients who respond to treatment – shown to reduce the incidence of brain metastasis (common after treatment for SCLC due to inadequate penetration of chemotherapy agents through the blood–brain barrier) and prolong survival.

New developments
- Molecular markers and gene expression profiling may lead to targeted cancer treatments in the future.
- Lung cancer screening: RCTs of CXR and sputum cytology-based screening and non-randomized cohort studies of CT-based screening have been successful at detecting early stage asymptomatic lung cancer. However, considering the high rates of false positive results in these

studies and lead time bias it is unclear whether this will translate into a mortality benefit. Trials such as the National Lung Screening Trial are ongoing.

Useful websites

British Thoracic Society: http://www.brit-thoracic.org.uk (follow link to Clinical Information Then Lung cancer).

NICE guidelines: http://www.nice.org.uk/CG24.

Macmillan Cancer Support: http://www.cancerbackup.org.uk.

Superior vena cava obstruction

Symptoms
- Cough
- Dyspnoea
- Dysphagia
- Hoarse voice
- Headache (worse on bending forward or lying down)
- Presyncope/syncope (due to reduced venous return).

Clinical signs
- Facial and upper body oedema
- Facial plethora
- Cyanotic appearance
- Superficial vein distension of face and upper body
- Suffusion of eyes
- Hoarse voice
- Inspiratory stridor
- Elevated fixed JVP
- Dilated venous angiomata under tongue
- Pemberton's sign: worsening of listed features upon raising both arms above head simultaneously.

Investigations
- CXR: mediastinal widening, lesion at right hilum.
- Contrast enhanced CT: defines level and extent of blockage, presence of collateral vessels, may identify likely underlying cause.
- Conventional venography as a prelude to stenting.

Viva questions
What are the common causes of superior vena cava obstruction?
Invasion or external compression of the SVC can be caused by pathology involving the right lung, lymph nodes, mediastinal structures or thrombus. The commonest causes are:
- Lung cancer: 10% of SCLC, 1.7% of NSCLC.
- Lymphoma: more common in non-Hodgkin's lymphoma (NHL).

Other causes include:
- Thymoma.
- Primary mediastinal germ cell neoplasms.
- Solid tumours with lymph node metastases.
- Fibrosing mediastinitis due to untreated infection (commoner in pre-antibiotic era).
- Post-radiation fibrosis.
- Thoracic aortic aneurysm.
- Thrombosis: increasing incidence due to use of intravascular catheters e.g. central venous lines, pacemaker lines.

Describe the management of SVCO
Unless there is evidence of respiratory compromise or cerebral oedema (coma, confusion) the underlying cause of SVCO should be investigated

prior to commencing treatment as radiotherapy or steroids (in lymphoma) may obscure the diagnosis.

- Corticosteroids: may be helpful in steroid responsive malignancies.
- Endovascular stent: placed percutaneously under local anaesthetic appears to provide the most rapid relief of symptoms. Heparin may be used during placement. The benefit of anticoagulation following stenting is unclear.
- Chemotherapy and radiotherapy: a Cochrane review demonstrated similar rates of symptomatic relief for both treatments in SCLC and NSCLC.[1]

Reference

1. Rowell NP, Gleeson FV. Steroids, radiotherapy, chemotherapy and stents for superior vena caval obstruction in carcinoma of the bronchus. *Cochrane Database Syst Rev* 2001; **4**: CD001316. Available at: http://www2.cochrane.org/reviews/en/ab001316.html

Pneumonectomy and lobectomy

Clinical signs (correspond to side of surgery and restricted to involved area in lobectomy)

- Thoracotomy scar – do not forget to look laterally and posteriorly with the patient at 45° so that posterolateral scars are not missed
- Asymmetrical chest flattening or deformity (best seen from end of bed with patient at 45°).
- Tracheal deviation (towards lesion in pneumonectomy and *upper* lobe lobectomy; trachea may be central in other lobectomies).
- Displaced apex beat (towards lesion).
- Reduced chest expansion.
- Dull percussion note.
- Decreased/ absent breath sounds. However, in pneumonectomy, there may be transmitted bronchial breathing from deviated trachea appreciated in the upper zones.
- Look for underlying cause:
  - Old TB (supraclavicular scar indicating prior phrenic nerve crush).
  - Lung carcinoma (clubbed, nicotine stains, cachexia, radiation burns, lymph nodes).
  - Bronchiectasis (clubbed, productive cough, coarse crepitations).

❶ Top Tips

Try to identify underlying cause for pneumonectomy or lobectomy while examining patient

If a lobectomy or pneumonectomy is the focus of your respiratory station your examiners will expect you to identify any apparent underlying diagnosis (e.g. left-sided lobectomy secondary to old TB, if both a thoracotomy scar and a phrenic nerve crush scar are present).

♠ Common Pitfalls

The posterolateral 'thoracotomy' scar has 3 main causes:

- *Pneumonectomy:* empty unilateral cavity which fills with fluid giving dull percussion note and decreased/absent breath sounds; may be misdiagnosed as a unilateral pleural effusion.
- *Lobectomy:* compensatory hyperinflation of ipsilateral lobes occurs which may partially mask clinical signs making them difficult to appreciate.
- *Open lung biopsy:* if your clinical findings do not fit with pneumonectomy or lobectomy, the scar may be explained by an open lung biopsy scar which is shorter (usually between 3–4cm).

Symptoms

Patient usually asymptomatic or may have symptoms reflecting the underlying cause (➔ 'Viva questions', p.88).

Viva questions

List some reasons for performing a pneumonectomy or lobectomy

- Lung malignancy (common) and pulmonary metastasis (rare)
- Localized bronchiectasis with uncontrolled symptoms (e.g. recurrent haemoptysis)
- Old TB (prior to anti-tuberculous therapy)
- Fungal infections (e.g. aspergilloma)
- Traumatic lung injury
- Large emphysematous bullae (bullectomy)
- Congenital lung disease e.g. CF
- Bronchial obstruction with destroyed lung.

The resection of a 'solitary pulmonary nodule' is controversial, although it is considered in cases where there is a suspicion of an 'undiagnosed SCLC'. Alternatively, a 'wait and watch' approach with interval CT scanning is performed.

What are the chest radiographic features in a pneumonectomy/ lobectomy?

On PA CXR, the following features will be seen:

- 'White out' on one side (pneumonectomy).
- In lobectomy there may be volume loss in the ipsilateral hemithorax, increased transradiancy of the ipsilateral lung due to compensatory hyperinflation, the presence of surgical clips and evidence of rib resection.
- Deviated trachea or mediastinum towards the pneumonectomy or lobectomy.
- Compensatory hyperinflation (of opposite lung in pneumonectomy or other ipsilateral lobes in lobectomy).

What is the importance of preoperative evaluation in pneumonectomy?

Preoperative evaluation is vital in both pneumonectomy and lobectomy because of the significant loss of lung function that follows.

Additionally, because such interventions are usually performed in patients with underlying lung disease, it is essential to assess the patient's functional reserve and predicted pulmonary function following surgery.

In general:

- Preoperative FEV_1 >2L → low risk (no further testing in absence of pulmonary hypertension).
- Preoperative FEV_1 <2L → high risk (need to have predicted postoperative FEV_1 and gas transfer estimated following quantitative lung ventilation/ perfusion scanning).

Preoperative cardiopulmonary testing can also be performed: if pre-operative VO_2 max <10mL/kg/min (higher mortality risk >30%) versus those with preoperative VO_2 max >15mL/kg/min (lower mortality risk <15%).

Are you aware of any subtypes of pneumonectomy?

There are 2 main types of pneumonectomy:

- Simple – removal of affected lung.
- Extrapleural – removal of affected lung plus part of the diaphragm, parietal pleura and pericardium on the ipsilateral side. These linings are then replaced by surgical Gore-Tex®.

The primary use of extrapleural pneumonectomy (EPP) is in the treatment of malignant mesothelioma because this particular technique has been shown to produce the best survival rates.[1]

If this patient had a lobectomy secondary to lung malignancy, can you suggest a likely subtype of lung cancer?

Surgery has a greater role in the management of 'NSCLC' rather than 'small-cell carcinoma' which has poorer prognosis and is almost always unsuitable for surgical intervention by the time of presentation.

What proportion of 'non-small-cell lung cancers' are suitable for surgery?

Approximately one-quarter (25%) of NSCLC will be suitable for surgical resection.

Comment on operative mortality of (i) lobectomy and (ii) pneumonectomy? Are there any differences between the right and left sides?

Operative mortality for lobectomy is approximately 2–4% and for pneumonectomy this rises to 6%.

There is a marked difference in mortality risks between the right and left sides following a pneumonectomy – right-sided pneumonectomy is associated with higher overall mortality (10–12%) as compared to left-sided pneumonectomy (1–3.5%). Reasons are uncertain for this difference but are most likely due to life-threatening complications that are encountered at higher frequency following right-sided procedures such as post-pneumonectomy space empyema, pulmonary oedema and bronchopleural fistula.

What is the 'post-pneumonectomy syndrome'?

- This syndrome results from the extrinsic compression of the distal trachea and main-stem bronchus due to mediastinal shifting and compensatory hyperinflation that occurs in the remaining lung.
- Post-pneumonectomy syndrome occurs almost exclusively in patients with right-sided pneumonectomy, approximately 6 months post surgery, but can occur years after the procedure.
- The syndrome is characterized by progressive dyspnoea, cough, inspiratory stridor and pneumonia. Treatment includes surgical re-positioning of mediastinum and filling of post-pneumonectomy space with non-absorbable material ± possible stenting of bronchi. This condition can be fatal if left untreated.

Reference

1. Horn L, Johnson DH. Evarts A. Graham and the first pneumonectomy for lung cancer. *J Clin Oncol* 2008; **26**(19):3268–75.

Cor pulmonale

Although you are unlikely to have a case solely on cor pulmonale, as a common complication of respiratory disease it is important to be able to identify this complication of another respiratory pathology in order maximize your score in this case.

Definition

Cor pulmonale can be defined as the alteration in structure and function of the right ventricle and fluid retention due to pulmonary hypertension caused by disease affecting the lung and its vasculature.

Pathophysiology

In order to understand the various clinical features of cor pulmonale it is useful to consider its pathophysiology. This is complex, involving many different mechanisms; however, the key points are explained as follows:

Fluid retention

- Hypoxia and secondary polycythaemia are sensed within the kidney and carotid body resulting in increased sympathetic activity and renal vasoconstriction which lead to increased retention of salt and water. When vascular permeability increases for example with raised pCO_2 this fluid accumulates in dependent tissues.
- Hypercapnia results in increased bicarbonate reabsorption in the kidneys which promotes passive reabsorption of salt and water.

Pulmonary hypertension

- Hypoxia induces pulmonary vasoconstriction and chronically induces smooth muscle cell proliferation and vascular endothelial changes that result in increased pulmonary vascular resistance and pulmonary hypertension.
- Interstitial lung disease and emphysema result in destruction of the pulmonary vascular bed as a result of fibrosis and loss of lung parenchyma.
- Secondary polycythaemia contributes to the resistance in blood flow through the pulmonary vasculature.

Right ventricular dysfunction

- The listed changes lead to increased work of the right ventricle (RV) and, when it is unable to compensate, RV failure.

Symptoms

- Dyspnoea
- Fatigue
- Lethargy
- Exertional chest pain
- Orthopnoea
- Hoarseness of voice (due to compression of left recurrent laryngeal nerve by dilated main pulmonary artery).

Clinical signs

- Bounding pulse, peripheral vasodilatation and flapping tremor (CO_2 retention).
- Ruddy facial appearance and suffused conjunctivae (polycythaemia).
- Central cyanosis.
- Raised JVP: prominent a wave due to right atrial hypertrophy and large v wave due to tricuspid regurgitation (TR).
- Left parasternal heave (RV hypertrophy; may not be palpable due to hyperinflated lungs).
- Palpable 2nd heart sound (pulmonary hypertension).
- Wide splitting of 2nd heart sound, loud P2 (pulmonary hypertension).
- Pansystolic murmur at left sternal edge loudest in inspiration (TR due to RV dilatation).
- Early diastolic murmur loudest in pulmonary area (functional pulmonary incompetence).
- 4th heart sound (RV hypertrophy).
- Hepatomegaly (may be pulsatile in TR).
- Sacral and ankle oedema.

Investigations

- Pulse oximetry.
- ABG: type I or II respiratory failure. Assess requirement for long-term oxygen therapy (indicated in presence of cor pulmonale if pO_2 <8kPa)
- CXR: increased cardiothoracic ratio, enlarged pulmonary arteries with attenuated peripheral vessels.
- ECG: right axis deviation, prominent p waves (p pulmonale) due to right atrial enlargement, right bundle branch block.
- Echocardiogram: dilated or hypertrophied RV, paradoxical interventricular septum movement, TR, raised pulmonary artery pressure (estimated from TR jet using Doppler technique).
- Right heart catheterization: remains gold standard in diagnosing pulmonary hypertension.

Viva questions

What is the definition of pulmonary hypertension?

- Mean pulmonary artery pressure >25mmHg with a pulmonary capillary or left atrial pressure <15mmHg.
- Caused by an increase in pulmonary blood flow, increase in pulmonary vascular resistance or elevated pulmonary venous pressure.

Name the common causes of cor pulmonale

- COPD (10–40% of patients, poor prognostic indicator)
- Interstitial lung disease
- Obstructive sleep apnoea
- Hypoventilation disorders including obesity-related hypoventilation, neuromuscular disorders, kyphoscoliosis.

The causes of pulmonary hypertension have been classified by WHO as follows:

1. Pulmonary arterial hypertension – includes idiopathic pulmonary hypertension, familial pulmonary hypertension, disease related to collagen vascular disease, HIV and drugs.

2. Pulmonary venous hypertension – due to left-sided heart disease.
3. Pulmonary hypertension associated with hypoxaemia.
4. Pulmonary hypertension due to chronic thrombotic or embolic disease, including pulmonary embolism and sickle cell disease.
5. Pulmonary hypertension associated with miscellaneous disorders- including sarcoidosis, Langerhans cell histiocytosis.

Describe the management of patients with cor pulmonale

- Optimize management of underlying condition.
- Consider long-term oxygen therapy.
- Consider overnight NIV for hypoventilation syndromes and OSA.
- Diuretics (judicious use required as excessive diuresis can reduce filling pressure and reduce RV output).

Abdomen

Behdad Afzali
Rupert P. M. Negus

Introduction

The abdominal station in MRCP PACES should be a 'set piece' that can be approached with confidence. You are likely to encounter patients with chronic stable disease such as chronic liver disease, haematological malignancy with associated hepatosplenomegaly and chronic kidney disease, particularly those undergoing some form of renal replacement therapy, for instance dialysis or transplantation. Signs in the abdomen are generally straightforward to elicit and the commonest obstacles to passing are poor presentation or a failure to put the features together in a logical fashion.

General principles behind abdominal examination

Many diagnostic findings in the abdominal station can be identified by inspection alone, so particular attention should be paid to adequate exposure and the identification of extra-abdominal signs (e.g. multiple spider naevi of chronic liver disease, telangiectasia of hereditary haemorrhagic telangiectasia and xanthelasmata in primary biliary cirrhosis). Do not forget to have a good look at the back as important signs may be restricted there (e.g. spider naevi or posterior nephrectomy scars).

During the observation phase, attention should be paid to the nutritional status of the patient and to any other available clues (for instance, one of the authors, BA, diagnosed bilateral adrenalectomies from a medic alert bracelet at the bedside in his MRCP exam). The presence of abdominal scars (Fig. 3.1) is very useful as they usually overlie the organs that have been surgically handled. Whist surgery is frequently concerned with resecting parts or the whole of organs, remember that organs, including kidneys, pancreas and liver, may also be transplanted. As a result of a detailed end-of-the bed examination, sufficient information may be garnered to allow a diagnosis to be formulated, with subsequent palpation, percussion and auscultation, simply confirming the suspected diagnosis. Keep to a well-practised order to produce a fluid display which you should be able to complete in around 5 minutes.

Summary of suggested order of examination

1. Introduce yourself to the patient and lie them down if this has not already been done. Ask if there is pain or tenderness anywhere.
2. Inspect the patient from the end of the bed. Ensure that you look for any additional clues, such as those around the bedside.
3. Examine the nails, hands and arms for signs of abdominal disease.
4. Feel the pulse and ask for the blood pressure (BP).
5. Check the face and eyes, looking for jaundice and at the conjunctivae for anaemia. Check the lips and look in the mouth at the tongue, mucous membranes and teeth.
6. Examine the back and neck, particularly the supraclavicular fossae.
7. Now moving towards the abdomen itself, palpate the breast tissue for gynaecomastia in men.
8. Inspect the abdomen at rest.

9. Perform superficial, then deep, palpation of the abdomen, palpating for:
   - Liver and spleen
   - Kidneys
   - Bladder
   - Abdominal aorta.
10. Test for shifting dullness.
11. Auscultate the abdomen.
12. Check for ankle oedema.
13. Thank the patient and cover them up.
14. Tell the examiner how you would complete your examination.

1. Introduction and positioning

Introduce yourself to the patient and ask their permission to proceed with the abdominal examination. Ask them if they have any discomfort or pain anywhere at the outset, which will avoid forgetting this at a later stage.

Positioning of the patient with adequate exposure is key to the abdominal examination. Whilst the upper body down to the knees is the minimum exposure required not to miss any physical signs, in the PACES exam, always maintain the patient's dignity with suitable bedclothes and undergarments. Lay the patient flat. This position ensures that the abdominal wall muscles are relaxed, so deeper structures can be palpated with ease.

2. Inspection from the end of the bed

Spend 30 seconds inspecting the patient from the end of the bed. In the vast majority of cases, the value of standing at the exact centre of the end of the bed for this 30-second examination cannot be underestimated and is frequently sufficient to establish the likely diagnosis. For example, the patient with an arteriovenous fistula in the arm and a surgical scar in an iliac fossa is likely to have end-stage renal disease due to diabetes mellitus, adult polycystic kidney disease or chronic glomerulonephritis.

Next look carefully for environmental clues (including under the bed or behind the chair). These may reveal special shoes for patients with diabetic feet, limb prostheses for arteriopaths (associated with renovascular disease), walking aids (required for osteoporotic fractures from prolonged undernourishment or steroid therapy), medic alert bracelets, glucose meters, artificial tears/saliva (autoimmune disease associated with Sjögren's syndrome), insulin pumps and inhalers (these look like large versions of asthma inhalers).

Ask yourself whether the patient appears comfortable. Discomfort could indicate tenderness in the abdomen or respiratory compromise from abdominal pathology (pulmonary oedema or pleural effusion from kidney disease, diaphragmatic splinting from massive ascites, pleural see page from peritoneal dialysis or ascites).

Assess the nutritional status of the patient. The body mass index (BMI), a 19th-century estimate of the appropriateness of a subject's weight for their height, can be calculated by the formula:

$$BMI = weight\,(in\,kg)\,/\,height^2\,(in\,m)$$

A BMI of 20–25 is taken as normal; >25 indicates that the subject is overweight and >30, obese. A BMI significantly <17.5 denotes gross undernourishment and may indicate starvation, including that due to an eating disorder, malabsorption, malignancy or other chronic disease.

From the end of the bed, look at the arms for an arteriovenous fistula or a haemodialysis catheter (usually internal jugular – note that the line goes *over* the clavicle). Abdominal scars, stomas, fistulas, gastrostomy feeding tubes and peritoneal dialysis catheters will all also be obvious as will the more florid signs of chronic liver disease such as ascites and dilated superficial abdominal veins.

Surgical scars in the abdomen
The commonest surgical scars in the abdomen are shown in Fig. 3.1. The following points summarize operations that can be performed through these incisions (note that with the increasing use of laparoscopic surgery, which includes single-port surgery through the umbilicus, 'classical' surgical scars will become increasingly rare and the site of the port scar may not help determine the nature of the operation):

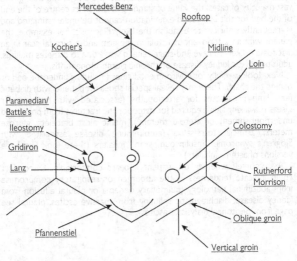

Fig. 3.1 Surgical scars in the abdomen.
(Courtesy of Mr S. Purkayastha and Mr B. Paraskeva, St Mary's Hospital, London.)

- Midline laparotomy:
  - All emergency surgery, especially if the diagnosis before laparotomy is unclear (e.g. perforated duodenal ulcer).
  - Elective general and vascular surgery.
- Paramedian/Battle's:
  - General abdominal surgery e.g. colectomy.
- Rooftop incision:
  - Upper gastrointestinal surgery (e.g. gastrectomy).
  - The Mercedes Benz scar (vertical extension of the rooftop incision) is often used for liver transplantation.
- Kocher's incision:
  - Right subcostal incision for open cholecystectomy.
- Gridiron and Lanz incisions:
  - Open appendicectomy.
  - The gridiron incision uses a muscle splitting (between the muscle fibres) rather than cutting approach (transversely across the muscle fibres).
- Loin incision:
  - Open renal procedures.
- Rutherford Morrison:
  - Renal transplant (left- or right-sided).
- Groin incisions:
  - Vertical for vascular surgery and oblique for hernia repairs and varicose vein stripping.
- Pfannenstiel:
  - Pelvic access for gynaecological and obstetric operations.
  - Other pelvic surgery.
- Stomas:
  - Left- and right-sided iliac fossa (LIF/RIF) stomas are positioned a third to halfway between the umbilicus and superior anterior iliac crest.
  - Transverse colostomies are sites 5–8cm below the lower rib cage.
  - RIF stomas are usually loop or end-ileostomies.
  - LIF stomas are usually loop or end-colostomies.
- Gastrostomy feeding tubes:
  - These are usually inserted percutaneously in the epigastric region.

3. Examining the nails, hands and arms

Examine the hands carefully before proceeding to the arms. Start with the nails, then the back of the hand, the palm, wrist and then forearm and arm.

- Note any alterations in pigmentation in the hands as they are classically affected by vitiligo (which should be symmetrical) and also hyperpigmentation of the palmar creases, indicative of Addison's disease. NB Palmar crease pigmentation is a normal finding in darkly pigmented races.
- Signs of chronic liver disease including leuconychia and palmar erythema (➋ Table 3.2, p.106 which summarizes those signs of chronic liver disease that may be visible in the hands and arms).
- Look for features of end-stage or chronic renal disease. Nail changes such as leuconychia, half and half nails (proximal half of the nails white, the rest darker with a sharp demarcation between then), absent lunulae,[*] leuconychia striata, Mees' lines (transverse white lines across the fingernail without pitting) and Beau's lines (transverse pitted lines

across the fingernails) can all indicate renal disease (Table 3.1). An arteriovenous fistula may be present in patients on haemodialysis. (*The word lunula comes from the Latin word 'luna' (literally, moon) and refers to the white crescent-shaped part of the proximal nail.)

• Make sure you do not miss a medic alert bracelet.

Table 3.1 Causes of common nail changes

Nail clubbing[a]	Leuconychia	Koilonychia
Idiopathic	Hypoalbuminaemia of any cause (malnutrition, malabsorption, protein-loosing enteropathy, urinary loss)	Chronic iron deficiency
Familial (autosomal dominant)	Idiopathic	Idiopathic
Congenital cyanotic heart disease	Familial	Familial (e.g. nail patella syndrome)
Subacute bacterial endocarditis	Sulphonamide antibiotics	Physiological (in neonates)
Lung carcinoma	Arsenic poisoning[e]	Occupational (exposure to solvents)
Pulmonary fibrosis	Heavy metal poisoning[e]	Poor peripheral circulation
Chronic suppurative lung disease (bronchiectasis, chronic lung abscess, cystic fibrosis)		Altitudinal
Cirrhosis		
Chronic inflammatory bowel disease (Crohn's disease, ulcerative colitis)		
Coeliac disease		
Arteriovenous fistulae[b]		
Infected PTFE grafts of the aorta[c]		
Hyperthyroidism[d]		

[a] Nail clubbing was probably first described by Hippocrates; the first 3 listed are the commonest causes of clubbing.

[b] A cause of asymmetrical clubbing (unilateral clubbing present on the side of the fistula and not the contralateral hand or in the feet).

[c] A cause of clubbing in the feet but not the hands.

[d] Thyroid acropachy.

[e] These 2 tend not to cause uniform leuconychia but leuconychia striata instead.

❶ Top Tips

Make sure you can name at least 3–5 causes for common nail changes – these are shown in Table 3.1.

4. Feel the pulse and ask for the BP

Feel the patient's pulse briefly to determine whether there is any obvious abnormality. It is not necessary to time the pulse accurately here if it appears to be normal.

GI bleeding or hormone-secreting abdominal tumours e.g. phaeochromocytomas can cause tachycardia (and sweatiness). Bradycardia may be caused by beta-blockade, an Addisonian crisis or may be a feature of hyperkalaemia associated with advanced renal disease.

Hypertension can be either a cause (especially in the Afro-Caribbean population) or a result of kidney disease. Hypotension may indicate GI bleeding or anti-hypertensive drugs. If Addison's disease is suspected then offer to measure the BP lying and standing for evidence of postural hypotension.

5. Check the face, lips and mucous membranes for signs of abdominal conditions. Look at the conjunctivae for anaemia and jaundice

Start with the face and look for signs suggestive of underlying systemic conditions e.g. the taught skin and microstomia of systemic sclerosis.

Look at the eyes. Gently pull down the eyelid and look for anaemia with the patient looking up, then for jaundice with the patient looking down. It is sufficient to pull down only one eyelid!

- Anaemia can be a feature of many abdominal diseases other than blood loss, such as malabsorption, chronic inflammatory bowel disease, chronic kidney disease and abdominal malignancies.
- Remember that jaundice can be pre-hepatic, hepatic and post-hepatic. Absence of other features of chronic liver disease is instructive, suggesting a pre-hepatic cause such as vitamin B12 deficiency.
- Examine the lips and mouth:
  - Oral ulcers are associated with inflammatory bowel disease, but also occur in general systemic conditions such as SLE.
  - Hyperpigmentation of the mucous membranes occurs in Addison's disease, whereas pigmented macules, particularly on the lips, are indicative of Peutz–Jeghers syndrome (hereditary intestinal polyposis syndrome). The telangiectasia of Osler–Weber–Rendu syndrome may appear on the lips or tongue.

- Examine the size of the tongue (macroglossia can be caused by amyloid and acromegaly, whereas a pale, smooth tongue may be associated with iron and vitamin B12 deficiency). Tonsillar enlargement may indicate malignancy or abscess if unilateral or a generalized lymphoproliferative disease or infection if bilateral.
- Note if the patient has oral candidiasis or hairy leucoplakia (strongly associated with HIV infection but not, in itself, AIDS-defining).
- Poor dentition is traditionally associated with diverticular disease.
- Gum hypertrophy is now only rarely caused by transplant immunosuppression, usually in the context of ciclosporin. Gum disease may indicate vitamin C deficiency and bushy loops vasculopathy (capillary overgrowth) associated with dermatomyositis.

6. Examine the back and neck

Ask the patient to sit forwards. Spider naevi are generally located in the distribution of the superior vena cava, so look at the upper back (>5 spider naevi is usually considered to be pathological). Spider naevi on the back may be the only sign of chronic liver disease. Remember that there are other causes of spider naevi (see below); all of them supposedly arise from an excess of oestrogens.

> **Causes of spider naevi**
>
> - Normal in childhood
> - Pregnancy
> - Oral contraceptive pill
> - Chronic liver disease
> - Thyrotoxicosis.

NB Spider naevi were first described by Sir Erasmus Wilson, a surgeon and specialist in skin diseases, who was responsible for the importation of 'Cleopatra's Needle' from Egypt to London during the reign of Queen Victoria.

Look further down the back and note if there are any abnormalities of the spine, such as kyphosis secondary to osteoporosis or overlying scars which may indicate surgical correction of spina bifida, which may be associated with bladder and post-renal kidney disease.

Look for posterolateral renal scars that may indicate a previous open nephrectomy.

Palpate the left supraclavicular fossa from behind for enlarged lymph nodes. An enlarged node here (Virchow's node) can be due to metastatic proximal upper GI malignancy (frequently adenocarcinoma of the stomach). This is known as Troisier's sign.

- Virchow was an eminent 19th-century German pathologist.
- Troisier was a 19th-century French pathologist who also described, with others, Troisier–Hanot–Chauffard syndrome, which is better known as haemochromatosis (➔ p.126).

7. Palpate the axillary lymph nodes and, in men, the breasts

Ask the patient to lay back down. Look at both axillae. Is there acanthosis nigricans?

Causes of acanthosis nigricans

- Insulin-resistant diabetes mellitus type 2
- Paraneoplastic
- Hypo- and hyperthyroidism
- Acromegaly
- Cushing's disease
- Obesity:
  - Idiopathic
  - Familial.

In men, palpate the breast tissue for gynaecomastia, an increase in breast tissue which has to be palpated, rather than a generalized increase in fatty tissue ('pseudogynaecomastia') around the breasts.

Causes of gynaecomastia

- Idiopathic
- Chronic liver disease
- Chronic renal disease
- Drugs (e.g. spironolactone)
- Thyrotoxicosis
- Secretory malignancies (producing hCG in particular):
  - Neonatal (from maternal hormones)
  - Adolescent
  - Congenital (e.g. Klinefelter syndrome).

---

8. Inspect the abdomen at rest

Although you would already have done this during your inspection from the end of the bed, you will nevertheless be expected to look at the abdomen 'close-up'. Ensure that you look laterally in both flanks for 'nephrectomy' scars. (NB The 'classical' nephrectomy scar may indicate ureteric surgery.) In particular look for:

- Abdominal scars (Fig. 3.1)
- Obvious abdominal distension (remember the 5 Fs: Fat, Fluid, Flatus, Faeces, Fetus)
- Caput medusae
- Peritoneal dialysis catheter, past or present
- Visible masses.

Ask the patient to raise their head a little and see if any obvious hernias or divarication of the recti are present.

9. Palpate the abdomen

Tell the patient you are about to feel their abdomen and that if there is any tenderness they should tell you at which point you will stop. Palpate the abdomen in all 9 areas. Kneel down when doing this and *always look at the patient's face*. Palpate gently at first to elicit any tenderness, then more deeply for masses. Note the characteristics of any masses (size, location, consistency, mobility, tenderness).

Examine the liver and spleen

Having completed the general examination, move on to examining the liver and spleen. Assess the liver by palpation using the edge of the hand from the RIF to the right hypochondrium. Ask the patient to breathe in and out, moving the leading edge of the hand up to feel downward motion of the liver edge during inspiration. If the liver is palpable, determine whether the border is smooth or 'craggy', pulsatile or tender. The left lobe of the liver may be enlarged alone in alcoholic hepatitis and will be felt as a mass in the epigastrium.

Palpate the spleen from the RIF to the left hypochondrium. Use the tips of the fingers for palpation, advancing them on inspiration. If the spleen is enlarged, make a note of how far below the costal margin it extends. The characteristics of an enlarged spleen are described later in this section.

If the spleen is impalpable in the supine position, ask the patient to roll towards you and palpate again. It is recommended that feeling for mild splenomegaly is done after having elicited for shifting dullness (➲ Elicit shifting dullness, p.103), whilst the patient still in the right lateral position, as this will require you to roll the patient only once.

Percuss for both the liver and spleen:

- Percuss upwards from the RIF in the midclavicular line until you reach liver dullness. Percuss downwards in the right midclavicular line until you reach liver dullness. The upper border of the liver is usually at the level of the 5th intercostal space. Measure the distance between the 2 points of dullness with a tape measure or by the number of fingerbreadths. The normal liver is usually not larger than 12–15cm in the midclavicular line. The liver scratch test is not acceptable for the purposes of the exam.

- Percuss for the spleen from the RIF diagonally to the left hypochondrium. In normal individuals the percussion note should remain resonant throughout. Then either percuss in Traube's semilunar space or try to elicit Castell's sign, but not both:

  - Traube's semilunar space* – a crescent-shaped space, ~12cm in size, made up of the left anterior axillary line, 6th rib and left costal margin. This area is usually tympanic (due to the air in the stomach or the splenic flexure) but becomes dull to percussion due to splenomegaly or a pleural effusion. It may also be dull following a heavy meal! (* Of note, Traube himself never reported this sign. It first appeared in the medical literature in a publication from one of Traube's pupils.)

  - Castell's sign* – percuss the anterior axillary line on the left in the lowest intercostal space (but not over the rib) with the patient supine. Resonance on expiration (gastric air) changes to dullness on inspiration if there is splenomegaly. (* Castell was a naval gastroenterologist in the United States in the mid-20th century.)

Palpate the kidney, bladder and abdominal aorta

Ballot the kidneys on either side of the midline. Remember that the kidneys are much closer to the midline than most people think. As a rough rule, you should not be more lateral than the lateral border of the rectus muscles on either side. Put the hand in the costophrenic angle anteriorly and palpate downwards with the hand on the anterior abdominal wall. A ballotable kidney will usually indicate renal enlargement.

It is important to feel for an enlarged/obstructed bladder. After palpating the suprapubic area for a mass, don't forget to percuss for dullness in this area as well.

The abdominal aorta should always be palpated when examining the abdomen. The aorta is palpable in most individuals between the umbilicus and the epigastrium, slightly to the left of the midline. The umbilicus is classically the surface marking for the bifurcation of the aorta into the common iliac vessels. Estimate the width of the aorta, which should be no more than 2 fingerbreadths. Be gentle as aortic aneurysms can be inflamed and tender, not to mention the risk of rupture. Note that an abdominal aortic aneurysm may be associated with renovascular disease (especially if it bridges the renal arteries, when there is a risk of renal artery occlusion).

10. Elicit shifting dullness

Percuss in the midline, which should be resonant due to underlying gas-filled small bowel and one flank which should be correspondingly dull. It is usually more natural to percuss towards the patient's left-hand side. It is not necessary to percuss too laterally (i.e. beyond the posterior axillary line) because the extremes of the flanks will be dull to percussion anyway. Now roll the patient towards you and wait for about 15 seconds while keeping your hand over the position of dullness. This is to allow fluid to drain down and bowel to float up. Percuss again over the position of previous dullness; resonance confirms 'shifting dullness' and, by inference, the presence of ascites.

Remember to check for mild splenomegaly before asking the patient to roll back to the supine position. This 'all in one' manoeuvre of eliciting shifting dullness and splenomegaly is not possible if shifting dullness is elicited by rolling the patient onto their left-hand side i.e. away from you).

In order to detect ascites clinically, at least 1500mL will need to be present. Ultrasound will reliably detect smaller volumes (down to ~500mL).

Causes of ascites are discussed on ➔ p.112.

NB Attempting to elicit a fluid thrill will probably be unnecessary in the exam as patients with large-volume tense ascites are unlikely to be suitable to attend the PACES exam. Similarly, the Puddle test is not in general use.

11. Auscultate the abdomen

A variety of physical signs may be elicited by auscultation in the abdomen and include:

- Bowel sounds which are most reliably heard in the RIF over the ileocaecal valve.
- The venous hum associated with portal hypertension (usually best heard between the umbilicus and xiphisternum). Arterial bruits over the liver may indicate a large haemangioma, alcoholic hepatitis or primary liver cancer. Rubs can occur in the presence of hepatic abscesses and peri-hepatitis (Fitz–Hugh–Curtis syndrome).

- A rub over the spleen which may indicate a splenic infarct or subcapsular haematoma.
- Renal artery bruits should be auscultated anteriorly ~4cm diagonally above the umbilicus. Whilst renal bruits are not very sensitive or specific signs of renal artery stenosis, the examiners will expect you to auscultate for this sign.

12. Check for ankle oedema

Having completed the examination of the abdomen, all that remains is a brief examination of the extremities.

Press over the shins for pitting oedema. If there is oedema, note if it is unilateral (venous or lymphatic obstruction) or bilateral (heart failure, renal failure, hypoalbuminaemic conditions, nephrotic syndrome) and demarcate the extent of the oedema by determining the proximal extent in the legs by pressing on the skin of the thighs, then the lower back and then the chest wall. Total body oedema is known as anasarca in the United States, although 'generalized oedema' is a better term for the PACES examination.

Note that 'myxoedema', typically from hypothyroidism or Grave's disease, is classically non-pitting as the pathology is due to deposition of excess extracellular material and not accumulation of fluid. With that said, hypothyroidism can also cause cardiac failure and pericardial effusion, in which case pitting oedema from an accumulation of fluid in the dependent areas may be present.

13. Thank the patient and cover them up

In general, human beings feel vulnerable when physically exposed. It is both considerate and good practice to thank the subject and cover them up with a blanket before facing the examiner. Not only will this satisfy the examiner but this manoeuvre will also provide a few extra seconds to think.

14. Tell the examiner how you would complete your examination

Whilst one would complete a full abdominal examination by assessing the hernial orifices, the external genitalia, performing a rectal examination and looking at the observations chart, you should tailor your completion of examination according to the condition that you have examined, for instance, start by asking to dipstick the urine for glycosuria and looking at the fundi if the patient has features of end-stage renal disease (ESRD) as type 2 diabetes mellitus is the commonest cause of ESRD in the UK.

The urine dip is used to detect the presence of blood, protein, glucose, nitrites and white blood cells, and may also detect bilirubin and urobilinogen.

Finally, gather your thoughts *before* presenting the case; be confident and speak fluently.

Presentation of findings

If you are confident of the diagnosis, it is far more impressive to state the diagnosis first and justify it by presentation of the relevant positive and negative physical signs. A list of all examination findings to preface the diagnosis is not necessary and may waste valuable time, particularly in the event of an incorrect diagnosis.

When presenting an abdominal system examination, the following order should be adhered to: diagnosis (with justification), likely aetiology (with 2 or 3 differential diagnoses) and any complications of the disease or its treatment. Additional differential diagnoses should also be thought through at this stage so that they can be quickly volunteered if questioned. It is important to state the commonest causes of a particular condition first and reserve rare aetiologies for instances when the patient has clear implicating signs, such as hearing aids in Alport's syndrome.

For example, 'this gentleman has end-stage renal disease with evidence of renal replacement therapy in the form of a functional left brachiocephalic arteriovenous fistula and right renal allograft. The commonest causes of end-stage renal failure (ESRF) in this Caucasian gentleman are diabetic nephropathy, adult polycystic kidney disease and chronic glomerulonephritis. The palpably enlarged native kidneys suggest polycystic kidney disease. This gentleman also shows trophic changes of chronic immunosuppression and a left hemiparesis which may be related to a previous ruptured berry aneurysm'.

Chronic liver disease

Liver disease is a major cause of death in the UK and is increasing, unlike heart disease, cerebrovascular disease, cancer and respiratory disease. The prevalence of alcohol-induced liver disease (the most common cause of cirrhosis), has increased steadily since the 1970s, rising to above that seen in continental Europe, where the frequency has fallen over the same time period.

Presentation

Patients may present in a number of ways:
- Asymptomatic, referred following routine blood tests or abnormal physical examination.
- Symptomatic with:
  - Complication of chronic liver disease (jaundice, ascites, oedema or even upper GI tract bleeding).
  - Pruritis, lethargy or symptoms of underlying disease.
- Emergency presentation with complications of chronic liver disease (haemorrhage, encephalopathy, abdominal pain, fever) or underlying disease (alcohol withdrawal, for example).

Clinical signs

- Undernourishment may be evident.
- Peripheral stigmata of chronic liver disease e.g. leuconychia, Dupuytren's contracture, spider naevi, gynaecomastia (see Table 3.2).
- There may be tattoos or needle track marks from IV drug abuse.
- Asterixis.
- The abdomen may be distended if there is ascites.
- A liver biopsy scar may be found.

Table 3.2 Stigmata of liver disease in the limbs

More common	Less common
• Nails: • Leuconychia • Nail clubbing • Hands: • Palmar erythema • Dupuytren's contracture • Arms: • Jaundice[a] • Bruising • Excoriations from pruritis • Spider naevi[b] • Tattoos	• Nails and hands: needle track marks • Asterixis[c] • Xanthelasma • Skin bronzing (haemochromatosis) • Terry's nails[d] • Cutaneous abscesses at the site of IV drug injection • Paper money skin[e]

[a] Generalized.

[b] SVC distribution; mainly upper arms.

[c] See p.107 for a special note regarding asterixis.

[d] Proximal 2/3 of nails appear white, the rest red; frequently seen in patients with cirrhosis.

[e] Multiple superficial capillaries visible in the upper arm.

- There may be an upper abdominal scar if the patient has received a liver transplant or portocaval shunt surgery (➔ Fig. 3.1, p.96).
- Hepatomegaly – if present then note if there are any palpable irregularities in the liver.
- Splenomegaly – splenomegaly usually indicates portal hypertension but the spleen may return to normal size following adequate treatment of portal hypertension. Remember that the spleen is 2–3 times enlarged before it becomes palpable.

Signs of portal hypertension

- Splenomegaly
- Caput medusa
- Oesophageal varices on endoscopy
- Ascites

---

❶ Top Tips

- Asterixis, if mild, can sometimes be better felt with gentle pressure than visualized.
- In cirrhosis, the liver is usually small, especially if the aetiology is alcoholic liver disease. Whilst the liver can be large or of normal size in chronic liver disease (CLD), if you feel an enlarged liver with signs of CLD, be suspicious of malignancy.
- Always look for an underlying cause. The 3 commonest causes of CLD in the Western world are excessive alcohol intake, chronic viral hepatitis (C or B; look for tattoos) or non-alcoholic hepatic steatosis (usually overweight).
- Spider naevi are located in the distribution of the SVC. Always make sure you've looked at the upper back thoroughly because in some cases spider naevi are the only visible signs of CLD and may only be present on the back.
- Specify whether the patient has compensated or decompensated CLD.
- NB Jaundice is also a sign of acute liver disease so don't feel that it always has to be CLD if the patient is jaundiced.

Special points regarding asterixis

- Remember that asterixis (from the Greek *a* ('not') and *sterixis* ('fixed position') is a form of myoclonus due to intermittent loss of muscle tone (hence named negative myoclonus).
- Therefore it should be tested while the patient carries out a tonic muscle contraction (wrist dorsiflexion).
- Asterixis can affect different sites (wrists, metacarpophalangeal and hip joints are commonest) and is bilateral in metabolic conditions. Unilateral asterixis is usually a sign of a focal cerebral lesion.
- Asterixis is very unlikely to be present in the exam but you should describe to the examiner that you would ordinarily test for it for 30 seconds after demonstrating how to elicit the sign.
- Asterixis was first described by Adams and Foley in 1949.[1]

Causes of chronic liver disease

- Alcohol – by far the commonest cause of chronic liver disease in the UK.
- Chronic viral hepatitis:
  - Hepatitis C – frequently associated with IV drug use.
  - Hepatitis B – often contracted abroad.
- Non-alcoholic steatohepatitis. This is less common (although increasing) and may progress to cirrhosis. It is associated with obesity and the metabolic syndrome.
- Autoimmune causes including chronic active hepatitis and primary biliary cirrhosis (PBC). PBC should be particularly considered in middle-aged women.
- Metabolic conditions e.g. haemochromatosis.

❧ Common Pitfalls

- Failure to identify the extra-abdominal signs (e.g. radiotherapy scars, telangiectasia) may result in failure to diagnose CLD, especially if no abdominal signs are present.
- The lateral border of the rectus sheath in a thin patient may feel like a liver edge and is a common error in routine medical practice. Lack of dullness to percussion and absence of other signs should exclude hepatomegaly.
- It is tempting to fabricate signs and describe an enlarged liver when extra-abdominal signs of CLD are present – this should be avoided at all costs. The liver is often not palpable in cirrhosis and therefore, CLD can occur in the presence or absence of hepatomegaly.
- During the presentation there is a tendency to describe uncommon conditions as causes of CLD. The most important thing is to present the 3 commonest causes i.e. alcoholic liver disease, chronic hepatotrophic virus infection (commonly hepatitis B and C) and non-alcoholic hepatic steatosis, unless there is obvious evidence for another cause.

Viva questions

Can you name some complications of CLD?

Complications of CLD include:

- Portal hypertension
- Haemorrhage, usually upper GI (gastric ulcers and erosions still occur more frequently than variceal bleeding)
- Ascites
- Spontaneous bacterial peritonitis
- Hepatic encephalopathy
- Hepatorenal syndrome
- Hepatopulmonary syndrome.

What do you understand by decompensated CLD? What are the precipitating factors which can lead to decompensated CLD?

- The liver can compensate for a significant amount of hepatocyte injury but can decompensate as a result of ongoing liver injury

(continued alcohol intake or untreated chronic active viral hepatitis) or additional stress (e.g. GI bleeding, large salt intake, sepsis, constipation, dehydration).
- Clinically, decompensated CLD will present with a combination of ascites, encephalopathy, hepatorenal or hepatopulmonary syndrome in an acute setting.
- It is unlikely that decompensated CLD will be present in the exam.

How do you grade severity of hepatic encephalopathy?

Hepatic encephalopathy is graded according to the West Haven criteria:
- Grade 0: clinically normal but with small changes in memory or mentation.
- Grade 1: mild confusion, euphoria or depression; short attention span and impaired mental tasks such as addition; disordered sleep patterns.
- Grade 2: drowsiness, lethargy, mild disorientation mainly for time but also sometimes for place; inappropriate behaviour and personality change; impaired mental tasks such as subtraction.
- Grade 3: somnolent but rousable, usually with verbal stimuli sufficing; grossly confused and disorientated; speech may be incomprehensible; amnesia often present.
- Grade 4: comatose; no response to verbal or painful stimuli.

How do you grade the severity of cirrhosis?

- The most commonly used grading system for grading the severity of cirrhosis is the modified Child–Pugh system which scores clinical and biochemical parameters out of three to obtain a composite score (Table 3.3).
- Severity is classified according to the Child–Pugh score into Class A (5–6 points), Class B (7–9 points) or Class C (10–15 points) corresponding to 1-year survivals of 100%, 80% and 50% respectively.

Table 3.3 Child–Pugh score for grading severity of cirrhosis

Parameter	1 point	2 points	3 points
Encephalopathy	None or Stage 0	Stages 1–2	Stages 3–4
Bilirubin (micromol/L)[a]	<34	34–50	>50
INR	<1.7	1.7–2.3	>2.3
Ascites	None	Mild	Severe
Albumin (g/L)	>35	28–35	<28

[a] Sclerosing cholangitis or primary biliary cirrhosis are characterized by higher levels of bilirubin. Therefore, in these conditions, the criteria for bilirubin (micromol/L) are modified as follows: 1 point for bilirubin <68; 2 points for bilirubin 68–170; and 3 points for bilirubin >170.

How do you classify causes of jaundice?

Jaundice can be classified as:
- Pre-hepatic – due to excessive breakdown of red blood cells e.g. autoimmune haemolytic anaemia, malaria, hereditary haemoglobinopathies (e.g. sickle cell disease).

- Hepatic – due to hepatocyte injury e.g. acute viral hepatitis, paracetamol, alcohol, hypoxic/ischaemic.
- Post-hepatic – due to obstruction to the normal flow of bile e.g. gallstone obstruction, pancreatic head malignancies.

What do you know about hepatorenal syndrome?

Hepatorenal syndrome results from inadequate hepatic breakdown of vasoactive substances, leading to excessive renal vasoconstriction. It can develop rapidly (type I) or slowly (type II) and mimics pre-renal renal impairment. As the kidneys attempt to conserve maximum salt and water in response to perceived hypovolaemia, the patient produces low volumes of highly concentrated (high osmolar) urine that is low in sodium. It is usually a diagnosis of exclusion, having given a fluid challenge and ruled out obstruction, sepsis and nephrotoxic drugs. You will not be required to know the major and minor diagnostic criteria that can be used to establish the diagnosis for the exam. It is difficult to reverse without hepatic transplantation unless the patient has spontaneous recovery of liver function (e.g. post-ethanolic hepatitis).

The kidneys of patients with hepatorenal syndrome are usually normal and in the acute setting may be salvaged (and if transplanted into another patient with ESRF would function – this is not, however, routinely done in clinical practice!). In general, if the GFR is <30mL/min in the pre-morbid state, combined liver and kidney transplantation is usually undertaken in favour of single liver engraftment as perioperative injury and postoperative immunosuppression usually lead to loss of the remaining kidney function.

How do you manage ascites in association with CLD?

- A no-added-salt diet should be started (90mmol or 5.2g salt/day).
- Spironolactone from 100–400mg/day, in all patients able to tolerate the drug without excessive hyperkalaemia.
- Loop diuretics should be initiated next, usually furosemide from 40–160mg/day.
- If these measures fail or if the patient has significant symptoms related to the ascites, therapeutic paracentesis should be carried out.
- Radiological procedures such as transjugular intrahepatic portosystemic shunt (TIPS) procedure may help to relieve portal hypertension but the risk of encephalopathy is increased as nitrogenous waste effectively bypass the liver with a resultant increased concentration in the systemic circulation.
- Surgical measures (portosystemic and peritoneovenous shunts) are much less frequently used these days but still play a role in recurrent ascites. Liver transplantation is a curative procedure for end-stage liver disease when medical management fails.[2]

References

1. Adams RD, Foley JM. The neurological changes in the more common types of severe liver disease. *Trans American Neurology Association* 1949; **74**:217–19.
2. Dawwas MF et al. Survival after liver transplantation in the United Kingdom and Ireland compared with the United States. *Gut* 2007; **56**(11):1606–13.

Ascites

Ascites is a common medical finding. It comes up with surprising frequency in the exam, usually in association with CLD.

Presentation

Patients may present:
- Asymptomatically, having been referred with another condition, e.g. CLD, nephrotic syndrome.
- Symptomatically with:
  - Abdominal swelling or discomfort.
  - Complication of ascites (e.g. peritonitis, respiratory embarrassment) or the underlying condition (e.g. hepatic encephalopathy, symptomatic acute/chronic renal failure).

Clinical signs

- The patient may be malnourished if there is underlying malignancy, severe cardiac failure, alcoholic cirrhosis or nephrotic syndrome.
- Leuconychia or signs of chronic liver disease may be present.
- Lymphadenopathy secondary to underlying malignancy.
- Raised JVP from right-sided cardiac failure.
- Pleural effusion may result from either right-sided cardiac failure or from movement of ascitic fluid through the diaphragm (usually right-sided).
- There may be abdominal scars from previous tumour resection.
- Recent paracentesis or evidence of diagnostic taps may be visible.
- Abdominal distention and umbilical eversion may be seen in severe cases.
- Shifting dullness is the classical feature and is pathognomonic of ascites.
- Abdominal masses of underlying malignancy which may be impalpable due to the presence of ascites.
- Peripheral oedema.

---

❶ Top Tips

- Ensure that you look for the extra-abdominal signs. If present, they will usually be obvious!
- One useful examination technique is to roll the patient to the right-hand side when eliciting shifting dullness so as to permit palpation for a mildly enlarged spleen immediately after examining for ascites. This will avoid moving the patient twice.
- Ascites in the absence of stigmata of CLD is usually due to malignancy. Make sure you feel for an enlarged spleen, lymph nodes and any other masses.
- Make sure you ask for the urine dipstick, especially with respect to proteinuria.
- NB Gynaecomastia, if present, may be due to CLD, spironolactone or both.

☞ Common Pitfalls

- Percussing too laterally and finding dullness in the flanks. Note that if you percuss laterally enough, the flanks will always be dull. This does not indicate the presence of ascites
- Remember that ascites is not a diagnosis and that you need to state the likely underlying cause.

Causes of ascites

Ascites can be classified either into common and uncommon causes or into transudative and exudative aetiologies. In the scheme which follows, exudative causes are highlighted.

Common causes

- Cirrhosis with portal hypertension (usually alcoholic or chronic hepatitis virus disease).[*]
- Malignancy e.g. metastatic GI tract, liver, ovarian, mesothelioma of peritoneum (exudative).
- Congestive cardiac failure (due to raised portal pressure).
- Nephrotic syndrome (due to reduced oncotic pressure and salt and water overload).

([*] In the exam, CLD with portal hypertension will be the commonest cause of ascites. In this setting, signs of CLD will be present.)

Uncommon causes

- Budd–Chiari syndrome
- Portal vein thrombosis
- Constrictive pericarditis
- Malabsorption syndromes
- Peritoneal mesothelioma (exudative)
- Tuberculous peritonitis (exudative)
- Myxoedema
- Ovarian diseases e.g. ovarian hyperstimulation syndrome and Meigs disease (ovarian fibroma with ascites and pleural effusion) (exudative or transudative).

Viva questions

What are the causes of ascites formation in CLD?

- Relative renal hypoperfusion causes increased renin from the juxtaglomerular apparatus.
- Renin activates aldosterone.
- Deficient hepatic metabolism reduces aldosterone and ADH breakdown.
- Hypoalbuminaemia decreases oncotic pressure.
- Third-spacing of volume exacerbates renal hypoperfusion.

The combination of salt and water retention (from secondary hyperaldosteronism and high anti-diuretic hormone) with high portal pressure causes net ultrafiltration of fluid into the abdominal cavity resulting in ascites.

*How would you distinguish between transudative and exudative ascites
in patients with low serum albumin?*

- Use the serum:ascites albumin gradient (SAAG). A low gradient
  (<11g/L) indicates loss of protein into the ascites and is a sign of an
  exudate whereas a high gradient (≥11g/L) indicates a transudate.[1]

*What methods do you know for assessing for the presence of ascites?
What are their relative sensitivities and specificities?*

The publication of Cattau *et al.*[2] addressed this very question. The overall
accuracy of the various manoeuvres is shown in Table 3.4.

Table 3.4 Sensitivity and specificity of physical signs for ascites

Test	Sensitivity	Specificity
Bulging flanks	0.78	0.44
Flank dullness	0.94	0.29
Shifting dullness	0.83	0.56
Fluid wave	0.50	0.82
Puddle sign	0.55	0.51

Candidate would not be expected to have memorized these figures

References

1. Paré P et al. Serum-ascites albumin concentration gradient: a physiologic approach to the differential diagnosis of ascites. *Gastroenterology* 1983; **85**(2):240–2.

2. Cattau EL et al. The accuracy of the physical examination in the diagnosis of suspected ascites. *JAMA* 1982; **247**:1164–6.

Hepatomegaly

Worldwide, hepatomegaly is a very common finding, usually in association with infectious diseases (e.g. malaria, hepatitis virus, leishmania) or malignancy. In the PACES exam, it will normally be present in the non-infectious setting.

Presentation

Patient may be referred:

- Asymptomatically:
  - With an incidental finding of large liver on physical examination.
  - Patient notices a mass in the abdomen.
- Symptomatically with:
  - Features of underlying malignancy (weight loss, lethargy, symptoms related to site of primary disease e.g. altered bowel habit).
  - Abdominal pain – usually due to rapid enlargement, necrosis of an enlarging tumour or heart failure. Pain may be referred to the right shoulder.
  - Jaundice with enlarged liver (e.g. malaria).

Clinical signs

- There may be signs of acute or chronic liver disease e.g. malnourishment, peripheral stigmata of liver disease, jaundice and ascites.
- Signs associated with an underlying carcinoma may be present, such as cachexia, tobacco-stained fingers or scars from previous chest or abdominal resections.
- Look for features to suggest right or biventricular failure, including a raised JVP, pulsatile hepatomegaly and peripheral oedema.
- More rarely, infiltrative conditions such as amyloidosis may cause hepatomegaly. Look for a classic heliotrope rash, signs of rheumatoid arthritis, ankylosing spondylitis, multiple myeloma and chronic ulceration.
- Sarcoidosis may cause hepatomegaly associated with hepatic granulomas. Look for lupus pernio (purple/red indurated papules/ plaques, usually affecting the ears, nose and cheeks). If sarcoidosis is suspected ask to examine for associated respiratory signs.
- Lymphoproliferative disorders are associated with anaemia and lymphadenopathy.

---

❶ Top Tips

- The surface marking of the upper border of the liver is the right 5th interspace and is best determined by percussion.
- The liver may be palpable in normal subjects on deep inspiration.
- The liver may be transiently enlarged in acute alcoholic hepatitis. This can cause hepatomegaly affecting either the whole of the liver or occasionally only the left lobe. The latter presents as an epigastric mass.

❧ Common Pitfalls

- Hepatomegaly in the absence of stigmata of CLD is unlikely to be due to cirrhosis. Consider a malignancy instead.
- Chronic myeloid leukaemia may present with jaundice secondary to an autoimmune haemolytic anaemia. The jaundice is pre-hepatic, giving the sclera a lemon yellow tinge.
- Take care not to confuse the rectus sheath with a liver edge! Avoid this by palpating just lateral to the rectus sheath.

Top 3 causes of hepatomegaly

- Congestive cardiac failure
- Malignancy
- Lymphoma

Viva questions

What scoring systems may help in the evaluation of a patient presenting with an acute alcoholic hepatitis?

- *Maddrey's discriminant function test* was described by Maddrey et al. in 1978[1] to predict prognosis in alcoholic hepatitis:
  - It is calculated by:
    4.6 × [prothrombin time:control value (seconds)]
    + serum bilirubin (mg/mL)
  - During the episode, a score >32 carries a 50% mortality rate and is an indication for treatment with steroids, whereas >90% of patients with a score <32 will survive.
- *The Mayo End stage Liver Disease (MELD)* score has been applied to alcoholic hepatitis.[2,3] This is a composite score derived from the serum bilirubin, creatinine and INR and predicts survival probability over 90 days. In one study, patients with a score ≤11 had a 30-day survival of 96% whilst the 30-day survival in those with a score ≥11 was 45%.
- *The Glasgow alcoholic hepatitis score* on day 1 has an overall accuracy of 81% when predicting 28-day outcome.

How would you manage a patient with acute alcoholic hepatitis?

- The mainstays of management are supportive and include: abstinence from alcohol, adequate nutrition and treatment of any intercurrent infections.
- Liver biopsy may be indicated to confirm the diagnosis.
- Maddrey's discriminant function score of >32 is an indication for treatment with steroids. 40mg oral prednisolone is frequently used. Other drugs which may be useful include pentoxifylline.

What are the histological features of alcoholic liver disease?

- Hepatic steatosis – accumulation of fat in liver cells. This is not related to the total alcohol exposure alone.
- Alcoholic hepatitis – acute inflammation and hepatocyte necrosis (usually hepatocytes affected by steatosis).
- Hepatic cirrhosis – fibrosis of liver tissue.

While cirrhosis is irreversible and if progressive can lead to liver failure, both steatosis and hepatitis are potentially reversible following abstinence from alcohol.

What clotting factor abnormalities may be associated with hepatic amyloidosis?

Hepatic amyloidosis is characteristically associated with loss of the clotting factors IX and X. In addition, infiltration with amyloid protein contributes to vascular fragility. There is a significant risk of bleeding if percutaneous liver biopsy is performed and spontaneous hepatic rupture has been described.

References

1. Maddrey WC *et al.* Corticosteroid therapy of alcoholic hepatitis. *Gastroenterology* 1978; **75**(2):193–9.
2. For models of end-stage liver disease (MELD), please see http://www.mayoclinic.org/meld.
3. The on-line calculator for 90-day mortality from alcoholic hepatitis is found at http://www.mayoclinic.org/meld/mayomodel7.html.

Splenomegaly

Isolated splenomegaly is not common, either in the exam or in general medical practice. In developed nations, malignancy (lymphoproliferative) is the most likely setting for isolated splenomegaly; in developing nations, it is most common in the context of infectious diseases.

Presentation

Patients may present as follows:
- Asymptomatic, referred with an abdominal mass.
- Fever.
- Anaemia or consequences of thrombocytopenia (bruising or bleeding) e.g. in haemolytic disorders.
- Pancreatitis (splenic vein thrombosis).
- Traumatic rupture or haemorrhage. (NB Pain from the spleen may be referred to the left shoulder.)

Clinical signs

- The patient may be malnourished if splenomegaly occurs in the context of malignancy or chronic infection.
- Lymphadenopathy secondary to lymphoproliferative disease or infection.
- Look for signs of RA.
- Start palpation for the spleen in the RIF using the finger tips/pulps and work up towards the left hypochondrium. Ask the patient to inspire; as they do so move the palpating hand in towards the left hypochondrium to 'tip' the spleen.
- The spleen is on a vascular pedicle and is relatively mobile. Use the non-palpating hand (usually the left) to 'fix' the spleen by pulling the patient's rib cage anteriorly along the line of the left 10th rib, the normal long axis of the spleen.
- If the spleen is still not palpable, roll the patient 1/3 of the way towards you and repeat the procedure. This should be carried out during the same manoeuvre looking for the shifting dullness of ascites (➔ see p.111).
- The differential diagnosis of an enlarged spleen is usually a palpable left kidney. The spleen cannot be balloted, is dull to percussion, has a notch and you should not be able to 'get above' it.
- Look for ascites which may be present in the context of malignancy and portal hypertension.
- Look for signs of underlying carcinoma which may be associated with splenic vein thrombosis.

❶ Top Tips

- Worldwide, the commonest causes of splenomegaly are: chronic malaria, kala-azar and schistosomiasis. Always consider the ethnic background of the patient with splenomegaly, as well as the possibility of travel abroad to endemic areas.
- Splenomegaly is nearly always present in chronic myeloid leukaemia (CML) and myelofibrosis and may be massive (>20cm).
- Enlargement to 4–8cm is found in lymphoma, chronic lymphocytic leukaemia (CLL) and cirrhosis with portal hypertension as well as CML and myelofibrosis.
- If the spleen is just palpable again consider CML, myelofibrosis, lymphoma and CLL, cirrhosis in addition to acute infections such as Epstein–Barr virus, cytomegalovirus and subacute bacterial endocarditis.
- 'Left-sided' (sinistral) portal hypertension is commonly caused by splenic vein compression or thrombosis as a result, for instance of a pancreatic tumour. Compression causes increased pressure in the left portal venous system leading to gastric varices.

❦ Common Pitfalls

- Rough handling can be uncomfortable; seriously rough handling can result in splenic rupture!
- Distinguish the spleen from other epigastric masses. Enlargement of the left lobe of the liver can occur in isolation in alcoholic hepatitis and Budd–Chiari syndrome.

Causes of isolated splenomegaly

Common causes

- Chronic malaria
- Kala-azar
- Schistosomiasis
- Lymphoproliferative diseases (but usually also includes lymphadenopathy ± hepatomegaly)

Uncommon causes

- Felty's syndrome
- Chronic haemolytic anaemia
- Infective endocarditis
- Left-sided portal hypertension – portal vein or splenic vein thrombosis (e.g. due to pancreatic malignancy or pancreatitis).

Viva questions

What is the characteristic chromosomal abnormality in CML and what signal transduction pathway abnormality is this associated with?

- The Philadelphia chromosome is the hallmark of CML, where it is found in >90% of cases. Cytogenetically it usually results from a chromosomal translocation: t(9;22)(q34;q11).

- This molecular rearrangement expresses a *bcr-abl* hybrid mRNA transcript that encodes an altered bcr-abl protein with enhanced *in vitro* tyrosine kinase activity.
- The fused bcr-abl protein interacts with the interleukin 3 receptor subunit. The transcript is continuously active and does not require activation by other cellular messaging proteins. Bcr-abl activates proteins which control the cell cycle, speeding up cell division and inhibiting DNA repair.

Tell me about Felty's syndrome

- Felty's syndrome is defined by the presence of 3 conditions: rheumatoid arthritis, splenomegaly and neutropenia. It affects <1% of patients with RA.
- The cause of Felty's syndrome is unknown. The frequency of Felty's syndrome increases with the duration of rheumatoid arthritis.
- People with this syndrome are at risk of infection (lung and skin mainly) on account of neutropenia.
- Complications of Felty's syndrome include recurrent infection, hypersplenism causing anaemia and thrombocytopenia, skin hyperpigmentation and cutaneous ulceration.

Why might the platelet count be reduced in alcoholic liver disease?

- Splenomegaly associated with portal hypertension results in platelet sequestration and thrombocytopenia.
- In addition there is a direct toxic effect of alcohol on production, survival time and function of platelets. Folate deficiency may contribute.
- Platelet counts may begin to rise after 2–5 days' abstinence from alcohol.
- A platelet count of $<50 \times 10^9$/L is an indication for platelet transfusion in the presence of bleeding, particularly from varices.

How would you differentiate between a splenic and renal mass?

- The 4 characteristics of a splenic mass are as follows:
  - Dull to percussion
  - Not ballotable
  - Palpable splenic notch
  - The palpating finger cannot get above a splenic mass
- These features are absent with a renal mass.

Hepatosplenomegaly

Hepatosplenomegaly is a common case in the exam. In clinical practice, it is common to see patients with enlargement of both the liver and spleen in many diverse specialties, so a working knowledge of the causes should be well rehearsed.

Presentation

- Asymptomatic, referred with abdominal masses or detected on routine examination or abnormal blood results on routine phlebotomy; rarely referred from ophthalmology with abnormal slit-lamp examination.
- Symptomatic with:
  - Lethargy, fatigue, breathlessness (anaemia) or easy bruising/bleeding (thrombocytopenia).
  - Abdominal pain (may be referred to left or right shoulder).
  - Febrile illness (infectious disease or lymphoproliferative illness) with or without weight loss and/or night sweats (symptoms of lymphoproliferative conditions).
  - Tremor, dysarthria, falls, impaired co-ordination or performance of fine motor tasks (parkinsonian features).
  - Intense itch (primary biliary cirrhosis).

Clinical signs

- There may be signs associated with cirrhosis and portal hypertension e.g. spider naevi, bruising, jaundice, ascites
- The liver and spleen are both palpably enlarged
- Signs relevant to specific diseases associated with hepatosplenomegaly are listed in Table 3.5.

Causes of hepatosplenomegaly

Common causes of hepatosplenomegaly

- Infective (➔ 'Viva questions' below.)
- Myeloproliferative and lymphoproliferative diseases
- Cirrhosis with portal hypertension.

Uncommon causes of hepatosplenomegaly

- Wilson's disease
- Haemochromatosis
- Glycogen storage disorders.

Viva questions

Worldwide what would you consider to be the most common causes of hepatosplenomegaly?

- Malaria. Chronic malaria is seen in both *Plasmodium vivax* and *P. ovale* because they have hepatic lifecycles, but not in *P. falciparum* which does not have a lifecycle outside of the circulation. Nevertheless, *P. falciparum* may also be associated with hepatosplenomegaly.
- Visceral leishmaniasis. Known also as kala-azar, this is the most severe form of leishmaniasis. Leishmaniasis is caused by protozoan parasites of the *Leishmania* genus and is the second-largest parasitic killer in the world (after malaria). The parasite is spread by sandflies and migrates to the internal organs such as liver, spleen and bone marrow and, if

Table 3.5 Clinical signs and conditions associated with hepatosplenomegaly

Sign	Condition
Anaemia	Myeloproliferative disorders (e.g. chronic myeloid leukaemia and myelofibrosis)
Lymphadenopathy	Lymphoproliferative disorders; infective causes (e.g. Epstein–Barr virus, TB); sarcoidosis
Parkinsonism, dysarthria, Kayser–Fleischer rings on slit lamp examination, neuropsychiatric manifestations	Wilson's disease
Xanthoma and xanthelasma	Primary biliary cirrhosis
Arthropathy	Haemochromatosis
Yellow-brown skin pigmentation; pingueculae,[a] eye movement disorders, myoclonus, early dementia	Gaucher's disease (lysosomal storage disease)
Learning difficulties	Niemann–Pick disease (sphingomyelinase deficiency); Wilson's disease

[a] From the Latin 'pinguis', meaning fat or oily – a yellow-white pigmentation of the conjunctiva usually adjacent to the limbus of the eye.

❶ Top Tips

- If other stigmata of chronic liver disease are present, the diagnosis is likely to be cirrhosis with portal hypertension.
- Ascites does not usually occur in myeloproliferative and lymphoproliferative disorders.
- Lymphadenopathy elsewhere makes the diagnosis of lymphoproliferative disorder more likely.
- Glycogen storage diseases are rare causes of hepatosplenomegaly.

❧ Common Pitfalls

- It is crucial to distinguish hepatosplenomegaly from bilateral renal enlargement due to adult polycystic kidney disease. Uraemia may confound the picture by making the patient appear subtly jaundiced. It should be possible to get above enlarged kidneys and they may be ballottable.
- Jaundice associated with hepatosplenomegaly may be due to haemolysis rather than hepatitis or cholestasis.

left untreated, will almost always result in the death of the host. Signs and symptoms include fever, weight loss, anaemia and substantial swelling of the liver and spleen.

- Schistosomiasis (bilharzia). This parasitic disease is caused by several species of fluke of the genus *Schistosoma*. Schistosomiasis is often a chronic illness with a low mortality rate but high morbidity relating to irreversible damage to internal organs such as the liver and urinary tract. Chronic infection causes granulomatous reactions and fibrosis in affected organs, resulting in portal hypertension with hepatosplenomegaly (particularly with *S. mansoni* and *S. japonicum*). Schistosomiasis is readily treated using a single oral dose of the drug praziquantel.

What is meant by pre-sinusoidal portal hypertension?

In schistosomiasis caused by *S. mansoni* and *S. japonicum*, schistosome eggs become trapped in the portal tracts where there cause a granulomatous reaction and subsequent fibrosis. Since this involves the last branches of the portal veins, portal hypertension ensues. However, the liver sinusoids are not affected. Thus liver synthetic function is unaffected.

What is the genetic basis of Wilson's disease?

- The genetic abnormality in Wilson's disease is a mutation of the adenosine triphosphatase 7B (*ATP7B*) gene.
- This gene is a key element in the transport of copper into the secretory pathway of the cell for incorporation into copper-containing enzymes and excretion of excess copper in the bile.
- Mutation of this gene therefore leads to accumulation of free copper in hepatocytes, followed by eventual 'spill-over' into the serum and thence to the urine.
- Simultaneously, the levels of copper-containing enzymes, such as caeruloplasmin, decrease.

What are the biochemical features of Wilson's disease and what are the limitations of these tests?

- Low serum caeruloplasmin and high urine copper levels are the cardinal features of Wilson's disease.
- Both copper and caeruloplasmin are acute phase reactants and their levels increase in the presence of an acute phase response. Therefore, levels should be interpreted in the context of the patient's overall condition.

What are the clinical manifestations of Wilson's disease?

- Accumulation of copper in the liver is at first an asymptomatic process. Most patients therefore present from the 2nd decade of life onwards.
- The disease can affect most organ systems as shown in Table 3.6.

Table 3.6 Clinical manifestations of Wilson's disease

Gastrointestinal	Chronic active hepatitis
	Fulminant hepatitis
	Chronic liver disease with cirrhosis
Neurological	Resting or intention tremor
	Parkinsonism [a]
	Dysdiadochokinesia
	Dystonias
	Choreoathetosis
	Ataxia
	Epilepsy
Psychiatric	Personality change
	Emotional lability
	Intellectual impairment
	Psychosis and affective disorders
Ophthalmological	Kayser–Fleischer rings in Descemet's membrane[b]
	Sunflower cataracts
Musculoskeletal	Osteopenia
	Arthropathy
	Chondrocalcinosis
Renal	Fanconi syndrome
	Renal stone disease and nephrocalcinosis [c]
Cardiac	Cardiomyopathy
	Sudden cardiac death
Haematological	Haemolytic anaemia (rare)

[a] Hence the reason why Wilson's disease is also known as hepatolenticular degeneration.

[b] Not pathognomonic of Wilson's disease as it can also be caused by other conditions, notably chronic obstructive jaundice due to primary biliary cirrhosis and primary sclerosing cholangitis; slit lamp examination required.

[c] Thought to be due to the renal tubular acidosis and hypercalciuria arising from proximal tubular dysfunction.

Primary biliary cirrhosis

The incidence of this condition is higher in the UK, than worldwide, where it affects approximately 20–30 per 100,000 of the population (combined for male and female; 5 per 100,000 worldwide). Like other autoimmune diseases, the prevalence is higher in females and it occurs more frequently than would be expected in the PACES exam.

Presentation

- Asymptomatic, referred following routine examination or routine blood tests (abnormal liver function tests and abnormally high cholesterol).
- Symptomatic with intense pruritis and excessive lethargy.
- Abdominal pain, usually in the right upper quadrant, but may be referred to the right shoulder.

Clinical signs

- Patients with PBC are likely to be female (90%) and between 40–60 years of age.
- Scratch marks are frequently present.
- The patient will be jaundiced.
- Orbital xanthelasmata are characteristic and skin xanthomas develop frequently.
- Both liver and spleen are likely to be enlarged.
- There may be stigmata of CLD.
- Look for stigmata of other associated autoimmune diseases.

Top Tips

- Look for stigmata of other autoimmune conditions that may be associated with PBC e.g. systemic sclerosis and autoimmune thyroiditis (20%).
- Differentiation from autoimmune hepatitis may be difficult. The presence of xanthomas should prompt you to consider PBC as the more likely diagnosis.
- Anti-mitochondrial antibodies (AMAs) are found in virtually all patients with PBC.[1]
- Antibodies associated with autoimmune hepatitis include anti-nuclear antibodies in 80%,[2] anti-double-stranded DNA[3] and smooth muscle (actin) antibodies.[4]

Common Pitfalls

- The most common error is to correctly notice the signs of CLD without appreciating that the underlying diagnosis is PBC. In female patients of the appropriate age, the differential diagnosis of CLD should include PBC for the purposes of the exam.

Viva questions

What are the most frequent presenting complaints of PBC?

- PBC is asymptomatic in many patients and is diagnosed incidentally
  e.g. at cholecystectomy.
- In those who present with symptoms, pruritis and fatigue are the
  commonest presenting features.
- Some patients experience right upper quadrant pain.
- Impaired bile production leads to impaired absorption of fat-soluble
  vitamins and easy bruising in some subjects.

What is the natural history of PBC?

- The female:male ratio in PBC is approximately 9:1. AMAs are directed
  against the mitochondrial enzyme complex M2. The antigen itself is the
  pyruvate dehydrogenase complex E2 found on the inner mitochondrial
  membrane. AMA is positive in 90% of patients with PBC.
- In many cases disease progression is so slow that lifespan is unaffected
  and PBC may be diagnosed incidentally e.g. at cholecystectomy.
  However, symptomatic patients are unlikely to survive >2 years.

Can you name some conditions that might mimic PBC?

- The most common differential diagnoses for PBC are autoimmune
  hepatitis and primary sclerosing cholangitis.
- PBC can occasionally be mistaken for Wilson's disease as Kayser–
  Fleischer rings may occur as a result of impaired copper excretion.
- Granulomas in the liver may suggest cholestatic sarcoidosis but AMAs
  are usually absent in this condition.

What treatment options are currently available for PBC?

- General measures include avoidance of alcohol and supplementation of
  the diet with the fat soluble vitamins (A, D, E, K).
- Ursodeoxycholic acid reduces cholestasis and improves liver function
  tests. However, it has little effect on symptoms or prognosis.
- Pruritis is generally assumed to be caused by circulating bile acids and
  may be helped by the anion exchange resin cholestyramine. There is,
  however, evidence that the itch may have a central component.
- In advanced cases, a liver transplant may be successful. Functional
  decline, uncontrolled itching, hepatic encephalopathy, bleeding varices
  and recurrent infections are all indications for transplantation.

Who described PBC?

PBC was first described by Thomas Addison, ~100 years before it was
officially given the name primary biliary cirrhosis.

References

1. Walker JG et al. Serological tests in diagnosis of primary biliary cirrhosis. Lancet 1965; **1**:827–31.
2. Czaja AJ et al. Patterns of nuclear immunofluorescence and reactivities to recombinant nuclear
   antigens in autoimmune hepatitis. Gastroenterology 1994; **107**(1):200–7.
3. Enomoto N et al. Mutations in the nonstructural protein 5A gene and response to interferon in
   patients with chronic hepatitis C virus 1b infection. NEJM 1996; **334**(2):77–81.
4. Muratori P et al. Smooth muscle antibodies and type 1 autoimmune hepatitis. Autoimmunity.
   2002; **35**(8):497–500.

Haemochromatosis

Haemochromatosis is actually a very common condition, with a carrier frequency estimated to be ~10% in the Caucasian, particularly Celtic, northern European population. The clinical sequelae are more prevalent in male patients.

Presentation

- Asymptomatic presentation with abnormal blood tests.
- Symptomatic presentation with the classical triad of fatigue, arthralgia and gonadal/sexual dysfunction.
- Later presentation with complications of haemochromatosis include the following:
  - Hepatic cirrhosis (◑ CLD, p.106)
  - Type I diabetes mellitus
  - Skin discoloration (classically 'bronze')
  - Cardiomyopathy, often dilated, often with arrhythmias.

NB Haemochromatosis is recognized as a potent risk factor for hepatocellular carcinoma. Estimates vary greatly but a 200-fold increased risk has previously been reported.[1]

Clinical signs

- Slate grey pigmentation of skin.
- The liver will be enlarged, firm and may be tender. Other stigmata of chronic hepatocellular failure are not usually present.
- The spleen may be mild or moderately palpable.
- Physical signs relating to organ systems involved are shown in Table 3.7.

Table 3.7 Organ system involvement in haemochromatosis

Physical features	Pathological process
Skin pigmentation	Skin deposition of iron
Heart failure	Dilated cardiomyopathy
BM stix marks, peripheral neuropathy, diabetic retinopathy, evidence of large-vessel disease	Type 1 diabetes from pancreatic endocrine failure
Hepatomegaly	Liver deposition of iron
Chronic liver disease	Liver cirrhosis
Liver mass	Hepatocellular carcinoma
Small testes	Hypogonadism, usually from pituitary involvement[a] and less commonly from direct gonadal involvement
Features of hypothyroidism	Hypothyroidism from pituitary involvement[a]
Arthropathy, especially of the metacarpophalangeal joints and knees	Joint involvement[b]

[a] The anterior pituitary is commonly affected in haemochromatosis.

[b] Chondrocalcinosis is very common but this is a radiological entity.

❶ Top Tips

- Look for complications of diabetes as this condition occurs in 2/3 of patients with haemochromatosis.
- Anterior pituitary function is impaired in 2/3 patients and results in hypogonadotrophic pituitary failure; pan-hypopituitarism is much rarer.
- The presence of ascites raises the possibility of hepatocellular carcinoma.
- Pigmentation of skin may be caused by haemochromatosis, amiodarone therapy for cardiac complications *or both*.

✦ Common Pitfalls

- The commonest error is to miss the association between features of liver disease and evidence of diabetes. Ensure that you always ask to perform fundoscopy and to dipstick the urine for glucose at the end of your examination. It is always good practice to examine the pulps of the fingers for blood glucose monitoring marks – this is of relevance to patients who clearly have ESRF as well.
- Remember that haemochromatosis, as a disease of iron accumulation, can take years to manifest. The peak incidence occurs in middle-age, so be careful if considering the diagnosis in younger patients, in whom diabetes mellitus not related to haemochromatosis is more likely.

Early features of haemochromatosis
- Fatigue
- Arthralgia
- Gonadal dysfunction

Late features of haemochromatosis
- Diabetes mellitus type I
- Skin bronzing
- Progressive liver disease
- Other features as described in Table 3.7

Viva questions

What is the typical genetic abnormality found in haemochromatosis?

- Haemochromatosis is one of the most common heritable genetic conditions in people of northern European extraction with a prevalence of ~1 in 200.
- The disease has a variable penetration. About 1 in 10 people carry a mutation in one of the genes regulating iron metabolism, the most common allele being the C282Y allele in the *HFE* gene.
- Another common mutation is H63D; however, this usually results in biochemical iron overload only without the other phenotypical features of the disease. Mutations of the *HFE* gene account for 90% of the cases of non-transfusional iron overload.

Can you name a cause of accelerated iron accumulation in patients with primary haemochromatosis?

Alcoholism may accelerate iron accumulation in patients with genetic haemochromatosis for reasons that are not well known. It is far more likely for those who develop cirrhosis from haemochromatosis to have a history of higher alcohol consumption.[2]

What are the difficulties with screening for haemochromatosis?

- Serum ferritin, iron and % saturation may be increased in other causes of cirrhosis, particularly alcohol and hepatitis C. The underlying diagnosis can be resolved by liver biopsy.
- Ferritin is also an acute phase reactant and increases in many inflammatory conditions.
- Phenotypically, females have milder (and later onset) disease than males due to menstrual losses of iron and due to sex differences in iron regulatory proteins.
- More than one mutation in the *HFE* gene and mutations in other genes have been described leading to haemochromatosis. Care must be taken when interpreting a negative genetic screen in a patient who has clinical haemochromatosis.

How would you treat someone with primary haemochromatosis?

- Given the organ systems involved, a multidisciplinary approach with input from other specialties is strongly recommended.
- The mainstay of treatment for patients is to avoid alcohol and iron supplementation in their diet.
- Weekly phlebotomy is still the most reliable way of reducing body iron stores.
- Desferrioxamine, an iron chelator, can be used as injections to reduce iron stores.
- In those with advanced liver cirrhosis or with hepatocellular carcinoma, a liver transplant is indicated if the patient is fit enough to undergo the procedure.

References

1. Kowdley KV. Iron, hemochromatosis and hepatocellular carcinoma. *Gastroenterology* 2004; **127**; 5(S1):S79–86.
2. Scotet V et al. Hereditary hemochromatosis: effect of excessive alcohol consumption on disease expression in patients homozygous for the C282Y mutation. *Am J Epidemiol* 2003; **158**(2):129–34.

Liver transplantation

In the UK, 600–700 liver transplants are carried out annually. In the exam, however, the frequency of a liver transplant in the abdomen station is surprisingly high.

Presentation

Patients with liver transplants will present as follows:
- Asymptomatic presentation with another unrelated condition.
- Symptomatic with a complication of immunosuppression:
  - Infectious disease, either typical (lower respiratory tract infection or skin) or atypical (including *Pneumocystis jiroveci* (*carinii*), cytomegalovirus, varicella and herpes zoster).
  - Malignancy, either solid organ (e.g. bowel), lymphoproliferative (e.g. post-transplant lymphoproliferative disease), skin (e.g. squamous cell or basal cell carcinoma).
  - Metabolic complication, such as post-transplant diabetes mellitus and hyperlipidaemia.
  - Cardiovascular disease e.g. ischaemic heart disease, cerebrovascular disease, hypertension.
- Transplant dysfunction e.g. from recurrent disease (e.g. alcohol-related hepatitis) or acute rejection.
- Surgical complications in the early postoperative period e.g. hepatic vein/portal vein thrombosis and biliary leak.

Clinical signs

- There may be residual stigmata of chronic liver disease.
- A 'Mercedes Benz' type incision scar will be present (→ Fig. 3.1, p.96).
- There may be other residual scars associated with postoperative intensive care, such as from a tracheostomy, central line insertion and abdominal drains.
- Usually, no mass is palpable in the right upper quadrant as the 'new' liver is placed in the same place as the old one. Occasionally, a liver edge may be palpable, although hepatomegaly is uncommon in a healthy liver transplant.
- A mass in the left loin may represent a concurrently transplanted renal allograft (e.g. for combined liver and kidney failure following paracetamol overdose).

> **❶ Top Tips**
>
> - It is important to appreciate that a liver transplant is usually not palpable and that the liver is usually not enlarged.
> - If there is a mass in the left loin, it is more likely to be the renal allograft of simultaneous kidney–liver transplantation.

◆ Common Pitfalls

- It is very easy to be confused by an unusual abdominal scar in the exam. Remember that surgeons are simple creatures and tend to operate on organs directly underneath where they put their incision.
- A Mercedes Benz scar should indicate a large upper abdominal operation. The differential diagnosis for these operations would include a liver transplant, radical gastrectomy and Whipple's procedure. Don't forget that bilateral adrenalectomies can also be carried out through a Mercedes Benz scar.

Causes of end-stage liver disease

Common causes
- Chronic alcohol abuse
- Viral cirrhosis

Uncommon causes
- Autoimmune (e.g. PBC)
- Cryptogenic cirrhosis

Viva questions

What is the commonest indication for liver transplantation?
Alcoholic liver disease.

Is a liver transplant indicated for cirrhosis from chronic hepatitis C infection?
Yes, this is now accepted as an indication for liver transplantation.

What is the overall survival following liver transplantation?
There are many estimates but the overall survival is ~60% over 15 years.

What are the criteria for referral to a liver unit for transplantation?
In the context of liver failure, the King's College Hospital (KCH) criteria identify patients at particular high risk of death who should be discussed with a liver transplant unit.[1]

The KCH criteria divide patients into those with paracetamol-induced acute liver failure and those with non-paracetamol-induced liver failure:
- Paracetamol-induced:
  - Arterial lactate >3.5 4 hours after resuscitation
  - Or pH <7.3 or arterial lactate >3.0 12 hours after resuscitation
  - Or any 3 of: INR >6.5, creatinine >300, encephalopathy (grade III or IV).
- Non-paracetamol-induced:
  - Arterial lactate >3.5 4h after resuscitation
  - Or INR >6.5
  - Or any 3 of: INR >3.5, age<10 or >40 years, serum bilirubin >300 micromol/L, jaundice >7 days, aetiology being a drug reaction.

What immunosuppressive drug regimens are currently in use?
- Current immunosuppressive regimens use corticosteroids in combination with a calcineurin inhibitor such as tacrolimus or ciclosporin and an antiproliferative agent such as mycophenolate mofetil.

- The first patient to receive a liver transplant and survive to 1 year was performed by Dr Thomas Starzl in 1967. However, it was not until the introduction of ciclosporin in the early 1980s that long-term survival became possible.

What other forms of liver support are available?

- A number of devices exist to try and bridge the gap between liver failure and recovery or transplantation. Probably the best know is the molecular adsorbents recirculation system (MARS), which consists of 2 circuits. In the first, the patient's blood is exposed to albumin via a semipermeable membrane, allowing toxins such as ammonia, bile acids and bilirubin to be bound. The second circuit serves to remove these bound toxins from the albumin.
- Newer support systems include ECLAD (extracorporeal liver assist devices) and Demetriou, which incorporates hepatoblastoma cell lines attached to semipermeable membrane columns.
- Heterotopic liver transplantation is the implantation of a lobe of allogeneic liver while leaving the native liver *in situ*. This is carried out when there is potential for the native liver to recover. The donor liver lobe is rejected with time, leaving the recovered, functioning liver.

Reference

1. O'Grady JG et al. Early indicators of prognosis in fulminant hepatic failure. *Gastroenterology* 1989; **97**(2):439–45.

Inflammatory bowel disease

Inflammatory bowel disease (IBD) is common. It is particularly prevalent in developed nations in comparison to developing countries. Estimates of prevalence suggest that approximately 250 people per 100,000 are affected in the West.

The genetic associations of IBD mean that these conditions have higher prevalence in 1st-degree relatives of affected individuals.

Presentation

- Most patients present with symptoms, particularly abdominal pain and diarrhoea.
- Vomiting and weight loss are also common and anaemia is almost a universal feature.
- Bowel inflammation may cause rectal bleeding and this may be the precipitating symptom for presentation.
- IBD is often associated with extra-abdominal symptoms and signs including arthritis, skin lesions (e.g. erythema nodosum). Ulcerative colitis is associated with sclerosing cholangitis (⊃ 'What is sclerosing cholangitis?', p.135).

Clinical signs

- The patient may be malnourished.
- Cushingoid features suggest steroid therapy.
- Oral ulceration may be present in Crohn's – look for apthous ulceration both in and around the mouth.
- Extra-abdominal signs of IBD (see below).

Extra-abdominal features of IBD

- Finger clubbing
- Uveitis
- Large and small joint arthropathies and sacroiliitis (often unilateral)
- Skin disease – pyoderma gangrenosum, erythema nodosum
- Peripheral oedema from hypoalbuminaemia.

Cushingoid changes may be a complication of steroid therapy.

- Operative scars (⊃ Fig. 3.1, p.96) frequently seen include those from:
  - Right hemicolectomy, bowel resection and stricturoplasties in patients with Crohn's.
  - Colectomy in ulcerative colitis.
- Stomas positioned in:
  - The RIF suggest an ileostomy.
  - The LIF suggest a colostomy.
- There may be a palpable mass in the RIF in an acute exacerbation of Crohn's.
- There may be fistulating perianal disease (remember that Crohn's disease can affect the entire GI tract from the mouth to the anus).

❶ Top Tips

- Clubbing is indicative of extensive small bowel Crohn's disease.
- Anterior abdominal wall fistulae in Crohn's occur after previous surgery.

❦ Common Pitfalls

- Arthropathy, does not necessarily correlate with the severity of intestinal disease.
- An ileostomy may be left after resection for ulcerative colitis.

Viva questions

How do you differentiate between Crohn's disease (CD) and ulcerative colitis (UC)?

- The main differentiating factors between CD and UC are the sites of inflammation and the extent of inflammation across the bowel wall.
- CD affects any part of the intestinal tract from the mouth to the anus and is characterized by 'skip lesions' (intervening areas of normal bowel) whereas UC exclusively affects the colon. A dilated terminal ileum (termed 'backwash ileitis') may be seen in UC.
- CD characteristically causes transmural inflammation (full thickness of the bowel) whereas UC causes predominantly superficial inflammation in the mucosa. Histologically, CD causes granulomas, while UC is more likely to cause crypt abscesses.
- Evidence of fat malabsorption (steatorrhoea, fat-soluble vitamin deficiencies (A, D, E and K) usually points more towards CD than UC, as CD frequently affects the small intestine.
- Physical signs that suggest CD more than UC include a right lower quadrant (terminal ileal) mass and significant peri-anal disease (ulceration or multiple peri-anal fistulas).
- In ~10% of cases, it is impossible to distinguish CD from UC and the term 'indeterminate colitis' is used instead.

How might a patient with IBD present to the emergency department?

- A typical exacerbation is usually characterized by diarrhoea worsening over several days, which is bloody in both ulcerative and Crohn's colitis.
- *De novo* presentations of IBD are unusual via the A&E department but are important to recognize. They may be difficult to distinguish from a bacterial gastroenteritis, although these latter episodes will usually have a highly suggestive history e.g. take-away food 24–72 hours prior to the onset of symptoms or a history of recent travel abroad.
- Symptoms of bacterial gastroenteritis are usually of sudden onset.
- IBD may present with pain or obstructive symptoms alone.

What are Truelove and Witts criteria?

- Mild: <4 stools per day (with or without blood), no systemic disturbance and a normal ESR.
- Moderate: >4 stools per day, with minimal systemic disturbance.

- Severe: >6 stools per day with blood and evidence of systemic disturbance as evidenced by fever, tachycardia, anaemia or an ESR >30.

What are the current treatment strategies for the management of Crohn's disease?

Ileal and colonic disease

High-dose aminosalicylates (e.g. mesalazine 4g/day) may be sufficient in mild disease, whilst oral or IV steroids (prednisolone 40mg or hydrocortisone 400mg/day) are used for more severe disease. Elemental diets have a role in selected patients. If concomitant infection is suspected during an exacerbation of CD, metronidazole should be given. Azathioprine (AZA) may be used as a steroid-sparing agent and infliximab (5mg/kg) in refractory disease. Surgery will need to be considered if medical therapy fails.

Perianal and fistulating disease

Antibiotics may be effective in simple disease (metronidazole and/or ciprofloxacin). Similarly, AZA (1.5–2.5mg/kg/day) may be effective where infection has been controlled or excluded. Persistent or complex disease may require the use of surgery and/or infliximab.

Maintenance therapy

Smokers should be advised to stop smoking and offered referral to a smoking cessation clinic. When required, remission can be maintained with AZA, methotrexate or infliximab.

How would you manage acute colitis?

- In the acute presentation, the goal is initially to induce remission. This requires a period of therapy with high-dose agents. When remission has been achieved, the focus changes to maintenance therapy, directed at preventing relapses.
- The mainstay of treatment for mild to moderate disease (by the Truelove and Witts criteria) is corticosteroid therapy.
- Mesalazine (5-aminosalicylic acid, 5-ASA) is an effective topical agent for the management of distal disease.
- Severe acute disease requires intensive therapy with IV steroids and close monitoring. Approximately 30% of subjects progress to requiring colectomy (➔ 'When would you consider surgery?', p.135).
- Toxic megacolon is now a rare presentation of UC.
  - This life-threatening condition is characterized by a very dilated colon accompanied by abdominal bloating, pain and systemic features consistent with sepsis or severe inflammation.
  - Untreated, there is a high mortality rate from perforation and sepsis; therefore, treatment with IV steroids to reduce inflammation and decompression of the bowel is required urgently.
  - The patient should be kept nil by mouth, IV fluids used for resuscitation and to replenish losses into the bowel and antibiotics administered to treat sepsis.
  - A colectomy needs to be performed for patients who fail to respond to conservative therapy as the morbidity and mortality of the procedure is less than the condition itself.

When would you consider ciclosporin in a patient with a severe exacerbation of UC?

IV hydrocortisone (400mg/day) remains the mainstay of treatment for a severe exacerbation of UC. The use of IV ciclosporin at a dose of 2mg/kg/day should be considered if there is no improvement in the first 3 days.

When would you consider surgery?

- Immediate referral for a surgical opinion is indicated if there is toxic dilatation (colon >5.5cm or caecum >9cm diameter).
- Following 3 days of intensive treatment, in patients with a stool frequency of >8/day or a CRP >45, approximately 85% require colectomy.
- Surgery is probably indicated in cases of exacerbation of UC that have failed to respond after 10 days of intensive treatment.
- Great vigilance must be taken to ensure not to miss perforation during the management of exacerbations, which may occur with minimal clinical signs in patients receiving steroid therapy, even in those whose initial presentation did not appear severe.

What is sclerosing cholangitis?

- Inflammation of the bile ducts leading to progressive scarring and biliary obstruction.
- Untreated, this condition progresses to CLD and eventual liver failure.
- It can occur either as a primary condition with an autoimmune aetiology (primary sclerosing cholangitis) or in association with IBD, particularly UC.
- This condition is associated with the presence of autoantibodies, notably perinuclear anti-neutrophil cytoplasmic antibodies (p-ANCAs), antinuclear antibodies (ANA) and anti-smooth muscle antibodies, although none of these antibodies are specific to the disease.
- As with other chronic biliary obstruction diseases, treatment options are limited to supplementation of fat-soluble vitamins, stenting of the bile duct (if possible) and, if indicated, liver transplantation. In the longer term, patients require screening for cholangiocarcinoma, which is a serious complication of sclerosing cholangitis.

When would you initiate a patient with CD on anti-TNF therapy?

Anti-TNF is indicated in steroid refractory and fistulating disease. The NICE guidelines for starting a patient on anti-TNF therapy are as follows (all 3 criteria need to be fulfilled):

- Severe active CD.
- Disease refractory to steroids and steroid-sparing agents or intolerant of these drugs.
- Patients for whom surgery is inappropriate (diffuse disease or short bowel).

ℰ Useful website

NICE guidance: http://www.nice.org.uk/nicemedia/pdf/Nicecrohns40guidance.pdf.

Abdominal masses in the epigastrium and iliac fossae

In the real world, abdominal masses are common findings. It would be entirely reasonable for the examiner to ask for a differential diagnosis of masses in the abdomen, irrespective of the anatomical localization. NB Renal transplants will not be discussed here (➔ p.141).

Presentation
- Asymptomatic presentation and incidental palpation of an abdominal mass is common.
- Occasionally the patient has non-specific symptoms, such as lethargy or weight loss, but it is rare for them to present complaining that they have noticed a lump.
- Symptoms suggestive of IBD (➔ Inflammatory bowel disease, p.132) are another mode of presentation in patients with abdominal masses.
- Presentation with jaundice or itch may result from biliary obstruction due to sinister abdominal masses which should always be taken seriously.

Clinical signs
- The patient may be undernourished (malignancy or inflammatory bowel disease, chronic infection/inflammation).
- Jaundice suggesting tumour in the head of the pancreas, biliary obstruction, paraneoplastic haemolytic anaemia.
- Anaemia of chronic disease (IBD, malignancy, lymphoma).
- Cushingoid features are suggestive of steroid therapy (IBD).
- Lymphadenopathy, splenomegaly and/or hepatomegaly may be present (lymphoma, malignancy).
- Presence of surgical scars or a stoma (malignancy, IBD).
- There will be a palpable mass in either iliac fossa or epigastrium.
- Ascites (advanced malignancy or portal obstruction).

❶ Top Tips
- The key is to pay particular attention to the patient's general status and any extra-abdominal signs.
- Virchow's node (left supraclavicular fossa) should be sought particularly in the presence of an epigastric mass.
- Always make sure you tell the examiner that you'd like to do a rectal examination.
- It is important to know at least 3 causes of masses in each area of the abdomen.
- An enlarged caudate lobe of the liver may be palpable as an epigastric mass. This is sometimes seen with alcoholic hepatitis where it may have an associated bruit.

◆ Common Pitfalls

- Not being able to volunteer a differential diagnosis for the mass. Stay calm and consider the anatomy – what structures are directly beneath your palpating fingers?

Viva questions

Can you name some causes of an epigastric mass?

- Carcinoma of the stomach or pancreas
- Abdominal aortic aneurysm (pulsatile)
- Lymphoma
- Caudate lobe of liver.

Can you name 5 causes of a right iliac fossa mass?

- Crohn's disease
- Caecal carcinoma
- Ileocaecal mass including amoebic abscess, ileocaecal tuberculosis, appendicular mass, ileal carcinoid and lymphoma
- Ovarian tumour (benign or malignant)
- Renal transplant (➔ p.141).

Can you name 5 causes of a left iliac fossa mass?

- Carcinoma of the sigmoid colon
- Diverticular mass/abscess
- Faecal mass
- Ovarian tumour (benign or malignant)
- Renal transplant (➔ p.141).

Enlarged kidneys

Adult polycystic kidney disease (APCKD) is one of the top causes of ESRF in the UK. This condition affects the population worldwide and is the commonest cause for palpable kidneys in the exam.

Knowledge regarding APCKD and the other important causes of renal enlargement would be expected from a PACES candidate.

Presentation

- Asymptomatic presentation with abnormal physical examination, BP, urine dipstick or blood tests noted during routine examination.
- Family members of patients with APCKD may be screened for the condition.
- Abdominal pain or recurrent urinary tract infections are another mode of presentation.
- On occasion, a patient presenting with subarachnoid haemorrhage will be found to have APCKD.

Clinical signs

- The patient may have a hemiparesis from a previous stroke or a ruptured berry aneurysm.
- Anaemia.
- Hypertension.
- Signs of complications of chronic kidney disease, evidence of renal replacement therapy and, if appropriate, side effects of immunosuppressive therapy (→ Renal allograft p.141).
- Fullness in one or both flanks.
- Nephrectomy scar if one or both kidneys have been removed for recurrent infection/intractable pain/space occupying symptoms or malignancy. Note that sometimes large kidneys have to be removed through an anterior approach through a midline laparotomy. Conversely, the frequency of laparoscopic nephrectomies is increasing, so bear in mind that even large kidneys can be removed through keyhole surgery by skilled surgeons.
- One or both kidneys will be palpably enlarged, possibly massive and ballotable.
- Hepatomegaly (irregular and firm) from associated hepatic cysts.
- An audible bruit over the enlarged kidney.

❶ Top Tips

- Palpably enlarged kidneys are usually quite obvious. You don't need to press too hard to palpate them.
- Remember that you can't get above nor ballot an enlarged spleen. Splenic notches may also help to identify the mass.
- In bilateral renal enlargement, one side is usually easier to feel than the other. If the patient has ESRF, it is very likely that they have polycystic kidney disease, so both kidneys should be enlarged!
- An audible bruit might reflect increased renal perfusion or a vascular tumour e.g. angiomyolipoma and is not necessarily due to renal artery stenosis.

Causes of renal enlargement

Unilateral renal enlargement

- Autosomal dominant polycystic kidney disease (ADPKD) – usually one side is easier to feel than the other in the early stages. (The left kidney is lower in the abdomen than the right.)
- Hydronephrosis – rarely palpable; can be due to ureteric obstruction.
- Renal tumour (benign or malignant) with or without a systemic cause (e.g. von Hippel–Lindau disease or tuberous sclerosis).
- Congenital renal anomalies e.g. fusion anomalies (horseshoe kidney).

Bilateral renal enlargement

- ADPKD.
- Hydronephrosis – an enlarged bladder may be the only sign.
- Bilateral renal tumours.
- Amyloidosis.
- Congenital renal anomalies e.g. fusion anomalies (horseshoe kidney).

Viva questions

How is ADPKD inherited and how and when would you recommend screening?

- ADPKD is phenotypically inherited in an autosomally dominant manner. In fact, the mutated gene is recessive to the normal allele and cysts form only in renal tubular cells where a stochastic event has lead to a mutation of the normal allele (in the same way as is the case with childhood retinoblastoma).
- The usual screening test, for those who wish to have it, is an ultrasound scan of the kidneys. However, as renal cysts develop with ageing, a negative ultrasound scan below the age of 30 does not exclude the disease.
- When to screen a patient is a question of considerable clinical debate. As there is no specific treatment for ADPKD, it can be argued that regular BP checks and treatment is preferable to ultrasonic confirmation of the condition. Others argue that the diagnosis of ADPKD should be established in everyone who is of childbearing age for the purposes of genetic counselling and for exclusion of berry aneurysms which, if sufficiently large, can be treated angiographically and reduce the long-term risk of subarachnoid haemorrhages.
- The ultrasonic criteria for a diagnosis of ADPKD are as follows:
  - 15–39 years of age: 3 or more cysts in the kidneys (unilaterally or bilaterally).
  - 40–59 years of age: 2 or more cysts in each kidney.
  - >60 years of age: 4 or more cysts in each kidney.
- Remember that there are 2 types of ADPKD, type 1 and type 2. The latter usually presents with a milder phenotype.

Can you name some extrarenal manifestations of ADPKD?

- Cysts in other organs (see following question)
- Intracranial berry aneurysms
- Polycythaemia (excess erythropoietin release)
- Hypertension (excess renin release)
- Cardiac valve disease (usually mitral valve prolapse but can also cause MR, AR and TR)

- Diverticular disease
- Aortic aneurysm (thoracic or abdominal) or thoracic coarctation
- Abdominal wall hernias.

Can you name some organs that may contain cysts in ADPKD?
- Common sites: kidneys (!), liver (2nd commonest site), pancreas, arachnoid cysts.
- Uncommon/case reports: spleen, thyroid, lungs, ovaries, testes, seminal vesicles, bladder, broad ligament, uterus.

Patients with ADPKD often present with abdominal pain. Can you name some causes?
- Infected cyst
- Haemorrhage into a cyst.

The following conditions occur with higher frequency than the general population in patients with ADPKD and also cause abdominal pain:
- Diverticulitis/diverticular perforation
- Nephrolithiasis (higher incidence than general population)
- Strangulated/incarcerated hernia
- Ruptured AAA
- Tuberous sclerosis complex (TSC) – the gene for ADPKD type 2 is very close to the gene for TSC, hence certain mutations may affect both genes, causing both ADPKD and TSC.

Renal allograft

Approximately 2500 kidney, pancreas or combined kidney-pancreas transplants are carried out in the UK every year. The demand from potential transplant recipients, however, far outweighs the donor availability.

Patients with renal transplants present to A&E departments with both complications of the transplant and also with general medical conditions, which require an understanding of transplant immunosuppression.

Presentation

Patients with renal transplants will present as follows:
- Asymptomatic presentation with another unrelated condition.
- Symptomatic with a complication of immunosuppression:
  - Infectious disease, either typical (lower respiratory tract infection or skin) or atypical (e.g. *Pneumocystis jiroveci* (*carinii*), cytomegalovirus, varicella-zoster).
  - Malignancy, either solid organ (e.g. bowel), lymphoproliferative (e.g. post-transplant lymphoproliferative disease), skin (e.g. squamous cell or basal cell carcinoma).
  - Metabolic complication, such as post-transplant diabetes mellitus and hyperlipidaemia.
  - Cardiovascular disease e.g. ischaemic heart disease, cerebrovascular disease, hypertension.
- Transplant dysfunction e.g. from recurrent disease or acute rejection.
- Surgical complications in the early postoperative period e.g. urinary leak from the surgical anastomosis (of ureter to bladder), urinary tract infection (which may be complicated by pyelonephritis, especially if the transplant ureteric stent becomes infected).

Clinical signs

- Scar (usually oblique) in the iliac fossa.
- Palpable mass directly underneath it.
- The patient may have signs of chronic immunosuppression:
  - Increased skin pigmentation.
  - Multiple skin warts.
  - Prematurely aged skin.
  - Evidence of skin malignancies (BCC or SCC) or previous excised skin malignancies.
  - Fine tremor of ciclosporin toxicity (demonstrated with arms outstretched).
  - Surgical or radiotherapy scars suggestive of treatment of other malignancies (e.g. lymphoma).
  - Gingival hypertrophy – rare these days due to meticulous dental care (patients now have hypertrophic gums trimmed).
  - NB Transplanted patients are usually not cushingoid.
- Signs of ESRF (➋ p.97) and/or renal replacement therapy (RRT; either peritoneal dialysis or haemodialysis) and/or complications of chronic kidney disease (CKD; ➋ p.142).
- Signs of ESRF (➋ p.97) including:
  - Complications of CKD.
  - Renal replacement therapy (RRT; either peritoneal dialysis or haemodialysis).

- Evidence of aetiology of native kidney disease:
  - ADPKD (◆ p.138).
  - Diabetic nephropathy – BM stick marks on fingertips, lipodystrophy at sites of insulin injection (abdomen, thighs; expose thighs anteriorly if wearing shorts).
  - Hearing aids could suggest Alport's disease or aminoglycoside induced nephrotoxicity plus ototoxicity.
  - Facial lipodystrophy associated with mesangiocapillary glomerulonephritis type 2.
  - In the absence of evidence indicating the underlying pathology of the native kidney (e.g. ballotable renal masses), the likely underlying cause for ESRF is chronic glomerulonephritis.
- Functioning status of renal transplant:
  - Hypertension (may also be due to side effect of immunosuppressant).
  - Fluid overload (raised JVP, peripheral/sacral oedema).
  - Current evidence of dialysis.
  - Phosphate binders by bedside.

❶ Top Tips

- On the right side, abdominal scars below McBurney's point usually indicate a transplanted organ.
- Make sure you have looked very carefully for polycystic kidneys as this is a common cause of ESRF.
- Patients may receive pre-emptive renal allografts (before reaching ESRF) and will therefore not have evidence of previous RRT.
- Remember that 'kidney transplant' is not a diagnosis. You need to say 'ESRF with a renal transplant' and volunteer a likely cause for the ESRF.

Complications of Chronic Kidney Disease

- Anaemia.
- Parathyroidectomy (for poorly controlled hyperparathyroidism – look carefully for scar as these are frequently hidden in a neck crease).
- Pseudoclubbing (shortened terminal phalanges from tertiary hyperparathyroidism; if present, usually indicates long-standing renal disease as calcium homeostasis is monitored more closely nowadays).
- Scratch marks.
- Uncontrolled hypertension.
- Atherosclerotic disease (median stenotomy scar with venous harvesting scars and stroke).

Signs of Renal Replacement Therapy

- Tunnelled dialysis catheter scars.
- Arteriovenous fistula/arteriovenous graft.
- Peritoneal dialysis catheter scar.
- Previous renal allograft.
- Skin changes of chronic immunosuppression including premature ageing, malignancies, skin warts.

Chronologically the complications of CKD occur before RRT. However, the signs of RRT are apparent to the candidate first.

❶ Top Tips

In a patient with a renal transplant, state in chronological order:
- What happened to the native kidneys e.g. ADPKD.
- What previous RRT was used.
- Whether the graft is functioning (no current RRT in use).
- What current immunosuppressive therapy is suggested:
  - Steroids (cushingoid appearance).
  - AZA (seborrhoeic warts).
  - Ciclosporin (tremor, gum hypertrophy).
- Complications of disease e.g. hypertension, fluid overload, uncontrolled hyperparathyroidism (pseudoclubbing or parathyroidectomy scar) or anaemia in later stages due to reduction in renal erythropoietin production.

Viva questions

What are the commonest causes of ESRF?
- Diabetes mellitus
- ADPKD
- Chronic glomerulonephritis
- Hypertension in Afro-Caribbean patients. (NB The causative association between hypertension and ESRF in other ethnic groups is not very well established.)

What are the complications of transplanting a patient with Alport's syndrome?

Patients with Alport's syndrome have a defect in type IV collagen, so a new transplant exposes them to antigens they have not encountered before. The subsequent antibody response against this antigen may result in some patients developing anti-glomerular basement membrane disease (the antibody responsible for Goodpasture's disease).

Can you offer some differential diagnoses for that mass in the right iliac fossa?
- Common:
  - Caecal carcinoma
  - CD
- Uncommon:
  - Ovarian tumour (in a female)
  - Ileocaecal abscess (e.g. with *Yersinia* sp.).

Can you name some opportunistic infections associated with renal transplantation?
- Cytomegalovirus
- *Pneumocystis jiroveci (carinii)*
- Epstein–Barr virus (particularly in patients with post-transplant lymphoproliferative disease)
- BK* virus (a common polyomavirus which lies dormant in the renal tract after primary infection and can be reactivated by immunosuppression. Complications of BK virus in transplant patients include ureteric stenosis and interstitial nephritis)

- JC virus (another polyomavirus which causes progressive multifocal leucoencephalopathy) is being reported more and more in chronically immunosuppressed renal transplant recipients.

(* BK virus is named after the initials of first patient in whom the virus was described.)

Why are kidney transplants placed in the pelvis?
- Good blood supply.
- There is sufficient space for the kidney.
- Proximity to the bladder for the ureteric anastomosis.
- Easy access to perform renal biopsies or nephrostomies (in the event of a ureteric stricture) without having to puncture the peritoneum or risk abdominal viscerae.
- Note that a kidney can be transplanted on either side of the pelvis, depending on the quality of the vascular supply and venous drainage. As many patients with ESRD have diabetes, vasculopathy is common, therefore an assessment of the arterial supply during transplant work-up is important.

What is the commonest cause of death in a patient with a renal transplant?
- The commonest cause of death in all patients with renal disease is cardiovascular. Accelerated cardiovascular disease (CVD) is a feature of all patients with renal disease as a result of both generic (hypertension, hyperlipidaemia, chronic inflammation) and renal-specific (calcium/phosphate/PTH abnormalities, chronic anaemia, chronic calcineurin inhibitor therapy) risk factors.
- After CVD, the commonest causes of death are malignancy and infections. Both are related to chronic immunosuppression.

Combined kidney–pancreas transplant

Approximately 2500 kidney, pancreas or combined kidney–pancreas transplants are carried out in the UK every year. Kidney–pancreas transplantation can be performed, simultaneously or successively (either kidney or pancreas first), to treat type I diabetes with either end-stage or near end-stage, renal failure.

Complications occur more frequently following whole pancreas transplantation (as opposed to pancreatic islet cell transplantation) than after kidney transplantation. This is largely due to the digestive juices contained in the pancreas and the less solid consistency of the pancreas relative to the kidney.

NB This case highlights clinical features unique to kidney–pancreas transplant as opposed to renal allograft (➋ p.141)

Presentation

Patients with combined kidney–pancreas transplants will present in the same manner as those with renal transplants, although peri-pancreatic collections and pancreatitis are additional complications seen in the early postoperative period.

Clinical signs

- There are 2 scars (frequently oblique), one in each iliac fossa.
- Typically each of the 2 scars has a palpable mass directly underneath it.
- The patient may have signs of chronic immunosuppression
  (➋ p.141).
- Evidence of chronic or end-stage renal failure and/or RRT.
- Diabetic complications include:
  - Retinopathy which is strongly correlated with diabetic nephropathy.
  - Peripheral neuropathy.
- Functioning of the pancreas transplant is indicated by the absence of:
  - Bruising from insulin injection.
  - Fingertip pinprick marks of glucose monitoring.
  - Glycosuria on dipstick testing.

❶ Top Tips

- Always make sure you ask to dip the urine for proteinuria and glycosuria and perform fundoscopy after examining the abdomen.

☞ Common Pitfalls

- Remember that a transplant on each side may either be 2 kidney transplants (performed at different times – failed transplants are usually not removed unless there is a problem with leaving them in e.g. recurrently infected, malignant disease) or combined kidney–pancreas transplantation.
- It is surprisingly common when asked the cause of the ESRF in this scenario for the candidate to struggle. Clearly, the patient has ESRF due to type 1 diabetes.

Viva questions

How is the pancreas drained? Do you know any complications of this route?

Old pancreatic transplants were bladder drained (the pancreatic duct was anastomosed to the bladder). In this way, urinary amylase levels could be monitored and act as an early sign of graft pancreatitis or pancreatic rejection.

However, this route of drainage is complicated by reflux pancreatitis, persistent haematuria, recurrent urinary tract infections and metabolic acidosis (pancreatic bicarbonate loss, particularly during episodes of dehydration). These complications often necessitated enteric conversion of the pancreatic exocrine drainage at a later date.

Many units now perform pancreatic transplants with primary enteric drainage to avoid these complications.

Can you name some complications of post-transplant immunosuppression?

- Infections (➲ p.143 Renal allograft)
- Malignant disease:
  - Solid organ tumours
  - Post-transplant lymphoproliferative disorder
  - Skin malignancy
- Metabolic diseases:
  - Hypertension
  - Hyperlipidaemia
  - Post-transplant diabetes mellitus (PTDM)
  - Post-transplant anaemia (PTA)
- CVD
- Chronic transplant injury (ciclosporin and tacrolimus are both nephrotoxic)
- Morphological changes:
  - Cushingoid changes
  - Acne vulgaris
  - Hirsutism
  - Gingival hypertrophy.

Hereditary haemorrhagic telangiectasia

Hereditary haemorrhagic telangiectasia (HHT) is a more common condition than is recognized, affecting ~1 in 5000 of the population.

Presentation

- Epistaxis is the most frequent presentation.
- Chronic GI bleeding can lead to presentation with symptoms of anaemia. Melaena and haematemesis are not common modes of presentation.
- Others may present for cosmetic reasons due to the distressing appearance of telangiectases.

Clinical signs

- The patient may have anaemia.
- Koilonychia occurs only rarely.
- The salient signs are telangiectasia affecting the skin and mucous membranes without the features of systemic sclerosis.
- Typical sites for telangiectasia are the fingers, face, lips, tongue, buccal mucosa, conjunctiva and nose.
- Listen for hepatic bruit (rarely present).
- High output cardiac failure as a result of a large arteriovenous malformation (AVM) is rare.

❶ Top Tips

- This is a hereditary condition. The examiner may allow you to ask the patient some questions in which case you should enquire about other affected family members.

❖ Common Pitfalls

- It is common to mistake HHT for Peutz–Jeghers syndrome (PJS). Note that in HHT the lesions are telangiectases while in PJS the visible lesions are pigmented macules.
- Avoid mistaking HHT for systemic sclerosis (there is no skin thickening in HHT).

Viva questions

What is the eponymous name for HHT and why is it given that name?
Osler–Weber–Rendu syndrome. All 3 doctors described the condition independently over a 40-year period.

What are the complications of HHT?
- Recurrent epistaxis.
- GI haemorrhage resulting from telangiectases and AVM in the bowel.
- Anaemia.
- Complications of AVM in internal organs, especially strokes and subarachnoid haemorrhage (SAH) (from cerebral AVM) and haemoptysis (lung AVM).

What are the common sites for AVM in HHT?
- Brain
- Lung
- Liver
- Bowel
- Spine.

What is the genetic basis of HHT?
The condition is inherited as autosomal dominant. However, a number of mutated genes have been described, most involving components of TGF-β signalling. The most commonly affected gene maps to chromosome 9.

What is Heyde's disease?
- The association between aortic valve stenosis and colonic angiodysplasia.
- Patients with Heyde's disease have a mild form of von Willlebrand disease and are therefore prone to blood loss. Sheer stresses around the aortic valve increase the breakdown of the large molecular size of von Willebrand factor (vWF) resulting in a consumptive deficiency.
- This condition is not related to HHT and often improves after aortic valve replacement.
- It was first described by Edward Heyde in 1958 who was an American physician.

What was so special about William Osler?
Osler was a remarkable and highly educated man. He was nominally a pathologist who made immense contributions to the practice, study and teaching of medicine. The scholar of medicine will recognize his name in the following:
- Osler's nodes (painful, vasculitis nodules associated with bacterial endocarditis).
- Osler–Weber–Rendu syndrome (HHT).
- Osler's manoeuvre (palpable radial pulse with sphygmomanometer cuff inflated above arterial pressure. This is a sign of pseudohypertension as a result of arterial calcification).
- Osler's syndrome (Ball-valve gallstone – recurrent biliary colic due to a gallstone in Vater's diverticulum).
- Osler's triad (a triad of pneumonia, meningitis and endocarditis, usually caused by disseminated *Pneumococcus*).
- Osler–Vaques disease (polycythaemia rubra vera).
- Osler–Libman–Sacks endocarditis.
- Filaria osleri (*Strongylus canis* bronchialis).
- *Sphryanura osleri* (a nematode in the gills of newts).

Peutz–Jeghers syndrome

Peutz–Jeghers syndrome (PJS) is characterized by the appearance of benign hamartomas in the GI tract which are accompanied by mucocutaneous pigmented macules over the hands, feet and lips. Although it is a rare condition (and therefore unlikely to appear in the exam), it is an important condition to diagnose accurately because of the malignant potential of the hamartomas.

Presentation

- Usually patients are asymptomatic and the diagnosis is made based on family history and screening or during routine examination for something else.
- Usually patients with affected family members are asymptomatic and diagnosed following screening or during a routine examination.
- The GI lesions can cause intussusception, which may be the first presenting feature.
- Presentation with malignant disease in those previously undiagnosed.

Clinical signs

- There is characteristic mucocutaneous pigmentation (circumoral, hands and feet).
- There may be clinical signs of anaemia.
- There may be abdominal operative scars from bowel resection.

❶ Top Tips

- Whilst Peutz–Jeghers polyps may occur anywhere in the intestine, malignancy is rare except in the stomach and duodenum.
- Both gastroduodenal and colonic polyps may bleed resulting in iron deficiency anaemia.

✦ Common Pitfalls

- Do not confuse PJS for HHT. PJS is characterized by pigmentation whereas HHT is made up of telangiectatic vessels.
- Always include Addison disease in your differential diagnosis of pigmented lesions in or around the mouth.

Viva questions

What is Peutz–Jeghers syndrome?

- Hamartomatous polyps in the GI tract and hyperpigmented macules on the lips and oral mucosa.
- These lesions are benign but there is an increased lifetime risk of developing cancers in solid organs not related to the polyps.
- In early life, intussusception may occur, leading to presentation to a paediatrician.

What is the inheritance of PJS?

- Autosomal dominant with a prevalence of between 1 in 100,000–200,000 births.
- The mutation is in a gene known as *STK11* which is a tumour suppressor gene.

Normal abdomen

In the exam, subjects with normal abdomens may be used. This is to ensure that candidates do not make up signs that are not there. Although rare as an abdominal case in the exam, the normal abdomen is by far the commonest examination finding in real life.

Presentation

These patients may well have abdominal symptoms, although no cause is found, possibly after exhaustive investigation.

Clinical signs

- No abdominal signs.
- The patient may have unrelated diseases, so extra-abdominal signs may be present.

> **① Top Tips**
>
> - Don't panic!
> - Make sure you don't make up signs that aren't there.
> - Ensure you palpate the lower abdomen as there may be a gravid or tumorous uterus (e.g. fibroid) instead of a normal abdomen.
> - Sometimes unilaterally enlarged kidneys are hard to feel.
> - Look out for signs of blood-borne infections (tattoos, piercings, etc.).

Viva questions

Are you sure you couldn't feel anything?

Yes!

Can you name some causes of a distended abdomen?

- Fat
- Faeces
- Fetus
- Flatus
- Fluid.

Where would you palpate next?

In the lower abdomen feeling for any evidence of a gravid uterus.

Can you name the surface markings of the aorta, gallbladder and kidneys?

- The aorta lies in the epigastrium, just to the left of the midline. It bifurcates at the level of L4/5, i.e. at the level of the umbilicus. In obese patients this is less reliable.
- The surface markings of the gallbladder are where the right midclavicular line crosses the right costal margin (i.e. the 9th right costal cartilage).
- The hila of the kidneys lie on the transpyloric plane of Addison. This is a line joining the lowest points of the left and right costal margins and is at the level of L1.

History taking

Robert H. Thomas
Rupa Bessant

Introduction

Welcome to station 2, history taking. We would like to start by saying that having worked very hard to pass the written papers you deserve to be sitting this prestigious exam and PACES is an opportunity to perform as a clinician and formally demonstrate your unique clinical skills that make you an excellent physician.

History taking is traditionally an area of the PACES exam that candidates find very difficult. Taking a good history from a patient is the most fundamental skill of a training physician and PACES candidates often feel that their general daily work practice is adequate preparation for this station. This is not the case, despite most candidates being well skilled in clerking a patient from A&E or clinic where few limitations apply. Unfortunately, faced with strict time constraints, exam anxiety and often deliberately unusual scenarios, poorly prepared PACES candidates may demonstrate a fundamental weakness in what should be a basic part of physician training. Do not devalue your chance of success in the PACES examination by poor preparation or anxiety. The practice needed in order to succeed in the history taking station should not be underestimated.

As well as running out of time, a candidate's main concern is the broad range of scenarios that can be chosen as an examination topic and this can easily unsettle and panic even the best prepared. This chapter offers a structured approach that will help to alleviate this fear. The stopwatch begins once a candidate has been handed the scenario (usually in the form of a letter addressed to the candidate from another healthcare practitioner).

The time allowed for this station is as follows

- 5 minutes private preparation – candidate then called into the exam room.
- 14 minutes with the patient being observed by examiners.
- 1 minute of personal reflection time.
- 5 minutes for questions from the examiners.

The initial preparation period is of huge importance and when sitting PACES, we would suggest using the structured template in Fig. 4.1 which can be adapted to any scenario given to a PACES candidate in the exam. We would encourage you to memorize this template for reproducibility during this preparation time. Even in the most esoteric of scenarios when anxiety is high, this structured template can guide panicked candidates to a satisfactory pass by helping elicit the key facts that demonstrate competency and safety. The 12 scenarios which follow have been written in accordance with the template described, each with a different clinical or psychosocial challenge. We recommend that you either read the cases individually or practise them as an exam scenario with a colleague. This chapter provides an insight into how an examiner scores this station and key points to address to optimize your chances of passing. Either reading by yourself or working through the individual scenarios with a colleague may help to reinforce the issues encountered.

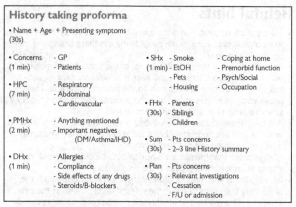

History taking proforma

- Name + Age + Presenting symptoms
  (30s)

• Concerns (1 min)	- GP - Patients	• SHx (1 min)	- Smoke - EtOH - Pets - Housing	- Coping at home - Premorbid function - Psych/Social - Occupation
• HPC (7 min)	- Respiratory - Abdominal - Cardiovascular	• FHx (30s)	- Parents - Siblings - Children	
• PMHx (2 min)	- Anything mentioned - Important negatives (DM/Asthma/IHD)	• Sum (30s)	- Pts concerns - 2–3 line History summary	
• DHx (1 min)	- Allergies - Compliance - Side effects of any drugs - Steroids/B-blockers	• Plan (30s)	- Pts concerns - Relevant investigations - Cessation - F/U or admission	

Fig. 4.1 History taking proforma. DHx, drug history; FHx, family history; HPC, history of presenting complaint; PHMx, personal medical history; SHx, social history. (Reproduced from PassPACES Courses Ltd.)

Helpful hints

- Take a small stopwatch into the exam and place it on the table in front of you, explaining to the patient why it is there and asking their permission to do so.
- Immediately ask if the patient has a list of their prescribed medication with them. If so, ask to see it and keep it to reference during the history. Do not forget to return it to the patient at the end. This provides an invaluable insight into the patient's past medical history and saves valuable time when eliciting the drug history.
- Ask the patient about non-prescribed medication (e.g. St John's wort) which would not necessarily be included in the drug list which may have been printed out by the pharmacist.
- Always check that the patient is not on beta-blockers, steroids or statins as important negatives in the drug history.
- At the start of your history taking station, always address both the presenting complaint raised in the referral letter as well as the patient's concerns. This will help to identify the number of problems you will need to deal with during this station and therefore help with the time to be allocated to each issue, rather than discovering additional unexpected problems at a later stage.
- Practise being able to quickly determine cigarette and alcohol consumption in pack-year history and weekly units respectively.
- Re-address the patient's concerns in the summary. This demonstrates to the examiners that every opportunity has been given for the patient to clarify their main worries.
- Keep the summary relevant and succinct.
- Talk slowly and enjoy this PACES platform to demonstrate your skills.

Case 1

Dear Doctor

I would be grateful if you could review this patient. Sharon Tesdale presented last night to the emergency department with left arm weakness and slurred speech. A head CT out of hours was normal. We observed her overnight and her symptoms have subsequently resolved today. We would be grateful for your advice.

Yours sincerely,
Dr Vithya Murphy FY1

History to elicit

Sharon Tesdale, 41 years old. Inpatient referral following a self-limiting episode of neurological deficit.

- Doctor's concerns: 41-year-old with possible transient ischaemic attack (TIA).
- Patient's concerns: the patient is scared she will have another stroke.

HPC

Mrs Tesdale retired to bed feeling well, but woke up at 3 a.m. with heaviness to her right upper limb. She had difficulty raising the arm from the bed and was unable to move her fingers. Her left lower limb was unaffected by any new weakness. She woke her husband up who noticed some slurring of her speech and he immediately bought her to hospital. Her symptoms were self-limiting with return to her pre-morbid functioning by mid-morning.

Mrs Tesdale had a thrombotic stroke 5 years ago and despite a prolonged hospital stay with aggressive physiotherapy, has a residual left-sided hemiparesis. Since discharge from hospital there have been no subsequent episodes of neurological deficit until today.

The patient denies recent head trauma, sudden onset headache, fit or aura.

PMHx

- *DVT* Whist rehabilitating from her previous stroke, Mrs Tesdale developed a painful swollen right calf muscle and was diagnosed with a deep vein thrombosis (DVT). She was anticoagulated with low-molecular-weight heparin (LMWH) and discharged on warfarin. She remains anticoagulated for life.
- *Important negatives the candidate should ask about*: hypertension, diabetes mellitus, ischaemic heart disease, migraine, epilepsy, recurrent miscarriage, pulmonary embolisms, arthritis, skin rash, ulceration of mucous membranes.

DHx

- Aspirin 75mg OD.
- Warfarin 5mg nocte. (Preferred INR 2–3.)
- Paracetamol PRN.
- No known drug allergy (NKDA).

- No non-prescription medication.
- Compliant with all medication and regular INR checks.
- No concerns about side effects of current medication.
- No oral contraceptive pill (OCP), steroids, statins or beta-blocker medication.

SHx

- **Smoking** No.
- **EtOH** Never.
- **Pets** Nil.
- **Occupation** Former hairdresser – unable to work due to residual hemiparesis.
- **Home** Lives with husband in a privately owned house. Comfortable and independent with housing modifications made including a stair lift, bath rails and sit/stand shower.
- **Functioning** Mrs Tesdale requires a walking stick to support her left side on mobilization. She cannot stand for prolonged periods of time.
- **Psych/social** Is a positive person denying any low mood.

FHx

- **Parents** Mother and father both in good health.
- **Siblings** 1 sister in good health.
- **Children** No children.

Summary

Mrs Tesdale is a 41-year-old female with a previous history of thrombosis including a stroke and a DVT. She presents today with self-limiting neurological deficit consistent with TIA despite adequate anticoagulation with warfarin.

Plan

Patient's concerns

Reassure the patient that she probably has had a 'mini' stroke despite anticoagulation therapy and further assessment is needed to reduce future risks.

Investigations should include:

FBC, U&E, LFTs, CRP, ESR, clotting profile including INR, fasting glucose and cholesterol. Lupus anticoagulant/anticardiolipin antibody. An unenhanced head CT has already been performed.

Cessation advice

None recommended here other than healthy lifestyle.

F/U or admission

- Mrs Tesdale is already on the short stay unit.
- Requires haematological review.
- Anticoagulant optimization and risk stratification before discharge.

Differential diagnosis

- Acquired thrombophilia including antiphospholipid syndrome (APLS) and Behçet's Dx.
- Iatrogenic progesterone (e.g. OCP).
- Congenital thrombophilia including Factor V Leiden deficiency, protein C and S deficiency, antithrombin III deficiency.

Discussion related to the case

This is a classic PACES example, with a relatively easy and benign history of thrombotic stroke. The more unusual presentation in a young patient on anticoagulation therapy should be detected. Clinicians should treat a TIA as a medical emergency as it represents a warning of possible impending fatal or disabling stroke. NICE has issued guidance on TIA management.[1]

- The candidate should ask important negative questions to exclude the possibility of acquired thrombophilia, especially APLS with a background of SLE. Although many patients with APLS do not have concurrent lupus, thrombosis may be the presenting feature with subclinical disease including glomerulonephritis or anaemia.
- The significant history of a TIA should not be underestimated (the patient's main presenting concern) – further investigation and treatment (e.g. regarding anticoagulation) needs to be carried out urgently.
- A cranial CT study is required to exclude the possibility of stroke mimics particularly with concurrent warfarin administration. The majority of CT studies are normal in these patients.
- An MRI and diffusion-weighted imaging (DWI) to make the diagnosis of a thromboembolic event should be considered (as recommended by NICE). If negative, this raises the possibility of a functional or psychological cause of her neurology and increasing her INR would have no therapeutic effect.
- Candidates should also refer the patient for an ultrasound scan of her carotid arteries. Any patient with recent neurological symptoms and a severe (>70%) stenosis at the internal carotid artery can benefit from surgical referral for a endarterectomy in accordance with the North American Symptomatic Carotid Endarterectomy Trial (NASCET).[2]
- Although it is highly likely that Mrs Teasdale has a thrombophilia, other causes of TIA must be excluded. An echocardiogram to exclude a cardiac cause of embolic stroke (both septic or thromboembolic) should be performed.
- Medical therapy should be initiated to optimize cardiovascular risk factors and aim to improve long-term vascular protection.
- The anticoagulation booklet (usually yellow in colour), which details a chronological anticoagulation profile, should be reviewed to ensure whether a consistent therapeutic INR has been maintained. Any drug interactions with warfarin administration must be considered (e.g. St John's wort).
- An urgent inpatient referral to the haematologists should be requested for the following specialist advice:
  - Whether an increase in the INR to >3 is warranted.
  - Further investigations to exclude congenital causes of thrombophilia.
- The psychosocial well-being of the patient must be addressed and support for patients with any chronic disease must be offered.
  - Whilst Mrs Teasdale appears psychologically intact, establish her normal pre-morbid functioning as this will have a direct impact for future attendances.

- Despite her age, a candidate should recognize that Mrs Teasdale is married but does not have any children. Thrombophilic patients often suffer recurrent miscarriages, which can have significant psychological morbidity. This should be explored sensitively. If appropriate, further obstetric advice or advice regarding other options e.g. adoption, can be sought.
- Prior to discharge, a new home assessment by social services should be carried out to try and improve her quality of life living with disability.
- Support may also be required for her husband as the main carer and there may be potential for financial support through the benefit system.

❶ Top Tips

- In the acute setting, the PACES patient is highly likely to be a simulated patient with a contrived history. There may be higher expectations on the candidate to elicit the salient points.
- With any patient on warfarin, candidates should always refer to their anticoagulation (yellow) booklet to see the trend of their INR.
- With respect to drugs that have a narrow therapeutic window (e.g. warfarin), accuracy of alcohol and drug history is essential to identify possible interaction.

Viva questions

What cerebral vascular distribution is most likely to be involved?

Mrs Teasdale has right upper limb proximal and distal weakness. In the acute setting, a flaccid paralysis is seen with the classical upper motor neuron spasticity developing with time. Blood supply to the cerebral hemispheres is via the cerebral arteries. The circle of Willis allows contralateral flow from the basilar and internal carotid arteries to supply the anterior (ACA), middle (MCA) and posterior (PCA) cerebral arteries. The ACA supplies the medial aspect of the frontal and superior parietal lobe, while the PCA perfuses the occipital lobe. The majority of the cerebral cortex is supplied by the MCA, which perfuses the motor cortex located anterior to the central sulcus. Due to long track decussation within the brainstem, Mrs Teasdale has suffered a vascular insult to the left MCA leading to symptoms in the right upper limb.

What is a stroke mimic and can you give any examples of one?

Although neurological deficit is most commonly caused by stroke, there are non-vascular causes that can be indistinguishable in clinical presentation. Termed 'stroke mimics', they can be due to a primary CNS problem or sequelae of systemic disease. CT is used in the first instance to differentiate between a haemorrhagic or ischaemic event and a stroke mimic. Stroke mimics include:

- Subdural or extradural haemorrhage
- Bleeding from vascular malformations
- Normal pressure hydrocephalus
- Multiple sclerosis

- Mass lesions including tumour and abscess
- Seizure disorder and post ictal states
- Metabolic derangement including hypoglycaemia and hyponatraemia
- Migraine
- Functional and psychological hemiparesis.

What would you expect the CRP and ESR to show in SLE?

ESR is a useful but non-specific marker of inflammation or infection. Dependent on the variables of haematocrit, serum immunoglobulin and fibrinogen levels, it is commonly elevated in active RA, polymyalgia rheumatica, crystal arthropathies and SLE. CRP is arguably a more acute reflection of inflammation or infection. Driven by the cytokines interleukin-1 and interleukin 6, CRP is independent of complications that commonly affect the ESR (e.g. anaemia). In active SLE without serositis, the CRP is usually normal or low and this helps distinguish patients from those with active RA, a disease generally marked by elevated CRP. The findings of significant CRP precipitins in SLE patients may suggest the presence of superimposed infection.[3]

References

1. NICE. *Diagnosis and initial management of acute stroke and transient ischaemic attack (TIA)*. London: NICE, 2008. Available at: www.nice.org.uk/CG68.
2. North American Symptomatic Carotid Endarterectomy Trial Collaborators. Beneficial effect of carotid endarterectomy in symptomatic patients with high-grade carotid stenosis. *NEJM* 1991; **325**(7):445–53.
3. Honig S et al. C-reactive protein in systemic lupus erythematosis. *Arthritis Rheum* 2005; **20**(5):1065–70.

Case 2

Dear Doctor

Thank you for seeing Mr Abdul Ibiez who has recently registered with my practice. He attended for a repeat prescription for his oral hypoglycaemic agent and routine bloods have revealed unexpectedly high random cholesterol of 6.2nmol/L. I would be grateful for your advice with his continued management.

Yours sincerely,
Dr Ethan Smith

History to elicit

Abdul Ibiez, 48 years old. Presented today following advice from his GP about high cholesterol.

- GP's concerns: high cholesterol in a diabetic middle-aged Asian gentleman.
- Patient's concerns: his father had high cholesterol and recently died of a heart attack aged 68.

HPC

Mr Ibiez was told his cholesterol was high whilst living in Pakistan about 8 years ago. Following advice from his doctor, he modified his diet and tried to eat healthily, although he found this more difficult when eating meals with his family. His diet mainly consists of rice and vegetables but does admit that his wife used a lot of oil when cooking meat. Mr Ibiez has not had his lipid profile monitored for several years. He remembers his father being on tablets to control his high cholesterol and to stop the 'skin around his eyes turning yellow'.

Mr Ibiez is not known to have ischaemic heart disease but in the last few months he has noticed being increasingly short of breath when playing with his children. He has never had any associated chest pain, cough or any stigmata of systemic infection. He is not limited by shortness of breath when walking regularly in order to keep his weight down.

PMHx

- *Diabetes* Mr Ibiez has been on metformin for 10 years. His blood sugars, which he monitors daily, are around 6.5mmol/L although he has not had his HbA1c checked recently. His eyes were last tested 5 years ago. He has no symptoms of peripheral neuropathy and has never been admitted to hospital with a diabetic related problem.
- *Asthma* Mr Ibiez was diagnosed with asthma many years ago. He has never been admitted to hospital or required steroids following an asthma attack. He has not used his salbutamol inhaler for many years.
- *Important negatives the candidate should ask about*: hypertension, ischaemic heart disease, thyroid disease, TB.

DHx

- Metformin 500mg BD.
- Salbutamol PRN.

- NKDA.
- No non-prescription medication.
- Compliant with his medication.
- No concerns about side effects of current medication.
- No statin or beta-blocker medication.

SHx
- *Smoking* Yes 10/day for 30 years (15 pack-years).
- *EtOH* Never.
- *Pets* Nil.
- *Occupation* Shop keeper in East London.
- *Home* Lives with his mother, wife and 3 children in a 2-floor house that he owns. His house is in good condition and he has a strong support network with friends and other family members in the local community.
- *Functioning* Mr Ibiez is pre-morbidly very well with no disability.
- *Psych/social* He is sad about the death of his father and expresses worries about being able to look after his family and his long-term health related to high cholesterol.

FHx
- *Parents* Father recently died aged 68 – heart attack. Mother alive with no significant illness.
- *Siblings* 2 brothers and 1 sister – all in good health.
- *Children* 3 children aged 7–15 all in good health.

Summary
Mr Ibiez is a 48-year-old Asian male who has been referred by his GP following an unexpectedly high lipid profile. His cardiovascular risk factors include diabetes, smoking and a positive family history in a 1st-degree relative. He has new stigmata of CVD with shortness of breath but no chest pain and has concerns regarding his health and the future management of this complaint.

Plan

Patient's concerns
Address the patient's concerns directly, stating that a full examination and further investigations are appropriate for risk stratification of CVD.

Investigations should include:
Bedside tests of BP, urine dipstick and an ECG. Blood tests including a FBC, U&E, random/fasting glucose and full lipid profile including cholesterol, HbA1c and TFTs. A CXR is required.

Cessation advice
Mr Ibiez should be encouraged to stop smoking and lose weight. He should be provided with information leaflets on the different approaches that your hospital has to offer. This advice should also be recommended in the letter to his GP.

F/U or admission

- Mr Ibiez can be managed in the community.
- An outpatient appointment should be given to him to reassess the situation following the test results.

Differential diagnosis

- Primary hyperlipidaemia with possible familial tendency.
- All causes of secondary hyperlipidaemia.

Discussion related to the case

Mr Ibiez has a high cardiovascular risk. Although his dyslipidaemia needs to be addressed, the need for full cardiovascular risk stratification to minimize future ischaemic heart disease-related problems should be recognized. Candidates are encouraged to have a holistic approach to patient care and single risk factors should not be addressed individually, but as a multifactorial cardiovascular issue.

- As attempted lifestyle modification has not had the required therapeutic effect on Mr Ibiez's lipid profile, he will probably require HMG-CoA reductase inhibitors.
  - Ensure there are no risk factors e.g. warfarin, St John's wort and excess alcohol consumption.
  - 2nd-line/adjunct therapy may be required.
- Other causes for his dyslipidaemia must be excluded e.g. hypothyroidism, chronic kidney disease or ethanol excess.
- A multidisciplinary approach is essential with involvement of the following:
  - A dietician for advice on his BMI and diet.
  - Diabetic nurse for optimization of his diabetic regime.
- Address any complications of diabetes:
  - Examination and investigations can exclude common sequelae of diabetes e.g. peripheral neuropathy and renal function.
  - Diabetic eye clinic for the assessment of diabetic retinopathy.
- If the BP is high, antihypertensive medication should be commenced. Candidates should highlight the difficulties of:
  - Beta-blockers with respect to past medical history of asthma.
  - Angiotensin-converting enzyme (ACE) inhibitors in the face of potential diabetic nephropathy.
- Counselling for gastric protection should aspirin be introduced.

There is a strong emphasis on psychosocial implications of disease in the exam scenarios. The patient's mood in this chronic cardiac disease and recent bereavement with the loss of his father must be addressed.

❶ Top Tips

- Have a cultural understanding when taking a history and do not be limited in your questions by your own lifestyle and beliefs.
- With CVD, always address the 5 major preventative measures and do not limit yourself to 1 single risk factor.
- Always look for drug interactions or contraindications in simulated PACES cases.

Viva questions

How would you approach management of Mr Ibiez's cardiovascular well-being?

- CVD is a multifactorial and dynamic disease with well-established risk factors which should be addressed systematically.
- Risk factors that cannot be altered in a patient include: age, gender (oestrogen is cardiovascular protective and hence heart disease is lower in women) and family history of CVD. Recognizing these in 'at-risk' individuals however, allows for earlier intervention leading to improved survival.
- Variable risk factors can be classified as major or minor, with an initial approach focusing on the major risks.
  - *Major risk factors include*: BP, dyslipidaemia, diabetes and smoking.
  - *Minor risks factors include*: weight loss, alcohol intake, regular exercise, stress and behavioural modification in type A personality types. Recreational cocaine usage should be avoided. Although these have less influence on the cardiovascular profile, they should still be addressed for optimal cardiovascular well-being.

What are the recommended treatment targets for hyperlipidaemia?

The British Heart Society (BHS) and Joint British Society 2 (JBS2) guidelines recommend that total cholesterol should be lowered by 25% or LDL cholesterol by 30% to reach <4.0mmol/L or <2.0mmol/L respectively or whichever is the greater. A total cholesterol concentration <5.0mmol/L or LDL concentration <3.0mmol/L however, provides the minimal acceptable standard.

These guidelines are also consistent with WHO criteria[1] (NICE have not stated cholesterol targets specifically for primary prevention of CVD).

What is the appropriate further management of Mr Ibiez's hyperlipidaemia?

According to the NICE guidelines,[2] treatment for primary prevention of CVD should be initiated with simvastatin 40mg. If there is potential drug interaction, then alternative preparations such as pravastatin should be used. Higher intensity statins should not normally be used. Fibrates, nicotinic acids or anion exchange resins should not be routinely offered as a primary prevention of CVD, but ezetimibe can be considered in those people with primary hypercholesterolaemia (heterozygous familial and non-familial).

References

1. World Health Organization (WHO): http://www.who.int/cardiovascular_diseases.
2. NICE. *Lipid modification*. London: NICE, 2010. Available at: http://www.nice.org.uk/CG67.

Case 3

Dear Doctor

I would be grateful for your advice with Emma Graham who I have been seeing over the past 2 weeks with intractable diarrhoea following a holiday in Egypt. Despite conservative management she reports a worsening in symptoms, opening her bowels up to 5 times per day. Emma now complains of non-specific abdominal pain and occasional blood in her stool. She is pyrexial today at 37.9. I have sent a stool sample for microbiology/culture and requested an abdominal radiograph as an outpatient. She is a non-smoker and has a past medical history of gallstone disease only.

Yours sincerely,
Dr Catherine Giles

History to elicit

Emma Graham, 25-year-old female. Presented today following GP referral to A&E.

- *GP's concerns* Non-resolving episode of diarrhoea following recent travel to Egypt.
- *Patient's concerns* Emma feels very unwell and is due to start a new job next week.

HPC

Emma Graham is 25 years old and has recently finished university and celebrated her success with a holiday to Egypt with some friends. She decided to stay in a 4-star hotel and ate in the hotel restaurant every night. On her last day, she felt non-specifically unwell with fatigue and abdominal pain, but related her symptoms to over indulgence during her last evening and travelled home the following day. Since the holiday 2 weeks ago, Emma has been opening her bowels several times each day with increasing frequency, now up to 10 times each day. Her stools are very loose, of a normal brown colour and yesterday had some fresh red blood mixed with the stool. Her GP felt that is was 'something she ate' and encouraged maintenance of oral fluids and a follow-up appointment for review. Her abdominal pain is diffuse and colicky with no exacerbation or relief following defecation. There is nausea but no vomiting. Over the last week Emma has felt feverish and fatigued. Her holiday friends have all remained well since their travels.

Emma's bowel habits are usually regular, but has she had a similar episode of diarrhoea with an associated fever during the exam revision period. She had required a few days of rest. Her symptoms, which resolved spontaneously after 1 week, were felt to be stress-related. No medical guidance was sought. Emma is usually fit and healthy and has not had any recent courses of antibiotics. She is usually 10 stone and, although she is trying to maintain a normal diet, has lost over a stone in weight since her exam period. Her only other complaint is a rash on the front of both her legs, which is painful to touch and was thought to be sunburn. On more direct questioning, Emma mentioned that it started a few days before her trip to Egypt.

PMHx

- *Gallstones* An ultrasound scan ordered by her GP following an episode of abdominal pain 1 year ago demonstrated multiple small gallstones, but nothing else of note. These symptoms did not persist.
- *Emma has no other relevant past medical history* and there is no risk of her being pregnant at the moment.
- *Important negatives the candidate should ask about:* previous abdominal surgery, radiation therapy, peripheral migratory arthritis or spinal pain, uveitis, thrombotic episodes, mucosal ulceration, dysphagia/ordonophagia, nephrolithiasis, recurrent cystitis, asthma, eating disorders.

DHx

- Microgynon® oral contraceptive pill – once daily.
- NKDA.
- No non-prescription or recreational drugs.

SHx

- *Smoking* Never.
- *EtOH* Socially at university, but more recently (8–10U per day) while on holiday.
- *Pets* Nil.
- *Occupation* Contracted to start as a trainee solicitor shortly.
- *Home* Emma has just moved back home with her parents in London, but was living in halls of residence at Leeds University.
- *Functioning* Pre-morbidly very well with no disability.
- *Travel* Emma has not been on another holiday outside of the UK for >2 years.
- *Psych/social* Emma is concerned about the impact of her symptoms on her new training contract. She denies feeling depressed or any concerns with her body image.

FHx

- *Parents* Emma's mother has mild RA and her father is in good health.
- *Siblings* 2 sisters – both in good health.
- *No children*.

Summary

Emma is a sensible 25-year-old university graduate who has a 2-week history of worsening bloody diarrhoea associated with generalized abdominal pain and systemic symptoms of fever, fatigue and skin rash. There has been associated weight loss and a probable previous episode, which was self-limiting. Recent travel history to Egypt is noted.

Plan

Patient's concerns

Address the patient's concerns directly and tell her that this is an unusual presentation for 'traveller's diarrhoea'. Further investigations are required and her future employers can be notified officially if symptoms do not resolve.

Investigations

FBC, U&E, LFT, CRP, ESR. Urine and faeces samples should be sent for MC&S and faecal occult blood. An abdominal and chest radiograph should be performed.

F/U or admission

- Emma requires admission for further investigation and management of her systemic symptoms on a background of GI illness.
- She has a significant risk of deterioration and should not be managed as an outpatient.

Differential diagnosis

- Inflammatory bowel disease (IBD) – Crohn's disease or ulcerative colitis (UC).
- Infective colitis – pseudomembraneous, amoebiasis, *Shigella*, *Camylobacter*, CMV, cryptosporidium (esp. immunosuppressed patients).
- Less likely – irritable bowel syndrome, coeliac disease, thyrotoxicosis.

Discussion related to the case

Emma has IBD and her recent trip to Egypt is coincidental to her symptoms. Candidates need to recognize the presence of symptoms before travel (e.g. diarrhoea during exam period and rash on shins suggestive of erythema nodosum) and the fact that none of the friends who accompanied her to Egypt have been affected with diarrhoea.

Differential diagnosis:

- An important infective cause is entamoeba histolytica (amoebiasis):
  - This has a worldwide distribution and is commonly seen in countries with a warm climate like Egypt and India.
  - Its presentation can mimic that of IBD.
  - It can demonstrate similar significant complications including toxic megacolon.
- Other differentials can be easily excluded with no history of exposure to radiation or immunosuppression.
- Irritable bowel syndrome is a diagnosis by exclusion made in the absence of organic bowel pathology.
  - The presence of blood in Emma's stool disregards this differential.

With respect to IBD, although a formal diagnosis between Crohn's disease and UC cannot be made during the history station, clinical and histological knowledge of these conditions would be expected from candidates.

- It is important to note that:
  - Both diseases present at approximately the same age.
  - Both Crohn's disease and UC have similar sex predominance.
  - A lack of extra-intestinal manifestations can make it difficult on history alone to differentiate between the two.
- Candidates should be able to risk stratify Emma depending on her investigations: emphasize the need to exclude fulminant disease and toxic megacolon, which if present, would require resuscitation and an early surgical review.

Examiners would expect discussion on basic treatment plans.

It is best to systematically subdivide the immediate from the longer-term management.

- Immediate management includes:
  - Symptom control.
  - Steroid therapy as a priority.

- Cross-sectional imaging studies (CT/MRI).
- Inpatient referral to gastroenterology for possible OGD (and duodenal biopsy) and flexible sigmoidoscopy.
- IBD is a pro-thrombotic state and the indication for anticoagulation in the acute setting should be considered.

Long-term, Emma's management requires a multidisciplinary approach:
- Emma should be counselled with regard to intestinal complications:
  - Stricture
  - Fistulation
  - Adenocarcinoma
  - Lymphoma
  - The possibility of future surgery.
- Knowledge on extra-intestinal manifestations would also be expected from a candidate.
  - In this case, Emma has early onset gallstone disease (usually after 3rd decade).
- A strong support network should be encouraged for regular follow-up both through her GP and a specialist doctor. Support groups can be offered and educational reading is easily obtainable.
- As with all chronic disease, it should be impressed upon Emma that there is easy access to psychological support should the need arise.

> **❶ Top Tips**
> - A chronological history is extremely important.
> - Discuss treatment in subdivisions of immediate and longer-term management.
> - GP letters can be both helpful and misleading. They may insinuate misleading disease in PACES!

Viva questions

Where is the commonest intestinal site for Crohn's disease?
The small bowel is involved in up to 80% of cases, with regional enteritis of the terminal ileum, either alone or in combination with the remaining ileum or jejunum. Macroscopically, there is thickening and nodularity of the circular folds, with apthous ulceration causing a cobblestone appearance to the mucosa. Affecting anywhere from the mouth to anus, other sites involved, in order of decreasing frequency, include: the colon (25–55%), rectum (50%), duodenum (10%), oesophagus (3%) and stomach (2%).

In Crohn's disease, what types of perianal fistulas can occur?
Crohn's disease is the third most common cause of fistulation. Although enterocolic and enterocutaneous fistulas have been described, 33% of patients suffer from perianal disease. Dependant on its relationship to the internal and external muscles of the anal sphincter, the fistula is characterized according to Park's classification and can be supra-sphincteric, inter-sphincteric, extra-sphincteric, trans-sphincteric or superficial.

What are the common extra-intestinal manifestations of Crohn's disease?

- Hepatobiliary:
  - Fatty liver
  - Gallstone disease
  - Pancreatitis
- Genitourinary:
  - Urolithiasis
  - Renal amyloidosis
  - Focal cystitis
- Musculoskeletal:
  - Clubbing
  - Hypertrophic osteoarthropathy (HOA)
  - Erosive arthritis
  - Avascular necrosis (AVN)
  - Muscle abscess
- Erythema nodosum
- Uveitis
- Growth retardation (childhood onset).

Case 4

> Dear Doctor
>
> Please could you see Mr Kevin Trawney, a 47-year-man who was found by his daughter at home, living in squalid conditions and unable to cope? He has a background of excess alcohol consumption and has only been home from hospital for 5 weeks following a period of detoxification. I found him to be jaundiced today and with a temperature of 38.1 degrees.
>
> Yours sincerely,
> Dr Chloe Lumb

History to elicit

Kevin Trawney, 47-year-old male. Presented today following GP referral to A&E.
- GP's concerns: Mr Trawney has deteriorated since discharge and is now pyrexial. He is unable to cope at home.
- Patient's concerns: fell back into his routine of drinking again.

HPC

Mr Trawney recently had an acute admission for decompensated liver disease secondary to alcohol consumption. During his inpatient stay he was medicated through withdrawal and detoxification with a significant improvement in his health. Unfortunately, during his acute admission, Mr Trawney's wife left their home in response to his continued drinking and moved in with their daughter who lives nearby. In an effort to resolve this issue, Mr Trawney absconded from the ward 5 weeks ago and returned home without a suitable discharge plan in place. His family and GP were informed.

Mr Trawney initially abstained from alcohol consumption and made regular efforts to see his daughter. His wife, however, remained upstairs during his visits and refused to see him. Despite making a concerted effort to remain sober and reassure his wife of his changed ways, he found himself getting increasingly bored and frustrated at home. 2 weeks into his abstinence, Mr Trawney learnt that his wife left to go on holiday for an indefinite period. In response to this and despite his best intentions, Mr Trawney attended his local pub where he drank 3 pints of lager and then bought a bottle of whisky on his way home.

For the following 3 weeks, Mr Trawney has maintained a significant alcohol intake. Most days he would start drinking in his local pub around lunchtime, spend the afternoon sleeping at home and watch television in the evening with a bottle of whisky. His daily alcohol intake included 4 or 5 pints of premium strength lager and approximately 1/3 of a litre of whisky (2 bottles a week). Until a recent argument, Mr Trawney's daughter had brought a hot meal to him on alternate days. Over the past week Mr Trawney's health has deteriorated with a gradual loss of appetite and the onset of right upper quadrant pain which is achy and throbbing in nature. His stomach has begun to swell again. He has felt increasingly nauseous and has occasionally vomited. He denies haematemesis. He has also noted a change in his bowel habit with episodes of diarrhoea, opening his bowels 3–5 times per day, but was uncertain whether his stool had changed in colour. The last few days, he has become increasingly shaky and found it difficult to cope at home. He could not remember coming to hospital, although his daughter since informed him that she found him unrousable on the floor at home.

PMHx

- **Alcohol excess** Mr Trawney has drunk heavily since he lost his job following an accident 5 years ago. He has been diagnosed with early liver cirrhosis and has had increasingly frequent admissions to hospital during the last 2 years.
- **Important negatives the candidate should ask about**: peptic ulcer disease, GI haemorrhage, anaemia, blood transfusions, pancreatitis, diabetes, palpitations, cognitive impairment, seizures and tremor.

DHx

Mr Trawney does not take any regular prescription medication. He used to take a multivitamin tablet and oral thiamine, but as he absconded from hospital, a repeat prescription was not initiated.

Mr Trawney has also previously been trialled on antidepressant medication with little effect.

- NKDA.
- No non-prescription or recreational drugs.

SHx

- **Smoking** 10 per day for 30 years (15 pack-year history).
- **EtOH** Varies up to a maximum of 100 units per week, with approximately 3–5 pints of lager per day and a litre of whisky per week.
- **Occupation** Unemployed. Formerly a roof tiller but suffered a fall from height 5 years ago and was subsequently unable to work due to chronic back pain. He is on incapacity benefit for depression.
- **Home** Recently separated from his wife, Mr Trawney lives in a ground-floor council flat in Crystal Palace.
- **Functioning** Pre-morbidly Mr Trawney has an exercise tolerance of <100m due to back pain. He is self-caring at home, although he has relied on his daughter to fulfil some of his activities of daily living, such as shopping and cleaning. She lives near by with her partner and 2 children.
- **Psych/social** Mr Trawney has been diagnosed with clinical depression but has been non-compliant with antidepressant medication. He admits to low mood but has no intentions or previous history of self-harm. He finds relief in alcohol but is aware of the adverse effects it has on him. He finds his inability to abstain from alcohol depressing.

FHx

- **Parents** He has had little contact with his parents over the last 4 years, but remembers them being well previously.

- *Siblings* None.
- *Children* Mr Trawney has a 27-year-old daughter who is in good health.

Summary

Mr Trawney is a 47-year-old man with known alcohol-related liver cirrhosis, admitted with symptoms consistent with decompensated liver disease related to increased alcohol consumption. He has had several admissions to hospital for withdrawal and detoxification, the most recent of which was 5 weeks ago. There is a background of clinical depression and full psychosocial review and support is required.

Plan

Patient's concerns

Reassure him that he is in place of safety but will need mutual cooperation to address the current issues. The immediate management will need to focus on his acute medical needs. Although previous attempts to overcome his alcohol problems have failed, long-term supportive measures will need to be revisited to achieve a life of alcohol abstinence. The social issues relating to his wife need to be addressed at a later time.

Investigations

FBC, U&E, LFT, CRP, ESR, GGT, amylase, vitamin B12, folate and ferritin. Blood culture. ECG. Urine samples should be sent for MC&S. A CXR should be performed. An abdominal ultrasound scan should be organized as a matter of urgency and, if present, ascitic fluid should be tapped for culture.

F/U or admission

- Mr Trawney will require admission for both medical and social reasons.
- He is unwell, requiring assessment for possible sepsis and continued management of alcohol withdrawal.
- A full psychosocial assessment is also necessary.

Differential diagnosis

- Decompensated liver disease related to alcohol consumption on a background of alcohol related liver cirrhosis.
- Spontaneous bacterial peritonitis or hepatitis.
- Sepsis.

Discussion related to the case

The topic of alcohol in a PACES exam is an examiner's favourite, as it tests a candidate's knowledge of acute medicine in relation to decompensated liver disease, the pathophysiology of chronic alcohol consumption and the significant psychosocial sequelae of alcoholism both to the patient and to their relatives. As alcohol-related problems are common in an acute hospital take, candidates should be fully familiar with these management issues. Candidates coming from abroad or working in a demographic area of low alcohol abuse, are encouraged to prepare for this scenario.

Mr Trawney is an alcohol abuser, defined in DSM-IV as 'repeated use despite recurrent adverse consequences'.[1] He is withdrawing from alcohol and candidates should discuss the management of alcohol withdrawal methodically by structuring the answer into acute, intermediate and long-term treatment options.

- In the acute setting:
  - Symptoms of tachycardia, hypotension and recurrent fitting episodes may occur.
  - Qualify the use of IV rehydration – Mr Trawney may be chronically hyponatraemic in relation to his liver cirrhosis.
  - Persistent hyponatraemia may contribute to his intercurrent fitting episodes and reduced conscious level.
  - Fitting may necessitate benzodiazepine administration, although this may worsen any hypotension.
  - If pushed by the examiner, recognize the limitations of your knowledge and acknowledge that more senior help may be required.
- In the intermediate management:
  - Address the importance of vitamin replacement to prevent the long-term neurological sequelae of Wernicke's encephalopathy and Korsakoff's syndrome. Many hospitals provide IV vitamin replacement followed by long-term oral replacement therapy.
  - Mr Trawney will also require a reducing course of benzodiazepines to prevent withdrawal fits and tremor.
  - As a result of liver cirrhosis, Mr Trawney will be chronically immunosuppressed putting him at increased risk of community-acquired infections requiring antibiotic therapy.
  - A septic screen including CXR and urine dip would be expected.
  - An urgent abdominal ultrasound scan can locate any ascites to be sampled to address his risk of spontaneous bacterial peritonitis (SBP).
  - Any ascitic drain inserted should only remain in for a few hours to minimize the risk of further infection.
  - Mr Trawney is not on an aldosterone antagonist (e.g. spironolactone), the addition of which may reduce the rate of ascites recurrence.
  - Be aware that exact withdrawal policies vary between hospital trusts.
- Long-term, without complete abstinence from alcohol, Mr Trawney is at risk of further disease. The effects of alcohol abuse should be discussed in relation to the systems involved. For example:
  - *Cardiovascular* Alcoholic cardiomyopathy, arrhythmias, hypertension, coronary heart disease.
  - *Gastrointestinal* Gastric erosions, peptic ulcer disease, portal hypertension, oesophageal varices, pancreatitis.
  - *Haematology* Autoanticoagulation, anaemia, raised MCV related to bone marrow depression.
  - *CNS* Alcoholic dementia, optic atrophy, cerebellar disease, proximal myopathy, peripheral neuropathy.
- The psychosocial implications of disease related to alcohol are significant.
  - Addressing these psychosocial issues should begin on admission. Most hospitals offer a drugs and alcohol service and Mr Trawney should be referred immediately.
  - Hospital policy changes between trusts. An introduction to this service may happen at discharge with the onus of responsibility placed on the patient.
- A multidisciplinary approach should be adopted to encourage continued abstinence:
  - A physiotherapy referral is essential to assess Mr Trawney's mobility and dependence.

- Occupational therapy assessment should include a home visit before discharge.
- Some hospital trusts offer 'half-way' housing for recovering alcoholics or private institutions can provide continued detoxification at the patient's expense.
- Mr Trawney's GP can prescribe pharmacological alcohol deterrents such as Antabus®.
- Candidates should involve Mr Trawney's daughter in all discussions, as her insight into her father's expectations will be invaluable.
- Mr Trawney's mood should be addressed before discharge:
  - The former diagnosis of depression should be recognized and that a trial of antidepressants had 'little effect'.
  - A referral to a psychiatrist should be offered.
  - Continued abstinence may be having a significant effect on Mr Trawney's mood.
  - As the departure of his wife appeared to encourage his demise since his last admission, it may be prudent to address this issue directly, offering support mechanisms through formal counselling or group therapy.
- Finally . . . alcohol misuse is often a recurrent problem in the life of an individual and it should be reminded that every patient be treated with the respect they deserve. A candidate should never appear sceptical of the patient's intentions.

❶ Top Tips

- Be aware that PACES simulated scenarios can involve taking a collateral history from a friend or member of the family.
- Never appear sceptical of a patient's intentions in recovery from alcohol- or drug-related issues.
- When discussing investigations to be done, candidates should ensure they can justify the need for each investigation.

Viva questions

What is meant by a unit of alcohol?

The strength of an alcoholic drink depends on how much pure ethanol it contains and this is represented on the label as a percentage of alcohol by volume (%ABV). In the UK, one unit equates to 10mL or 8g of pure alcohol, but the %ABV is complicated by the following matters:

- A small glass (125mL) of 9% wine is equal to 1 unit, but wines are regularly now over 11%.
- A half pint of 3.5% lager is equal to 1 unit, but continental and premium lager advertise 5% ABV.
- A standard 25mL single measure of 40% spirit is equal to 1 unit, but many pubs serve 50mL measures.

Be aware that a 'gentleman's measure' or 'a whisky' referred to by an individual often contains several units.

It is estimated that a healthy liver takes 1 hour to clear 8g of ethanol and government recommendations advise a maximum weekly intake of 21 units for men and 14 units for women to avoid long-term organ damage.

Why does Mr Trawney develop ascites?

Ascites is accumulation of free fluid within the peritoneal cavity. This occurs for many reasons but the most common cause in the UK is as a transudate from the sequelae of liver cirrhosis. Transudates classically demonstrate low protein (<30g/dL), low LDH, low pH and low glucose. In Mr Trawney, the ascitic fluid occurs as a result of increased pressure in the portal vein (>8mmHg) raising hydrostatic pressure in the splanchnic capillary bed. The liver has also lost endogenous function and there is a reduced oncotic pressure due to hypoalbuminaemia. As a result, fluid moves out of the vasculature and is sequestered in the peritoneal cavity. Subsequent stimulatory effects on the BP and renal flow can lead to the feared hepatorenal syndrome (➔ Chronic liver disease, p.110).

Define the difference between Wernicke's encephalopathy and Korsakoff's syndrome

Both Wernicke's encephalopathy and Korsakoff's syndrome occur due to a deficiency in thiamine either through poor intake or absorption. Thiamine (vitamin B1) is absorbed in the jejunum and ileum. Absorption when in large concentrations within the bowel is via passive diffusion, with active transport required when bowel concentrations are low. Alcohol ingestion inhibits active transport making alcoholics, who may already have poor dietary thiamine intake even more susceptible to thiamine deficiency.

The clinical features of Wernicke's encephalopathy come on abruptly and have a classical triad of ophthalmoplegia, ataxia and encephalopathy. If treated early the signs and symptoms are reversible.

If untreated, Korsakoff's syndrome develops with cortical atrophy and irreversible damage to the mammillary bodies and thalamus. Clinically the patient gradually develops severe antegrade and retrograde memory loss, whilst demonstrating confabulation and lack of insight. Coma and death are soon to follow.

Reference

1. VandenBos GR (ed) *APA Dictionary of Psychology*. Washington, DC: American Psychological Association, 2007.

🕸 Useful websites

Alcoholics Anonymous: http://www.alcoholics-anonymous.org.uk
Alcohol Concern: http://www.alcoholconcern.org.uk
National Association for Children of Alcoholics: http://www.nacoa.org.uk

Case 5

Dear Doctor

I would be grateful for advice on further management of Jack Whitehead. He presented by ambulance this morning accompanied by his mother who heard a loud bang in the bathroom and found her son shaking uncontrollably on the floor. This continued for approximately 5 minutes and spontaneously resolved. He has been slightly drowsy ever since. We would appreciate your advice before discharge.

Yours sincerely,
Dr Navine Tomlinson
Accident and Emergency SHO

History to elicit

Jack Whitehead, 22-year-old male. Presented to A&E today.
- A&E SHO's concerns: fit, healthy, young man presenting for the first time with a probable seizure.
- Patient's concerns: Jack is worried he may have epilepsy.

HPC

Jack went to bed after returning from work and at 2 a.m. the previous day. Following a good night's sleep, he woke up naturally at 11 o'clock this morning feeling well. He had to be back at work in the early afternoon and remembers going to the bathroom to brush his teeth. He is unable to recall anything further from that point until he found himself in the A&E department.

His mother, aware that Jack had woken up, heard a loud 'thud' from upstairs. The bathroom door was open and she found Jack lying on the floor, shaking violently with his knees bought up to his stomach. Jack did not respond to his mother as she called out to him. She describes him to have been 'in a trance' with his eyes open but not recognizing her. He was breathing and appeared red faced. The toothpaste dribbling from Jack's mouth had been blood stained. Jack had cut his forehead on the edge of the bathroom sink. His mother rang for an ambulance immediately and kept Jack warm with a blanket. The ambulance came within 10 minutes by which time the shaking had completely resolved although Jack remained very drowsy and non-communicative.

Since his arrival in the A&E department, Jack's consciousness gradually returned to normal. He cannot recall what happened and complains of a frontal headache. He noted his tongue to be painful and swollen on the left side. He has not been incontinent at any time. Jack does not give a history of previous seizures but had an episode about 2 weeks ago when he 'blacked out' for about 30 minutes whilst watching television. He had also bitten his tongue then and felt disorientated when he came round. He had not reported this episode to anyone previously.

PMHx

- *Appendicectomy* Aged 15 following 3 days of right-sided abdominal pain.
- *Head injury* 3 years ago Jack was assaulted when he was drunk on a night out. He was admitted for observation overnight and discharged the next morning with no follow-up.

- *He has no other relevant past medical history.*
- *Important negatives the candidate should ask about*: recent trauma, previous head and neck surgery, alcohol abuse, diabetes, renal dysfunction, SLE, stigmata of infection.

DHx

- Paracetamol 1g PO QDS PRN (occasionally taken).
- He has never taken any previous anti-epileptic or neuroleptic medications.
- NKDA.
- No non-prescription drugs.
- Jack used to smoke cannabis regularly, but denies any misuse for >1 year. Other recreational drug use is denied.

SHx

- *Smoking* 10–15 per day since aged 15 depending on work (~5 pack-year history).
- *EtOH* Not a regular drinker but can binge once a month (up to 20U).
- *Pets* Nil.
- *Occupation* Having finished his apprenticeship, he has been recently appointed as a lighting technician for the BBC. His job involves high-wire rigging of production lights on sound stages and regular driving between venues.
- *Home* Jack lives at home with his mother and father. His sister is on a gap year.
- *Functioning* Pre-morbidly very well with no disability.
- *Travel* Jack has not been on holiday outside of the UK for >4 years.
- *Psych/social* Jack denies feeling low in mood.

FHx

- *Parents* Mum and dad are in good health with no significant medical history.
- *Siblings* 1 sister – in good health.
- *No children*.

Summary

Jack is a 22-year-old lighting technician who presented following a self-resolving, witnessed seizure lasting approximately 5 minutes. It was associated with tongue biting and a post-ictal period but no obvious preceding aura. He has not had any previous witnessed seizures but gives a suspicious history of a similar episode 2 weeks previously. He has a past history of head injury, recreational drug misuse and occasional alcohol binge drinking.

Plan

Patient's concerns

Address the concerns of both Jack and his mother directly, reassuring them that this could be a fitting episode, but further investigations are required to determine the exact aetiology.

Investigations

FBC, U&E, LFT, serum calcium, CRP, ESR. A CXR should be performed and a head CT scan should be requested if not performed by A&E.

F/U or admission

- Jack should be admitted for basic investigations and neurological monitoring.
- Reassure Jack that admission should be short.
- If all the investigations are normal he can be further managed as an outpatient.

Differential diagnosis

- Grand mal tonic–clonic epilepsy seizure
- Complex partial seizure
- Pseudo-seizure.

Discussion related to the case

An epilepsy scenario tends to concern many PACES candidates as they have had little exposure to epilepsy outside of the emergency management of uncontrolled seizures seen in A&E departments. The terminology of fits, seizures, convulsions or epilepsy are often used interchangeably. It is important that candidates have a clear understanding of what epilepsy is and how to differentiate it from the other causes of seizure:

- Epilepsy is a common chronic neurological disorder, characterized by recurrent unprovoked seizures due to excessive or synchronous neuronal activity.
- A patient presenting with a first ever episode of seizure should not be presumptively diagnosed with epilepsy.
- There are numerous causes for seizure episodes.
- The social and occupational ramifications of labelling a patient as epileptic are enormous. The diagnosis of epilepsy should therefore only be made after excluding all other reversible causes of seizure. A history of aura preceding symptoms can strengthen a diagnosis.

Jack Whitehead has had a seizure. This history suggests that there was an impairment of consciousness with generalized tonic–clonic movements that were not attributable to a particular cerebral hemisphere. A similar unwitnessed episode 2 weeks earlier makes a diagnosis of epilepsy likely. Reversible causes of seizure should be excluded:

- A cranial CT scan should already have been performed in accordance with NICE head injury guidance to exclude large intracranial causes of seizure:[1]
  - With a history of a previous head injury, the discovery of any low attenuation encephalomalacia may be the foci for abnormal neuronal activity.
  - An EEG is also recommended.
  - As this appears to be his second seizure episode, an outpatient MRI scan should be considered.

- Metabolic precipitants of seizure include:
  - Hypo/hyperglycaemia.
  - Hypo/hypernatraemia.
  - Hypocalcaemia.
- There is nothing in the history to suggest sepsis or encephalitis.
- Candidates should have a clear differential list and structure answers in order of probability.

Candidates require a holistic understanding to this disease. The legal constraints with respect to driving are significant – note there is cross-over here with similar scenarios in the communication station.
- Jack is required to inform the DVLA of his change in medical fitness.[2]
- Because this is his first documented seizure, Jack will not be able to drive for 6 months.
- His licence will be fully restored to age 70 if no further episodes take place.
- If Jack has subsequent seizures and is diagnosed with epilepsy, his license is revoked for at least 1 year.
- There is a different legal standing for Group 2 licence holders.
- Loosing his licence will have a significant impact on Jacks occupation:
  - He should also be encouraged to inform his employers of this A&E attendance.
  - Jack should stop working at height on the lighting rigs.
  - Alternative arrangements need to be made with his employers should he wish to return to work.
  - Such radical lifestyle changes may necessitate the psychosocial support, which should be offered.

The treatment of epilepsy is complicated. No definitive diagnosis can be made in this scenario and a candidate would not be required to commence Jack on antiepileptic medication. Examiners would expect a candidate to discuss the aims, contraindications and types of commonly used antiepileptic agents as well as the treatment of status epilepticus.
- The objective of treatment is to prevent further seizure occurrence by maintaining an effective dose using either a single agent or combination therapy in situations of 1st-line failure.
- In this scenario of probable tonic–clonic seizure, the most appropriate medications include:
  - Sodium valproate.
  - Carbamazepine.
  - Lamotrigine.
- Note that plasma half-life of anticonvulsant drugs differ and may require a once- or twice-daily regimen.
- Antiepileptic medications have narrow therapeutic windows which increases the risk of drug interactions related to hepatic enzyme induction or inhibition (e.g. St John's wort and alcohol ingestion).
- Be aware of drug teratogenicity and breastfeeding complications in female pregnant patients.

❶ Top Tips
- All candidates should have an understanding of DVLA guidance with respect to medical illness.
- Candidates should be aware of the social and occupational ramifications of labelling patients with a particular disease, especially in the case of epilepsy.
- Always be able to discuss the treatment of medical emergencies associated with common disease presentations.

Viva questions

What is Todd's paralysis?
Following a partial seizure involving the motor cortex, ~13% of patients develop a unilateral weakness usually localized to the upper or lower limbs. Other neurological deficits of speech, sensation and visual disturbance have been described. The symptoms originally described by Robert Todd (1809–1860) are transient and last <48 hours requiring supportive treatment only. The aetiology of Todd's paralysis is unknown but several hypotheses exist.

What is electroencephalography?
An electroencephalography (EEG) machine records electrical brain activity from firing neurons, by placing ~25 electrodes in a specific distribution along the scalp. Signals obtained are amplified and filtered to monitor brain wave patterns in response to different external stimuli. Its most frequent application is in identifying abnormal electrical activity in epileptic patients, although additional indications include assessing brain death in comatosed patients and differentiating between psychiatric syndromes. EEG can localize likely areas of pathology within the brain parenchyma and it is a useful adjunct to conventional MRI.

Why is it important to identify and treat status epilepticus?
Status epilepticus is defined as single or multiple seizures lasting >30 minutes without the patient regaining consciousness. It is usually seen in patients previously diagnosed with epilepsy and is strongly associated with structural brain disease. Status epilepticus is a life-threatening condition and although cerebral perfusion is preserved, the increase in cerebral metabolic demand causes hypoxic and ischaemic central nervous system insult. Without termination of the seizure, irreversible neuronal damage carries a mortality of 20%.

This patient previously smoked cannabis. Can you tell me about cannabis and some of the other commonly used recreational drugs?
Cannabis is the most widely used illegal substance in the world today. Made from the *Cannabis sativa* plant, its buds, leaves and resin contain THC (9-delta-tetrahydrocannabinol) which has short duration psychoactive effects. Cannabis is usually smoked in a rolled cigarette or 'joint', but can also be ingested orally and is commonly mixed with home baking. Its 'street' names include pot, weed, hydro, grass and bud. Its long-term use is associated with paranoia, anxiety, learning difficulties and infertility.

Other commonly used recreational drugs include:

- *Cocaine* Is a potent central nervous system stimulator. The substance can be smoked, snorted or injected. In its hydrochloride crystal salt form termed 'crack cocaine' its efficacy and addictive qualities are increased. Street names include coke, snow, nose candy, flake, blow, big C and snowbirds.
- *Ecstasy* In its pure form, MDMA (3,4-methylenedioxy-N-methylamphetamine) is a variation of mescaline and amphetamine. Considered a designer drug it leaves users with a strong 'feel-good' factor, eliminating anxiety and tiredness with a combination of extreme relaxation. It suppresses eating, drinking and sleeping therefore being favoured as a 'party' drug. Taken orally, preparations are rarely pure and often cut with household chemicals. Street names include E, Hug drug, speedballs, ice, X and 69's. Several high-profile cases associating Ecstasy with sudden death have been reported.
- *Ketamine* Is marketed as an anaesthetic for human and veterinary use and can be injected, smoked or consumed as a liquid. It has psychoactive effects similar to other hallucinogenic agents including LSD (D-lysergic acid diethylamide) and PCP (phencyclidine) although its effects are longer lasting. The user has feelings of euphoria, anaesthesia, relief of tension and it intensifies sexual experiences. Street terms are Ket, Special-K, Candy Raver and vitamin-K.

References

1. NICE. *Head injury*. London: NICE, 2007. Available at: http://www.nice.org.uk/GC56.
2. Driver and Vehicle Licensing Agency (DVLA): http://www.dft.gov.uk/dvla.

Case 6

Dear Doctor

Please can you see Margaret Collins, a 51-year-old patient who I have been seeing recently? She complains of epigastric pain that has had a gradual onset over the past 2 months with a partial response to antacid medication. She is a very anxious lady and I would appreciate your help with this matter. Of note, she is an ex-smoker.

Yours sincerely,
Dr Jilly Charlesworth

History to elicit

Margaret Collins, 51-year-old female. Presented today following GP referral to upper GI outpatient department (OPD).

- GP's concerns: non-resolving epigastric pain despite antacid medication.
- Patient's concerns: Mrs Collins is extremely anxious as her father died of gastric cancer.

HPC

Mrs Collins first noticed some discomfort about 6 weeks ago with occasional pain in the middle of her stomach. There has been a progressive worsening, with a gradual onset of achy pain that can sometimes be felt in her back. Although initially every few days, she is now suffering daily and more recently has been woken at night. Her pain is worse just before meal times and she has taken to snacking during the day, as eating and drinking milky tea alleviates her symptoms rapidly. Mrs Collins has stopped taking the antacid tablets which her GP prescribed for her last month as they have had little effect recently. She denies any associated symptoms of nausea or vomiting and has never had any episodes of haematemesis or dysphagia. Her bowel habit is unchanged and she denies any darkening of her stool. Despite exercising regularly Mrs Collins' weight has increased slightly.

Mrs Collin's father died aged 72 from complications related to gastric cancer. She remembers him complaining of stomach pains for months and being reluctant to see his doctor. Unfortunately his disease was metastatic at presentation and he deteriorated rapidly and died 2 weeks after diagnosis.

PMHx

- *Rheumatoid arthritis* Mrs Collins began with symptoms in her hands at the age of 45. Her rheumatologist increased some of her medication 2 months ago and she feels that the swelling and stiffness have improved over the past few weeks.
- *She has no other relevant past medical history.*
- *Important negatives the candidate should ask about*: gallstone disease, previous peptic ulcer disease, hiatus hernia, pancreatitis, aneurysmal abdominal aorta, anaemia.

DHx

- Diclofenac 50mg TDS; previously on ibuprofen 400mg TDS (since age 46).
- Paracetamol 1g PRN, methotrexate 17.5mg weekly (Mondays), folic acid 5mg weekly (Thursdays), omeprazole 20mg nocte (sometimes forgotten).
- NKDA.
- No non-prescription or recreational drugs.

SHx

- **Smoking** Ex-smoker following the birth of her daughter 17 years ago. 2.5 pack-year history.
- **EtOH** Occasional wine in the evening. Max. 10 units per week.
- **Pets** Nil.
- **Occupation** Market research analysis for a perfume company.
- **Home** Mrs Collins lives with her husband and daughter in a privately owned house kept in good condition.
- **Functioning** Pre-morbidly Mrs Collins is reasonably well. She has slight restriction to her activities in the morning e.g. with writing or using her house keys. This subsides within a couple of hours with normal functioning throughout the remainder of the day.
- **Psych/social** Mrs Collins is greatly concerned about the pain and its possible relation to the disease that killed her father. She still misses him greatly and continues to wonder if things would be different had he seen a doctor earlier.

FHx

- **Parents** Father died aged 72 years. Mum aged 77 years has mild osteoarthritis but remains well.
- **Siblings** 1 brother and 1 sister – both in good health.
- **Children** 1 daughter – in good health.

Summary

Mrs Collins is a 51-year-old female with a 6-week history of increasing epigastric pain relieved by food. There is no associated weight loss. She has a history of RA, currently well controlled with methotrexate and diclofenac. Anxiety-related issues related to her father's death may be confounding to these symptoms.

Plan

Patient's concerns

Address the GP's and patient's concerns directly. Reassure her that her epigastric pain will require further investigation but the history is more in keeping with a benign process and not indicative of gastric cancer.

Investigations

FBC, U&E, LFT, CRP, ESR, amylase. A CXR should be performed. The patient will require an abdominal ultrasound scan and an OGD.

F/U or admission

- Mrs Collins can be managed as an outpatient assuming that her biochemical profile is within normal limits.
- There are government initiatives for a maximum 2-week wait on endoscopy.

Differential diagnosis

- Gastritis or peptic ulcer disease related to NSAID medication.
- Biliary colic.
- Less likely – malignancy, pancreatitis, expanding aortic aneurysm.

Discussion related to the case

This scenario highlights the importance of addressing the patient's concerns directly. The referral letter states Mrs Collins has epigastric pain but fails to mention the past medical history of RA. In a history of possible peptic ulcer disease the following points should be addressed:

- Enquire about risk factors e.g. NSAID usage and alcohol consumption.
- Try to differentiate between types of ulcer disease:
  - Duodenal ulcers (DUs) are directly related to excess gastric acid and NSAID usage.
  - Duodenal ulcers can be differentiated from gastric ulcers (GUs) in relation to food.
  - Eating should alleviate the symptoms related to a duodenal ulcer leading to continued eating and weight gain.
  - Food usually exacerbates gastric ulceration leading to food avoidance and weight loss
  - Both are strongly related to *Helicobacter pylori* infection.
  - Nausea and vomiting make GU disease more likely.

Candidates should elicit a history of NSAID medication and note the recent change to medication and dose. The response to NSAID varies between patients with arthritis and clinicians may change drug types to achieve greater symptomatic control. Diclofenac has a stronger association with peptic ulcer disease than ibuprofen. Mrs Collins' admission that she forgets to take her omeprazole occasionally may in fact indicate a more significant non-compliance with this and other drugs.

- It would be advisable to discontinue diclofenac and start acid reduction therapy.
- The rheumatology team should be informed as there may be exacerbation of Mrs Collins' rheumatoid symptoms.
- The recently increased dose of methotrexate may allow a reduction in the dose of diclofenac.
- Mrs Collins may restart NSAID therapy following ulcer recovery.
- Addition of protective medication (e.g. misoprostol) should be considered.
- Alcohol should also be avoided short term.

The anxiety related to the death of her father may be an important discussion point during the interview.

- Anxiety and stress have been implicated in peptic ulcer disease.
- Mrs Collins' symptoms are not indicative of gastric cancer despite risk factors for malignant disease.
- An OGD with biopsy and abdominal ultrasound will allow direct visualization of the stomach to completely reassure Mrs Collins.
- The candidate should acknowledge Mrs Collins' feeling of responsibility towards her father's death.

- Psychological support may have significant effects on her current epigastric symptoms.
- This could be in the form of individual or group counselling or more formal psychological assessment should there be associated feelings of low mood or self-worth.
- Referral can be made via her GP or independently through the British Society of Counselling and Psychotherapy.[1]

❶ Top Tips
- Importance of addressing the patient's concern. Would have missed anxiety related to her fathers death if not asked directly.
- Simulated patients may have a very binary history to help differentiate disease (e.g. DU vs. GU), but in reality it is not as clear cut.
- Compliance: patient may be feeling guilty as the GP advised her to take medication which she did not do.

Viva questions

How does NSAID therapy predispose to peptic ulcer disease?

Gastric acid is required for the efficient breakdown and nutritional absorption of ingested food, but is a direct irritant to the gastric mucosa. Mucous is secreted by gastric mucosal cells to line the stomach and act as a physical barrier against gastric acid induced erosion. Mucous secretion is under the control of prostaglandin, produced along the arachadonic acid pathway by cyclo-oxygenase enzymes (Cox-1 and Cox-2). Most NSAIDs inhibit Cox-1, reducing prostaglandin production and putting the gastric mucosa at risk of gastritis, erosion and ulceration. The more selective Cox-2 inhibitors have been shown to be more gastro-protective.

What is the commonest histological subtype and location of gastric carcinoma?

The majority of gastric carcinoma (95%) is adenocarcinoma, but patients can occasionally present with squamous cell or adenocanthomatous change. Gastric carcinoma is most commonly seen in either the cardia or the distal 1/3 of the stomach, with the lesser curve associated in 60% of episodes and the greater curve in 10%.

What possible extra-articular manifestations of rheumatoid arthritis may Mrs Collins suffer from?

- Felty's syndrome: RA + splenomegaly + neutropenia.
- Sjögren's syndrome: xerostomia + keratoconjunctivitis.
- Pulmonary manifestations: rheumatoid nodules, pleural effusions, lower lobe interstitial fibrosis, Caplan's syndrome.
- Subcutaneous nodules over extensor surfaces.
- Cardiovascular involvement: pericarditis, myocarditis or aortits.
- Neuropathy related to rheumatoid vasculitis.

Reference
1. British Society of Counselling and Psychotherapy: http://www.bacp.co.uk.

Case 7

Dear Doctor

Please could you see Maureen Paterson, a 64-year-old lady who has recently been discharged from your hospital following admission for a chest infection. She has struggled this winter with increasing shortness of breath and has required 2 courses of oral antibiotics. She is a life-long smoker. Following this admission I feel that a respiratory review would be helpful.

Yours sincerely,
Dr Thomas Peele

History to elicit

Maureen Patterson, 64-year-old lady. Presented in respiratory OPD following GP referral.
- GP's concerns: recurrent chest infections requiring antibiotics.
- Patient's concerns: Maureen feels her breathing is getting worse and restricting her activities.

HPC

Mrs Paterson was discharged from hospital 2 weeks ago following admission for a chest infection. For 4 days prior to her admission, she had experienced symptoms of gradually worsening shortness of breath, wheeze and cough productive of green sputum. She felt increasingly unwell with fever and sweating. Her breathlessness was no longer helped by taking her puffers and she had noted shortness of breath even whilst walking indoors. An ambulance was called following a panic attack as she tried to ascend her stairs to use the toilet. She responded rapidly to treatment with 3 days of IV antibiotics, nebulized salbutamol, a course of oral steroids and oxygen therapy. She was discharged home with 5 days of oral medication. Mrs Paterson has continued to improve and was followed up by her GP last week who felt that an outpatient respiratory review was appropriate.

Mrs Paterson was diagnosed with asthma by her GP 3 years ago when she was started on inhalers. She felt that her breathlessness was reasonably well controlled. During the last year she has suffered with more chest infections and on 2 occasions needed to visit her GP because of sputum production. He prescribed a course of oral antibiotics for her and these helped to improve her symptoms. Her shortness of breath is not related to posture and she denies any chest pain. Her current exercise tolerance has deteriorated over the last few years and she is now restricted to walking approximately 150m on the flat. She can climb 2 flights of stairs but admits to feeling a little wheezy. Currently she uses her inhaler 2–3 times per day.

PMHx

- **Asthma** Mrs Patterson was diagnosed with asthma 3 years ago and has been on different colour inhalers since. She recently had her first hospital admission for exacerbation of shortness of breath induced by a chest infection. She does not regularly take steroid tablets.

- *Hypertension* Mrs Patterson was diagnosed with high BP 10 years ago and has been on antihypertensive medication since. She has 3-monthly checks with her GP and her BP has remained stable.
- *Important negatives the candidate should ask about:* ankle or calf muscle swelling, chest pain, diabetes, pulmonary fibrosis, TB or atypical infections, weight loss, haemoptysis. Establish any occupational hazards and pets.

DHx

- Atenolol 50mg OD.
- Seretide 250, 2-puffs BD.
- Salbutamol 2-puffs PRN.
- Prednisolone 5mg OD. (Has been on a reducing dose – compliant with instructions.)
- NKDA.
- No non-prescription or recreational drugs. No sedative medication.

SHx

- *Smoking* 20 per day for 40 years (40 pack-year history).
- *EtOH* Never.
- *Pets* Nil.
- *Occupation* Mrs Patterson took formal retirement from her position as a school teacher at age 60, but still marks GCSE papers during exam periods. She denies ever working with respiratory irritants.
- *Home* Mrs Patterson lives in a privately owned 2-bed house with her husband who is visually impaired, set on 2 floors with the bathroom upstairs. She has a small garden.
- *Functioning* Pre-morbidly, Mrs Patterson had an unrestricted exercise tolerance until 3 years ago, but since her diagnosis with asthma her breathing has left her increasingly restricted in normal activities with a deterioration during the last year.
- *Travel* No relevant travel history.
- *Psych/social* Mrs Patterson does not admit to any feelings of low mood. She is a positive person, but does feel panicked occasionally when she struggles to catch her breath. She has good neighbours and family who visit regularly.

FHx

- *Parents* Mum died of lung cancer related to smoking aged 62. Dad died of a heart attack aged 73.
- *Siblings* 1 brother – in good health.
- *Children* 2 boys and 1 girl. All in good health.

Summary

Mrs Patterson is a 64-year-old lady presenting in outpatients today for review of her respiratory system following a recent admission for a chest infection. There has been a gradual deterioration in her respiratory symptoms over the past few years and she has suffered from increasing chest infections more recently. She is an asthmatic, an active longstanding smoker and the main carer for her visually impaired husband.

Plan

Patient's concerns

Reassure Mrs Patterson that her breathlessness could be for several reasons that will require further investigation. Independent of the diagnosis, her smoking habit will need to be addressed.

Investigations

FBC, U&E, LFT, CRP. These need comparison with her recent inpatient blood results. ECG and echocardiogram looking for evidence of ischaemic heart disease and/or cor pulmonale. A CXR should be performed. Serial PEFRs should be measured and compared to baseline. Full lung function tests including DCLO (diffusion transfer factor) need to be performed 6 weeks after resolution of symptoms. Airway hyper-responsiveness and a definitive diagnosis of asthma should be confirmed with histamine or methacholine challenge tests.

F/U or admission

- Mrs Patterson can be treated as an outpatient with clinic review following necessary tests.
- A referral should be made to members of the multidisciplinary team including the respiratory nurse specialist, occupational therapist and physiotherapist with all communications copied to her GP.

Differential diagnosis

- Chronic obstructive pulmonary disease (COPD) or asthma.
- Left ventricular failure.
- Less likely – bronchogenic carcinoma, pulmonary embolism, bronchiectasis, alpha-1 antitrypsin deficiency.

Discussion related to the case

The diagnostic dilemma between asthma and COPD is a continued favourite with PACES examiners. This history scenario is in keeping with one diagnosis rather than the other but in practice, both conditions commonly coexist:

- COPD is defined as a combination of chronic bronchitis and emphysematous change, frequently in association with a smoking history.
- Asthma is commonly diagnosed in adolescence but can also have onset in later life. Symptoms of wheeze and dyspnoea, demonstrate diurnal variation and are often exacerbated by cold weather or a specific allergen trigger.[1]

Mrs Patterson probably has COPD and requires full lung function studies for diagnosis. These should be carried out following a full recovery period (e.g. 6 weeks) after her recent infective exacerbation.

- Measuring the FEV_1:FVC ratio differentiates between restrictive and obstructive conditions.
- There is an increase in the total lung capacity (TLC) and RV in COPD patients due to air trapping.
- Transfer factors (DLCO and KCO) will help differentiate asthma from COPD in complicated patients.
- Flow volume loops will localize the obstructive pattern to large or small airways.

- Reversibility should be assessed with salbutamol therapy.
- Patients should be encouraged to keep a peak flow diary:
  - This may show diurnal variation.
  - Demonstrate baseline PEFR in COPD to set clinical expectations in acute exacerbations.
  - Respiratory physicians generally tell patients to double reliever dose if PEFRs are <80% of their normal value.
  - If <60%, patients are encouraged to attend A&E for assessment.

Mrs Patterson has brittle emphysematous lungs and mild chest infections can result in severe disability. Good community treatment is essential to prevent recurrent admissions to hospital. Treatment plans are dependant on the extent of her disease and its reversible nature.

- The mainstay of treatment is short- and long-acting B2 agonists with the addition of inhaled steroid therapy.
- Respiratory nurse referral can ensure that good inhaler and PEFR measurement techniques are addressed.
- Some practitioners provide 'rescue packs' containing a short course of oral antibiotics and oral steroids to be started when PEFRs decrease below a certain percentage compared to normal.
- Preventative measures are of great importance in COPD patients who demonstrate limited reversibility.
- Smoking cessation is essential and patients must be encouraged to give up smoking.
  - Mrs Patterson should be offered a referral to the smoking cessation clinic.
  - Treatment options include nicotine replacement therapy and nicotine receptor antagonists (e.g. Zyban®).
  - Adjunct treatments include psychological support groups and hypnotherapy.
- If Mrs Patterson continues to smoke, the strong risk of further deterioration to her already compromised respiratory function must be highlighted to her. Any future hospital admissions may require invasive ventilation techniques.
- Long-term oxygen therapy (LTOT) at home can help in pulmonary rehabilitation to reduce the risk of cor pulmonale and improve survival.
  - There are strict eligibility criteria for LTOT related to PaO_2 and FEV_1 levels with an acceptable small rise in PCO_2.
  - LTOT at home is contraindicated on safety grounds to those who continue to smoke.
- The beta-blocker therapy for hypertension is a relative contraindication in reversible airways disease. An alternative antihypertensive agent in line with national hypertensive guidelines is recommended.[2]
- With a strong correlation between smoking and malignancy, mitotic disease should always be considered should symptoms not improve.

COPD, like many other chronic diseases, requires a multidisciplinary approach.

- A social services and an occupational therapy review are recommended to ensure home safety and to optimize her activities of daily living.
- Although Mrs Patterson is her husband's main carer at present, this role may change as care requirements alternate in the future.

❶ **Top Tips**
- Know all members of a multidisciplinary team and their role in different scenarios.
- When asked to define an illness (e.g. bronchitis), use the opportunity to answer the question but also guide and control the direction of the viva.
- It is important to know national guidelines for disease treatment and not rely solely on local institutional policy where you work.

Viva questions

Define chronic bronchitis

Chronic bronchitis is defined clinically, in contrast to emphysema which is a pathological diagnosis. Chronic bronchitis requires a patient to have a daily cough, productive of sputum for a minimum of 3 months consecutively over at least 2 years. All other causes need to have been excluded.

What are the eligibility criteria for long-term oxygen therapy (LTOT)?

LTOT decreases the long-term mortality from vascular complications related to chronic hypoxaemia in COPD, but does not affect the overall progression of disease. Inclusion criteria can vary between institutions, but candidates should be aware of the NICE guidelines for national recommendations of oxygen therapy in COPD.[3] For safety reasons, patients who continue to smoke are refused delivery of pressurized oxygen cylinders at home. LTOT is clinically indicated in patients who have the following:
- Arterial oxygen saturation <92% on room air.
- PaO_2 <7.3kPa when stable.
- PaO_2 >7.3kPa but <8.0kPa when stable with concomitant polycythaemia, nocturnal hypoxaemia, pulmonary hypertension or peripheral oedema.
- Severe obstructed air flow with FEV_1 <30% predicted.

Note that LTOT should be administered for at least 15–20 hours per day and, when assessment criteria are boarder line, patients should be denied LTOT and reassessed in 3 months.

What are common radiological features of COPD on CXR?

COPD is a clinical diagnosis and cannot be made from image interpretation. Features on a CXR suggestive of COPD are:
- Flattened hemidiaphragm: <1.5cm distance between the line connecting the costo- and cardiophrenic angles.
- Hyperinflated lungs.
- Barrel-chest appearances.
- Right heart enlargement.
- Presence of bullae.
- Pulmonary vascular pruning.

References
1. Chotirmall SH et al. Diagnosis and management of asthma in older adults. *J Am Geriatr Soc* 2009; **57**(5):901–9.
2. NICE. *Hypertension*. London: NICE, 2006. Available at: http://www. nice.org.uk/CG34.
3. NICE. *Chronic obstructive pulmonary disease*. London: NICE, 2010. Available at: http://www.nice. org.uk/CG10121.

Case 8

Dear Doctor

I would be very grateful if you could please see this 25-year-old female patient who presents today with intractable thigh and arm discomfort. Her symptoms started this morning, with a gradual onset of achy pain in all her limbs and she continues to be uncomfortable despite simple analgesia. She has had multiple previous attendances for similar symptoms at her local hospital in Manchester. She is known to have sickle cell disease.

Yours sincerely,
Dr Millie Udezui

History to elicit

Ezinne Oji, 25-year-old female. Presented to A&E today as a GP referral.
- A&E concerns: uncontrolled pain possibly related to a sickle cell crisis.
- Patient's concerns: Ezinne is not attending her local hospital and worries about her standard of care.

HPC

Ezinne was woken early this morning with a diffusely achy, deep discomfort in her right thigh. Recognizing the symptoms of sickle bone pain, Ezinne got up to take paracetamol and hydrate with tap water. She noticed the gradual onset of a similar diffuse achy pain in her left thigh and both shoulders a few hours later and supplemented her repeat paracetamol dose with codeine she had been prescribed for such occasions with some relief. Her pain was more marked proximally than distally, was not exacerbated by movement, position or palpation. Despite rest, the pain deteriorated. There was no limb swelling or rash. Ezinne denies any chest pain, shortness of breath or fever. Ezinne has noticed some burning when passing water and frequency of micturition over the last few days. She has not experienced abdominal pain or diarrhoea.

Ezinne is Nigerian and usually lives in Manchester. She is known to be homozygous for the sickle cell gene and has a close relationship with her haematologist and chronic pain consultant at her local hospital. Although previously a frequent attender to hospital with episodes of uncontrolled sickle pain similar to her current symptoms, her condition has been well managed over the last 2 years. With early appropriate use of her paracetamol and codeine 'rescue packs' at home, Ezinne successfully manages many crises at home. Occasionally she attends her local A&E for oral opiate supplementation, where her pain relief requirements are documented. She has had 3 sickle bone crises requiring admission over the last 2 years but denies ever having a chest or abdominal crisis.

Despite her 'rescue pack', Ezinne's pain deteriorated at lunchtime today and as she felt the need for supplemental analgesia, decided to attend the A&E department today.

PMHx

- **Anaemia** Ezinne is anaemic with regular FBCs demonstrating a haemoglobin count between 7–9g/dL. This does limit her in exercise, but not in activities of daily living. She has required 2 transfusions over the last 2 years, both following previous sickle cell crises.
- **Osteoarthritis** Ezinne experiences pain and reduced movement of her right hip following sickle crises in this joint over the past 3 years. She has been told a hip replacement will be required in the future.
- **Gallstones** Diagnosed on ultrasound at the age of 17 with gallstone disease, Ezinne had an elective cholecystectomy at 23 years old following multiple episodes of biliary colic.
- **Past medical history** She has no other relevant past medical history.
- **Pregnancy status** There is no risk of her being pregnant at the moment.
- **Important negatives the candidate should ask about:** jaundice, previous osteomyelitis, renal impairment or nephrolithiasis, leg ulcers, cellulitis, thrombotic episodes, cardiomyopathy, constipation.

DHx

- Paracetamol 1g PRN QID.
- Codeine phosphate 60mg PRN QID.
- NKDA.
- No non-prescription or recreational drugs.
- Ezinne is compliant and up-to-date with her vaccination status.

SHx

- **Smoking** Never
- **EtOH** Never.
- **Pets** Nil.
- **Occupation** A trainee beauty therapist studying part-time due to her illness.
- **Home** Usually lives in Manchester with her boyfriend, but is visiting her sister here in London.
- **Functioning** Pre-morbidly Ezinne is independent at home and work. Her hip does limit her exercise tolerance but does not restrict her normal daily functioning.
- **Travel** Ezinne visited Nigeria over a year ago with no international travel since.
- **Psych/social** As a strong Christian, Ezinne tries to remain positive about her disease but worries about her long-term health. Her boyfriend is supportive, but being estranged from her family, especially in times of crisis makes her feel low in mood.

FHx

- **Parents** Both her parents are alive and well and are recognized to have sickle trait.
- **Siblings** 1 sister – in good health but known sickle trait. 1 brother – deceased 2 years ago in Nigeria from a chest infection.
- **No children.**

Summary

Ezinne is a sensible 25-year-old sickle cell patient with a short history of intractable bone pain in all limbs. As the current episode has been resistant to prescribed 'rescue pack' medication, she attends today for analgesic control of her symptoms.

Plan

Patient's concern

Address the patient's concerns directly and reassure Ezinne that despite her attendance here, there will be close communication with her base hospital in Manchester to optimize her analgesic control.

Investigations

FBC, blood film (sickle and target cells, increased reticulocyte count), U&E, LFT, CRP, ESR, blood cultures and G&S to allow the cross match of blood for potential transfusion at a later date in her admission. ECG. ABG to consider. Urine should be dipped and samples sent for MC&S. A CXR should be performed to exclude a respiratory cause of sepsis.

F/U or admission

Ezinne has an acute medical condition that requires immediate hospitalization and treatment.

Differential diagnosis

- Thrombotic sickle crisis with bone marrow infarction.
- Malingering.
- Less likely – myositis and in cases of single limb pain fractures should be excluded.

Discussion related to the case

In this PACES scenario, it would be expected that a candidate make the diagnosis of sickle cell crisis, but given that this disease has a wide spectrum of phenotypic presentations, be aware that simulated PACES patients may have variable symptomatology. Recognize the urgency of the situation and relay this to the examiner, establishing immediate-, short- and long-term management plans to demonstrate knowledge of the disease.

- In the immediate management:
  - Establish the extent of the crisis where possible and aim to shorten the discomfort she experiences.
  - Analgesia and anxiolytic relief is required in the form of opiates, with confirmatory guidance from her local hospital in Manchester being of additional value.
  - IV hydration, oxygen therapy (if PaO_2 reduced or oxygen saturation <95%) and re-warming blankets demonstrate an understanding to the pathophysiology of her symptoms.
  - Consider the transfusion of blood products in aplastic crises.
  - Prescribe broad-spectrum antibiotics (e.g. augmentin) to cover encapsulated bacterial infection.
  - In simulated PACES scenarios, a precipitating factor is often to be found. In this case, recognizing the symptoms of a urinary tract infection may guide treatment decisions.
- The short-term management is associated with adequate analgesia:

- Sickle and non-sickle patients who have developed dependency to opiates can present complaining of clinical symptoms requiring analgesia.
- Allergies to morphine have been described and the need for stronger substitutes is recognized in severe crises.
- It can be difficult to assess the genuine need for opiate administration.
- Acknowledge the risk of malingering but never to appear critical or sceptical of a patient's intentions.
- Ezinne has information relating to her analgesic requirements easily accessible and her local hospital should be contacted to review her normal opiate requirements and her individualized analgesia regimen.
- Long-term management includes:
  - A haematology referral for expert opinion.
  - Hydroxycarbamide can reduce the rate of painful attacks by increasing the concentration of fetal haemoglobin.
  - Splenic autoinfarction in sickle patients requires the need for annual pneumococcal vaccinations and daily prophylactic doses of penicillin.[1]
  - As Ezinne is estranged from her usual healthcare provision, a comprehensive discharge summary is important for continued patient care.

Ezinne acknowledges her chronic anaemia and a previous history of transfusion, which carries with it long-term complications associated with multiple transfusions. The two primary goals of transfusion are:
- To correct the low oxygen carrying capacity in severe anaemia.
- To increase microvascular perfusion by reducing the proportion of sickle red cells in the circulation. In the clinical setting, transfusions are often used to address both indications (see Table 4.1).

Table 4.1 Transfusion in sickle cell disease

Episodic transfusion	Chronic transfusion	Non-indications	Complications
Acute splenic sequestration	Stroke prevention	Steady state anaemia	Volume overload
Transient red cell aplasia	Pulmonary hypertension	Uncomplicated crisis	Acute/chronic haemolytic reaction
Acute chest syndrome	Vital organ failure	Infection	Haematogenous infection
Stroke	Debilitating pain	Minor surgery	Iron overload
Pre-anaesthetic	Priapism	Aseptic avascular necrosis	
	Pregnancy	Uncomplicated pregnancy	
	Leg ulcers		

Other issues a candidate should consider:

- Ezinne is of child-bearing age and in a stable relationship. Should she wish to have children, a planned pregnancy with frequent obstetric follow-up is essential. Genetic counselling should be offered.
- Sickle patients often require surgery for hip replacements secondary to AVN and being a high anaesthetic risk, Ezinne would require optimization to prevent a hypoxic sickle crisis.
- Ezinne is also exposed to hypoxic sickle risks when flying and pre-warning an airline of intended travel is recommended.
- Should a simulated PACES patient be of male gender, priapism is a recognized complication that needs to be addressed sensitively.

As sickle cell disease is the most common monogenetic disorder world-wide affecting an estimated 30 million people, the disease pathway is well established and is associated with significant morbidity and early mortality. The median survival for homozygous women is 48 years and 42 years for men. The psychosocial implications of this chronic disease are enormous. Professional support may be most appropriate to commence when home in Manchester, but the offer of early support through the hospital Chaplin in line with her strong faith demonstrates a good holistic approach.

❶ Top Tips

- Never appear sceptical of a patient's intentions in an exam scenario.
- Control the pace of the viva by structuring answers in a methodical manner.
- Always make efforts to continue patient care wherever possible and maintain communication with other hospitals/clinicians.

Viva questions

Describe the haemoglobin abnormality in sickle cell disease

In normal adults, the majority (>95%) of haemoglobin is HbA, a tetrameric compound comprising of two alpha and two beta peptide chains ($\alpha 2$, $\beta 2$) attached to a common heam molecule. In sickle cell, a single nucleotide gene mutation on the γ-globin gene, causes an amino-acid substitution of glutamate by valine at position 6 on the short arm of chromosome 11. Patients with a single gene mutation are heterozygous (HbAS) and are termed sickle 'trait', while homozygous patients have sickle cell disease and HbSS is seen on electrophoresis.

What is the significance of erythema infectiosum in sickle cell disease?

Erythema infectiosum is better known as 'slapped cheek syndrome' and is caused by the single-stranded DNA parvovirus B19. Transmitted by respiratory droplets it infects red blood cell precursors in the bone marrow and causes arrest of erythropoiesis. In HbSS where haemoglobin turnover is higher than in unaffected adults, this can have devastating effects and cause a life-threatening aplastic crisis. The effects of parvovirus B19 last for 3–5 days and treatment is supportive with the potential requirement for blood transfusion.

What are the common radiological features of AVN of the hip?

- The joint space may be widened due to cartilage thickening and the presence of joint effusion.
- The femoral head may be smaller and more sclerotic than the contralateral side.
- There may be femoral head fragmentation.
- As the hip regenerates, remodelling of the femoral head causes it to become flatter and wider ('coxa magna').
- If plain radiographs are normal, MRI scanning may be useful in detecting early changes.

Reference

1. Davies JM et al. Update of guidelines for the prevention and treatment of infection in patients with an absent or dysfunctional spleen. *Clin Med* 2002; 2:440–3.

Case 9

Dear Doctor

I would be grateful for your advice regarding Mr Fields who is a 36-year-old man presenting to A&E today with difficulty in walking. His symptoms started approximately 2 days ago with swelling of his right knee causing severe pain and discomfort. He has been off work recently feeling generally unwell. His temperature today is 38.1.

Yours sincerely,
Dr Christopher Burkstead

History to elicit:

Mr Robert Fields, 36-year-old male. Referred to medical registrar on-call today from A&E.
- A&E concerns: deteriorating monoarthropathy with systemic stigmata of infection.
- Patient's concerns: Mr Fields cannot walk and feels extremely unwell.

HPC

Mr Fields is an insurance broker who has been feeling generally unwell for approximately 1 week. He has been off work for the last few days describing his symptoms as 'flu-like'. Despite over-the-counter remedies he has continued to deteriorate with increasing episodes of sweating and fever, which are mainly occurring during the night. He denies any cough, shortness of breath, headache, dysuria or GI upset.

Mr Fields noted the onset of swelling and pain in his right knee 2 days ago which has now become difficult to bend. He denies any recent trauma and despite ice packs and elevation, the knee swelling has not resolved. Since this morning Mr Fields has experienced an achy pain in his right groin. He is now having difficulty walking and feels he cannot cope at home feeling so unwell and immobile. No other joints are affected and he denies ever having these symptoms previously.

PMHx
- **Mr Fields has no relevant past medical history**, having never been admitted to hospital or had any surgery.
- **Important negatives the candidate should ask about:** gout, pseudogout, psoriasis, haemochromatosis, IBD, previous tropical infection (e.g. Whipple's disease), recent diarrhoea, urethritis, conjunctivitis.

DHx
- No regular prescription medication, past or current.
- NKDA.
- Following direct questioning, Mr Fields reluctantly gave a 4-year history of occasional recreational IV drug usage. He injects heroin every few months when his wife is away. He has a 'reliable' supplier who also provides a sterile syringe and needle. He has never shared a needle, denies regular usage and is adamant he is not addicted. His wife is

aware of his habit and he promised her he would stop using IV drugs following the birth of their first daughter. In a moment of weakness, he last injected heroin 1 week ago.

SHx

- **Smoking** Yes, 10/day for 15 years (7.5 pack-years).
- **EtOH** Socially when out with friends but does not drink at home with his wife.
- **Pets** Nil.
- **Occupation** Insurance broker for 10 years. Stable income.
- **Home** Mr Fields lives in a terraced house in Croydon. It is privately owned with his wife and in good condition.
- **Functioning** Pre-morbidly very well with no disability.
- **Travel** Mr Fields has not been on holiday outside of the UK for over 2 years.
- **Sexual** Married monogamous relationship for 8 years, denying extramarital affairs.
- **Psych/social** Denies any suggestions of mood disruption.

FHx

- **Parents** Both Mr Fields' parents are alive with no significant morbidity.
- **Siblings** 1 brother (38 years) in good health.
- **Children** Mr Fields has a daughter of 8 months who is in good health.

Summary

Mr Fields is a 36-year-old man with a 1-week history of symptoms in keeping with systemic infection and a 2-day history of large joint monoarthropathy with right knee erythema, pain and swelling. He is an infrequent recreational IV drug user, last injecting heroin the weekend before his symptoms started.

Plan

Patient's concerns

Mr Fields is worried his illness is related to his recent IV drug usage and is concerned about the repercussions if his wife were to find out.

Investigations

FBC, U&E, LFT, CRP, ESR. Blood cultures. Mr Fields requires HIV screening as per hospital protocol. ECG and echocardiogram. Synovial tap will be required and sent for MC&S. A right knee and CXR should be performed.

F/U or admission

- Mr Fields is at high risk of septic arthritis.
- This is a surgical emergency and would require inpatient review and treatment with IV antibiotics post lavage.

Differential diagnosis

- Septic arthritis.
- Large-joint seronegative monoarthropathy (psoriatic arthritis, pseudogout, Reiter's syndrome, haemochromatosis, Wilson's disease, PVNS).
- Reactive arthritis (*Yersinia, Salmonella, Shingella*, HIV, Whipple's disease).

Discussion related to the case

This case of a potential septic arthritis ordinarily referred to the orthopaedic team, highlights the subtlety of asking the right questions during the history taking station. Focusing solely on seronegative differentials, without asking questions regarding illicit drug abuse may have resulted in missing a surgical emergency in a young man.

- Septic arthritis is most often caused by *Staphylococcus aureus* infection.
- It is essentially indistinguishable by history from rarer causes e.g. TB, *Brucellosis* or *Salmonella*.
- The commonest cause is by haematogenous spread from bacteraemia.
- Contiguous dissemination from focal osteomyelitis or direct trauma needs to be excluded.
- Commonly non-specific inflammatory markers are raised, whilst acute radiographic findings are normal in the acute phase.
- Microscopy of synovial fluid demonstrating leucocytosis is highly suggestive.

Mr Fields is not a stereotypical IV drug user. Without adequate preparation in asking personal questions, candidates may feel awkward and appear weak when asking questions related to recreational habits or sexual history. Important sensitive history to be elicited in this case include urethral discharge, previous STIs, sexuality, sexual partners and HIV risk. A direct, professional and succinct approach is best and if needed, reassuring the patient that any information obtained will be treated confidentially.

The clinical consequences of Mr Fields' use of IV drugs are far greater than an acute case of septic arthritis.

- The history suggests bacteraemia with haematogenous spread to the right knee and Mr Fields is at risk of bacterial endocarditis and its sequelae:
  - During the viva, risks of cardiovascular compromise (new heart murmurs/heart failure) or any vasculitic stigmata of disease (e.g. Roth spots, Janeway lesions) need to be mentioned.
  - Knowledge of Duke's clinical criteria in the diagnoses of infective endocarditis would be expected (➔ Table 5.10, p.260).
- There should be a low threshold for further appropriate investigations to exclude venous thrombosis with the potential risk of subsequent pulmonary emboli.
  - Paradoxical arterial embolization with cerebrovascular stoke can occur in young adults with previously undiagnosed AVM, PDA, ASD or VSD.

Despite the intermittent use of IV drugs, referral for specialized drug cessation advice is required for both education and support with recovery from possible addiction. Mr Fields has also put himself at significant risk of HIV infection which requires further investigation.

- Pre-test HIV counselling is mandatory.
- Many hospitals have specialized nurses to discuss the possible ramifications of a positive result with patients prior to testing.
- It is recommended that candidates research the practices of their local hospital and adapt those for use in the examination.

There are significant psychosocial and legal consequences to this case that should be considered. Lateral thinking may also score highly at viva.

- Marital counselling may be required, particularly with view to Mr Fields' concerns regarding the effect his presentation at hospital will have on the relationship with his wife.
- It would be recommended that both Mrs Fields, and potentially their daughter, be screened for HIV if Mr Fields tests positive.
- Abstinence from unprotected sexual intercourse should be sought until a second negative HIV result is confirmed 3–6 months following this hospital presentation.
- Legally, advice on police involvement should be taken which may raise the possibility of social services and child protection issues.
- A police record may impact on Mr Fields' employment and limit his social opportunities long-term with regards to future holidays as certain countries (e.g. USA) have strict boarder control policies with respect to criminal records.

> **❶ Top Tips**
> - In all scenarios, there is often the opportunity for cessation advice (e.g. EtOH/smoking). This can be a useful lifeline if struggling with the viva.
> - Never assume appearances dictate social class and recreational activities. Confidently ask direct and sensitive questions if clinically relevant.
> - Knowledge and reference to local institutional policy will identify those candidates who are experienced in the daily practices of hospital life.

Viva questions

What are the possible radiological features of septic arthritis?
- *Acute setting:*
  - Initial radiographs may be normal.
  - There may be soft-tissue swelling and joint distension.
  - Some periarticular osteoporotic changes may be seen.
- *Subacute setting (8–10 days):*
  - There may be marginal and central erosions of the articular cortex with reactive bone sclerosis.
  - Subchondral bone destruction may be seen.
  - Bony ankylosis can occur if there is cartilage destruction.

What are the common pathogens associated with Reiter's syndrome?
Reiter's syndrome is a seronegative HLA-B27-linked spondyloarthropathy precipitated by GI (postdysenteric) or genitourinary (venereal) infections. Common pathogens include:
- Venereal Reiter's syndrome:
  - *Chlamydia trachomatis.*
  - *Neisseria gonorrhoea.*

- Post-dysenteric Reiter's syndrome:
  - *Salmonella* spp.
  - *Shigella* spp.
  - *Campylobacter* spp.
  - *Yesinia* spp.

Describe Duke's criteria for the diagnosis of bacteria endocarditis

Major criteria:
- Bacteraemia by an organism know to cause endocarditis.
- Endocardiographic evidence of abscess, vegetation or prosthetic valve dehiscence.
- New valvular regurgitation on clinical examination.

Minor criteria:
- Fever.
- Bacteraemia by an organism not known to cause endocarditis.
- Immunological stigmata (Janeway lesions/Roth spots/Osler's nodes).
- Predisposing conditions e.g. IV drug user, prosthetic heart valves.
- Evidence of vascular embolic phenomenon.
- Positive echocardiogram that does not meet major criteria.

To meet the modified Duke criteria for definitive diagnosis of bacterial endocarditis, patients must reach 1 of the following:
- 2 major criteria
- 1 major & 3 minor criteria
- All 5 minor criteria.

Case 10

Dear Doctor

Please could you review Mrs Dutta who has come from Bangladesh to visit her daughter in the UK? Since her arrival she has been complaining of a persistent cough. Examining her today she has right-sided basal crepitations. I would appreciate your help with this matter and further treatment.

Yours sincerely,
Dr Emily Millison

History to elicit

Mrs S. Dutta, 61-year-old female. Presented today following GP referral to A&E.

- GP's concerns: signs and symptoms of pneumonia.
- Patient's concerns: has a cough but does not want to spend time in hospital away from her daughter.

HPC

Mrs Dutta lives in Bangladesh and has come to the UK 4 days ago to support her daughter who is heavily pregnant. Her daughter noted her mother's cough since her arrival and hears her coughing at night. Mrs Dutta has become very chesty and describes the cough to have gradually deteriorated since it begun as a tickle in her throat 2 weeks ago. She has had green/brown sputum production over the last week, which has been streaked with fresh red blood on coughing. Mrs Dutta feels that the plane flight from Dhaka has made her symptoms worse. She has become increasingly dyspnoeic with breathlessness on minimal exertion. She has experienced pain in her ribs during deep coughing fits and has felt panicked when she struggles to catch her breath during these episodes. She denies fever, but her daughter has noticed unusual amounts of sweating and has changed the bed sheets twice since her mother's arrival. Mrs Dutta accompanied her daughter for a routine pregnancy check today. Having mentioned her own symptoms to her daughter's GP, she referred Mrs Dutta to the accident and emergency department for assessment.

PMHx

- *Diabetes* Mrs Dutta has type 2 diabetes mellitus, diagnosed 8 years ago. Although initially diet controlled, she has been on metformin for the last 5 years. She has successfully lost significant weight during the last 2 months. Her monthly blood glucose measurements usually run between 5.5–6.5. She has never experienced hypoglycaemia or required hospitalization for her diabetes. She has never had her fundi examined.
- *Hypertension* Mrs Dutta was diagnosed with hypertension 12 years ago and has been treated with a beta-blocker ever since. Recently, her doctor in Bangladesh commenced an additional new drug to achieve tighter control of her BP.
- *Gout* Mrs Dutta was diagnosed with gout 2 years ago following episodes of bilateral ankle pain and swelling. She has had 2 acute

attacks in the last year, both controlled with simple analgesia. She is on prophylactic medication.

- **Important negatives the candidate should ask about**: myocardial infarction, stroke or TIA, asthma, calf swelling, previous pulmonary embolisms, previous pneumonia, previous TB infection.

DHx

- Atenolol 50mg OD.
- Ramipril 2.5mg OD.
- Allopurinol 300mg OD.
- Metformin 500mg BD.
- The patient has never been prescribed immunomodulating medication.
- NKDA.
- No non-prescription or recreational drugs.

SHx

- **Smoking** Never.
- **EtOH** Never.
- **Pets** Nil.
- **Occupation** Housewife.
- **Home** Mrs Dutta lives with her husband and parents-in-law in Bangladesh. In the UK she is staying with her daughter and her son-in-law in Plaistow in their 3rd-floor flat with a lift.
- **Functioning** Pre-morbidly well with no disability.
- **Travel** This is her first visit to the UK. She has had no other travel experiences.
- **Psych/social** Denies low mood.

FHx

- **Parents** Both parents in good health.
- **Siblings** 3 sisters and 2 brothers – 1 of her brothers died of a heart attack aged 58. Two of her sisters have type 2 diabetes mellitus. Her other 2 siblings are in good health.
- **Children** She has 1 daughter who is healthy and pregnant and 1 son who remains in good health.

Summary

Mrs Dutta is a 61-year-old foreign national from Bangladesh who presents with a 2-week history of productive cough and haemoptysis, with associated night sweats and exertional dyspnoea. She has a background of diabetes, hypertension and gout.

Plan

Patient's concerns

Acknowledge the patient's wishes to care for her daughter, but emphasize that the management of her current medical situation should take priority.

Investigations

FBC, U&E, LFT, CRP, ESR, fasting cholesterol. Sputum MC&S especially looking for AFB. Early morning urine sample for AFB. ECG. A CXR should be performed.

F/U or admission
- It would be prudent to treat as an inpatient.
- Isolation should be considered in the short term until a formal diagnosis is made.

Differential diagnosis
- Pulmonary *Mycobacterium* TB.
- Community-acquired pneumonia.
- Less likely, bronchogenic carcinoma (e.g. alveolar cell), sarcoidosis or pulmonary embolism.

Discussion related to the case

Mrs Dutta's symptoms, as well as her recent arrival from Bangladesh where TB is pandemic, makes pulmonary TB highly likely. A community-acquired pneumonia would be the commonest differential diagnosis in a UK resident.
- The Department of Health recognized 8000 cases of TB in the UK in 2008.
- There is strong disease prevalence in heavily populated areas, most commonly London and other inner cities.
- These demographics should also encourage candidates to consider TB in atypical presentations of pulmonary disease.
- We advise that candidates taking the PACES exam outside of their usual catchment area should research the demographics of their exam hospital with respect to common diseases.

TB can present as a spectrum of disease:
- It can be asymptomatic in the early stages, although this would be unlikely in a PACES exam.
- Mrs Dutta has a classic presentation with open pulmonary symptoms, haemoptysis, dyspnoea, weight loss and night sweats.
- Most cases are primary in aetiology, with 1% of cases being post primary reactivation.
  - Assess the patient's HIV risk and ask about previous immune modulation therapy.
  - Remember the use of steroids in asthma and disease-modifying agents in RA.
- Investigations to consider include:
  - A CXR which may demonstrate lobar consolidation, hilar lymphadenopathy or a Ghon focus in the anterior apical segments of the upper and lower lobes.
  - A pleural effusion may account for Mrs Dutta's recent exertional dyspnoea and, if present, should be tapped looking for AFB.
  - A pleural biopsy could also be considered but has a low sensitivity for diagnosis.
  - Remember to exclude extrapulmonary manifestations of TB.
  - Cross-sectional imaging can exclude differentials of pulmonary embolism or other parenchymal abnormalities and should be requested if indicated.

In the acute setting Mrs Dutta requires inpatient management.
- There is a possibility of open TB and preventative measures should be taken immediately:

- Facemask protection.
- Negative pressure isolation on the ward if available.
- The treatment for pulmonary TB is complicated and would ideally involve the input from an infectious disease consultant.
- Combination therapy of rifampicin, isoniazid, ethambutol and pyrazinamide would be recommended, although this regimen may change depending on local disease demographics and demonstrated drug resistance:
  - The importance of regimental compliance with anti-TB medication should be stressed.
  - Note possible drug interactions as Mrs Dutta's gout may be exacerbated by the addition of pyrazinamide.
- If Mrs Dutta returns to Bangladesh during her treatment, issues related to drug availability and completion of the treatment course will need to be addressed.
- The side effects of ramipril may be a contributory culprit in the worsening cough.
- The diagnosis of TB requires consultant advice with regards to communicable disease notification:[1]
  - Contact tracing is essential.
  - Close family members should be screened and their BCG status ascertained.
  - Her pregnant daughter raises radiation protection complications and TB transmission risks with regards to the unborn fetus.

Although the strong cardiovascular risk factors are not the main focus of this case, they should none the less, be addressed in due course.
- Risk stratify Mrs Dutta and aim to minimize her potential long-term complications of disease.
- Whilst an inpatient:
  - Monitor blood glucose and BP profiles.
  - A fasting cholesterol level should be screened.
- Mrs Dutta has not undergone retinal screening, which is an annual requirement for all diabetic patients in the UK.
- Retinal examination would also be required with the presumptive addition of ethambutol to her medication.

It is a doctor's duty of care to highlight Mrs Dutta's non-UK resident status to the accounts department. Her acute treatment would be covered by reciprocal arrangements between Bangladesh and the UK healthcare policy. Long-term treatment and recuperation would need either negotiation or insurance cover. This may complicate healthcare provision both here and in Bangladesh.

> **❶ Top Tips**
> - When candidates learn of their exam location, they should make an effort to research hospital specialities and local disease demographics.
> - Candidates should always consider medication side effects as a possible cause of symptomology.
> - Never hypothesize on expert advice, admit a short fall in knowledge and offer to find an answer to the question and relay this to the patient.

Viva questions

What are the main side effects of the common anti-TB medications?

- *Rifampacin:*
  - Alterations to liver function
  - Coloured bodily secretions (orange/red)
  - GI symptom
  - Renal failure.
- *Isoniazide:*
  - Dry mouth
  - Optic neuritis and vertigo
  - Erythema multiforme
  - Drug-induced lupus.
- *Ethambutol:*
  - Red/green colour blindness
  - Optic neuritis
  - Peripheral neuritis.
- *Pyrazinamide:*
  - Hepatotoxicity
  - Photosensitivity
  - Sideroblastic anaemia.

What are the common extrapulmonary manifestations of TB?

- Tuberculus lymphadenitis – most commonly seen in the cervical chain, but inguinal and axillary have also been described.
- Spinal TB (also known as Potts disease) – commonly affects the thoracic spine with vertebral body destruction and anterior wedging. There is a strong association with paraspinal and psoas abscess.
- Skeletal TB – most commonly seen in weight-bearing joints with associated osteomyelitis.
- Cranial TB – tuberculous meningitis most commonly manifests with cranial nerve palsies and communicating hydrocephalus if arachnoid extension. Seizures are also seen in intracranial tuberculoma formation.
- Abdominal TB – a spectrum of disease causing enteritis, peritonitis and intra-abdominal lymphadenitis and can be easily misdiagnosed as Crohn's disease.
- Genitourinary TB.

What are the commonest UK pathogens for community acquired pneumonia?

- *Streptococcus pneumoniae*
- *Haemophilus influenzae*
- *Mycoplasma pneumoniae*
- *Legionella pneumophilia*
- *Klebsiella pneumoniae*

Reference

1. http://www.infectioncontrolservices.co.uk.

Case 11

Dear Doctor

Thank you for seeing Ms Lillian Anderson, a 56-year-old female with a previous diagnosis of type 2 diabetes mellitus. She has noticed worsening symptoms in keeping with peripheral vascular disease over the last year. Her HbA1c today is 9.8% with a random glucose of 10.2%. We would be keen for your advice and management with a view to optimal glycaemic control.

Yours sincerely,
Mrs Margaret Tetlow
Vascular Surgical Team

History to elicit

Lillian Anderson, 56-year-old female. Outpatient consultation following referral from the vascular surgery team.
- Surgeon's concerns: worsening peripheral vascular disease due to poor glycaemic control.
- Patient's concerns: a recent change in lifestyle has made glycaemic control much harder.

HPC

Ms Anderson, a former District Nurse, was diagnosed with type 2 DM 15 years ago, when she was commenced on metformin. GI side effects of bloating and nausea led to poor compliance with metformin. Her diabetic regime was supplemented with subcutaneous insulin 2 years ago. Ms Anderson believed that her blood glucose was subsequently well controlled for a period of time.

With a change in lifestyle following her redundancy last year, Ms Anderson has struggled to keep tight glycaemic control. Her diet has deteriorated and her home monitoring has shown her blood glucose to vary from 3.6–16. She is aware of the complications of poor glycaemic control and therefore increased her once-daily insulin regimen on her own accord. She denies ever having any hypoglycaemic episodes and has never been admitted to hospital with a diabetic-related disorder. Her last retinal assessment 2 years ago was normal.

Over the past 6 months Ms Anderson has also had increasing pain in her left calf muscle, which restricts her walking to <100m. She has developed an ulcer on the left ankle, which is not healing despite self-management. For the last few months, she also complains of a progressive burning sensation in both feet. Unfortunately, she has not been attending her GP for regular visits, but has asked for a vascular assessment of her worsening symptoms.

PMHx
- **Diabetes** Long standing diabetic history as previously described.
- **Dyslipidaemia** Her GP noticed elevated fasting cholesterol 2 years ago. Ms Anderson is compliant with her statin therapy.
- **Important negatives the candidate should ask about**: hypertension, ischaemic heart disease, diabetic nephropathy, hypoglycaemic episodes.

DHx

- Metformin 500mg BD.
- Lantus 25U mane.
- Simvastatin 40mg nocte.
- NKDA.
- Poor metformin compliance due to GI side effects.
- No non-prescription medication.
- No beta-blocker medication.

SHx

- **Smoking** Never.
- **EtOH** Since her redundancy, she has increased her social alcohol intake but drinks <10U per week.
- **Pets** Nil.
- **Occupation** Former District Nurse.
- **Home** Ms Anderson lives alone in a 2-bed house. She is 18 years divorced and her only son is away at university.
- **Functioning** Ms Anderson is pre-morbidly very well with no disability. Since retirement, she is less active than she was previously.
- **Psych/social** Following her redundancy, Ms Anderson has struggled to cope with the change in lifestyle and despite good neighbours, she finds herself alone for long periods of time. She is worried about her mood.

FHx

- **Parents** Mother and father both died of 'old age'.
- **Siblings** 1 sister – in good health, lives in Norfolk.
- **Children** 1 son in good health.

Summary

Ms Anderson is a type 2 diabetic patient on a suboptimal once-daily insulin regimen due to non-compliance with oral hypoglycaemic agents. There is rapid worsening of macrovascular complications and a full diabetic assessment and optimization of treatment is necessary. Ms Anderson is also struggling psychologically to adapt with her change in her lifestyle following her redundancy.

Plan

Patient's concerns

The importance for a change to her diabetic treatment (including insulin regimen) must be stressed in order to minimize the progression of macro/microvascular complications. Address the psychosocial reasons for a recent deterioration in glycaemic control.

Investigations

Bedside tests including BP monitoring, urine dipstick, albumin creatine ratio (ACR) and an ECG. Blood tests including FBC, U&E, HbA1c, fasting glucose and cholesterol, B12, folate and TFT. A CXR is recommended, ankle brachial pressure indexes (ABPIs) should be measured and a request for CT angiogram (CTA) be made if renal function is satisfactory.

Cessation advice

The patient should be reminded of the risks of drinking alcohol with a history of diabetes and a dietician referral made to optimize dietary influences on blood sugar levels.

F/U or admission

- Ms Anderson should be managed in an outpatient capacity.
- There should be regular follow-up by the multidisciplinary team including her GP.

Discussion related to the case

Peripheral vascular disease (PVD) is related to atherosclerosis of peripheral arteries causing symptoms of claudication, rest pain, ulceration with delayed healing and potential gangrenous infection. ~15% of Westernized individuals >70 years have PVD and its risk factors are similar to those of ischaemic heart disease, with the 2 conditions commonly coexisting. Diabetes is a major contributory factor with 1 in 3 diabetics over the age of 50 suffering from PVD. Whilst the long-term management of PVD is surgical, the initial treatment and risk factor modulation should be medical:

- Diabetes is a dynamic disease and requires continued appraisal and titration of treatment for optimal glycaemic control.
- Without any change to Ms Anderson's current regimen she is at risk of CVD, progressive neuropathy, retinopathy (she is out of date with the recommended annual screening) and nephropathy.

Candidates should have a full understanding of the management of type 2 diabetes mellitus, its deterioration to insulin dependence and the macro/microvascular complications of the disease.

- There is suboptimal insulin treatment and poor metformin compliance.
- Conversion to a modified-release preparation may reduce GI side effects:
  - In some institutions, changing a patient's insulin regimen is discouraged unless done by a specialist endocrinologist.
  - In this PACES scenario a candidate should however discuss the option of a twice-daily insulin regimen (e.g. NovoMix® 30 BD).
  - It is important to ensure hypoglycaemic management is discussed appropriately with the patient when contemplating insulin alteration.
- Gabapentin or pregabalin should also be considered for the management of painful diabetic neuropathy although the pain may be due to vascular insufficiency.
- A change to Ms Anderson's lifestyle has manifested in poor glycaemic control and a rapid deterioration in the associated complications.
- The importance of a multidisciplinary team approach is essential and includes the following:
  - An endocrinologist.
  - Diabetic nurse specialists.
  - Dieticians.
  - Multidisciplinary foot clinics (including doctors, podiatrists and orthotics) are increasingly common practice. Regular foot examinations are essential for all diabetic patients because the circulatory and neuropathic sequelae of diabetes can turn minor breakdowns into severe ulcerations. ~15% of all people with

> diabetes will develop an ulceration and about half of all
> amputations start with a simple ulcer.
> - Patient's own GP.

Ms Anderson's redundancy was the catalyst for her recent deterioration. Consideration of the following points in relation to her psychological decline will show a holistic approach to patient care.

- Recognizing her age with acknowledgment that early retirement and the unplanned nature of her redundancy did not allow her to adapt her lifestyle sufficiently (e.g. by taking part-time retirement in the first instance).
- Whether there are any intercurrent health issues or a non-clinical problem that had limited her ability to work.
- Alcohol consumption can be related to a patient's mood and Ms Anderson admits to increasing her recent intake.
  - Excessive alcohol consumption with diabetes mellitus should be discouraged.
  - The recommended weekly alcohol intake is 21 units for men and 14 units for women.
  - One unit equates to 10mL by volume and is approximately half a pint of ordinary strength beer (3–4%) or a small glass (125mL) of ordinary strength wine (12%).
- The offer of support through information leaflets or more formal psychological routes is encouraged.

Diabetes mellitus is recognized by the DVLA as a potential risk with respect of road safety.

- Any significant hypoglycaemic episodes can result in licence suspension until tighter glycaemic control is obtained.
- There may be significant social and occupational implications.
- There is clear DVLA guidance available for medical conditions.[1]

> **❶ Top Tips**
> - Recognize the difficulty in treating medical professionals as patients.
> - Be aware of topical medical issues. For example, recommendations on alcohol intake for women and men.
> - Commonly encountered clinical scenarios expect a high-quality and proficient viva performance.

Viva questions

HbA1c is a marker of glycaemic control over what period of time?

Depending on the amount of glucose available, haemoglobin is glycosylated in a non-enzymatic process during the lifecycle of a red blood cell. Higher plasma glucose concentrations increase the availability for glycosylation. Red blood cells have a life span of ~120 days and therefore, measuring the HbA1c level reflects the average blood glucose concentration over the last 3 months. Lower than expected levels of HbA1c are seen in people with shortened red blood cell lifespan, such as haemolytic anaemia (including glucose-6-phosphate dehydrogenase [G6PD] deficiency and sickle-cell disease) or any other condition causing premature red blood cell death.

On the converse, higher than expected levels can be seen in people with a longer red blood cell lifespan, such as with vitamin B12 or folate deficiency.

How would you advise a patient regarding hypoglycaemia management?

Patients should be advised that hypoglycaemia occurs when their blood glucose falls below 4mmol/L, the most common symptoms of a 'hypo' include: feeling light headed/dizzy, feeling hungry, a change in mood (often irritability), feeling sweaty, trembling and difficulty with concentration. This should be managed by administering glucose (ideally 3 glucose tablets or 50mL of Lucozade®) and then waiting for 15 minutes before eating a light snack, such as a biscuit, fruit juice, glass of milk, fruit or cereal bar, to maintain blood glucose levels. Fatty foods (including chocolate) should be avoided as they delay the absorption of blood glucose.

Describe likely measures taken by a chiropodist for continued foot care in a diabetic patient

Diabetic patients with microvascular disease and distal neuropathy do not have the normal sensory response to avoid trauma to their feet. Once damage has been sustained, coexistent macrovascular disease delays or prevents healing, with increased risk of infection related to an impaired immune system.

NICE has published guidelines on foot management in type 2 diabetic patients. The following recommendations are included:

- Regular 1–3-monthly reviews by the foot protection team.
- Patients should be educated in self-inspection.
- Specialist footwear with insoles should be provided to avoid ulcer formation.
- Skin and nail care is essential.
- Non-healing progressive ulcers should be debrided and systemic antibiotics should be initiated in the presence of signs of infection.

What should be considered in diabetic patients requiring contrast enhanced CT scans?

Diabetic patients often have a degree of nephropathy in relation to their disease. For contrast-enhanced CT studies, satisfactory endogenous renal function is required for contrast excretion. Serum urea and creatinine (Cr) measurements are essential prior to contrast instillation. Although institutional guidelines vary, on average a Cr >150mmol/L requires renal protection through the use of an alternative contrast media. Most hospitals use a Cr of 250mmol/L as an absolute contraindication, unless a contrast enhanced study is essential in life-threatening situations. It is important to hydrate diabetic patients prior to any contrast study and monitor their renal function post scan to avoid the complications of worsening renal impairment.

Type 2 diabetics on metformin are encouraged to stop taking the oral hypoglycaemic agent for 48 hours post contrast study, to avoid the complications of hypoglycaemia and lactic acidosis related to metformin toxicity.

Reference

1. DVLA website: http://www.dft.gov.uk/dvla.

Case 12

Dear Doctor

Please can you review Anthony Carlson, a 32-year-old designer who I have been seeing over the past 2 weeks with increasing difficulty in swallowing? His symptoms have not been alleviated with anti-reflux medication. I have referred him for an outpatient endoscopy as he thinks he has lost a stone in weight.

He has a past medical history of well-controlled asthma.
I would appreciate your opinion.

Yours sincerely,
Dr Emily Allen

History to elicit

Anthony Carlson, 32-year-old Afro-Caribbean male. Presented today following GP referral to A&E.

- GP's concerns: non-resolving dysphagia in a young healthy man.
- Patient's concerns: great discomfort swallowing and now avoiding food.

HPC

Anthony first noticed a problem with dysphagia about 3 weeks ago when he experienced discomfort on swallowing his sandwich. He was just recovering from a 'head cold' he had caught from his niece, which had left him with blocked sinuses and a scratchy sore throat from coughing. His symptoms at this time were relieved by gargling aspirin. Despite his sinuses improving his throat did not, and over the next few days he found it increasingly uncomfortable to swallow any kind of solid food, particularly with solid boluses e.g. chicken and steak. He was able to drink freely at this time and it helped to wash the food down, although carbonated drinks were a little irritant too.

After about a week Anthony visited his GP who felt that he had oral candidiasis related to his combination asthma inhaler, prescribed some antacid medication and oral nystatin, and made an appointment to see him in 1 week's time.

Initially his symptoms improved significantly with the new medications. Although it became easier to swallow, Anthony felt that the food was getting stuck in the middle of his chest and he had an associated burning sensation when trying to get food to move down his gullet, which eased by drinking water. He never needed to regurgitate the food. Anthony's symptoms were very much worse last week, when he saw his GP, with searing pain in the centre of his chest on swallowing even semisolid food. Consequently, over the last few days, he has been eating tinned soups only to alleviate the hunger he feels. Anthony feels he has lost weight and has needed to put another hole in his belt buckle.

Generally, Anthony feels tired, but denies symptoms of fever or rigors. His bowels are working normally.

PMHx

- *Asthma* Anthony has been asthmatic since the age of 17. He was treated with a short course of steroids following an infective exacerbation of his asthma 3 years ago that required an overnight stay in hospital. He was followed-up by a respiratory doctor following his discharge home. His asthma has been well controlled on a combination of inhalers since then.
- *Anthony is usually fit and healthy* and apart from his 'head cold' 3 weeks ago, he did have one other episode of illness 7 months ago when his GP diagnosed glandular fever.
- *Important negatives the candidate should ask about*: symptoms related to systemic sclerosis including Raynaud's symptoms and gastro-oesophageal reflux (which may be the only symptom of oesophageal involvement) oral or genital ulceration, Crohn's disease, previous radiation exposure.

DHx

- Seretide 50/100 2 puffs BD.
- Compliant with asthma medication and washes mouth out after use.
- NKDA.
- Anthony does not take any non-prescription drugs. He has used cocaine occasionally prior to 2 years ago.

SHx

- *Smoking* Never, because of his asthma.
- *EtOH* Occasionally at parties, but never more than 5 glasses of wine per week (10U).
- *Pets* Nil.
- *Occupation* Clothing designer.
- *Home* Anthony lives with his partner in a flat in Hoxton. It is rented accommodation but kept in good condition.
- *Functioning* Pre-morbidly very well with no disability.
- *Travel* Anthony visited his mother in the Caribbean last summer, but has not had a holiday since.
- *Psych/social* Generally in good spirits and has a strong support network around him.
- *Sexual* Anthony is homosexual and lives with his partner of 9 months. This is first real relationship and prior to this had several sexual partners. He has always used protection until his current relationship. He has never been tested for STIs.

FHx

- *Parents* Mother lives in St Lucia and has heart disease. Anthony does not know his father.
- *Siblings* 1 brother – living in Sheffield in good health.
- *No children*.

Summary

Anthony Carlson is a 32-year-old homosexual male, with a 3-week progressive history of odynophagia and globus sensation. There is associated weight loss but no stigmata of systemic disease. He has a background of well-controlled asthma.

Plan

Patient's concerns

Reassure Anthony about the need for further investigation and control of his pain and nutritional parameters.

Investigations

FBC, U&E, LFT, CRP, CD4 count and viral load. Throat swab sent for MC&S. HIV test will need to be considered. A barium swallow and abdominal and chest radiograph should be performed.

F/U or admission

- Anthony requires symptom control, nutritional replacement and further investigation.
- This should be performed as an inpatient.

Differential diagnosis

- Infective oesophagitis (candidiasis, CMV, herpes).
- Reactive oesophagitis (reflux, Crohn's, Behçet's or drug-induced).
- Oesophageal stricturing conditions (systemic sclerosis, benign stricture, oesophageal carcinoma, oesophageal dysmotility).

Discussion related to the case

The incidence of dysphagia increases with age and is uncommon in the young. Candidates should elicit a history to differentiate between true dysphagia and odynophagia. Although the two can coexist, an examiner would expect a structured differential list prioritized on the merits of the predominant symptom, rather than a recited differential list for all causes of dysphagia.

By a process of elimination, an infective cause of Anthony's symptoms should be a candidate's top differential:

- Oesophageal cancer does affect men more than women and is seen in blacks more than whites, however:
  - The mean age at presentation of 55 years old.
  - There is usually a predisposing factor (e.g. reflux disease, coeliac disease or achalasia).
  - There is a strong association with smoking.
- Oesophageal dysmotility syndromes are seen in 5–10% of adults in the 5th–6th decades of life – they are usually associated with neuromuscular disease and diabetes mellitus.
- Progressive systemic sclerosis almost invariably has cutaneous manifestations before GI disease with a much longer history of dysphagia.
- Oesophageal involvement is an atypical presenting feature of Crohn's disease.
- Anthony has been trialled on anti-reflux medication with little effect and there are no irritant drugs in the history that can cause oesophagitis.

Candidates should have confidence in directly, but at the same time, sensitively questioning Anthony regarding his sexual history to establish his risk for retroviral disease. A good rapport needs to be built with the patient during history taking before the sexual history is obtained.

- It is likely that Anthony has HIV and is suffering from an AIDS defining illness in the form of oesophageal candidiasis.
- This causative agent is more likely than CMV or herpes because of the improvement in symptoms with nystatin.
- The pathogen cannot be entirely elicited by history alone:
  - Candida affects up to 80% of people with HIV.
  - It is one of the more common AIDS-defining illnesses along with PCP pneumonia, NHL, PML and Kaposi's sarcoma.
  - Oesophageal involvement requires systemic treatment as topical lozenges are subtherapeutic.

A multiorgan approach to HIV focusing on CNS, GI, pulmonary and retinal involvement is essential. Seroconversion can occur months or years before presentation. Anthony's previous episode of glandular fever may in fact have been a seroconversion illness and he therefore may have contracted HIV at the start of his relationship with his new partner.
- In reality, eliciting this chronological history is unusual, but in a simulated PACES exam this could easily be the case.

Anthony requires risk stratification with pre-test counselling for HIV.
- Most hospitals have a specialized nurse to whom Anthony should be referred.
- Expecting a positive result, it would be prudent to involve a sexual health consultant.

Should Anthony be found to be HIV positive:
- Combination therapy should be started as soon as the diagnosis of HIV is confirmed.
- Symptom control can be achieved through analgesia and IV antifungal agents.
- Remembering that Anthony is your patient at all times, it should be suggested that he discuss the new diagnosis with his partner and encourage him to undergo an HIV test.
- Candidates should extend psychosocial support to Anthony's partner, in the first instance, through local hospital resources in line with local policy.
- The importance of contact tracing other sexual partners should be strongly emphasized.

Despite the resilience of youth, HIV has a social stigma attached to it. A multidisciplinary approach is of paramount importance, as HIV usually requires an extra level of support over and above that of normal chronic diseases. With strong communication between specialists, Anthony's GP and good psychosocial support, it would be reassuring to think that Anthony's life expectancy would be no different to that of another person his age.

❶ Top Tips
- Shorter ordered differentials score higher than longer lists of unrelated differentials.
- Confidence and experience required prior to exam in asking sensitive questions e.g. sexuality.
- It is very trusting of patients to invoke parts of the history (e.g. use of condoms) and the information should be used sensitively and respectfully.

Viva questions

What is the pathophysiology of achalasia?

Achalasia is an oesophageal motility disorder with loss of normal organized peristalsis and failure of relaxation of the lower oesophageal sphincter. It is most commonly idiopathic in aetiology, but it has been hypothesized to an abnormality of Auerbach's plexus. A small proportion of secondary achalasia is caused by Chagas disease or gastric carcinoma at the stomach cardia.

Describe possible features seen on the barium swallow in this case

A barium swallow study is the gold standard investigation and demonstrates the following features:
- A dilated mega-oesophagus.
- Absence of primary peristalsis below the level of the cricopharyngeus.
- Tapering of the lower oesophagus with narrowing of the gastro-oesophageal junction, classically described as a 'rat-tail' deformity.
- Transit delay of contrast passage into the stomach.

What are the common retroviral drugs used for the treatment of HIV?

There are 3 main categories of retroviral drugs; these are nucleoside reverse transcriptase inhibitors (NRTIs), non-nucleoside reverse transcriptase inhibitors (NNRTIs) and protease inhibitors (PIs). Be aware of new drugs in development including T20 fusion inhibitors. A standard 1st-line regimen would be Combivir® (two NRTIs: zidovudine + lamivudine) boosted by a PI (nelfinavir). Should patients suffer greatly from the documented side effects of GI disturbance, lethargy, myalgia and lactic acidosis, more selective drugs are available although these are understandably more expensive. Please note: this treatment regimen is correct at the time of print and candidates are recommended to maintain knowledge of current drug policy in the treatment of HIV.

Cardiology

Tevfik F. Ismail
Mike Fisher

Introduction

A useful mnemonic for any examination routine is HELP. Every case should begin with:

- **H**ello: introduce yourself to the patient and explain what you are going to do.
- **E**xpose: expose the patient adequately for the proposed examination but with utmost care to preserve the patient's modesty and dignity. For the cardiovascular examination, you need to expose from the waist up as well as the arms, and the lower limbs. Once you have finished inspecting, cover the patient up to avoid exposing for an unnecessary length of time.
- **L**ighting: a spotlight should be shone upwards at the neck at 45° (90° away from your viewing angle) to enable you to maximize the chances of seeing any pulsations.
- **P**ain and **P**osition: always ensure that the patient is comfortable and is appropriately positioned at 45° to enable accurate assessment of the venous pressure.

Summary of suggested order of examination

1. Look at the patient from the end of the bed and don't forget to look around the bed for additional clues. Vital clues such as a raised JVP can be identified at an early stage with appropriate inspection.
2. Check hands, nails, lips, mouth and conjunctivae for peripheral signs of possible cardiac disease.
3. Feel the radial pulse noting the 5 features (rate, rhythm, character, volume and nature of the vessel wall, then feel both radial pulses simultaneously, eliciting for radial–radial delay or a difference in volume between the 2 sides. Then assess for radial–femoral delay. While you are doing this, look for the JVP at the same time.
4. Check for a collapsing pulse. (This is frequently forgotten by candidates.)
5. Palpate the apex, noting position and character – if you can't feel it, be honest, but remember to check on the right!
6. Listen at the apex remembering to time against the carotid pulse and while you are doing this note for any abnormality (slow-rising, bisferiens, jerky). If you hear a systolic murmur, check for radiation to axilla. If you don't hear a diastolic murmur, listen with the bell and if necessary perform the reinforcement manoeuvres described later.
7. Move diaphragm to the tricuspid, pulmonary and aortic areas. Again check for any radiation.
8. Ask your patient to sit forward and listen in expiration for an early diastolic murmur. Whilst your patient is still upright listen to lung bases and check for sacral oedema.
9. Check for ankle oedema, ask for the BP (if this has not already been requested) and any other additional features you would like to know.

With practice, this sequence can easily be completed within 3 minutes.

Inspection

- Start by looking for signs of syndromes with associated cardiovascular disease, for instance:
  - Down's syndrome (low-set ears, epicanthic folds, flat nasal bridge).
  - Ankylosing spondylitis (question-mark posture, restricted neck movements).
  - Marfan's syndrome (tall, arachnodactyly, arm span >height).
  - Turner's syndrome (webbed neck, cubitus valgus, short stature, infertility).
  - Noonan's syndrome (similar phenotype to Turner's syndrome, but may be present in men and both pregnant or non-pregnant women, as opposed to Turner's syndrome which is associated with infertility).
  - Williams syndrome (elfin facies).
  - Holt–Oram syndrome (triphalangeal thumb, radial hypoplasia).
- If you see any of these features, demonstrate this to the examiner, for example, ask the patient with marfanoid features to stand up and demonstrate their arm span or ask the ankylosing spondylitis patient to move their cervical spine thus revealing the restricted spinal movements.

❶ Top Tips
- Many candidates look but do not see. The chances of you ascertaining a sign are increased if you are looking for specific things actively rather than blindly inspecting.
- Start by standing right at the centre of the edge of the bed (avoiding parallax). If nothing else, this makes a show of the fact that you are inspecting (the first part of the examiner's marking scheme).

- Inspect the face for a malar flush (pulmonary hypertension with low cardiac output, typically in mitral stenosis) or a slate-grey rash in photo-exposed areas (adverse effect of amiodarone).
- Look for arterial (Corrigan's sign – AR) or venous pulsations (C–V waves – TR). Sometimes a slow rising pulse can be detected on inspection.
- Look for signs of current or previous central access or scars on the chest from tunnelled lines. These can be a source of endocarditis (particularly of the tricuspid valve) but may also have been used to administer long-term antibiotics giving a clue that the patient may have suffered endocarditis in the past.
- Inspect the praecordium for a sternotomy scar. If one is present, immediately glance at the legs to see if there are any scars from vein graft harvesting.

❶ Top Tips
- If there are such scars, then as part of your presentation at the end, regardless of what else you have found, you can say:
  - 'This patient has ischaemic heart disease and has had surgical revascularization with coronary artery bypass surgery.'

- Ask the patient to lift up his/her arms so that you do not miss a thoracotomy scar near the axilla or any other pertinent scars. For female patients, ask the patient to lift her breast up so that you can look for an inframammary scar (mitral valvotomy).
- Look for scars from current or previous devices such as a pacemaker or automatic implantable cardioverter-defibrillator (ICD).
- Note any gynaecomastia (e.g. from digoxin or spironolactone use or indeed both).
- Look for any obvious apical pulsation to determine the location of the apex beat.
- Listen for audible clicks from a prosthetic mechanical heart valve.

❶ Top Tips
- The *loudest* sound that you can hear from the edge of the bed is always the closure sound that the prosthetic valve makes. If you hear the click after the carotid pulse, the valve must be in the aortic position and if you hear it prior to the carotid pulse, it must be in the mitral position. If you hear 2 clicks, then think of a double-valve replacement (likely aetiology – rheumatic heart disease or endocarditis).
- Look for bruising or signs of over-anticoagulation in mechanical prosthetic valve patients and in patients who are in atrial fibrillation.

- Look at the nails for splinter haemorrhages, clubbing, peripheral cyanosis and Quinke's sign. Inspect the hands for Osler's nodes (tender, erythematous raised lesions on the pulps of the fingers), Janeway lesions (non-tender, flat erythematous macular lesions on the palms or soles of the feet). Look for evidence of a triphalangeal thumb or radial hypoplasia (Holt–Oram syndrome – associated with secundum atrial septal defects [ASDs], ventricular septal defects [VSDs] and rhythm disorders).

Palpation (Table 5.1)
- With both arms straight and stretched out, feel both radial pulses at the same time. If there is a volume deficit between the 2 sides, consider the presence of a Blalock–Taussig shunt and look for 2 additional scars: a thoracotomy scar on the side of the shunt from the palliative Blalock procedure and a sternotomy scar from the subsequent total correction operation. Other causes of a reduced/absent radial pulse include:
  - Cervical rib.
  - Subclavian stenosis.

- Radial artery injury e.g. from catheterization, cannulation or trauma.
- Congenitally absent or atretic radial artery.
- Radial artery harvesting for bypass graft surgery.
- Arteriovenous fistula.
- Takayasu's arteritis.
- Interrupted arch syndromes.
- Coarctation of the aorta with subclavian patch repair.

- Assess the heart rate and rhythm at the radial pulse, counting to at least 10 to ensure you are not missing atrial fibrillation. If the patient has a pacemaker, make sure that the heart rate is timed with precision in case it is firing exactly at its demand rate.

- Assess the character of the pulse at the brachial artery, determining whether it is normal, slow rising or collapsing. Holding the forearm by the wrist with one hand and supporting the elbow with the other, lift up the arm and forearm so that they are aligned, and straight above heart height. In so doing, you are straightening out the natural kinks in the brachial artery and in the axillary/subclavian junction that may mask a collapsing pulse. A collapsing pulse is present when there is a definite change of character on raising the arm from a merely prominent pulse to a definite tapping sensation.

---

❶ Top Tips

- Feel for the collapsing pulse with the flat parts of your fingers around the distal interphalangeal joints, rather than the tips, which are too sensitive. Hold the patient's wrist with your fingers over, not under, the wrist. This means that when you lift the wrist, you don't end up twisting your own body and looking awkward.
- When you have lifted, it is often necessary to wait a few seconds before the tapping or 'water-hammer' character of the pulse is felt.

- Look at the eyes for signs of anaemia, vasculitic lesions in both conjunctivae and jaundice (pre-hepatic from intravascular haemolysis around a leaking prosthetic valve or hepatic from cardiac cirrhosis). Look for corneal arcus and other periorbital stigmata of dyslipidaemia e.g. xanthelasma. If the patient has a marfanoid habitus then look at the eyes for ectopia lentis, the iris for iridodonesis (shimmering of the iris) and note the presence of blue sclerae.
- Look inside the mouth for evidence of poor dentition and also at the undersurface of the tongue for signs of central cyanosis. In severe AR, you may be able to see the uvula bobbing up and down (Muller's sign). The head may also be seen to bob up and down in the latter (de Musset's sign).
- Look at the side of the neck for signs of the typical plucked chicken skin suggestive of pseudoxanthoma elasticum, a cause of premature coronary artery disease and a classic exam case.
- Turn the head slightly to the left and use a spot light to visualize the JVP. Measure its vertical height above the sternal angle (normal ≤3cm). If the patient is in sinus rhythm, there should be

2 pulsations visible: a v-wave with or after the pulse and an a-wave preceding the pulse. Assess their prominence.

❶ Top Tips
- The rise and fall of the JVP with respiration is one of the quickest and easiest characteristics to look for when examining in a hurry. If you are unsure about the position of the JVP, check for hepatojugular reflux by first warning the patient and then gently pressing in the right upper quadrant. This will cause a transient rise in the JVP, often revealing its presence.

- Palpate the carotids once again to assess heart rate, rhythm, and character.
- Localize the apex beat and find the point of maximum impulse with one finger (demonstrating that you have done so for the examiner's benefit!). If it cannot be felt, check on the right side just in case there is dextrocardia. The apex is a pulse so assess its rate (especially if there is poorly rate controlled AF resulting in an apico-radial pulse deficit), rhythm and character, and feel for apical thrills. The apex may be normal, tapping (MS), heaving (pressure-loaded) or thrusting (volume-loaded).

❶ Top Tips
- If you cannot localize the apex beat, tilt the patient in the left lateral position. You then cannot comment on its position but you can still comment on the other factors mentioned earlier and this is particularly important when trying to determine the predominant pathology in mixed-valve disease: the compensatory response of the ventricle is the final arbiter.
- If you still cannot find the apex beat, make sure you are not missing dextrocardia. Feel the other side.

Table 5.1 Areas to palpate in the praecordium and possible findings and significance of these

Area to palpate	Possible findings
Apex	Position (heart clinically enlarged)
	Thrusting character (volume overloaded)
	Heaving character (pressure overloaded)
	Tapping (MS)
	Thrill (very severe MR)
Left sternal edge	RV heave (pressure overloaded RV indicating pulmonary hypertension)
	Thrill – VSD, very occasionally TR
Pulmonary area	Palpable 2nd heart sound (pulmonary hypertension)
Aortic area	Thrill (AS)

- Place your whole hand just to the left of the sternal edge slightly angled to the left in the direction of the right ventricular outflow tract (RVOT) feeling for thrills (either from TR, or by definition, a small VSD) and a RV heave (implying a pressure-loaded RV). Feel separately in the pulmonary area for thrills and a palpable 2nd heart sound. If the 2nd heart sound is palpable, by definition, it must be loud. Similarly, feel in the aortic area for thrills.

Auscultation

By now, you should already have a good idea of what the diagnosis is or at least of what it isn't and should be using auscultation only to confirm your suspicions (Table 5.2). The diagram of the cardiac cycle at the end of this section (Fig. 5.1) illustrates when murmurs will start and finish. Note especially the pansystolic murmurs of AV valve regurgitation will start at the 1st heart sound (when these close) and extend *beyond* the 2nd heart sound. Explaining this could well be a viva question!

❶ Top Tips

- Remember to time all murmurs against the carotid or subclavian pulse. Do not time against the radial pulse as there may be a delay especially with critical aortic stenosis, or some of the apical impulses may not reach the radial artery especially with rapid heart rates or irregular R–R intervals such as with AF.

- Mitral area:
  - Start with the bell in the mitral area. Listen initially just for the heart sounds. You need to decide whether the 1st heart sound is normal, loud (MS, hypertension) or soft (MR).
  - Listen also for the rumbling low-pitched mid-diastolic murmur of MS. If you cannot hear it, tilt the patient into the left lateral position, localize the apex and auscultate again. If you are still not sure, ask the patient to do some gentle exercise such as sit ups to increase transmitral flow and thereby accentuate the murmur. Remember to time all murmurs against the carotid or subclavian pulse.

❶ Top Tips

- When using the bell, remember to hold it off the chest slightly rather than pressing it on to the chest. Pressing too hard will turn it into a diaphragm, filtering out the very sounds you are trying to hear. If you are pressing too hard, you will leave a rim on the patient's skin and your fingernails will go pale making it obvious to any attentive examiner.

  - Switch to the diaphragm or, if using a stethoscope with a dual tuneable chest piece, press to ensure the diaphragm is engaged.

- Listen in the mitral area for murmurs. If you do hear a murmur, try and ascertain whether it is uniform in quality and/or timbre and if it extends throughout systole (MR). If there is a normal 1st heart sound and a gap before the murmur, it may represent mitral valve (MV) prolapse, in which case a mid-systolic click may also be present. Otherwise, make sure you are not missing mixed MV disease with MS.
- Remember the murmur of MR generally radiates to the axilla, but beware of the murmur of posterior MV prolapse. Because the jet is medially directed, it can strike the wall of the atrium close to the aortic valve and hence may be well heard in the aortic area. Conversely a loud aortic murmur may be heard all over the praecordium, but generally does not radiate to the axilla and does not extend to the 2nd heart sound.
- If you are not completely sure what you are hearing, ask the patient to breathe out slowly: this will accentuate mitral murmurs. If the murmur has a crescendo–decrescendo character, it could represent a very loud ejection systolic murmur from the aortic valve that is audible throughout the praecordium so do auscultate carefully.

❶ Top Tips

- The harsh barking crescendo–decrescendo murmur of AS may sometimes be heard best at the lower left sternal edge rather than in the aortic area (Gallavardin phenomenon/radiation).
- A muscular VSD may give rise to a crescendo murmur which may not extend for the whole of systole as the hole decreases in size during systole as opposed to a VSD in the membranous interventricular septum (the more common location), which generally will remain the same size throughout systole giving rise to a more uniform pansystolic murmur.

- Move to the left sternal edge (tricuspid area):
  - Listen with the bell at the left sternal edge for 3rd and 4th heart sounds or pericardial knocks.
  - If you hear a pan-systolic murmur, determine whether it is louder at the left sternal edge (TR or VSD) or in the mitral area (MR). If the murmur is louder at the left sternal edge, ask the patient to take a long deep breath in. TR, like other right-sided murmurs, gets louder during inspiration.
  - The intensity of a murmur from a small VSD will not usually change with respiration as ventricular filling will not be a major factor contributing to its propagation, particularly if the defect is small.
- Pulmonary area:
  - Listen initially only to the 2nd heart sound. Is it normal, loud (suggestive of pulmonary hypertension) or soft?
  - Listen for splitting of the 2nd heart sound if you are familiar with this; if not do not worry, it is not particularly important in the exam other than for assisting in the diagnosis of an ASD where there is fixed wide-splitting of the 2nd heart sound rather than increasing

physiological split with inspiration and decreasing split with expiration.
- If you hear a pulmonary ejection murmur, check whether it radiates to the back and whether it gets louder with inspiration to ensure you are not mistaking AS for pulmonary stenosis (PS).
- Aortic area:
  - Listen for the harsh barking ejection systolic murmur of AS over the right 2nd intercostal space. In the presence of an ejection systolic murmur, check for radiation to the carotids.
  - Also listen intently for the 2nd heart sound. A quiet 2nd heart sound may be a sign of severe AS. Again, expiration will accentuate the ejection systolic murmur of AS.

Diastolic murmurs

These are difficult! The clue to the correct diagnosis is in the other signs that have been gathered prior to auscultation, which is why it is so important to avoid the lemming-like rush to the stethoscope. Consequently if you hear an ejection systolic murmur at the base of the heart, but the pulse is collapsing, the heart clinically dilated as judged by the apex and the 2nd heart sound not quiet, even if you cannot hear an early diastolic murmur, the patient almost certainly has predominant AR. Likewise a patient with a malar flush, AF, a tapping apex and a loud 1st heart sound has MS, even if you can't hear the opening snap (which won't be present if the valve is calcified and rigid) or the mid-diastolic murmur.

- Now ask the patient to sit forward, take a deep breath all the way in and breathe all the way out, holding the breath at the end of expiration. Listen carefully for the high pitched blowing early diastolic murmur of AR first in the aortic area (with suspected aortic root disease) and then at the left sternal edge (for valvular AR).
- Auscultate the bases for the coarse late inspiratory crackles of pulmonary oedema. If there is extensive cardiac failure, there may be bi-basal effusions. Listen also for bruits from intercostal collaterals in aortic coarctation and, if this has not been corrected, an interscapular murmur from the coarctation itself. Look for the typical left thoracotomy scar of the requisite surgery.
- Tell the patient (and thereby also the examiner) that you are going to press in the sacrum for 5–10 seconds to check for pitting oedema. If necessary, do the same at the ankles (ensuring that you press with one finger in one place over the tibial plateau) and if there is bilateral pitting oedema, determine the proximal extent.
- If a patient had signs of TR and is able to lie flat, palpate for a pulsatile liver edge. If endocarditis is likely, offer to feel for splenomegaly. Do not palpate for hepatomegaly or splenomegaly routinely.

- Complete your examination by asking to dip-stick the urine for haematuria and proteinuria (endocarditis) and glycosuria (cardiac risk factor) and checking the temperature chart.
- Offer to measure the BP which may provide an important clue to the underlying diagnosis as well as helping to assess the haemodynamic effects of any lesion.

Table 5.2 Summarizing the discriminating features of the main valvular lesions. This table can also be used to determine which is the predominant lesion in mixed lesion cases

	Aortic		Mitral	
	Stenosis	Regurgitation	Stenosis	Regurgitation
Apex	Heaving (minimally displaced)	Displaced and thrusting	Tapping	Displaced
Pulse	Slow-rising	Collapsing (occasionally bisferiens)	AF	Perhaps AF
Heart sounds	2nd quiet	Normal	1st loud	Normal

Presentation

As a minimum, without having to be asked, you must be able to comment on at least 5 things:

- Which valve(s) and what lesion(s)?
- How bad is it? Or, for a prosthetic valve, is it functioning well?
- Is there any heart failure?
- Is there any evidence of endocarditis (assumed to be present until proven otherwise)?
- What caused it? If there is no obvious cause, speculate from your knowledge of general medicine.

Common Pitfalls

- If you don't tell the examiner that there were no stigmata of bacterial endocarditis, (s)he may just assume you didn't check.
- If you don't tell the examiners how severe you thought the AS was, they may justifiably assume you didn't assess it or were not interested.

The cardiac cycle

Fig. 5.1 shows the cardiac cycle and links the events with the pressure changes in the various cardiac chambers, shown in Fig. 5.2. Relate the timing of the different murmurs and how these relate to the heart sounds and the cardiac events.

The cardiac cycle

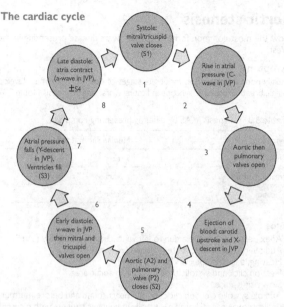

Fig. 5.1 The cardiac cycle.

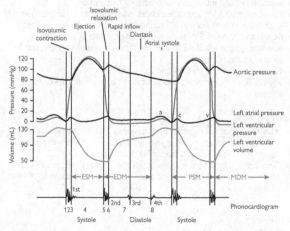

Fig. 5.2 Pressure events. ESM, ejection systolic murmur; EDM, early diastolic murmur; PSM, pan-systolic murmur; MDM, mid-diastolic murmur; Key: blue line: left ventricular pressure; grey line: left ventricular volume; top black line: aortic pressure; lower black line: left atrial pressure.

Aortic stenosis

Now the most common form of valvular heart disease presenting in the West.

Symptoms

Usually none in the mild to moderate stages of severity. Later may develop angina, breathlessness, or syncope indicating worsening prognosis (Table 5.3).

Table 5.3 Prognosis in AS by differing presenting complaint

Symptom	Median survival time
Chest pain	5 years
Breathlessness	2 years
Syncope	18 months

Signs

- Apex beat may be visible due to left ventricular hypertrophy (LVH).
- Audible murmur without stethoscope (very rare).
- Heaving, palpable apex (LVH).
- Ejection click and systolic thrill palpable in aortic area.
- Slow rising pulse.
- Audible systolic ejection click after 1st heart sound and before murmur (indicates valve is still pliable – usually in younger patients with bicuspid valves).
- Ejection systolic murmur, likely radiating to carotids.
- Reduced/absent 2nd sound (indicates valve is stiff and that stenosis is at least moderate. A normal 2nd sound makes severe AS very unlikely).
- Reverse splitting of 2nd sound due to late closure of aortic valve (unusual – generally if AS has reached this degree of severity, the second sound is absent).
- 4th heart sound due to LVH and stiff ventricle.
- Signs of left or right heart failure if caused by AS indicate very severe disease.

❶ Top Tips

- The volume of the murmur has no relationship to the severity of the stenosis, indeed the murmur may get quieter as the stenosis becomes severe and flow through the valve reduces.
- Severity is judged by the character of the arterial pulse, presence or absence of the 2nd heart sound and the presence or absence of signs of heart failure.

Aetiology

- Calcific degenerative is the most common.
- Congenital, usually associated with a bicuspid valve.
- Rheumatic (now quite rare).

Important differential diagnoses

- Aortic sclerosis: note that in practice, this overlaps with mild AS.
- PS: normal pulse character, aortic 2nd sound normal, although pulmonary component may be reduced. Murmur gets louder on inspiration.
- VSD: frequently very loud murmur, heard all over the praecordium. Murmur maximal at sternal edge, rather than aortic area. Much more likely to be associated with a thrill (Maladie de Roger).
- Hypertrophic obstructive cardiomyopathy: jerky pulse, murmur gets quieter if the patient crouches down due to increased afterload and consequent splinting open of the outflow tract. No ejection click, normal 2nd heart sound. Often in a younger person.
- Subaortic membrane (rare): no ejection click, normal 2nd sound.
- Supra-valvular obstruction (extremely rare): no election click, normal 2nd sound.

Investigation

- Echocardiography to confirm the diagnosis and grade the disease in terms of severity (Table 5.4). Very useful for following the progression of any stenosis. Note that valve area is the preferred method for grading the severity of AS, because this accounts for the fact that gradient will reduce if LV function is impaired, but measurement of valve area is more subject to error than other measures. Ideally valve area should be normalized to body surface area (BSA), with severe AS being $<0.6cm^2/m^2$.
- Stress echocardiography: can be very useful in the presence of poor LV function to decide whether the impaired LV is due to severe AS and therefore may benefit from surgery, or if the main problem is due to intrinsic myocardial disease with incidental and non-contributory AS, which does not improve with aortic valve replacement.
- Cardiac catheterization: coronary angiography will be necessary prior to surgery. A pullback gradient across the valve is rarely necessary in the modern era of echocardiography and getting a catheter across a severely stenosed valve is associated with radiological evidence of stroke in 22% of cases and clinical neurological deficit in 3%.[1] Likewise, right heart catheterization is rarely required.

Table 5.4 Common criteria for echocardiographic grading of severity of AS

	Mild	Moderate	Severe
Valve area	$>1.5cm^2$	$1–1.5cm^2$	$<1cm^2$
Mean valve gradient	<20mmHg	20–40mmHg	>40mmHg

Management

If asymptomatic, it is generally recommended that 6–12-monthly follow-up is sufficient.

Some would recommend surgery if the stenosis is severe, even in the absence of symptoms. The following criteria are typical:

- Consider operating if mean gradient >40mmHg and any of:
  - LV systolic dysfunction i.e. ejection fraction (EF)<45%

- Abnormal response to exercise (↓ BP)
- Ventricular tachycardia
- LVH >15mm
- Valve area <0.6cm^2
- Less invasive options for valve replacement are starting to become available. Percutaneous and transapical valve replacement is now being offered at several centres in the UK.
- Aortic balloon valvuloplasty has largely fallen out of favour as the results are poor, but is still occasionally used to try and tide a very sick patient over, when the expectation is that they will be fit for a more definitive procedure at a later date.

Viva questions

What are the common complications of AS?
- Endocarditis
- Heart failure
- AV block due to invasion of calcium from the valve ring into the His–Purkinje system
- Embolic events.

How would you differentiate sclerosis from stenosis?
Normal pulse character, normal 2nd heart sound, frequently in an elderly person. Note this overlaps with mild AS.

How would you differentiate between different grades of AS?
(Remember to start with clinical examination)
- In severe AS one sees slow-rising pulse, absent 2nd sound, possibly with evidence of heart failure clinically.
- Investigations – → Investigation, p.229. Remember to discuss the situation of apparently low gradient when LV is impaired.

What are the associated conditions?
- Coarctation of the aorta (remember to check for radio-femoral delay).
- Other valvular disease, particularly mitral in rheumatic valvular disease.
- Angiodysplasia of the colon and anaemia.

What are the indications for surgery?
- Symptomatic AS. This is particularly and urgently the case if the symptom is syncope, in which case the median survival is only 4 months.
- Asymptomatic AS where the gradient is 40mmHg or more and any of the following also apply:
  - LV systolic dysfunction i.e. EF <45%
  - Abnormal response to exercise (↓ BP)
  - VT
  - LVH >15mm
  - Valve area <0.6cm^2

Reference
1. Omran H et al. Silent and apparent cerebral embolism after retrograde catheterisation of the aortic valve in valvular stenosis: a prospective, randomised study. *Lancet* 2003; **361**:1241–6.

📖 Further reading
Bonow RO et al. Guidelines for the management of patients with valvular heart disease. *Circulation* 2008; **118**:e523–e661.

Aortic regurgitation

The causes of this lesion have changed significantly over the last 200 years. Previously syphilis was the commonest cause, but now it is more usually associated with bicuspid valves. As with other valvular regurgitation, a trivial degree of AR is common and may actually be normal.

Symptoms

The usual symptom is breathlessness as the degree of regurgitation becomes moderate. Chest pain is not uncommon. Patients may go on to experience other symptoms of heart failure as the condition progresses. It is not uncommon for AR to be asymptomatic, even in the presence of quite severe regurgitation.

Signs

> **❶ Top Tips**
> * AR is a lesion where a characteristic of the murmur does reflect severity. As the lesion becomes more severe, the murmur shortens. (❺ 'Viva questions', p.233 for a fuller explanation of this phenomenon.)

* Common:
    * Collapsing pulse (❺ Introduction, p.221 for notes on detecting this).
    * Wide pulse pressure.
    * Cardiac dilatation.
    * Early diastolic murmur, usually maximal at lower left sternal edge, but may be best heard in the aortic area, particularly if the aorta is significantly dilated for any reason.
    * Corrigan's pulse.
* Uncommon:
    * De Musset's sign – bobbing of the head with each pulse.
    * Durozier's sign – murmur heard over femoral arteries when the stethoscope is pressed over the vessel.
    * Quincke's sign – visible pulsing of the capillary filling of the nail bed.

Note there is a formal definition of a collapsing pulse, which is that the pulse pressure should be greater than the diastolic pressure. In other words, the systolic pressure will be more than twice the diastolic.

Aetiology

This should be considered depending on the pattern of onset as being acute or chronic AR.

Acute AR
* Infective endocarditis
* Aortic dissection
* Prosthetic valve failure
* Ruptured sinus of Valsalva (rare)
* Acute rheumatic fever (rare in the West, but not elsewhere)

Chronic AR
- Bicuspid aortic valve
- Marfan's syndrome
- Aorto-annular ectasia
- Rheumatic heart disease
- Endocarditis
- Seronegative arthritides
- Syphilis (now rare)
- Osteogenesis imperfecta (very rare)

Differential diagnosis
Pulmonary regurgitation (PR). The murmur may be similar but is not maximal at the lower left sternal border, and none of the other signs are present.

Associated conditions
Remember to look for other features of the possible aetiologies i.e. coarctation of the aorta, endocarditis, features of Marfan's syndrome (→ Marfan's syndrome, p.277), typical patterns of seronegative arthritis, ankylosing spondylitis (listen to the lung apices), syphilis etc.

Investigation
- As with all valvular heart disease, echocardiography is the mainstay of investigation to confirm the diagnosis and to grade it. See Table 5.5 for parameters that are considered to determine severe AR.
- MRI is gaining an ever greater place in the assessment of valvular disease, but particularly regurgitation, as it is able to accurately quantify EF, LV dimensions, and particularly regurgitant fraction.
- Coronary angiography may be necessary as a prelude to surgery to check for coronary disease, but otherwise does not add anything to the above modalities.

Table 5.5 Commonly used echo criteria for severe AR

Width of AR jet on colour flow	RF	LVEDD (corrected for BSA)	LVESD (BSA corrected)	Pressure half-time of Doppler slope of AR
>65% of LVOT	>50%	>70mm (>35mm/m²)	>50mm (>25mm/m²)	<200ms

LVEDD, left ventricular end-diastolic diameter; LVESD, left ventricular end-systolic diameter; RF, regurgitant fraction.

Management
- If AR is acute, then if the severity is anything more than mild, surgery is the treatment of choice.
- In chronic AR, if there are symptoms, i.e. anything worse than class I breathlessness or anginal chest pain, then again valve replacement should be offered.
- Generally in those with asymptomatic AR of whatever severity, the event rate is low and is less than that of surgery, so conservative medical management with ACE inhibitors and diuretics is indicated.

If AR is severe, even in the absence of symptoms, the following features would indicate valve replacement is appropriate:
- LV dilatation as defined in Table 5.5
- EF <50%
- Significant aortic root dilatation (maximal root diameter >45mm in Marfan's, >50mm with bicuspid valve or >55mm otherwise)
- Those undergoing any other cardiac surgery

Complications
- Endocarditis
- Heart failure

Viva questions

What are the possible aetiologies of AR?
Note the earlier discussion for a full list, but it is useful to remember to categorize the causes into acute and chronic types.

What are the indications for surgery?
- Symptomatic
- Dilated heart – see Table 5.5 for definitions
- EF <50%
- RF >50%. Note that rugurgitant fraction can be accurately determined by cardiac MR.

Does a longer murmur mean more or less severe AR and why?
A shorter murmur indicates more severe regurgitation. This is due to more severe flow of blood back into the LV, causing ever more rapid rise in the LV diastolic pressure. This results in the regurgitant flow diminishing much earlier in diastole as the gradient between aorta and LV diminishes.

What clinical findings would suggest severe AR?
- Clinically dilated heart
- Signs of left-sided heart failure
- Very wide pulse pressure
- Short murmur.

📖 Further reading
Bonow RO et al. Guidelines for the management of patients with valvular heart disease. *Circulation* 2008; **118**:e523–e661.

Mitral stenosis

The patient may present with symptoms consistent with heart failure (fatigue, exertional dyspnoea, orthopnoea, paroxysmal nocturnal dyspnoea, fluid retention) and AF (palpitations, decreased exercise tolerance, stroke), hoarse voice (Ortner's syndrome – compression of the left recurrent laryngeal nerve by the enlarged left atrium (LA) and/or pulmonary artery), haemoptysis (due to rupture of bronchial veins) or fever (due to endocarditis but more common in mixed MV disease).

Signs

- Note the age, gender and ethnic origin of patient (2:1 female:male ratio, Caucasian patients tend to be older because of declining incidence of rheumatic fever in the UK).
- Malar flush – dusky red discoloration of the maxillary eminences sparing the nasal bridge, due to a combination of severe pulmonary hypertension, low cardiac output and elevated venous pressures.
- Inframammary/left thoracotomy scar from previous mitral valvotomy.
- Stigmata of endocarditis (➔ p.262).
- Bruising from warfarin for AF, a complication of MS.
- Pulse may be regular or irregularly irregular suggestive of AF.
- JVP may be elevated suggesting right heart failure. There may be a prominent A-wave in the presence of sinus rhythm and pulmonary hypertension and/or a prominent systolic CV wave in the presence of secondary TR.
- Apex – usually undisplaced unless there is mixed MV disease. The apex may be tapping in character reflecting a loud S1. The LV has to generate a slightly higher pressure earlier in systole to exceed the raised LA pressure and close the mitral valve. Although the edges of the rheumatic leaflets are thickened and rigid, the scallops themselves, particularly of the anterior leaflet, remain mobile and bulge more briskly towards the LA causing a loud S1 and apical tap.
- Left parasternal heave due to RV pressure overload or a palpable forceful atrial contraction when the LA is grossly enlarged (rare as most patients are in AF by this stage). The latter can be distinguished from a RV-heave as it precedes the apical impulse whereas the RV heave is synchronous with it.

❦ Common Pitfalls

- The apex may appear heaving if the RV is so enlarged that it displaces the LV posteriorly and appears to form the apex. This may thereby give a false impression of the underlying lesion.

- Palpable P2 (suggestive of pulmonary hypertension and by definition implying a loud P2 on auscultation)
- On auscultation:
  - Loud S1 – 'closing snap'.
  - Loud S2 (due to loud P2 in the context of pulmonary hypertension). A2 and P2 may fuse with severe pulmonary hypertension resulting in loss of splitting of S2. This occurs because the high pulmonary

pressures force the pulmonary valve to close earlier. In addition, there may be a decrescendo early diastolic murmur from PR (Graham Steell murmur) heard loudest in the pulmonary area.

• Opening Snap (OS): this occurs shortly after P2 and is due to diastolic doming of the anterior leaflet of the MV. The rheumatic process causes thickening of the leaflet tips and edges as well as commissural fusion but leaves the main scallops of the anterior leaflet free. Also, as well as being much larger than the posterior leaflet, the chordae tendineae are attached mainly to the outside of the leaflet (unlike the posterior leaflet) leaving it free to snap open and dome towards the LV cavity in diastole generating the OS.

❶ Top Tips

• As the leaflets themselves become more thickened and scarred over time, the opening snap may be lost.
• It is also often absent in patients with congenital mitral stenosis where the leaflets are dysmorphic to begin with.

• Mid-diastolic murmur – low pitch rumbling sound heard immediately after the OS and best in the left lateral decubitus position at end-expiration with the bell.
• Signs of heart failure (pitting pedal or sacral oedema, coarse basal late inspiratory crackles).

❶ Top Tips

• If you cannot hear the murmur, ask the patient to perform a few sit-ups or to cough repeatedly to accentuate transmitral flow.
• If the patient is in sinus rhythm, the murmur may get louder towards the end of diastole as the transmitral flow is transiently augmented by atrial contraction. This is termed pre-systolic accentuation and by definition will be absent in AF.
• If the patient is in AF, listen for long gaps between heart beats. If during such gaps, the mid-diastolic murmur is long and extends up to S2, the MS is likely to be severe as the murmur only occurs when the pressure gradient between LA and LV is above 3mmHg. The longer this takes to dissipate, the more stenosed the valve must be.
• ~40% of patients with rheumatic mitral stenosis have multivalvular heart disease with the aortic valve being the most commonly involved second valve. Mixed MV disease is also very common, also affecting ~40% of patients, so do not miss this or the involvement of other valves.

❧ Common Pitfalls

• Other causes of mid-diastolic murmurs include flow in patients with severe MR, and the coincidence of atrial contraction and rapid passive LV-filling in patients with complete heart block but these can readily be differentiated by identifying associated features.

Severity
- Severe MS is suggested by:
  - The presence of AF.
  - Signs of pulmonary hypertension.
  - A short gap between S2 and the opening snap. This is because the LA pressure is very high in severe MS and therefore LA pressure exceeds ventricular pressure earlier, so opening the valve earlier.
  - A long mid-diastolic murmur (LA–LV gradient takes longer to equalize with increasing severity).
  - Signs of pulmonary congestion and right heart failure.
- Mild MS is suggested by the presence of sinus rhythm, absence of signs of pulmonary hypertension, absence of signs of pulmonary congestion or right heart failure and a short mid-diastolic murmur.
- Moderate MS is suggested by mixed features of either mild or severe MS. Reliable assessment of severity can be difficult even with investigations and can be significantly influenced by changes in physiological demand for instance due to pregnancy or an intercurrent infection.

Aetiology
- Rheumatic fever (>90% of cases).
- Degenerative: severe mitral annular calcification.
- Non-valvular: LA myxoma, ball-valve LA thrombus, large vegetations in infective endocarditis.
- Congenital:
  - Isolated
  - Cor triatriatum (division of one of the atria into 2 by a membrane)
  - Shone's syndrome (supravalvular mitral membrane, parachute MV, subaortic stenosis and aortic coarctation)
  - Mucopolysaccharidosis
  - Left-sided carcinoid syndrome (metastatic or bronchial carcinoid).
- Methysergide or ergot alkaloid valvulopathy (e.g. cabergoline).

Investigations
- 12-lead ECG – may reveal P-mitrale or AF.
- CXR to identify pulmonary congestion and haemosiderosis, and to assess LA size (splaying of subcarinal angle, loss of pulmonary bay).
- Transthoracic echocardiogram (TTE) to assess severity – mean gradient and mitral valve area (MVA); suitability for percutaneous balloon mitral valvuloplasty (PBMV); pulmonary pressures and RV function.
- Transoesophageal echocardiogram (TOE) for detailed assessment of valvular and subvalvular anatomy and to assess LA appendage for thrombus prior to PBMV.
- Right and left heart catheterization to assess coronary anatomy as part of work up for surgery, assess MVA and to assess pulmonary artery systolic (PASP) and wedge pressures (PAWP).

Viva questions

What are the indications for anticoagulation?

Those in AF (paroxysmal or sustained) should be on warfarin as the risk of thromboembolism is high and >3-fold higher than in non-rheumatic AF. Warfarin should be considered in those with LA >55mm even if in sinus rhythm.

How often should patients with MS be followed up?

Patients who are asymptomatic and have mild MS (MVA >1.5cm^2 or mean gradient <5mmHg) should be subject to annual follow-up.

Which patients should be offered percutaneous balloon mitral valvuloplasty/surgery?

- Patients who are asymptomatic but have moderate (MVA 1.0-1.5cm^2, mean gradient 5–10mmHg) or severe (MVA <1.0cm^2, mean gradient >10mmHg) MS should have their valve assessed for suitability for PBMV. If unsuitable, the patient should be followed up annually. If the valve is amenable, then pulmonary pressures should be evaluated. If the PASP is <50mmHg, does not rise above 60mmHg on exercise or the PAWP on right heart catheterization is <25mmHg, then the patient should be followed up annually.
- If, however, the PASP is >50mmHg, rises to >60mmHg with exercise, the PAWP is >25mmHg, or there is new onset AF, provided that the valve is suitable, either PBMV or surgery should be offered.
- Symptomatic patients with New York Heart Association (NYHA) II dyspnoea and moderate/severe MS should be offered PBMV if the valve is amenable. If unsuitable, surgical repair or replacement should be considered if there is severe pulmonary hypertension (PAP >60mmHg). Otherwise, the patient should be subjected to 6-monthly follow-up.
- Symptomatic patients with mild MS and NYHA II symptoms should be subjected to exercise testing. If the PAP rise to >60mmHg or mean gradient >15mmHg or the wedge pressure is >25mmHg, PBMV should be offered if the valve is suitable; otherwise the patient should be followed-up 6-monthly. Yearly follow-up and a search for alternative causes of breathlessness should be undertaken if these criteria are not met.
- Moderate or severe MS with NYHA III/IV dyspnoea is associated with a poor prognosis without intervention. PBMV should be offered if the valve is amenable, otherwise surgical repair or replacement should be undertaken. PBMV should be considered in any patient who is not fit for open heart surgery. Patients with mild MS and NYHA III/IV symptoms are managed as per similar patients with NYHA II dyspnoea (see above).

What determines suitability of a valve for PBMV?

- Leaflet mobility, thickening, subvalvular thickening and calcification are each separately assessed on a scale of 1–4 (Wilkins score).
- If the Wilkins score is ≤8, the valve is likely to be amenable.
- PBMV increases the severity of MR usually by one grade and therefore cannot be carried out if moderate or more severe MR is present.

- PBMV cannot be undertaken in the presence of LA thrombus due to the risk of embolization. If this persists despite anticoagulation, PBMV is *absolutely contraindicated*.

How do you manage MS presenting in pregnancy?

- Symptomatic patients with severe MS should be advised against pregnancy without prior treatment.
- Asymptomatic patients often present in the mid-trimester with symptoms as a result of the increased heart rate and intravascular volume associated with pregnancy.
- Patients with severe MS and NYHA III/IV symptoms that develop during pregnancy should be treated with PBMV with TOE guidance to minimize radiation exposure.

What is a normal MVA?

4–5cm^2 (depends on body size).

📖 Further reading

Bonow RO et al. Guidelines for the management of patients with valvular heart disease. *Circulation* 2008; **118**:e523–e661.

Mitral regurgitation

The patient may present with symptoms of heart failure (fatigue, exertional dyspnoea, orthopnoea, paroxysmal nocturnal dyspnoea, fluid retention) and atrial fibrillation (palpitations, decreased exercise tolerance, stroke). Those with ischaemic mitral regurgitation may also suffer from angina. Symptoms suggestive of endocarditis (unexplained fever) may be a cause for or a complication of MR.

Signs

- Sternotomy: potentially suggesting paravalvular MR in a malfunctioning prosthetic valve; vein graft harvesting scars (suggestive of ischaemic MR); or lateral thoracotomy (MR as part of mixed MV disease or as a complication of surgical valvotomy).
- Features of Marfan's syndrome or connective tissue disorders associated with MV prolapse.
- Stigmata of endocarditis (e.g. pyrexia, clubbing, splinter haemorrhages).
- Bruising from warfarin for AF, a complication of MR.
- Pulse regular or irregularly irregular suggestive of AF, rapid jerky upstroke due to short LV-ejection time when LV performance is good (LV empties rapidly into aorta and LA).
- JVP may be elevated due to right-heart failure in severe MR or functional MR. Additionally, there may be systolic CV waves due to secondary pulmonary hypertension leading to raised RV pressures and functional TR.
- Apex: may be readily visible, displaced owing to volume overload, and *thrusting* in character. Occasionally an apical systolic thrill (murmur grade 4/6 or louder by definition) may be felt. Assess apical rate if patient is in AF.
- Left parasternal heave due to RV pressure overload or a palpable forceful atrial contraction when the LA is grossly enlarged (rare as most patients are in AF by this stage). LA contraction can be distinguished from a RV-heave as it precedes the apical impulse whereas the RV heave is synchronous with it.
- Palpable P2 suggestive of pulmonary hypertension and by definition implying a loud P2 on auscultation.
- On auscultation:
  - Soft S1 (if loud or preserved, consider mixed rheumatic MV disease or MV prolapse).
  - High-pitch pansystolic murmur loudest at apex and radiating to axilla and increasing in intensity with expiration.
  - Widely split S2 especially with severe MR (A2 occurs earlier due to decreased ejection time of LV).
  - S3 due to rapid early filling of the LV from the engorged LA.
  - S4 due to forceful atrial contraction against a less compliant, dilated LV (rare, as usually by this stage the patient is in AF).
  - Diastolic rumble (rare – occurs as a result of high flow in severe MR and can be differentiated from MS by the presence of a soft S1 and the absence of an OS).
- On auscultation with MR due to MV prolapse:
  - Normal intensity S1.

- Single or multiple mid-systolic clicks as the myxomatous leaflets and the chordae snap shut.
- Soft high-pitch mid-to-late systolic murmur occurring as leaflets prolapse and LV size decreases towards the end of systole.
- Normal S2 but may develop S3 and S4 and loud P2 with increasing severity.
- The murmur of MV prolapse is dynamic and this can be brought out by asking the patient to squat and stand (see Top Tips box).
- Signs of heart failure (pitting pedal or sacral oedema, coarse basal late inspiratory crackles).

> **❶ Top Tips**
> - MV prolapse gives rise to a dynamic murmur, the onset and duration of which can be changed with manoeuvres such as squatting and standing. Anything that makes the heart smaller will allow the myxomatous leaflets with their elongated chordae to billow and prolapse more, causing earlier and longer regurgitation.
> - When the patient squats, venous return is increased making the heart larger. Afterload is increased as the femoral vessels are clamped decreasing the amount of blood ejected with systole and therefore increasing the end-systolic volume. The heart therefore increases in size, the leaflets billow less and the murmur becomes quieter and later in systole.
> - As the patient stands, venous return and afterload drop suddenly causing the heart to become smaller and consequently the murmur to become longer, louder and earlier in systole.

Severity
- To identify severe chronic MR, look for AF (develops as LA enlarges), displaced volume overloaded thrusting apex beat, signs of pulmonary hypertension (parasternal heave, palpable P2, evidence of TR), signs of cardiac failure.
- Mild chronic MR is suggested by the presence of sinus rhythm, absence of LV dilatation and absence of signs of congestive cardiac failure, unless this is the aetiology of the MR.
- Moderate MR is characterized clinically by the absence of features of either mild or severe MR.

Aetiology
- Degenerative
- Functional (secondary to LV dilatation and causes thereof)
- Ischaemic
- MV prolapse (affects 1–2.5% of the population):
  - Hereditary (autosomal dominant, *MMVP1* and *MMVP2* genes on chromosomes 16 and 11 respectively)
  - Idiopathic
  - Marfan's syndrome
  - Connective tissue disorders
- Rheumatic

❖ Common Pitfalls

Auscultation

- Failure to time the heart sounds carefully can result in misinterpretation and lost marks. If a mid-systolic click in MV prolapse is erroneously interpreted as S2, the following soft systolic murmur may be misinterpreted as a diastolic murmur. This can be avoided by careful timing against a central pulse (not the radial pulse which may give a false impression particularly in AF when some beats may not be conducted to the wrist), use of dynamic manoeuvres to enhance the murmur, and appreciation of its high-pitch character.
- Missing a loud S1 which may be the only initial auscultatory clue to the concomitant presence of MS. When listening, consciously neglect any pansystolic murmur and concentrate on the heart sounds alone to begin with.
- Incorrectly attributing the pansystolic murmur of TR to radiation from MR or worse still, to MR when none is present. Remember to check if the murmur increases in intensity with inspiration, suggesting TR (Carvalho's sign).

Investigations

- 12-lead ECG (may reveal P-mitrale or AF).
- CXR to identify pulmonary congestion and assess cardiac size.
- TTE (to assess severity, mechanism (including leaflet anatomy), LV function and dimensions, pulmonary pressures and RV function).
- TOE (to definitively assess severity, define mechanism of MR, feasibility of repair and exclude/diagnose endocarditis) and where available, 3D-TOE.
- As part of preoperative assessment for surgery:
  - Right and left heart catheterization (to assess pulmonary pressures and coronary anatomy. If bypass grafts are needed these can be carried out at the same time as valvular surgery)
  - Carotid Duplex (to determine whether any carotid disease requires treatment prior to cardiothoracic surgery).
  - Orthopentomogram (dental radiograph taken prior to a dental check to ensure any dental extractions required are undertaken before surgery to minimize future risks of prosthetic valve endocarditis).

Viva questions

What are the indications for surgery?

- No medical treatments have been shown to alter the prognosis of MR. Patients with mild or moderate MR are subjected to annual clinical and echocardiographic follow-up. MV repair surgery, or failing this, replacement with chordal preservation is recommended for:
  - Asymptomatic patients with EF 30–60% and end-systolic LV dimensions >40mm.
  - Patients with chronic severe MR and new onset AF or pulmonary systolic pressures at rest of >50mmHg even with preserved LV function (EF >60%).

- Those with a severely dilated and impaired LV (EF <30%, end-systolic LV size >55mm), surgery is only recommended if chordal preservation with durable repair is likely in absence of serious comorbidity and provided medical therapy is optimal.
- Asymptomatic patients with chronic severe MR and EF >60% and end-systolic LV dimensions <40mm should be followed up 6-monthly with annual echocardiography.

Why is MV repair preferable to replacement?

Disconnection of the subvalvular apparatus can result in up to 20% decline in LV function so MV replacement without chordal preservation should be avoided when possible. Patients with chronic asymptomatic severe MR and preserved LV function may be recommended for surgery even if they do not meet the criteria, provided that the chance of successful repair is >90%. The threshold for surgery is likely to fall as surgical repair techniques and outcomes continue to improve.

How is ischaemic MR managed differently?

The prognosis of functional ischaemic MR (where leaflets are normal but MR results from restriction of their movement due to ischaemic injury or dysfunction to the subvalvular apparatus) has a worse prognosis than organic MR. The threshold for treatment and definitions of severity are lower. Severe functional ischaemic MR is defined as an effective regurgitant orifice area of >20mm^2 or regurgitant volume of >30mL. MV surgery should be considered if the patient is undergoing CABG or, if not undergoing CABG, if EF >30% and the patient remains symptomatic despite optimal medical therapy. Those with severe LV impairment (EF <30%) who are not surgical candidates should be assessed for dyssynchrony and offered biventricular pacing ± ICD and/or transplantation if appropriate.

Are prophylactic antibiotics necessary for dental surgery?

No. Endocarditis prophylaxis is no longer recommended for uncomplicated MR and MV prolapse.[1]

New developments

- Surgical ablation of AF at the time of MV surgery.
- Percutaneous transcatheter MV clip repair (for those with central MR due to MV prolapse who are not fit for conventional surgery).
- Assessment with 3D-TTE and TOE.

Reference

1. NICE. *Prophylaxis against infective endocarditis*. London: NICE, 2008. Available at: http://www.nice.org.uk/CG64.

📖 Further reading

Bonow RO et al. Guidelines for the management of patients with valvular heart disease. *Circulation* 2008; **118**:e523–e661.

Tricuspid regurgitation

Most cases of tricuspid regurgitation are due to pulmonary hypertension (either primary or secondary) and even more than with the other valves, a minor degree of TR is considered normal.

Symptoms

Frequently asymptomatic but the patient may complain of ankle swelling and breathlessness is seen, although in many cases this reflects an underlying condition which has given rise to pulmonary hypertension. Occasionally patients complain of 'pulsing' in the neck.

Signs

- Swelling pulsation of the neck – the CV wave – is characteristic and frequently visible from the end of the bed. If on inspection a very high JVP can be seen without other signs of right-sided heart failure, e.g. significant peripheral oedema, then the patient should be considered to have TR until proven otherwise!
- Parasternal heave indicates severe TR.
- Pansystolic murmur at the lower left sternal edge which gets louder on inspiration.
- Pulsatile hepatomegaly.

> **❶ Top Tips**
> - It is often stated that right-sided murmurs get louder on inspiration whereas left-sided ones get softer. Since the lungs interpose themselves between the heart and your stethoscope on inspiration, any murmur may get quieter on inspiration. If the murmur does get louder, however, this is a very good indication the lesion is right-sided.

Aetiology

As with aortic valve lesions it is useful to divide the causes into acute and chronic presentations, but in the case of TR, because of the relative lack of symptoms, it may be much more difficult to know the pattern of onset. Acute cases will virtually always be due to tricuspid endocarditis or very occasionally major trauma.

Chronic causes

- Pulmonary hypertension.
- Endocarditis – look for any evidence of IV drug use.
- Ebstein's anomaly – this is apical displacement of the tricuspid valve (TV), but particularly of the septal leaflet. The tricuspid valve is normally offset from the MV slightly towards the apex, but in Ebstein's this is grossly exaggerated. The result is a deformed TV which always is at least moderately regurgitant.
- Rheumatic valvular heart disease (rare as the right-sided valves are not usually involved in the rheumatic process).
- Carcinoid syndrome.

Management

Medical management with diuretics and treatment of any underlying condition which is giving rise to pulmonary hypertension is the mainstay of treatment. When peripheral oedema is uncontrollable or low cardiac output becomes a problem, valve replacement or repair is an option. Results are generally poor, however, and this is very much a last resort.

Viva questions

How would you differentiate TR from MR?

TR is associated with a CV wave and the murmur gets louder on inspiration. Signs of left-sided failure will be absent.

Why is the CV wave so-called?

Inspection of the diagram of the JVP shows that the C wave is the point of closure of the TV. If TR is present therefore, it will start at this point and continue throughout RV systole (i.e. the period of the V wave). Hence CV wave.

Why is tricuspid endocarditis more common in IV drug users?

There is no doubt that this is the case. Most series have found around a 4-fold excess of tricuspid endocarditis in IDU. Also *Staph. aureus* endocarditis is more common in these people.

Avoid the pitfall of saying that the excess of tricuspid involvement is due to the fact that bacteria are injected into the veins. Any bacteraemia will rapidly be present in both venous and arterial sides, whatever its source, so this is not a credible reason. The real reason is probably that particulate matter present in the materials used to 'cut' illegal drugs damage the TV as they flow through the heart after being injected, before being trapped in the lungs. This damage then predisposes the TV to being seeded from the frequent bacteraemias.

Tricuspid stenosis

This is a rare condition, but it is just possible that a case might appear in membership due to the association with carcinoid syndrome.

Symptoms

As with TR, the symptoms are those of right-sided heart failure. Remember to ask about possible symptoms of the carcinoid syndrome if you suspect that TS may be present i.e. flushing, diarrhoea etc.

Signs

- Raised JVP.
- Peripheral oedema.
- A mid-diastolic murmur is very rarely audible.
- If TS is suspected, ask to examine the liver for hepatomegaly due to back pressure or carcinoid.

> The echocardiographic appearance of the TV is quite distinctive in carcinoid syndrome. The leaflets are thickened, retracted and immobile. This gives rise to both TS and severe TR.

Aetiology

- Carcinoid syndrome.
- Rheumatic fever – this is unusual as right-sided involvement is rare in rheumatic valvular heart disease.
- Congenital – partial tricuspid atresia.

Management

If the right-sided symptoms are uncontrollable with diuretics, valve replacement can be performed.

Pulmonary stenosis

This is quite an uncommon lesion, comprising ~5% of all congenital heart disease. The stenosis is usually at valvular level, but may also be sub- or supravalvular. Mild to moderate cases are very stable and rarely require treatment. The condition does, however, crop up in PACES from time to time.

Aetiology

Virtually all of the cases will be congenital and may be the result of maternal rubella. Although the pulmonary valve is least frequently affected, PS can, in combination with other valvular lesions, be the result of rheumatic fever. PS can also rarely occur in carcinoid syndrome.

Symptoms

Frequently none, particularly in adult cases, which are likely to be relatively mild. Asthenia, syncope, and symptoms of right heart failure may be present in more significant PS.

Signs

- Ejection systolic murmur, best heard in the pulmonary area and louder during inspiration.
- Softening and/or delay of the pulmonary component of the 2nd heart sound.
- Pulmonary thrill is commonly palpable.
- Palpable pulmonary ejection click.
- Prominent a wave in the JVP in more severe cases, due to RV hypertrophy.
- RV heave, again indicating more significant stenosis.
- RV gallop rhythm.

Main differential diagnosis

The most important differential is AS. In milder cases there may be little to tell the 2 apart, but the location of the murmur and particularly the fact that the murmur of PS gets louder, not softer, on inspiration, are useful differentiating features. With more severe cases, the presence of the right-sided signs detailed above and the absence of any effect on the arterial character and pulse pressure allow the 2 conditions to be discriminated.

Associated features

As with any condition that is usually congenital, it is important to look for any other evidence of congenital heart lesions. If PS is suspected, it is particularly important to look for features of Fallot's tetralogy (➲ p.279).

Investigation

Echocardiography is usually all that is required both for the diagnosis and monitoring of the condition. If there are associated anatomical lesions, particularly supravalvular abnormalities, cardiac MR is excellent for demonstrating both the cardiac and pulmonary artery anatomy.

Management

Most of the cases seen in adulthood will be very mild, requiring no treatment, or will have already undergone a corrective procedure. Balloon valvuloplasty of the RVOT is frequently used in infants as a palliative procedure and, if the outflow obstruction is severe, then surgical reconstruction of the RV outflow, or surgical techniques including shunts from the vena cavae or the RA to the pulmonary artery have been used. Recently percutaneous valve replacement has become possible and indeed the pulmonary valve was the first to be replaced by this method, preceding the better known percutaneous aortic valve replacement.

📖 **Further reading**

Bonow RO et al. Guidelines for the management of patients with valvular heart disease. *Circulation* 2008; **118**:e523–e661.

Mixed and multivalvular heart disease

Mixed or multivalvular heart disease is common both in the exam and in clinical practice. The challenge is to ascertain which valves are involved and what, if any, is the predominant lesion. Frequent combinations are mixed MV disease, mixed aortic valve disease and aortic valve disease with MR. Candidates are referred to the individual sections on valvular heart disease to familiarize themselves with the main signs.

Aetiology
- Endocarditis
- Rheumatic
- Degenerative
- Congenital

❶ **Top Tips**
- In the setting of mixed valve disease, the dominant lesion can be determined by assessing the impact of any lesions on the pulse character, BP and apex beat.
- The response of the ventricle is a good final arbiter of the predominant lesion; try and determine if the ventricle is under a volume load (MR, VSD, PDA or AR) or pressure load (AS, HCM) or under no changed load at all (MS).
- Tricuspid regurgitation rarely occurs as an isolated pathology and is most commonly due to pulmonary hypertension from left heart disease.
- When it is not possible to state the main lesion, a more pragmatic approach is to focus on the severity of each lesion as this will dictate management.

Mixed mitral valve disease

The aetiology is rheumatic. The most useful discriminating factors are the apex beat and auscultatory findings (Table 5.6).

Table 5.6 Discriminating factors in mixed MV disease

Feature	Mitral regurgitation	Mitral stenosis
Pulse	Normal or jerky in character	Normal or low volume
Apex position	Laterally displaced	Undisplaced
Apex character	Thrusting ± thrill	Tapping in character
S1	Soft	Loud
S3	Occasionally present	Absent

✦ Common Pitfalls

- Severe MS can lead to significant pulmonary hypertension. This can cause the RV to enlarge and displace the LV apex laterally and posteriorly. This can also result in TR. The latter can produce a pansystolic murmur which in the dilated RV can appear to be loud at the apex and give the misleading impression that there is concomitant MR. This error can be avoided by careful inspection of the JVP for CV waves and performing respiratory manoeuvres (the pansystolic murmur of TR becomes louder with inspiration). Severe TR also often gives rise to a pulsatile liver edge. Note however that both severe MR and MS can give rise to TR confounding matters further!

Mixed aortic valve disease

Any or all of the causes of AS, particularly a congenitally bicuspid valve, can give rise to AR and mixed valve disease is common. The most discriminating factors are the pulse character, BP and apex beat (location and character) (Table 5.7).

Table 5.7 Discriminating factors in mixed aortic valve disease

Feature	Aortic regurgitation	Aortic stenosis
Pulse	Collapsing	Slow rising, anacrotic
Systolic BP	High	Low
Pulse pressure	Wide	Narrow
Apex position	Laterally displaced	Minimally displaced
Apex character	Thrusting	Heaving
A2	Usually normal	Soft

◆ Common Pitfalls

- Significant AR results in a large LV end-diastolic volume. As a result, to compensate for the AR, the LV ejects a large volume of blood in systole and this increased flow can give rise to an ejection murmur giving the impression of mixed valve disease when none is present. To avoid this pitfall, concentrate instead on the haemodynamic consequences of the aortic valve disease.

Mixed aortic and mitral valve disease

- AS is often seen in combination with MR. Often, the latter develops as a result of the former, so-called 'functional' MR (Table 5.8).

Table 5.8 Discriminating factors in mixed aortic and mitral valve disease

Feature	Aortic stenosis	Mitral regurgitation
Pulse rhythm	Normally regular	AF very frequent
Pulse character	Slow rising, anacrotic	Normal or jerky in character
Systolic BP	Low	Normal
Pulse pressure	Narrow	Normal
Apex position	Minimally displaced	Laterally displaced
Apex character	Heaving	Thrusting
S4	May be present	Usually absent

- AR and MR both cause a volume load on the LV. It can therefore be very difficult to determine what the predominant lesion is. The key feature to look at is the effect on BP. A high systolic BP with a wide pulse pressure particularly in the presence of a regular pulse would suggest that AR was the predominant lesion. In the absence of these features, it may be difficult to tell clinically and focus should then be on assessing the severity of each lesion in turn. Pragmatically, if either lesion is severe enough to need intervention, the other lesion would also need to be fixed unless mild.
- MS and aortic valve disease:
  - Severe MS significantly impairs LV filling and can thereby shield the LV from the effects of severe AR. Severe MS, by producing a low cardiac output state, may attenuate the signs of severe aortic stenosis. As a result, if AS or AR appears moderate, and there appears to be significant MS, the latter will be the most significant lesion clinically.
  - The corollary of this, however, is that evidence of severe AS or severe AR in the context of MS suggests that the MS is not so severe that it is able to mask the effects of the aortic valve disease. The aortic lesion is therefore likely to be the most significant clinically.

Heart failure

Although several of the conditions dealt with in this chapter can lead to heart failure, the syndrome is of such great importance that it merits consideration in its own right. The condition is becoming increasingly common, both in terms of prevalence (between 2–20 per 1000 of the population) and also as a reason for admission to hospital. Given that the incidence increases sharply with age, the aging population means that it will become ever more common.

Classification

There are many different ways that heart failure can be classified:
- Side of heart affected
- New York Heart Association (NYHA)
- Individual aetiologies
- Systolic or diastolic
- Chronicity of the condition.

One method is by the side of the heart affected:
- Left-sided, due to:
  - Ischaemic heart disease (IHD) or hypertensive heart disease (most common causes).
  - Valvular heart disease.
  - Cardiomyopathy.
  - Myocarditis.
- Right-sided:
  - Most commonly due to intrinsic lung disease causing pulmonary hypertension and secondary right-sided heart failure (cor pulmonale).
  - May be due to right-sided cardiomyopathy e.g. arrhythmogenic RV dysplasia (rare).
- Congestive or biventricular failure:
  - This is RV failure due to pulmonary hypertension and fluid overload caused by LV dysfunction.

Heart failure can also be classified by the functional class of the patient according to the NYHA system (see Table 5.9).

Table 5.9 NYHA classification of heart failure functional class

NYHA class	Symptoms
Class I	No effect on normal daily activities
Class II	Able to walk ~100m on the flat, breathless with greater levels of exertion
Class III	Breathless on walking around the house, comfortable at rest
Class IV	Breathless at rest or on minimal exertion.

The syndrome may also be classified by the individual aetiologies listed earlier, or alternatively may be considered to be systolic or diastolic.

Some estimates have stated that up to 40% of all cases of the heart failure syndrome are due to diastolic heart failure. Whilst diastolic dysfunction undoubtedly contributes to many cases with abnormal systolic function, pure diastolic heart failure, which is strictly defined as symptoms and signs consistent with heart failure, an LVEDP >14mmHg and preserved systolic function (EF >45%), is less common than this.

Classification is also possible depending on the chronicity of the condition, thus acute heart failure presents with symptoms and signs resulting from sudden reduction in cardiac output, most commonly following a myocardial infarction. There may therefore be signs of low cardiac output and acutely raised filling pressures, with breathlessness and orthopnoea and also of sympathetic activation (tachycardia, diaphoresis, anxiety). Chronic heart failure on the other hand, mainly presents with congestive symptoms due to the neurohumeral activation and consequent salt and water retention.

A full diagnosis of heart failure will make reference to all of these classifications and it is particularly important that a comment on the aetiology is included, since the treatment and prognosis will vary with the underlying cause.

Symptoms

May be considered to be due to pump failure or congestion.
- Pump failure:
  - Fatigue
  - Asthenia
  - Weight loss (cardiac cachexia due to high circulating interleukin levels)
- Congestive symptoms:
  - Breathlessness
  - Orthopnoea
  - Paroxysmal nocturnal dyspnoea
  - Ankle swelling

Signs
- Tachycardia
- Raised JVP
- Clinically displaced apex
- RV heave in RV failure
- 3rd heart sound or gallop rhythm
- Basal fine crepitations in the lungs (NB crepitations are a very non-specific sign of pulmonary oedema)
- Peripheral and or sacral oedema.

Investigations
- ECG (NB the ECG is normal in <10% of cases of genuine heart failure due to systolic dysfunction, so if the ECG is normal, be suspicious of the diagnosis).
- CXR: enlarged heart, upper lobe venous diversion, Kerley B lines, frank pulmonary oedema.
- Echocardiography: this is the mainstay of investigation, allowing both systolic and diastolic function to be determined and underlying aetiology to be diagnosed in many cases.

- Coronary angiography: may be required to rule out ischaemic heart disease, even in the absence of a history of myocardial infarction or angina.
- Exercise testing/cardiopulmonary exercise testing. This is not required for diagnosis, but can give very useful information on prognosis. An oxygen uptake of <15mL/kg/min is associated with a prognosis poorer than that of heart transplantation and is often used as part of the workup to judge suitability for a transplant.
- Myocardial viability testing: this is particularly important in LV dysfunction due to IHD as there may be significant areas of the myocardium which are dysfunctional but still viable (hibernating myocardium). In this case revascularization may result in restoration of function. There are at least 4 methods of looking for viability: thallium scanning, cardiac MRI, stress echo and PET, although a discussion of the full strengths and weaknesses of the different methods is beyond the scope of this book.

Management

The most crucial element of proper management is correct diagnosis of the underlying aetiology, since this may be reversible. If this is the case then management is directed to correction of the cause. If the underlying cause is not reversible then medical management consists of:

- Diuretics: these are the most effective treatment for congestive symptoms, but have no effect on prognosis.
- ACE inhibitors/angiotensin II receptor blockers: both relieve symptoms and improve prognosis in all grades of heart failure.
- Beta-blockers: improve prognosis and reduce hospital admissions in all grades of heart failure, there is also evidence that quality of life is improved.
- Spironolactone: in those with class III symptoms despite the medications listed above having been optimized, this inhibitor of the aldosterone receptor improves prognosis. In those who are post myocardial infarction, the more selective agent eplerenone has similar effects with fewer side effects.
- Exercise training: this has been shown to have beneficial symptomatic and prognostic effects in all grades of heart failure. Graded, aerobic exercise is recommended.
- Where these points have failed to control symptoms, selected patients may be suitable for biventricular pacing (→ 'Viva questions', p.253).
- Digoxin has been shown to improve functional class by an average of about 1 NYHA class, but does not improve prognosis.
- Cardiac transplantation may be appropriate in selected cases, but the limited availability of donor organs significantly limits its use. Mortality is 15% in the 1st year, but thereafter falls to about 5% per year. Consequently median survival is 8 years.
- When end-stage heart failure is reached, a palliative care approach can improve quality of life and reduce subsequent distressing symptoms.

New developments and less conventional management options

There has been much recent interest in the development of artificial ventricular support devices, such as the Jarvik implantable artificial heart. There are still significant technical problems to be overcome before these may provide anything more than a very short-term bridge to transplantation. Some groups have palliated the congestive symptoms using continuous peritoneal dialysis and others have attempted to improve symptoms by treating the anaemia that frequently accompanies severe heart failure with erythropoietin.

Viva questions

Discuss the neurohumeral changes that occur with chronic CCF

- Reduction in cardiac output leads to reduced glomerular filtration rate, which in turn reduces the delivery of sodium to the distal convoluted tubule. This is sensed by the juxtaglomerular apparatus, which releases renin, so converting angiotensinogen to angiotensin I. This is then converted to angiotensin II, which increases the afterload on the heart by causing vasoconstriction and also causes salt and water retention, worsening congestive symptoms. This dysfunctional response is reversed by ACE inhibitors.

- The acute response to a reduced cardiac output is activation of the sympathetic nervous system. When cardiac output remains depressed this becomes chronic with high levels of circulating adrenaline and noradrenaline originating from the adrenal glands. This also results in increased afterload (by vasoconstriction), tachycardia which increases myocardial oxygen demand and further salt and water retention by a direct action on the kidneys. Once again it can be seen that this is a counterproductive response and explains the beneficial effects of beta-blockers.

What are the indications for biventricular pacing?

- Patients who remain in class III or IV despite at least 1 month of optimal medical treatment and who have a QRS complex broader than 120ms, should be considered for biventricular pacing. In heart failure it has been observed that the LV frequently shows loss of synchronous contraction, as well as reduced overall function. The hypothesis therefore developed that if the LV could be 'resynchronized', this would improve overall performance. This is achieved by pacing both left and right ventricles, using a lead inserted through the coronary sinus to pace the outer surface of the free wall of the LV. It has now been shown that not only does this treatment produce an improvement in symptoms, but also confers substantial prognostic benefits[1].

Reference

1. Cleland JGF et al.; CARE-HF Study Investigators. The effect of cardiac resynchronization on morbidity and mortality in heart failure. *NEJM* 2005; **352**(15):1539–49.

Prosthetic valves

The patient with a prosthetic valve may present with symptoms of heart failure (fatigue, exertional dyspnoea, orthopnoea, paroxysmal nocturnal dyspnoea, fluid retention) or of dysfunction of the valve; symptoms of endocarditis (fever, rigors, lassitude, embolic phenomena, heart failure); bleeding from over-anticoagulation; anaemia and jaundice from intravascular haemolysis; and evidence of thromboembolism and its consequences due to under-anticoagulation in those with mechanical valves.

Signs

- Scars:
    - Median sternotomy (if vein graft harvesting scars are also present, this is indicative of coexistent ischaemic heart disease).
    - Small infraclavicular scar. This may suggest a tunnelled line as a source of endocarditis which may have necessitated valve replacement or the use of a tunnelled line for long-term IV-antibiotics for endocarditis, although the trend is now for use of percutaneous peripherally inserted central catheters (PICC lines). Remember, the ultimate treatment for endocarditis is valve replacement surgery.
- Stigmata of endocarditis (pyrexia, clubbing, splinter haemorrhages, Osler's nodes, Janeway lesions, Roth spots, splenomegaly, microscopic haematuria, neurological deficits and other signs consistent with embolic phenomena).
- Bruising from warfarin which may hint at either the presence of AF and/or a mechanical prosthetic valve.
- Anaemia (due to subacute bacterial endocarditis, or resulting from intravascular mechanical haemolysis through or around a dysfunctional prosthetic valve).
- Jaundice (pre-hepatic jaundice as a result of intravascular haemolysis).
- Look for signs of valve dysfunction especially valve regurgitation which may be due to endocarditis.
- Audible mechanical clicks:
    - Patients with mechanical aortic or MV prostheses, particularly of the tilting disc variety, may have audible clicks heard from the edge of the bed. These can be used to assess heart rate and rhythm.

❶ Top Tips

- The loudest click audible from the edge of the bed is always the *closure* sound of the valve. Time the clicks against the carotid pulse.

☛ Common Pitfalls

- Timing of peripheral pulses may not be an accurate indicator of the heart rate (especially with poorly rate-controlled AF).

- A click immediately preceding the carotid pulse (1st heart sound) indicates a MV replacement. A click following the carotid pulse (2nd heart sound) indicates an aortic valve replacement.
- Two audible clicks suggest that both mitral and aortic valves must be mechanical prostheses.

- Auscultatory features:
  - Biological valves do not produce clicks but the heart sounds they create have an abnormal timbre and are generally of a lower pitch than normal heart sounds. A soft systolic murmur across an aortic or pulmonary prosthesis may be normal in the absence of any other signs of stenosis which can occur as these valves degenerate over time. However, a regurgitant murmur is never normal and represents either a paravalvular or valvular leak and may raise the spectre of endocarditis.
  - Mechanical valves will often have a loud crisp 'metallic' closure click synchronous with S1 for a MV prosthesis and S2 for an aortic valve prosthesis. Starr–Edwards ('ball and cage') aortic valves often have a series of clearly audible additional systolic opening clicks which represent the rattling of the ball in the valve's cage. If they are muffled or even absent, this may suggest either a low cardiac output state or more ominously may represent clot formation on the ball or the cage struts which dampens the normal clicks. Single tilting disc or bileaflet mechanical valves may occasionally produce faintly audible opening clicks.
  - A soft systolic murmur across an aortic valve prosthesis can often be heard and represents innocent turbulent flow as the valve orifice area will never truly match that of the native valve.
  - A systolic murmur across a MV prosthesis represents a paravalvular leak. Even when severe, these may be barely audible and when suspected must be carefully sought all the way to the back of the chest as they can sometimes be conducted via the aortic root posteriorly. Small paravalvular leaks are not uncommon in patients with calcific degenerative valve disease as calcification at the mitral annulus or aortic root can make it difficult for all sutures to completely 'take'.
  - Bileaflet tilting-disc valves such as the St Jude are designed to allow very small jets of regurgitant flow ('washing jets') to reduce the risk of thrombosis. These are inaudible and not haemodynamically significant so if there are signs of aortic regurgitation present, a paravalvular leak and/or endocarditis should be suspected.

> **❶ Top Tips**
> - In a young patient with evidence of replacement of more than one valve, the aetiology is likely to be a pathology which affects more than one valve, i.e. rheumatic fever, endocarditis or congenital heart disease.

Investigations

- TTE to ensure that the valve is well-seated, functioning normally with normal pressure gradients and flow velocities across the valve, and to detect vegetations where these are suspected.
- TOE: this is indicated where endocarditis is suspected as well as to evaluate dysfunction of a prosthesis, especially a mitral mechanical valve. Acoustic shadowing created by the valve may render even substantial paravalvular leaks practically invisible on transthoracic views.

Viva questions

Discuss the merits of biological vs. mechanical valves

Biological valve

The principal advantage of bioprosthetic valves is the lack of need for long-term anticoagulation. Warfarin is usually prescribed for 3 months during which time the bioprosthesis becomes fully endothelialized. They are therefore the valves of choice in patients who have contraindications to anticoagulation. Their main disadvantage is a higher incidence of degeneration and structural failure requiring re-operation which has a higher risk than initial surgery. Bioprosthetic valves are generally therefore offered to patients over the age of 70 and those aged 60 or above who have significant comorbidity that may limit longevity to 10–15 years (30–60% failure rate over this period). Patients with these valves require lifelong clinical and echocardiographic follow-up, initially annually and then more frequently if signs of valve dysfunction develop. Aortic valve bioprostheses degenerate much more rapidly than prostheses in the mitral position, presumably related to the greater pressure swings the valve is exposed to. Patient preference may also play a part in that many people elect for bioprostheses in order to avoid the need for long term warfarin therapy.

Mechanical valve

Mechanical valves are significantly more durable than bioprostheses and are therefore the valves of choice in those <60 years where there are no contraindications to long-term anticoagulation. The risk of thromboembolism is higher in the mitral position than in the aortic position presumably because of the lower flow rates across the MV. However, this may be confounded by the comorbid presence of LA appendage thrombus from AF which is a common complication of chronic severe MR. In those with AF and other known risk factors for thromboembolism the use of warfarin may be indicated anyway (➲ p.480). Mechanical valves may therefore be preferable in such patients even if they are >65 as warfarin would already be indicated for these coexistent cardiac conditions.

Pregnancy or women of childbearing potential requiring valve replacement

This situation presents particular problems in that on the one hand a mechanical valve introduces the need for either warfarin, with the risk of fetal malformation or long-term heparin which risks osteoporosis for the mother. On the other hand bioprostheses are particularly likely to undergo calcific degeneration during pregnancy and require urgent re-operation.

Comment on the types and anticoagulant management of mechanical valves

Mechanical prosthetic valves have evolved in design from the early Starr–Edwards (ball-and-cage) valve which is no longer in clinical use, through single-leaflet tilting disc valves to the modern bileaflet tilting disc valves which have better haemodynamics and larger effective orifice areas than their predecessors. These valves are designed with small leaks or 'washing jets' which together with their less thrombogenic coatings allow use of less intense regimes of anticoagulation.

Patients with bileaflet tilting-disc prostheses in the aortic position can be anticoagulated to a target INR of 2.5. Patients with similar prosthetic valves in the mitral position or who have more than one valve or concomitant AF should be anticoagulated to a target INR of 3.0 (2.5–3.5). Thromboembolic risk is highest in a patient with a Starr–Edwards MV replacement, particularly if they are in AF.

How would you manage anticoagulation if the patient needed surgery?

- Patients with mechanical valves who are undergoing surgery must have their anticoagulation stopped, generally until the INR is <1.5 for most procedures.
- For patients with a bileaflet tilting disc valve in the aortic position who have no other risk factors for thromboembolism (AF, previous thromboembolism, LV dysfunction, >1 mechanical valve, hypercoagulable state), warfarin can simply be omitted for up to 72 hours and restarted again 24 hours after surgery. Heparin cover is not required.
- All other patients with mechanical valves should have their warfarin stopped 48 hours or more before surgery and be commenced on IV heparin once the INR falls below 2.0. The heparin can then be stopped 4–6 hours prior to the planned surgery and restarted as soon as practical after surgery and until the INR is 2.5 or above.

New developments

In those who are not candidates for conventional surgery because of pro-hibitively high operative risk:

- Percutaneous transcatheter MV clip repair for patients with central MV prolapse.
- Percutaneous and/or transapical aortic valve replacement surgery for patients with severe AS.

Further reading

Bonow RO et al. Guidelines for the management of patients with valvular heart disease. *Circulation* 2008; **118**:e523–e661.

Constrictive pericarditis

The patient may complain of breathlessness, orthopnoea, paroxysmal nocturnal dyspnoea, loss of appetite, fatigue, effort intolerance, abdominal and ankle swelling. They may also experience palpitations (sinus tachycardia or AF) and a chronic unproductive cough (pulmonary hypertension).

Signs

- Cachexia (secondary to undernutrition, protein-losing enteropathy or underlying malignancy).
- Anasarca (secondary to elevated right-sided pressures and cardiac cirrhosis).
- Leuconychia (low albumin due to cardiac cirrhosis and protein-losing enteropathy) and Terry nails (3mm brown band at edge of nail bed).
- Radiotherapy tattoo marks (stigmata of radiotherapy which may have been the original trigger for pericardial constriction).
- Stigmata of chronic liver disease from consequent cardiac cirrhosis including jaundice.
- Signs of old TB (thoracoplasty with drooping shoulder, thoracotomy for plombage/lobectomy, phrenic nerve crush scar in neck).
- Pulse: low volume with either a regular tachycardia to maintain cardiac output in the setting of a fixed stroke volume or irregularly irregular suggestive of AF (occurs in >30% of patients due to chronic biatrial enlargement).
- BP: low with exaggerated pulsus paradoxus. This is a >20mmHg fall in systolic pressure with inspiration due to increased filling of RV with inspiration, which in the absence of pericardial stretch can only be accommodated by the septum bulging into the LV cavity. This reduces the size and the filling of the LV and thereby reduces left-sided output. Pulsus paradoxus may be present in up to 1/3 of patients.
- JVP: markedly raised with a prominent Y-descent (fall in venous pressure immediately after opening of the TV). The JVP may paradoxically increase or fail to fall with inspiration as the constricted RV cannot accommodate the increased venous return that accompanies this at a normal filling pressure (Kussmaul's sign).

❶ Top Tips

- You may need to ask the patient to stand up to see this more clearly as the JVP is usually very high.

- Apex: usually impalpable/undisplaced. As the heart is encased in thick rigid pericardium, the apex does not move despite changes in position.
- On auscultation:
  - Normal S1.
  - Pansystolic murmur associated with TR.
  - Normal or widely split S2 (early A2 due to pulsus paradoxus).
  - Loud RV S3 or pericardial knock. The RV fills under high pressure and rapidly in early diastole. Filling of the RV is suddenly stopped by the stiff pericardium and this rapid deceleration in blood flow produces the pericardial knock. It is best heard at the left sternal edge and is accentuated by inspiration like all other right-sided sounds. It is higher in pitch than other types of S3.

- Abdominal examination may reveal:
  - Hepatomegaly
  - Ascites

Aetiology

- Post-irradiation
- Post-infectious (especially tuberculous)
- Post-surgical
- Idiopathic
- Uraemic
- Autoimmune (e.g. SLE)
- Drug-induced (e.g. hydralazine, clozapine, procainamide)
- Neoplastic
- Post-traumatic (haemopericardium).

Investigations

- 12-lead ECG: generalized low voltage, P-mitrale and P-pulmonale, sinus tachycardia or AF.
- CXR: pericardial calcification, pulmonary congestion, signs of inciting, illness e.g. old TB, interstitial changes from radiation pneumonitis.
- Echocardiogram: thickened pericardium, LA enlargement, septal bounce in early diastole, TR, >25% variation in tricuspid inflow velocities with respiration and >15% variation in mitral inflow velocities. Normal variation in these parameters is <10%.
- Right and left heart catheterization: this is used to assess the coronary anatomy prior to surgical pericardiectomy and also to assess the haemodynamics for diagnosis. Diastolic LV and RV pressures are characteristically raised and equal. Ventricular pressure falls to zero just at the onset of diastole (would normally be sustained at zero for a greater length of time). It then rises very rapidly due to elevated filling pressures but this rise is rapidly checked by the non-compliant rigid pericardium causing the pressure to plateau at a high level. This gives rise to the so-called square-root sign reflecting the shape of the tracing that results. Pulmonary pressures are not usually elevated unless there is a concomitant second pathological process.
- CT/MRI: pericardial calcification, often up to 1cm thick. CT is more sensitive but may require IV contrast.

Management

- Early diagnosis is crucial. Once the diagnosis is made, any underlying diseases should be treated if possible.
- Steroids have been shown to reduce the incidence of constriction after tuberculous pericarditis, but there is no evidence for their use in other aetiologies.
- Fluid overload can be treated with judicious use of diuretics. Beta-blockers and rate-limiting calcium channel antagonists should be avoided as a compensatory sinus tachycardia is often required to preserve cardiac output. AF should be rate-controlled with digoxin but aiming for a rate of 90 per minute rather than the rates of 70 or less that are typically targeted in most patients with AF.
- There is no successful long-term medical treatment. The avoidance of the long-term consequences of pericardial constriction can only be achieved by surgical pericardiectomy.

Infective endocarditis

Definition

Infective endocarditis (IE) is an endovascular infection of any part of the heart (e.g. native valves, ventricular or atrial endocardium) including endarteritis of the large intrathoracic vessels (e.g. in a patent ductus arteriosus) or of intracardiac foreign bodies (e.g. prosthetic valves, pacemaker or ICD leads, surgically created conduits).

Diagnosis

This is most commonly based on the Duke criteria (see Table 5.10). In order to make the diagnosis one must have 2 of the major criteria, 1 major and 3 minor or 5 minor criteria.

Table 5.10 Duke criteria for the diagnosis of infective endocarditis

Major criteria	Minor criteria
Positive blood culture: should either be 2 separate cultures with a typical microorganism (*Strep. viridans*, *Strep. bovis* or a HACEK[a] organism, or community acquired *Staph. aureus* or *Enterococcus* without an obvious focus) **Or** microorganism consistent with IE with persistently positive blood cultures (2 samples >12 hours apart or all of 3 or majority of 4 separate cultures, the first and last being at least 1 hour apart)	Serological evidence of active infection with an organism consistent with IE **Or** positive blood culture not reaching major criterion
	Vascular embolic phenomena: arterial emboli, septic pulmonary or intracranial emboli, splinter haemorrhages, conjunctival haemorrhage, Janeway lesions
	Immunologic phenomena: Roth spots, Osler's nodes, glomerulonephritis, positive rheumatoid factor
Evidence of endocardial involvement: either vegetation (must be independently mobile mass on echo), or an intracardiac abscess or new dehiscence of a prosthetic valve or new valvular regurgitation	Fever
	Predisposing heart condition or IV drug use.
	Echo findings that are suggestive but do not meet the major criterion

[a] HACEK refers to *Haemophilus* species (*H. parainfluenzae*, *H. aphrophilus*, *H. paraphrophilus*), *Actinobacillus actinomycetemcomitans*, *Cardiobacterium hominis*, *Eikenella corrodens* and *Kingella* spp.

Classification

The original classification of IE into acute and subacute has largely broken down due to a blurring of the lines between these originally distinct types, and also the increasing frequency of prosthetic valve and IV drug use-related cases, which do not easily fit into these categories. The European Society of Cardiology recommends that IE be classified under 6 different domains (see Table 5.11). This scheme is designed to reflect the different pathogenesis, treatment and prognosis which is attached to the different categories of endocarditis.

Table 5.11 European Society of Cardiology classification of IE

Classification domain	Subcategory
Disease activity	Active: current diagnosis of IE with positive blood cultures
	Healed: definite previous diagnosis of IE but now bacteriologically sterile
	Persistent: IE that has not become eradicated after appropriate antibiotic course
	Recurrent: recurrence of endocarditis after a definite cure of a previous episode. This is difficult to differentiate from persistent types, but carries a particularly grave prognosis
Certainty of diagnosis	Established: definite diagnosis by Duke criteria
	Suspected: IE strongly suspected clinically with definite infection but endocardial involvement has not been established
	Possible
Type of valvular involvement	Native valve (NVE)
	Prosthetic valve (PVE)
	Endocarditis related to IV drug use
Side of heart involved	Left-sided
	Right-sided
Culture status	Culture positive endocarditis – includes cases where a bacterial diagnosis has been made by serology or PCR
	Culture negative (CNE) – a definite diagnosis of IE has been made but all attempts to identify the organism have failed
Population type of patient – this is useful mainly for epidemiological purposes and differs from the other categories in that it does not particularly reflect the prognosis or treatment of the condition	Neonates
	Children
	The elderly
	Patients with congenital heart disease
	Nosocomial

Symptoms

These are generally non-specific with fever being a common finding but there is no specific symptomatology and the patient is just constitutionally unwell.

Signs

Signs may be categorized as being:
- Due to the infection itself:
  - Fever
  - Changing murmur due to progressive valve destruction
  - Heart failure due to severe valvular regurgitation
  - Hepatosplenomegaly
- Due to immune complex formation and dissemination:
  - Roth spots
  - Osler's nodes
  - Proteinuria or haematuria due to glomerulonephritis
- Due to embolic phenomena:
  - Janeway lesions
  - Splinter haemorrhages
  - Conjunctival haemorrhage
  - Signs due to the presence or rupture of mycotic aneurysms.

> #### Common Pitfalls
> - When looking for splinter haemorrhages, remember to examine the toenails as well.
> - When looking for conjunctival haemorrhage, ask the patient to look up and down to see the whole of the conjunctiva.
> - Osler's nodes are tender nodules in the pulps of the fingers, so palpate the finger tips and be seen to ask the patient if they are tender.

Investigations

When endocarditis is suspected, the first specific investigations should be blood cultures, with either 2 sets being taken 24 hours apart or 4 sets over at least 1 hour. These should be done before antibiotics are initiated. Generally antibiotics should not be started until the second set of blood cultures has been performed 24 hours after the first set unless the patient is severely septic. Thereafter investigation is designed to establish endocardial involvement and TTE is the imaging modality of choice. If this is positive, then TOE is not necessarily required, but is useful when TTE is negative but the diagnosis is still suspected. TOE is also helpful in cases of suspected PVE, where adequate pictures are rarely obtained by TTE, or in the diagnosis of complications of established IE, such as valve perforation or aortic root abscess formation. Once the diagnosis has been made, renal function requires regular monitoring with both blood tests and urine dipstick and in cases of definite or suspected aortic valve involvement, ECGs should be done every 2 days. A lengthening PR interval suggests aortic root abscess formation and implies early surgery is indicated.

Management

The initial treatment is with IV antibiotics, however, the exact cocktail and length of treatment is so dependent on the exact type and classification of IE, that a discussion of the multiple regimens is beyond the scope of this book. Aid should be sought from the bacteriologists and from the current guidelines for management, such as those from the European Society of Cardiology. While there are no randomized trials, many authorities believe that prognosis is better when there is a low threshold for recourse to surgery, and this is particularly the case in PVE, staphylococcal IE or complicated cases. See viva questions for further discussion.

Antibiotic prophylaxis

Recent NICE guidance has advised that routine antibiotic prophylaxis is not necessary for patients with high-risk cardiac lesions. They advise that these patients should be counselled that there is some risk of endocarditis in those with structural heart disease undergoing invasive medical or dental procedures; however, the guidance states that the risks of routine antibiotic prophylaxis outweigh any possible benefits and should no longer be offered. This policy has proved highly controversial with many cardiologists feeling that the guidance is incorrect.[1]

Viva questions

How is endocarditis diagnosed?

By establishment of systemic infection and endocardial or endovascular involvement. The candidate should know the Duke criteria and to be able to discuss something about the different subtypes, as detailed in the Tables 5.10 and 5.11.

What are the complications of endocarditis?

These may be considered to be due to:

- Direct tissue destruction – acute and subacute valve failure and extravalvular extension of infection with aortic root abscess, which may lead to increasing heart block, and occasionally septic pericarditis.
- Septic embolic phenomena with lung, brain or splenic abscesses and formation and possible rupture of mycotic aneurysms, potentially in any site.
- Renal failure due to systemic sepsis or immune complex glomerulonephritis.

What are the indications for surgical intervention?

These are debated, but most would agree that uncontrolled infection, haemodynamic instability due to valve failure or increasing heart block due to aortic root abscess are all indications for surgery. Some would include renal failure in this list and many would argue that surgery is virtually always necessary in PVE, apart from when the organism is an extremely sensitive *Streptococcus*. The outcome of surgery is better when surgery is performed sooner rather than later.

What are the indications for antibiotic prophylaxis?

As noted above, current guidance says that antibiotic prophylaxis should not be routinely offered in any form of cardiac defect even those with complex congenital heart disease or previous endocarditis. Nevertheless, given the controversy that this policy has produced it is probably a sufficiently topical subject to warrant some further reading prior to the exam.[1]

Reference

1. NICE. *Prophylaxis against infective endocarditis*. London: NICE, 2008. Available at: http://www. nice.org.uk/CG64.

Ventricular septal defect

A defect of the septum between the ventricles. This is the commonest congenital heart defect with estimates that it comprises 25–40% of all congenital heart disease. While the great majority of VSD is congenital, it can also be acquired, almost exclusively as a result of cardiac rupture post myocardial infarction. In the latter case the patients generally present with sudden haemodynamic collapse, 24–72 hours after myocardial infarction with a new, loud systolic murmur. Without early surgery, the prognosis is very grave, hence while it is absolutely crucial to recognize the condition in clinical practice, so that early surgery can be considered, it is extremely unlikely that an acquired VSD would be a PACES case.

A much rarer form of VSD occurs when there is a defect of the atrioventricular septum. This is the area of the ventricular septum which separates the LV and the RA, which exists because the tricuspid valve is slightly offset towards the apex of the heart. A defect here, known as a Gerbode defect, results in flow from LV to RA.

Symptoms

Frequently a VSD will present with no symptoms, although very large defects will present in infancy with heart failure. In adulthood the condition will present with high output cardiac failure, or more frequently, as an incidental finding.

Signs

- Pansystolic murmur with an ejection character, best heard at the left sternal edge, classically in the 4th intercostal space, frequently with an associated thrill. The murmur from a VSD in the muscular septum may not span the whole of systole due to closure of the VSD with contraction of the septal myocardium.
- If the shunt is severe there may be signs of RV overload with a parasternal heave.
- Signs of right-sided heart failure may be present. This is universally the case in the rare Gerbode defect where there will be very marked and relatively fixed elevation of the JVP.
- In rare uncorrected cases pulmonary hypertension may develop with reduction and ultimately reversal of the shunt giving rise to signs of Eisenmenger's syndrome.

The classic Maladie de Roger is an isolated finding of a very loud ejection pansystolic murmur with no other signs. This is indicative of a small VSD.

Aetiology and classification

Cases may be either congenital or acquired, as noted in the discussion above. In the case of congenital types these are further subdivided according to their exact embryology; however, a full discussion of this is beyond the scope of this book. Although VSD is most commonly an isolated finding, as with any form of congenital heart disease it is always important to be aware that it may be associated with other defects and these should be actively sought out.

Investigation

Echocardiography is the investigation of choice. This is both to confirm the diagnosis but also to check for any other associated defects.

Complications

In the case of small VSDs, complications are not common and the condition is usually detected incidentally. In the case of large defects presenting in adulthood apart from heart failure the principal complication is endocarditis.

Management

In most cases the only management that is required is reassurance of the patients that the condition is entirely harmless. In large defects or those presenting with complications, VSDs are most commonly closed surgically, however percutaneous catheter-based closure is now an option.

Viva questions

What is Maladie de Roger?

This is a very loud pansystolic ejection murmur heard at the left sternal edge, not uncommonly associated with thrill, but indicative of a small defect not requiring further treatment.

When should antibiotic prophylaxis be offered to somebody with VSD?

As noted earlier, the current official guidance is that prophylaxis is not offered in any form of structural heart disease including VSD. The NICE guidance does make it clear however that any active infection should always be treated appropriately.

Atrial septal defect

Lesions not recognized and dealt with in childhood usually present in the 3rd or 4th decade of life. Patients may present with dyspnoea (due to pulmonary hypertension and AF), palpitations (atrial rhythm disturbances), stroke (paradoxical embolism, AF), right-heart failure (peripheral oedema) or recurrent unexplained respiratory tract infections.

Signs

- Features of syndromes associated with ASD such as Down's syndrome (low set ears, prominent epicanthic folds, Brushfield spots in the iris, flat nasal bridge, glossoptosis, simian palmar crease, short inward curving of little finger) and Holt–Oram syndrome (hypoplastic triphalangeal thumb, radial hypoplasia, phocomelia, bradycardia due to congenital complete heart block, atrial and ventricular septal defects).
- Look for signs of previous stroke particularly in young patients that may have resulted from paradoxical embolization across the ASD.
- Pulse: regular or irregularly irregular consistent with AF.
- JVP: normal or raised if right heart failure has developed. Prominent CV waves if TR has developed as a consequence of RV volume overload. Giant A-waves may be seen if pulmonary hypertension develops.
- Left parasternal thrust due to RV volume overload. The RV is hyperdynamic and ill-sustained.
- On auscultation:
  - S1 is usually normal. With a large ASD, the tricuspid component may be accentuated. This occurs because the large flow in diastole from the large left-to-right shunt across the ASD pushes the TV leaflets further into the RV than usual. The volume-overloaded hyperdynamic RV then slams them further and closes them more vigorously.
  - Soft ejection systolic murmur (usually grade 2–3/6) loudest over the pulmonary area. The murmur results from increased and therefore turbulent flow across the otherwise normal PV. A louder harsher ejection systolic murmur in this area should however raise the suspicion of PS.
  - Pansystolic murmur loudest at the left sternal edge and accentuated by inspiration may be heard if there is TR secondary to RV overload.
  - S2: fixed and widely split. P2 is delayed because of the increased pulmonary flow. The effects of respiration on the degree of split are abolished by the direct communication between the atria. With inspiration, venous return to the right heart is increased and would normally delay P2 in the absence of an ASD. However, the increased RA pressure decreases the left-to-right shunt, increasing the amount of flow into LA and therefore the LV. The reverse happens in expiration.
  - P2 may be loud if pulmonary hypertension develops.
  - A soft low-pitch diastolic murmur can rarely be heard over the TV with large ASDs due to the increased blood flow across an effectively narrowed TV for the volume of blood.
- Signs of right-heart failure (pitting pedal and sacral oedema).

Severity

- Large (so-called non-restrictive) ASDs are suggested by evidence of RV volume overload, a diastolic flow murmur across the TV and pulmonary hypertension. AF developing as a result of LA enlargement (due to increased pulmonary venous return) also infers a large ASD.
- Less severe (non-restrictive) ASDs are characterized by an ejection murmur in the pulmonary area alone and absence of any signs of RV overload or failure, pulmonary hypertension or AF.

Types

- *Primum ASD* – now more properly called atrioventricular (AV) septation defect: results from abnormal development of the endocardial cushions and often associated with other defects such as a VSD.
- *Secundum ASD:* defect in fossa ovalis resulting from incomplete development of the septum secundum or excessive resorption of the septum primum.
- *Sinus venosus ASD:* results from defective folding of the atrial wall near the origin of the SVC. The result is a SVC that is in direct communication with both atria. Very frequently associated with anomalous drainage of the pulmonary veins into the RA.
- *Coronary sinus ASD:* these occur because of a defect in the wall separating the coronary sinus and the LA. The coronary sinus normally drains into the RA only. These defects are extremely rare.

Investigations

- 12-lead ECG (may reveal AF, 1st-degree AV-block, partial right bundle branch block, left axis deviation with primum defects, right axis deviation with secundum defects, unusual P-wave axis – especially with sinus venosus defects).
- CXR: cardiomegaly, atrial enlargement, dilated pulmonary arteries, pulmonary plethora.
- TTE: can be used to identify primum and secundum defects, assess the size of shunts and their effects on RV function. Bubble contrast may be needed to reveal these defects. Sinus venosus defects are difficult to visualize.
- TOE: used to define anatomy in more detail and assess suitability for deployment of percutaneous closure devices. Also used to diagnose sinus venosus defects and to identify any associated anomalous pulmonary venous drainage.
- Right and left heart catheterization: rarely necessary but can be useful for assessing pulmonary pressures and shunt ratio where this cannot be done with echocardiography. In those over the age of 40, simultaneous coronary angiography can be undertaken as part of pre-assessment for surgical closure if this is indicted. In patients with significant pulmonary hypertension (pressures >2/3 systemic), vasodilator testing can be undertaken to determine reversibility of pulmonary hypertension.
- Cardiac MRI: useful for detailed definition of anatomy and for assessment of shunt size and impact on RV function. Also useful for defining associated cardiac anomalies, particularly with sinus venosus and primum defects.

- Lung biopsy: this is undertaken in the rare patient in whom closure is being considered and right heart catheterization with vasodilator testing is equivocal about the reversibility of pulmonary hypertension when the histopathological features of irreversible pulmonary hypertension can be sought.

Management

In many cases no intervention is required in patients with ASD, however closure can be achieved surgically or more recently with percutaneous closure devices. This should be offered in the following circumstances:

- After paradoxical embolism.
- For symptomatic ASD.
- In asymptomatic patients who have evidence of a significant shunt (ratio pulmonary to systemic flow >1.5).
- In any patient, if there is evidence of significant pulmonary hypertension (pressures >2/3 systemic), closure should only be offered if this can be shown to be reversible on right heart catheterization with a vasodilator test and the shunt fraction (i.e. the ratio of pulmonary to systemic blood flow) is at least 1.5.

Viva questions

What is the Lutembacher syndrome?

This is the coexistence of a secundum ASD and rheumatic MS. The MS was mistakenly thought to be congenital when the syndrome was first described. Patients with rheumatic MS who are treated by percutaneous balloon mitral valvuloplasty can acquire the syndrome if they develop an ASD as a complication of the transseptal puncture required to get the valvuloplasty balloon into the LA via the RA.

Patent ductus arteriosus

Patients presenting in adulthood for the first time are often asymptomatic and are detected after a routine clinical examination or investigation for another indication. Small PDAs may not be haemodynamically significant but may become infected resulting in endarteritis (presenting as an unexplained fever). Moderate-sized PDAs pose a volume load on the left heart and may therefore present with palpitations (development of AF with LA enlargement) or symptoms of left heart failure (effort intolerance, orthopnoea, paroxysmal nocturnal dyspnoea). Large uncorrected PDAs can eventually present as Eisenmenger's syndrome but this normally develops in childhood.

Signs

- Differential cyanosis and clubbing: toes are cyanosed and clubbed whereas fingers are pink and normal. With a patent ductus arteriosus, oxygenated blood flows from the descending aorta into the low resistance lower pressure pulmonary artery. However, as pulmonary vascular resistance increases with large shunts over time, the shunt may reverse (Eisenmenger's syndrome), leading to the differential cyanosis and clubbing. If any desaturated blood enters the left subclavian artery (the ductus arteriosus is in closest proximity to this vessel) there may also be cyanosis and clubbing of the left hand, sparing the right.
- Pulse: collapsing in character with wide pulse pressure due to diastolic run-off from descending aorta to pulmonary artery via the PDA. Usually regular but may become irregularly irregular if AF develops as the LA enlarges secondary to chronic volume overload. The collapsing pulse may normalize if the shunt reverses and Eisenmenger's syndrome develops.
- JVP: usually not raised. There may be a prominent A-wave in the context of secondary pulmonary hypertension and CV-waves if TR develops.
- Apex: undisplaced with small PDAs. Displaced and volume overloaded (thrusting) with larger defects unless the shunt is reversed.
- Left parasternal heave due to RV-pressure overload from secondary pulmonary hypertension.
- Palpable P2 (suggestive of pulmonary hypertension and by definition implying a loud P2 on auscultation).
- Palpable thrill in the left infraclavicular area. This is systolic and extends part-way into diastole unless the shunt is large ('non-restrictive') or reverses.
- On auscultation:
  - Normal S1.
  - Loud systolic crescendo murmur that peaks just prior to S2 and is usually best heard in the left chest, more lateral to the pulmonary area.
  - Loud S2 due to loud P2 but often obscured by the loud murmur which can continue through S2 into diastole.
  - Loud continuation of systolic murmur in early diastole which then tapers off often giving rise to an uninterrupted murmur – the classic 'machinery' murmur. As pulmonary vascular resistance increases, the pressure gradient driving flow from the aorta to the pulmonary artery in diastole decreases and eventually the pressures may become equal resulting in loss of the diastolic component. Once the shunt reverses, the murmur disappears completely.

Severity

- Mild shunt (small PDA): continuous murmur but normal pulse character, no evidence of volume load on the LV and no signs of pulmonary hypertension.
- Moderate shunt (moderate PDA): continuous murmur, wide pulse pressure with collapsing pulse, volume-loaded LV and evidence of pulmonary hypertension.
- Severe shunt (large PDA with or without shunt reversal): In the later stages will often present as Eisenmenger's syndrome in the adult. If the shunt reverses, there is no murmur with evidence of differential cyanosis and clubbing. Very large left-to-right PDA shunts rarely present in adulthood and are usually diagnosed and corrected in childhood.

Aetiology

- Congenital.
- Neonatal Rubella syndrome (NB Rubella also causes peripheral pulmonary arterial stenosis).
- Prematurity, in which case the duct usually closes spontaneously.
- Birth at high-altitude.
- Prostaglandin E1 infusion (a temporizing measure to keep the ductus patent in patients with transposition of the great vessels).

Investigations

- ECG: biventricular hypertrophy, P-mitrale, AF. With shunt reversal, P-pulmonale and RV hypertrophy and strain pattern.
- CXR: ductus itself may be visualized especially if calcified, enlargement of left-sided chambers, pulmonary plethora.
- Echo: ductus can be identified and shunt fraction (ratio of pulmonary to systemic flow $Q_p{:}Q_s$) can be estimated. Effects of shunt on left and right heart can be assessed:
  - $Q_p{:}Q_s{<}1.5$ suggests a mild shunt.
  - $Q_p{:}Q_s$ of 1.5–2.2 suggests a moderate shunt.
  - $Q_p{:}Q_s{>}2.2$ suggests a severe shunt.

Management

- Tiny ducts which cannot be detected clinically are at very low lifetime risk of endocarditis and do not have any haemodynamic consequences. They can therefore be managed conservatively.
- Any duct which has been infected should be closed once infection has been resolved regardless of its size provided that there is no evidence of irreversible severe pulmonary hypertension.
- All other ducts should be closed unless there is evidence of shunt reversal or significant irreversible pulmonary hypertension. In borderline cases, closure should not be undertaken unless the $Q_p{:}Q_s$ >1.5 or unless pulmonary hypertension is at least partially reversible during vasodilator testing at right heart catheterization.
- Closure is achieved using a percutaneously deployed duct-closure device. If this is technically not feasible, surgical closure is performed.

Coarctation of the aorta

Patients presenting in adulthood may complain of fatigue, particularly of the lower limbs, intermittent claudication of the legs, symptoms of heart failure (exertional dyspnoea, orthopnoea, paroxysmal nocturnal dyspnoea and fluid retention), uncontrolled hypertension (epistaxis, headache, visual disturbances and stroke) or endarteritis (fever, rigors, splinter haemorrhages and other embolic phenomena). Patients can also present with chest pain due to atherosclerotic coronary disease, that develops at an accelerated rate with coarctation, and aortic dissection. The latter can also present with haemoptysis.

Signs

- Left lateral thoracotomy scar from surgical repair of the coarctation.
- Elevated left shoulder. This can be a complication of repair via a left lateral thoracotomy.
- Lower body is relatively underdeveloped compared to the upper body due to hypoperfusion. If the coarctation is preductal (proximal to the left subclavian artery), the left upper limb may be smaller than the right.
- Features of associated conditions such as Turner's syndrome (woman with short stature, webbed neck, low hairline, prominent epicanthial folds, hypertelorism, lack of pubic hair and other secondary sexual characteristics, shield-like chest with nipple hypoplasia, cubitus valgus, nail hypoplasia, short 4th metacarpals/metatarsals, numerous pigmented naevi, lymphoedema).
- Stigmata of endocarditis/endarteritis (pyrexia, clubbing, splinter haemorrhages, Osler's nodes, Janeway lesions, Roth spots, splenomegaly, microscopic haematuria, neurological deficits or other embolic phenomena).
- Pulse: normally brisk and forceful due to the attendant systolic hypertension. There may be a radio-radial pulse volume deficit if the coarctation is proximal to the left subclavian.
- Femoral pulses may be reduced or absent and there is radio-femoral delay – a delay in the arrival of the peak of femoral pressure relative to radial pressure.
- BP is significantly higher in the brachial artery than the femoral artery. The difference is usually proportional to the severity of the coarctation. There may also be a >20mmHg difference between left and right brachial systolic pressures.
- JVP: normal unless congestive cardiac failure develops.
- Apex: minimally displaced, sustained or heaving in character secondary to the pressure overload caused by the coarctation or aortic stenosis due to an associated bicuspid aortic valve.
- Systolic thrills may be palpable in the suprasternal notch. Aortic thrills may be palpable if there is coexistent bicuspid aortic valve stenosis.
- Auscultation:
  - Normal or loud S1 (reflecting hypertension).
  - Ejection click and/ejection systolic murmur in the aortic area due to stenosis of an associated bicuspid aortic valve.
  - Systolic murmur derived from the coarctation itself usually loudest over the thoracic spine or lower in abdominal coarctation.

Classically begins after the first 1/3 of systole. The murmur is short in mild coarctation and becomes progressively longer and may even extend into diastole with more severe defects.
- Continuous systolic-diastolic murmurs audible throughout the praecordium and at the back emanating from collaterals.
- S2 is often loud due to accentuation of the aortic component.
- S4 may be heard reflecting significant LVH.
- An early diastolic murmur may be heard if there is AR from an associated bicuspid aortic valve.

❶ Top Tips
- Routinely check for radio-femoral delay in young patients with unexplained hypertension. This is best appreciated by placing the right wrist next to the right groin and simultaneously palpating both pulses.

❧ Common Pitfalls
- The left radial artery should not be used as it can be weak or attenuated as well as delayed in some cases.
- The slow rising pulse of AS due to a bicuspid valve may be augmented by a significant coarctation. This can lead to underestimation of the severity of AS if the pulse alone is relied upon.
- Similarly, AR gives rise to a wide pulse pressure and can misleadingly give the impression that the femoral pulse is normal unless comparison is made with carotid or brachial pulses and checks are made for radio-femoral delay.

Associated diseases and complications
- Bicuspid aortic valve and its sequelae (85% of patients)
- VSD
- MV prolapse
- Patent ductus arteriosus
- Aortic dissection
- Turner's syndrome
- Neurofibromatosis type I
- Marfan's syndrome
- Subarachnoid haemorrhage (associated with berry aneurysms of the circle of Willis in 5% of patients)
- Shone's syndrome (supravalvular mitral membrane, parachute MV, subaortic stenosis, and aortic coarctation)

Investigations
- 12-lead ECG: LVH with strain pattern.
- CXR: rib notching due to formation of intercostals artery collaterals, classically over the posterior 3rd to 8th ribs. May also reveal aneurysmal post-stenotic aortic dilatation. The coarctation itself may be visualized as an indentation in the aorta giving rise to a '3'-shaped descending thoracic aorta.

- TTE allows identification of the coarctation, assessment of its effects on the LV, and identification of any associated lesions (◆ Signs, p.271).
- TOE can be useful for assessing the coarctation anatomy further as well as excluding dissection and infective complications.
- Cardiac MRI is a very useful modality providing exquisite detail of both anatomy and functional effects. Useful for planning repairs and assessing their outcomes.
- Cardiac catheterization is useful for assessing coronary anatomy when surgical repair is contemplated given the high incidence of premature coronary artery disease. It can also be used to estimate the gradient across the coarctation but this can be equally well assessed non-invasively.

Management

Where technically feasible, primary percutaneous endovascular stenting is now an option and is also used to treat restenosis developing after primary surgical repair.

- Surgical repair can be accomplished by resection of the coarctation and end-to-end anastomosis provided that the affected segment is small. Longer segments of disease may require placement of an interposition graft or a bypass graft. A subclavian flap repair technique can also be used in which case the left radial pulse may be weak.
- Medical therapy is directed at treatment of hypertension and aggressive risk factor modification given the high incidence of premature coronary artery disease.

Viva questions

What are the indications for intervention/surgery?

- All symptomatic patients with a gradient >30mmHg across the coarctation should be offered treatment. Similar asymptomatic patients should also be treated in the presence of hypertension or signs of LVH.
- Patients requiring cardiothoracic surgery for another indication such as a bicuspid aortic valve or aortic arch aneurysm.

What advice should patients be given about exercise?

Patients with both treated and untreated aortic coarctation should be advised to avoid extreme isometric exercise such as weight-lifting given the increased risk of aortic dissection. Other forms of exercise, however, are helpful in maintaining health and reducing BP.

Hypertrophic cardiomyopathy

Patients may present with symptoms of heart failure (fatigue, exertional dyspnoea, orthopnoea, paroxysmal nocturnal dyspnoea, fluid retention), syncope (due to LVOT obstruction or malignant ventricular tachyarrhythmias), AF (palpitations, decreased exercise tolerance, stroke), chest pain (hypertrophy increasing myocardial oxygen demand and exceeding supply or myocardial bridging — intramyocardial compression of coronary arteries) or sudden death.

Signs

- Infraclavicular scar with underlying device — permanent dual chamber pacemaker to decrease LVOT gradient or ICD for those at high risk of sudden death (➲ Management, p.275).
- Pulse is jerky or bifid/bisferiens. There is a rapid upstroke which briefly terminates in mid-systole as the outflow tract is obstructed and resumes again as the ventricle overcomes the obstruction. The stiff, hypertrophied, non-compliant ventricle requires high filling pressures. The resulting chronic elevation of LA pressure leads to LA enlargement giving rise to AF.
- JVP is normal or has a prominent A-wave reflecting the increased RA pressures required to fill the RV which can also be involved in HCM.
- Apex — minimally displaced and heaving in character. There may be a double apical impulse reflecting palpable atrial contraction prior to ventricular contraction. The first impulse is due to the forceful atrial contraction causing the heart to rotate and the apex to tap against the body wall.
- On auscultation:
  - S1 is usually normal or loud.
  - Pansystolic murmur due to MR. This can occur as a result of systolic anterior motion of the anterior leaflet of the MV which in turn is caused by a Venturi effect due to the rapid blood flow in the LVOT.
  - Ejection systolic murmur loudest at the left sternal edge. The murmur is made longer and louder by standing and short and quieter by squatting (see 'Top Tips' below).
  - S2 is usually normal (reflecting lack of any aortic valve abnormality).
  - S4 may be audible, reflecting the rapid and vigorous pre-systolic contraction of the atrium to fill the stiff, non-compliant hypertrophied LV. Disappears with AF.
  - Signs of heart failure (pitting pedal or sacral oedema, coarse basal late inspiratory crackles).

> **❶ Top Tips**
> - The ejection systolic murmur results from a combination of systolic anterior movement of the anterior leaflet of the MV and asymmetrical septal hypertrophy. Any manoeuvre that makes the heart smaller therefore increases LVOT obstruction. Standing does this by decreasing venous return. Squatting, by increasing venous return and by increasing afterload (clamping the femoral vessels and decreasing the amount of blood ejected from the LV) increases heart size and has the opposite effect. Aortic stenosis behaves oppositely.

Aetiology

Hereditary – autosomal dominant pattern of inheritance. Mutations have been found in at least 11 different sarcomeric protein genes. Phenotype and penetrance can vary considerably even with the same mutation in different related individuals. Prevalence of 1 in 500 of the general population.

Investigations

- 12-lead ECG can be normal but in the majority (>95%) is abnormal revealing P-mitrale, LVH, marked lateral T-wave inversion, deep septal Q-waves laterally, and/or AF. Occasionally associated with Wolff–Parkinson–White syndrome (short PR interval, delta-waves, SVT).
- 24-hour Holter monitoring – used to screen for ventricular tachycardia as part of risk assessment.
- CXR is often normal or may reveal evidence of LA or LV enlargement.
- Exercise tolerance test – used to assess BP response to exercise as part of risk assessment. Exercise stress echo is used to assess effect of exertion on outflow tract gradient as this is dynamic and resting assessments may be misleading.
- TTE is used to define the pattern of hypertrophy, to assess the severity of LVOT obstruction and the degree of systolic anterior movement of the MV as well as any associated MR.
- Cardiac MRI – provides exquisite anatomical detail and useful for identifying mimics such as amyloid.

Management

- Assess risk factors for sudden cardiac death:
  - Previous arrhythmic cardiac arrest.
  - Sustained ventricular tachycardia (>30 seconds by definition).
  - Non-sustained VT on Holter monitoring.
  - Family history of sudden cardiac death in a 1st-degree relative.
  - Unexplained syncope (especially if during exertion).
  - Abnormal BP response to exercise (hypotension or failure of BP to rise with exercise).
  - Massive LVH (wall thickness ≥30mm).
  - LV apical aneurysm.
  - Dilated end-stage heart failure with LV-systolic dysfunction.

Patients with any of these risk factors should be considered for an ICD.
- Medical treatments:
  - Symptomatic patients are treated with beta-blockers. These reduce heart rate (increasing myocardial perfusion and relaxation), reduce contractility (reducing myocardial oxygen consumption), and block the effects of catecholamines on LVOT gradient with exertion.
  - Verapamil enhances LV relaxation, reduces heart rate and LV filling. It is particularly useful in patients without a large LVOT-gradient.
  - Disopyramide is used for its negative inotropic properties as an adjunct to beta-blockers. It is particularly useful in patients whose symptoms are attributable to LVOT obstruction.
  - Disopyramide accelerates AV-conduction and so should be combined with a beta-blocker.

- Diuretics can be used to relieve pulmonary congestion but care must be taken to avoid overdiuresis as this can decrease LV cavity size and thereby worsen LVOT gradient.
- Digoxin is a positive inotrope and so should be avoided unless the patient is in AF and has not responded to a beta-blocker alone.
- Warfarin is used for AF. The threshold for its introduction is lower than for patients without hypertrophic cardiomyopathy.
- Treatment of LVOT obstruction:
  - Patients who are refractory to maximal medical therapy and who have NYHA III/IV dyspnoea due to LVOT obstruction (gradient ≥50mmHg at rest or on exertion) can be offered percutaneous alcohol septal ablation. This involves injection of ethanol into a septal branch of the left anterior descending coronary artery. This generates a controlled myocardial infarction of the hypertrophied septum which then scars and regresses relieving the LVOT obstruction due to septal hypertrophy.
  - Patients who are not candidates for alcohol septal ablation because of unsuitable anatomy or blood supply to the septum can be offered surgical myectomy. This involves surgical resection of myocardium from the basal septum. It has the advantage that it does not create a potentially arrhythmogenic scar (unlike alcohol septal ablation) and is complicated by a lower incidence of AV-block. The operative mortality may be lower than percutaneous strategies. It may therefore be a preferable option for those willing to undergo surgery.
  - Dual chamber pacing was previously advocated as a method for reducing LVOT obstruction. The ventricular lead of a dual chamber pacemaker is implanted in the RV apex. This alters the normal sequence of activation of the myocardium. Pacing induces dysynchronous contraction of the septum causing it to contract early and even paradoxically relative to the lateral LV wall. However, RCTs have not shown it to be more effective than placebo at improving symptoms therefore it can no longer be recommended in the absence of another indication for pacing.
- Screening of other family members should be offered both with echocardiography and in suitable cases with genetic testing.

Marfan's syndrome

Marfan's syndrome, first described in 1896, is an autosomal dominant complex of signs due to a number of defects in the fibrillin-1 gene, which is present on chromosome 15. The fibrillin protein is found in association with elastin, and amongst other things seems to be required for the proper formation of elastic fibres. The condition is fairly rare, with an estimated prevalence of 1 in 5000–10,000, but given the stability of those with the syndrome and the range of clinical manifestations, it occurs rather more frequently in PACES.

Diagnosis

The syndrome primarily manifests itself as defects in the ocular, cardio-vascular and skeletal system and additional abnormalities are noted in the skin and respiratory systems (see Table 5.12). The most recent diagnostic criteria are defined by the Ghent system and in order to make the diagnosis, major criteria must be present in 2 different systems with additional involvement of a third.

Symptoms

Initially none, but the syndrome is generally diagnosed either in the course of screening of the family of an index case, or when the individual presents with one of the component features.

Management

Once the syndrome has been recognized, management is mainly concerned with dealing with whichever of the various features are present in that particular individual. Two aspects require particular attention however: family screening with investigations to detect manifestations in relatives, particularly aortic dilatation and screening for aortic aneurysm in the individual themselves. Echocardiography is the investigation of choice and the aortic dimensions should be meticulously recorded, with measurements being taken at the aortic valve annulus, sinuses of Valsalva, sino-tubular ridge and ascending aorta. Relatives of a patient with aortic dissection are more likely to have aortic involvement as involvement of particular systems tends to run in the same family.

Beta blockers have been shown to reduce the rate of aortic dilatation and should be prescribed to anyone with abnormal aortic dimensions.

Indications for aortic root replacement

- Symptomatic AR.
- Asymptomatic AR meeting the criteria for surgery stated previously (◑ Aortic regurgitation, p.233).
- Dilation of the aortic root with a maximum diameter >45mm. Note this is less than the threshold of 55mm usually given for aortic root dilatation not associated with Marfan's.
- An aortic growth rate of 1cm or more in 1 year, particularly if there is a family history of aortic dissection.

Table 5.12 The Ghent system for diagnosis of Marfan's syndrome

Cardiovascular	Ocular	Skeletal	Respiratory	Skin and integumentary
Dilatation of the ascending aorta involving the sinuses	**Ectopia lentis**	**Pectus carinatum**	Spontaneous pneumothorax	**Lumbosacral dural ectasia on CT or MRI**
Aortic dissection	Abnormally flat cornea	**Pectus excavatum requiring surgery**	Apical blebs on CXR	Skin striae not due to weight changes
MV prolapse	↑ axial length of the globe	↓ upper to lower segment ratio or arm span/height ratio >1.05		Recurrent or incisional herniae
Mitral annular calcification occurring <40 years	Hypoplastic iris or ciliary muscle	**Hypermobility of wrist or thumb joints**[a]		
Dilatation of pulmonary trunk aged <40		**Scoliosis or spondylolisthesis**		
Dilatation or dissection of the descending aorta aged <50		**Reduced elbow extension**		
		Pes planus		
		Protrusio acetabulae		
		Lesser pectus excavatum		
		High-arched palate		
		Other joint hypermobility		
		Typical facial appearance		

Major criteria are shown in bold type. Diagnosis requires major criteria to be present in at least 2 systems, with involvement (major or minor) of a further system.

[a] Steinberg's sign occurs when the thumb flexed at the metacarpophalangeal (MCP) joint crosses the ulnar border of the hand.

Viva questions

How may Marfan's syndrome present acutely/what are the acute complications?

Aortic dissection. This is the most feared complication as the mortality rate is at least 50%, whereas the mortality of elective aortic root replacement is around 5%.

How should patients with Marfan's be followed-up?

The major objective of follow-up is to avoid acute aortic dissection. A yearly echo should be done to monitor the aortic root, and if there is a family history of aortic dissection or the aorta has started to dilate, this should be more frequently.

What is the mode of inheritance?

Autosomal dominant with complete penetrance but very variable clinical expression. Even within a given family the manifestations can be quite variable and between families there is great variation, due to different mutations in the fibrillin gene being present.

Fallot's tetralogy

The majority of adults seen in the exam will have had a complete repair procedure but may have been initially palliated with a shunt prior to the inception of modern cardiothoracic surgery or as a temporizing measure. Patients featuring in the exam will therefore have either a shunt and/or signs of complications of the repair procedure.

> **Key facts**
>
> The tetralogy comprises a non-restrictive (large) VSD, an overriding aorta, RVOT obstruction (which may be subvalvular, valvular, supravalvular, or any combination of these 3) and right ventricular hypertrophy. Cyanosis occurs because deoxygenated blood from the RV can pass readily across the VSD into the overriding aorta in preference to entering the obstructed RVOT. Prior to modern complete repair surgery, this was palliated by fashioning a direct shunt between the subclavian and ipsilateral pulmonary arteries (Blalock–Taussig shunt) or indirectly via an interposition GoreTex® graft (modified Blalock–Taussig shunt). This had the effect of bypassing the obstructed RVOT and increasing pulmonary blood flow.

Signs

There are a multitude of possible signs that may be present including a wide variety of different murmurs. The key to success is to recognize the syndrome and then to consider each of the features in turn, assessing whether it is present, and if so, what is the severity.

- Abnormal facies (long face, low set ears, evidence of previous cleft palate repair – part of the velocardiofacial or DiGeorge syndrome). The facial features are, however, usually normal in patients with tetralogy of Fallot, the majority of which are not associated with a syndrome.

- Unilateral pectoral hypoplasia (Poland's syndrome – associated with tetralogy of Fallot). One arm may be slightly underdeveloped relative to the other on the side of any shunt procedure – suggesting this was done in very early childhood.
- Sternotomy (from total correction surgery) and lateral thoracotomy (from original palliative surgery to fashion a Blalock–Taussig shunt).
- Corrigan's pulse suggesting AR: a complication following repair surgery or due to associated aortic root disease.
- Device: pacemaker or ICD: for sustained complete heart block postoperatively or for treatment of malignant ventricular arrhythmias.
- Radio-radial pulse volume deficit: pulse weaker on side ipsilateral to any shunt. May be irregularly irregular due to AF (present in >1/3 of patients). May be collapsing if AR is present.
- BP: ask to measure this in both arms. If you are trying to detect a wide pulse pressure to look for AR, the BP should be checked on the side contralateral to any shunt.
- JVP: may be elevated if right-heart failure is present. This may be secondary to pulmonary regurgitation, or giant CV waves may be seen due to tricuspid regurgitation secondary to RV dysfunction.
- Apex: usually minimally displaced but may be thrusting and displaced if AR is present or if secondary MR develops.
- Left parasternal heave may be felt suggestive of RV pressure overload.
- A systolic thrill may be felt along the left sternal edge from a residual VSD (failure of complete closure at the time of repair or subsequent partial patch dehiscence). The defect is usually very small and therefore gives rise to a loud systolic murmur which is palpable as a thrill.
- A further systolic thrill may be palpable in the pulmonary area if there is any residual RVOT obstruction or restenosis of a bioprosthetic PV prosthesis.
- Auscultation can reveal a plethora of abnormal heart sounds and murmurs depending on which complications are present. These can easily be deciphered with careful logical and systematic auscultation:
  - Pansystolic murmur loudest at the apex with expiration and radiating to the axilla due to MR.
  - Pansystolic murmur at the left sternal edge which increases in intensity with inspiration due to TR.
  - Loud pansystolic murmur at left sternal border due to residual VSD – the louder the murmur, the smaller the defect.
  - Early diastolic murmur at 3rd left intercostal space accentuated with expiration and leaning forward due to AR, which occurs due to deformity of the aortic valve due to the abnormal aortic anatomy.
  - Ejection systolic murmur in the pulmonary area due to RVOT obstruction or PS.
  - Early diastolic murmur in the pulmonary area due to PR (often in combination with stenosis giving rise to a to-and-fro systolic-diastolic murmur).
  - Early diastolic murmur in the aortic area due to AR. Soft systolic murmur across the aortic valve if the AR is significant and gives rise to increased systolic transaortic flow.
  - The 2nd heart sound is often soft due to PR and AR. If present, it is usually single due to absence of the pulmonary component.

- Signs of heart failure (pitting pedal or sacral oedema, coarse basal late inspiratory crackles).

❶ Top Tips

- If the patient has a Blalock–Taussig shunt, the radial and brachial pulses will be weak on the ipsilateral side. Identifying this sign together with an ipsilateral thoracotomy scar (for the shunt) and sternotomy scar (for the subsequent total correction) enables spot diagnosis of an otherwise apparently complicated case.

✴ Common Pitfalls

- Remember that when assessing pulse character and BP, check the normal arm, not the side of the Blalock–Taussig shunt. Ensure that you carefully and diligently palpate the praecordium for thrills as identifying these will make interpretation of any auscultatory findings easier.

Severity

Given the multitude of lesions which may be present, an integrated assessment of the severity of each must be performed as for isolated lesions. Concentrate on the effects on left and right ventricular function. Severe PR is a particularly significant complication of older repairs which required a patch of pericardium to repair the RVOT obstruction. Severe PR with signs of RV dysfunction indicates the need for PV replacement surgery.

Investigations

- ECG: right axis deviation, right bundle branch block (with R' >10mV) and right ventricular hypertrophy with dominant R-wave in V1 (>6mV). Look at the QRS duration. If this is >180ms, there is increased risk of sudden death.
- CXR: look for evidence of chamber enlargement, dilated aorta, attenuated/underdeveloped pulmonary vasculature, boot-shaped heart.
- Holter: used to screen for AF/atrial flutter and for non-sustained VT in at risk patients (those with severe PR, RV dysfunction, QT-dispersion/prolongation, or QRS duration >180ms).
- Echo: useful for assessing all valves, biventricular function, and for initial assessment of the aortic root.
- Cardiac MRI: best method of assessing RV dimensions and function as well as defining nature and severity of any other lesions that might be present.

Viva questions

Is endocarditis prophylaxis warranted in these patients for dental surgery?

No. There is little evidence to justify routine endocarditis prophylaxis. There is an inconsistent relationship between bacteraemia from dental procedures and subsequent endocarditis and even less evidence of a positive benefit for prophylactic antibiotics. Simply brushing teeth can cause significant bacteraemia. Accordingly, current guidelines recommend antibiotics in at-risk patients only if a gastrointestinal or genitourinary tract procedure is being undertaken at a site of active or suspected infection (in which cases antibiotics directed at treating that infection should cover organisms that can cause endocarditis). Patients with uncorrected tetralogy of Fallot are deemed to be high risk for endocarditis. Those with a complete correction are deemed at moderate risk.

What other shunts are sometimes used to palliate tetralogy of Fallot and when are these used?

The Waterston shunt is a direct anastomosis between the ascending aorta and the main/right pulmonary artery. It was used if the subclavian artery was too small to allow a Blalock–Taussig shunt to be fashioned, such as in neonates. The shunt has the advantage that it grows with the patient. However, the increased pulmonary flow may result in long-term pulmonary hypertension so this remains a palliative procedure. Such patients have a continuous loud murmur associated with the shunt identical to that of a PDA. The Potts shunt is a similar shunt between the descending aorta and the left pulmonary artery performed for similar indications but is associated with more complications and was therefore less popular.

Do these patients need genetic counselling?

Yes. Approximately 15% of patients have a deletion of chromosome 22q11. This can easily be detected by chromosomal analysis using fluorescence *in situ* hybridization (FISH). There is a 50% risk of transmission to offspring by definition.

What are the main late problems that these patients can experience after a complete repair and how are these tackled?

- PR in those who had a transannular patch placed across the pulmonary valve annulus to repair the RVOT obstruction. Treated by PV replacement with a homograft or xenograft.
- AR and/or aortic root dilatation. This occurs due to distortion of the aortic valve during VSD repair or as a consequence of root dilatation. Treated by aortic valve ± root replacement.
- Rhythm disturbances. Atrial flutter and scar-related tachycardias may be amenable to ablation. Ventricular tachycardia often originates from the RVOT. Risk of sudden death can be reduced by tackling causes of underlying RV impairment (e.g. PV replacement in those with severe PR) as well as by ablation and use of ICD where risk is particularly high. Patients with AF or atrial flutter should be anticoagulated with warfarin.
- Residual VSD. This should be closed if the shunt ratio (pulmonary:systemic flow) exceeds 1.5.

Why did young patients with uncorrected tetralogy of Fallot find squatting a helpful manoeuvre?

Squatting, by effectively clamping the femoral vessels increases aortic afterload. Blood therefore finds it easier (in relative terms) to pass down the RVOT instead. This together with the increased venous return encourages more blood to pass into the lungs, ameliorating cyanosis.

New developments

Stenting of the RVOT. This can be used as a temporizing palliative procedure in neonates not fit for surgery. Definitive surgery can then be undertaken when the patient recovers sufficiently.

Dextrocardia

This is an uncommon congenital heart disorder, accounting for only around 0.01% of live births, with 2/3 of cases occurring in males. As people with this condition would normally survive to adulthood, they may well appear in PACES.

Clinically one would suspect dextrocardia when the apex beat is not felt on the left and then is found on the right side. It should be noted that true dextrocardia is when the heart is located on the right side of the chest and the cardiac axis from base to apex, points towards the right. The heart can be shifted over towards the right due to a variety of conditions of the lungs or the chest wall. Sometimes this may result in the heart being more displaced to the right (usually as judged on a CXR), but this is not dextrocardia as the base–apex axis will still be towards the left.

Signs

- The cardiac apex is felt on the right.
- Heart sounds are much louder on the right-hand side and are reflected in a reversed left-to-right manner e.g. MV 5th intercostal position on the right-hand side.
- Situs inversus is a very common association and should be carefully sought, for example by percussing for the liver borders.
- In paediatric cases other complex cardiac defects are quite commonly associated with dextrocardia, but in adults who may end up appearing as a case in PACES, this is much less likely. Nevertheless, there is a reasonable chance that other, more minor, cardiac abnormalities might be present such as ASD and these should be specifically looked for in the examination.
- In patients with dextrocardia, but without other complex congenital heart defects, common cardiac pathologies occur with the same frequency as a patient without dextrocardia. Again the clinical findings would be reflected in a left-to-right manner.
- Examine the lungs for evidence of bronchiectasis. Kartagener's syndrome is the association of dextrocardia, situs inversus, bronchiectasis and infertility in males.

Investigation

- CXR to confirm the right-sided heart.
- ECG will show a diminution of the R waves going from V1 to V6 (i.e. the opposite of the normal R wave progression), unless the chest leads are placed on the right side.
- Echocardiogram, mainly to assess the presence of any other cardiac abnormalities.
- MRI may also be necessary to assess such things as ventriculo-arterial concordance or discordance. In addition, the venous drainage of the lungs needs to be defined, as partial or total anomalous pulmonary venous drainage is quite commonly present when there are other complex defects associated with the dextrocardia.

Management

Dextrocardia in isolation does not warrant any management, but the relatively frequent associated disorders may require treatment. This would be undertaken by congenital heart disease specialists and consideration of the management of complex congenital heart disease is beyond the scope of this text.

Viva question

What is Kartagener's syndrome?

The association of dextrocardia, situs inversus, bronchiectasis and infertility in males. This is a rare autosomal recessive condition characterized by dysfunction of the dynein arm of cilia. This results in dysfunction and dysmotility of the cilia. In fetal life the defect causes problems with folding and movement of developing organs, resulting in the dextrocardia and situs inversus. In post-natal life, the ciliary dysfunction causes failure of the mucociliary elevator in the lungs and consequent bronchiectasis and plugging of spermatic ducts resulting in male infertility.

Neurology

Gerry Christofi*
Guy Leschziner*
Robin S. Howard

* Joint first authors

Introduction

The neurology section of the PACES examination is often the major cause of (unnecessary!) anxiety for MRCP candidates. The key is to approach the patient in a logical fashion. Some neurology cases are simply an exercise in pattern recognition – noticing the frontal balding and ptosis of myotonic dystrophy, the distal wasting and pes cavus of Charcot–Marie–Tooth disease, for example. However, in those cases without obvious clues to the underlying diagnosis, a clear systematic approach will usually pay dividends.

Localizing the site of the lesion

When faced with a neurological problem, the first question that should be posed is the site of the lesion. During the course of the examination, identify signs that might help in localization:

- Cortex: signs of dysfunction of higher cognitive function.
- Subcortical: upper motor neuron (UMN) signs (hypertonia, pyramidal pattern of weakness, hyper-reflexia, extensor plantars), slowness of thought.
- Basal ganglia: cogwheel rigidity, resting tremor, bradykinesia, postural instability, dyskinesias, dystonias.
- Brainstem: cranial nerve abnormalities with contralateral UMN signs.
- Cerebellum: gait ataxia, nystagmus, finger–nose ataxia, past-pointing.
- Spinal cord: bilateral UMN signs, presence of a sensory level.
- Nerve root: lower motor neuron (LMN) signs (wasting, weakness, hyporeflexia, sensory loss) in a myotomal or dermatomal distribution.
- Single or multiple nerve/plexus: LMN signs that are focal, and are not consistent with a nerve root lesion.
- Polyneuropathy: LMN signs, more pronounced distally, affecting the legs more than the hands, diminished reflexes, sensory signs.
- Neuromuscular junction: weakness without sensory involvement or significant wasting, usually but not invariably proximal, which fluctuates (either with time of day or during the course of the examination).
- Muscle: wasting and weakness with normal reflexes and sensation.

Defining the aetiology of the lesion

Once the lesion has been localized, consider the disease processes that commonly affect that site. Clues may be obtained from the history, if you are permitted to ask questions. The most helpful aspect of the history is usually the speed of onset:

- Seconds: electrical disturbance (i.e. epilepsy), trauma.
- <5 minutes: infarction.
- >5 minutes: migraine, haemorrhage.
- Minutes–hours: infection, inflammation, drugs.
- Hours–days: infection, inflammation, nutritional, drugs.
- Days–months: inflammation, nutritional, chronic infection, neoplasia, drugs.
- Months–years: degenerative (including genetic disorders), neoplasia, occasionally chronic infection, drugs.

In the heat of the examination, this algorithm can be utilized to avoid 'meltdown' in the face of what, at first appearances, can seem like an impossible case. Remember, demonstrating a coherent approach to a neurological problem will often result in a passing mark, even if the final correct diagnosis is not achieved.

This chapter has been divided into two sections. The first provides the candidate both with an approach to common problems that will be encountered, as well as a suitable format to tailor the examination to the specific presenting features.

The second section targets specific conditions that tend to occur with high frequency in the examination, and presents background information that may be required for the 'viva'.

In the preparation for the PACES examination, we suggest that you develop a general approach to examination of neurology patients, but cross-reference to the appropriate disease-specific section.

Approach to the neurological examination

In normal neurological practice, the examination is performed in the context of the history in an attempt to localize the lesion. Within the PACES setting, the available history will be absent or extremely limited, and so the neurological examination must be tailored to make use of all available clues. The candidate will be asked to perform a particular aspect of the neurological examination, for example to examine a patient's lower limbs. Given the limitation of time, it is important that the physical act of the neurological examination is as automatic as possible, so that you can concentrate on picking up and interpreting the signs, rather than thinking about the examination itself – this can only be achieved through practice.

The examiners (and authors) assume that the candidate can perform a general examination and understands the rudiments of neurology. A full description of the neurological examination is beyond the scope of this book, but if necessary, it is suggested that candidates refer to a standard text on neurological examination (see ➲ Further Reading p.297).

General principles

- As with other systems, examine the patient in the standard, 'textbook' way, as an unorthodox approach is likely to be disapproved of by the examiners. In the neurological context, this means performing the cranial nerve examination in a systematic way, from cranial nerve I to XII, and for limb examination, examining tone, power, reflexes, coordination, and sensation in that order.
- Always stand back and observe the patient from a distance, looking around the bed for additional signs such as walking aids, spirometer, medication or steroid cards. When instructed to examine the limbs, ask the patient's permission to fully expose them, and remember to look at the trunk and back. Replace the patient's clothing or blanket after the examination and thank them.
- Examine what the instructions tell you to. Always start with the examination suggested in the scenario. For example, if told to examine the upper limbs in a patient with very clear parkinsonian

tremor, do not leap to assess the gait. Make a show of inspecting the tremor, demonstrating that it is worse at rest, and there are other extrapyramidal features in the arms, before then going on to demonstrate extrapyramidal gait and monotonous speech.

- Ask if the patient has any pain before examining. If you inadvertently cause discomfort or pain during the examination, apologize and continue, but try to avoid going to pieces as a result. This is not necessarily a 'fail'!

Specific aspects of the neurological examination are addressed later, and the format of this chapter aims to provide a focused examination to certain clinical scenarios and conditions. Below is a guide to the general neurological examination that should be used in conjunction with these specific sections later in the chapter.

General inspection

- Look around the patient for evidence of medication, a steroid card, spirometer (suggesting respiratory compromise), orthoses (e.g. ankle–foot orthosis suggesting a foot drop) or mobility aids (e.g. a wheelchair which should prompt you to ask if they are able to walk before asking the patient to get up!).
- Then look at the patient directly. Examine for:
  - Bracelets or necklaces alerting to a particular medical condition.
  - General habitus: cushingoid appearance of steroid treatment, or specific pattern of muscle wasting suggestive of a diagnosis e.g. wasted temporalis indicating myotonic dystrophy.
  - Limb deformity or abnormal posture e.g. pes cavus of Charcot–Marie–Tooth disease (place a flat rigid object over the sole – if you can see daylight between the foot and the object, then pes cavus is present), wasted small limb of old polio, extended plantar flexed lower limb and flexed pronated upper limb suggesting a contralateral UMN lesion.
  - Face: look for ptosis, dysconjugate gaze or facial weakness. If facial weakness is present, note whether or not the frontalis muscles are spared, thus determining between an upper and lower facial nerve lesion; this will help direct the further examination.
  - Skin: rashes of SLE, lupus pernio, erythema nodosum or livedo reticularis. Heliotropic rash and Gottron's papules of dermatomyositis. Dry skin of hypothyroidism. Dry, hairless discoloured skin resulting from autonomic dysfunction in small fibre neuropathy.
  - Scars: muscle biopsy scars over triceps, deltoid or quadriceps. Nerve biopsy scar over lateral aspect of the ankle (sural nerve). Sternotomy scar suggesting thymectomy in myasthenia gravis. Scars over anterior or posterior aspect of neck suggesting previous cervical decompression, or over lumbar spine (laminectomy). Examine the scalp and behind the ear for evidence of previous burrhole surgery or craniotomy (e.g. removal of cerebellopontine angle tumour in the latter position).
  - Wasting: look at the intrinsic muscles of the hand, muscles of the face and legs. There may be global, proximal or distal wasting. Look for the 'inverted champagne bottle' appearance in Charcot–Marie–Tooth disease.

- Fasciculations: suggest a LMN problem. If found on the tongue, a diagnosis of motor neuron disease (MND) is likely but always assess tongue fasciculations in a relaxed tongue resting on the floor of the mouth.
- Abnormal movements: tremor, dystonia (forced sustained contraction), chorea (increased fidgeting), myoclonus (irregular jerking of limbs or fingers). If a tremor is present, observe if worse at rest, movement or posture – this can be formally examined later.

Gait (→ p.297)

Assessment of gait frequently provides the strongest pointers to the neurological problem. If possible, when asked to examine the lower limbs, ask the patient to walk immediately after general inspection. Beware of patients who are unsteady or cannot walk unaided, and always ask if someone can walk before asking them to do so.

- Initially stand the patient, and ensure stability on standing. Assess the base – is it narrow or broad? The latter suggests a cerebellar problem.
- Ask the patient to walk, taking a few steps with them at first. Assess if normal or abnormal, and if abnormal, if symmetrical or asymmetrical. Different types of gait include:
  - Spastic (scissoring): narrow-based, stiff, toe-scuffing (spastic paraparesis).
  - Hemiparetic: circumducting with scuffing of one foot (stroke).
  - Extrapyramidal: shuffling, festinant (hurrying), with poor arm swing, or simply very slow (parkinsonian), in some patients with freezing and slow turning.
  - Apraxic: e.g. with gait ignition failure, or with walking difficulty ('marche à petit pas').
  - Ataxic: broad-based, unsteady (cerebellar syndrome).
  - High stepping (foot drop), myopathic, antalgic, neuropathic.
  - Unusual in any other way e.g. affected by disorders of movement, such as dystonia, chorea or myoclonus.
- If the gait appears to be normal, ask the patient to tandem-walk ('could you walk heel-to-toe, as if on a tight-rope?') – this may bring out subtle gait ataxia.
- Perform Romberg's test: ask the patient to stand with a narrow base. The test is positive if the patient is stable with eyes open, but become unsteady with eyes closed, suggesting that there is loss of joint position sense i.e. sensory ataxia.

⊕ Top Tips

- When examining gait remember to walk alongside your patient if they appear unsteady.
- If there is clear evidence that a patient is unable or unsafe to walk, e.g. a wheelchair or Zimmer frame, consider omitting the gait examination – it may become very evident that they are unable to walk due to severe spasticity, weakness or incoordination.

Cranial nerves

The cranial nerve examination is systematically detailed on → p.358. More than any other aspect of the neurological examination, this needs to be practised repeatedly, as it is all too easy to forget to examine some of the cranial nerves, particularly in the heat of the moment, and the systematic examination should be automatic.

Limbs

Examination orthodoxy is that the order of the examination is inspection, tone, power, coordination, sensation and reflexes, although examination of the reflexes immediately after power is also permissible. Beware, that any significant deviation from these two routines may alert, or even irritate, the examiners.

There are some simple screening tests that can be performed within the limb examination that can be extremely helpful:

• Inspect the limbs for scars, wasting, fasciculations, posture, abnormal movements, and other features as outlined in ➋ General inspection, p.288. Try to find clues as to whether there is an UMN or LMN problem, and if LMN, if the pattern of wasting or posture suggests any specific nerve or root lesion.

• After inspection, assess the hands for tremor at rest, then ask the patient to outstretch their supinated hands in front of them. Assess for the disappearance of a resting tremor, or the presence of a postural tremor:

  • Look for the slow pronation of one hand ('pronator drift') suggesting a pyramidal lesion – if absent, ask the patient to close their eyes and see if drift then occurs.

  • Slow drop of the arms may suggest the fatiguability of myasthenia.

  • With eyes still closed, assess for rebound phenomenon to identify a cerebellar syndrome – ask the patient to maintain arm position while pushing down hard on one arm, then suddenly releasing it. With cerebellar dysfunction, the limb will return to position after oscillations.

• Assess tone in each limb in turn, paying particular attention to the tone in each joint:

  • Anxious patients may give the impression of increased tone (paratonia). Ensure that the patient is as relaxed as possible.

  • In the arms, look for a 'pronator catch' (sudden increase in tone of the pronator muscles) by rapidly supinating the forearm – this suggests spasticity.

  • In the legs, the equivalent of the pronator catch is ankle clonus, elicited by the rapid dorsiflexion of the ankle, with the knee flexed.

  • In the legs, roll the leg at the hip, and look at the foot – reduced tone may result in increased floppiness of the foot, whilst increased tone results in the foot maintaining the same position relative to the leg. Lift the knee rapidly off the bed – if the heel does not come off the bed, this suggests normal or reduced tone, but if the foot lifts up high, this suggests increased tone; beware that this may also occur if the patient's legs are not properly relaxed.

  • Increased tone may be due to spasticity, secondary to pyramidal (corticospinal tract) damage, or may be due to extrapyramidal rigidity (implying the basal ganglia). Spasticity is velocity-dependent and thus increases in line with the rate of passive movement – hence the rapid stretch performed when eliciting a pronator catch or ankle clonus may demonstrate early spasticity before other UMN signs become apparent. By contrast, in extrapyramidal disease, the rigidity is detectable throughout the range of movement of a joint ('lead-pipe rigidity'), and is not velocity-dependent. Begin with the wrist, and take the hand through passive, slow, deliberate extension, flexion and rotation movements, so that the wrist joint is moved throughout its range. This elicits early signs of stiffness in forearm muscles and 'cogwheeling' (extrapyramidal rigidity with superimposed tremor).

- Assess power:
  - The 6-point MRC scale is used in neurological practice (adapted with 4+ and 4− to differentiate very mild to moderate weakness). In the PACES setting, however, a brief description, e.g. 'I could just overcome hip flexion' is often more helpful than the exact MRC grading. Describe the pattern of weakness elicited – proximal or distal, unilateral or bilateral (if bilateral, symmetrical or asymmetrical), pyramidal or LMN (if LMN, in myotomal or nerve pattern).
  - Remember to stabilize the most proximal joint when assessing power. So, when assessing elbow flexion at the biceps, support the upper arm in a fixed position, in order to stop the patient using their shoulder to pull the candidate's arm towards themself, thus giving a false impression of the power of elbow flexion. This method should be used throughout.
  - If the history or other signs are suggestive, remember to look for fatiguability (**Ɔ** p.379) or myotonia (**Ɔ** p.385).
- Proceed to examination of the reflexes:
  - Minor degrees of reflex asymmetry are common in normal people, as are relatively reduced knee jerks compared with ankle jerks, and vice versa.
  - Make sure the limb is properly relaxed, and that the tendon you are percussing is under some tension but not fully stretched. Percuss the tendon at least twice to ensure that the reflex that you have elicited (or not) is reproducible.
  - If the reflex is absent, assess with reinforcement, by asking the patient to clench their teeth or clench their hands. Areflexia without other physical signs is usually not pathologically significant.
  - An inverted supinator jerk, where the biceps jerk is absent but generates a supinator jerk with reflex flexion of the fingers, is indicative of cervical myelopathy with C5/6 nerve root damage.
  - Look for pathological reflexes such as Hoffman's jerk (flicking the distal middle finger and looking for reflex flexion of the thumb and index finger) and the plantar response.
  - When performing the plantar response, without touching the forefoot, stroke the lateral aspect of the sole, coming round to the ball of the foot; touching the arch of the foot is likely to generate a withdrawal response.

Power assessment

- When assessing power in each muscle group, candidates should always ask themselves:
  - Which muscle (or group of muscles) is being tested?
  - Which root is supplying this action?
  - Which nerve is innervating the muscle being tested?
- If weakness is detected consider if any other weak muscle groups are also supplied by:
  - The same myotome suggesting a root lesion.
  - The same nerve suggesting a nerve lesion.
- If the pattern of weakness suggests:
  - A root lesion, then is there a corresponding dermatomal loss in sensation?
  - A nerve lesion, then is there loss of sensation in the area supplied by the nerve?
- Muscle weakness without associated sensory deficit may indicate involvement of the anterior horn cell:
  - An individual or consecutive myotomes suggest old poliomyelitis ● p.302 and p.311 or progressive muscular atrophy (● p.355).
  - More diffuse weakness with mixed UMN and LMN signs suggests amyotrophic lateral sclerosis (● p.355).
  - Myopathies and diseases affecting the neuromuscular junction will also lead to weakness without sensory loss (which are generally more widespread and may follow a pattern of weakness e.g. proximal myopathy).
- Continually thinking about the root, nerve and associated sensory loss (which may be either dermatomal or follow the pattern of the nerve distribution) will enable a candidate to quickly determine the nature of the lesion.
  For example, weakness of shoulder abduction may be due to C5 or an axillary nerve lesion:
  - Associated weakness of biceps (C5, C6) with loss of the sensation of the lateral aspect of the upper arm suggests a C5 lesion; absence of sensory loss indicates a lesion at the anterior horn cell.
  - Associated loss of sensation of the regimental badge area suggests an axillary nerve lesion.

Tables 6.1 and 6.2 summarize the neurological examination, together with the common findings which may be associated with either a root or a nerve lesion.

- Examine coordination:
  - In addition to simple tests such as looking for rebound phenomenon (● p.290), there are further tests of cerebellar function.
  - Examine finger–nose movements, ensuring that the target is held at a distance at the extreme of the patient's reach. Look for past-pointing, and intention tremor (tremor that increases in amplitude the closer to the target the finger is). The finger–nose test should be undertaken slowly and carefully as carrying out the test rapidly tends to miss early cerebellar signs.

- Assess for dysdiadochokinesis – difficulties with making rapid alternating movements, such as pronation-supination (an early sign may be that the patient moves their hand as if they are turning the pages of a book).
- In the lower limbs, look for heel–shin ataxia – ask the patient to make a circular movement, with the heel raised off the shin once it has reached the ankle, before placing it on the knee again. Simply gliding one heel up and down the opposite shin will miss early ataxia.
- If evidence of incoordination is demonstrated, then remember to look for other cerebellar signs such as dysarthria, nystagmus and gait ataxia at the end of the examination.
- Finally, go on to assess sensation (Fig. 6.1; ➲ p.312):
  - Try to focus your sensory examination according to earlier findings. For example, if there is evidence of bilateral UMN signs, attempt to determine a sensory level, if there is foot drop, use the sensory examination to determine a L5 dermatomal or common peroneal nerve sensory impairment, and if you think this is a peripheral neuropathy, demonstrate the glove-and-stocking sensory loss.
  - Assess the spinothalamic pathways with pin prick, using a disposable pin. The sensation on the forehead should act as control (sensation over the sternum may be abnormal in a high cervical lesion). Chart areas of sensory loss or altered sensation. Move from the anaesthetic area to the area of normal sensation and ask the patient to tell you 'when it feels normal'. Temperature sensation can be examined with a tuning fork blade, but in the interests of time, do not do this unless asked, or you feel that it would significantly add to your findings.
  - Assess the posterior columns with vibration and joint position sense (VS and JPS). Test VS at the ankles using a 128-Hz tuning fork. Familiarize the patient with the test by placing the heel of the vibrating fork on the sternum. When testing JPS, remember to hold the digit at the sides so that pressure clues are not given to the patient. A patient should normally be expected to detect 5° of movement at the interphalangeal joint of the big toe. Start distally, and if JPS is absent proceed proximally, up to the hip or shoulder if necessary.
  - Test light touch with a finger tip or cotton wool. Avoid stroking or tickling; these are related to spinothalamic modalities.

Table 6.1 Correlation between muscle weakness and potential nerve or root lesions in the upper limbs[a]

Movement	Muscle(s)	Root (top line; main innervated root in bold)/Nerve (bottom line)	Area of sensory loss corresponding to root/nerve lesion[b]	Reflex (if impaired)
Shoulder abduction	Deltoid	**C5**, C6	Lateral aspect upper arm and forearm, thumb, index finger	None
		Axillary	Regimental badge area over deltoid muscle	None
Shoulder adduction	Latissimus dorsi, pectoralis major	C6, **C7**, C8	Lateral aspect of forearm and whole of hand (particularly middle finger)	None
		Thoracodorsal	None (purely motor)	None
Elbow flexion	Biceps	C5, C6	Lateral aspect of upper arm and forearm, thumb and index finger	Biceps
		Musculocutaneous	Lateral aspect of forearm (lateral cutaneous nerve of forearm)	Biceps
Elbow extension	Triceps	C6, **C7**, C8	Lateral aspect of forearm, all fingers of hand **particularly middle finger**, little finger and ulnar ½ of ring finger.	Triceps
		Radial	Extensor aspect of forearm, back of hand, dorsum of first 4 fingers	Triceps ± Brachioradialis
Wrist extension	Extensor carpi radialis longus, extensor carpi ulnaris	C5, C6, **C7**, C8	**Lateral (extensor) aspect of forearm** (via lateral cutaneous nerve (branch of musculocutaneous nerve)), **thumb and index finger**, radial fossa ('anatomical snuff box')	None
		Radial and posterior interosseous nerve	Lateral (extensor) aspect of forearm via posterior cutaneous nerve), thumb and index finger, radial fossa ('anatomical snuff box')	None

Action	Muscle	Nerve root / Nerve	Sensory	Reflex
Wrist flexion	Flexor carpi radialis, flexor carpi ulnaris	C6, C7 / *Median and ulnar*	Lateral aspect of forearm, thumb, first and middle finger / Thumb, index and middle finger	None / None
Finger extension	Extensor digitorum	**C7, C8** / *Posterior interosseous nerve (branch of radial nerve)*	Little finger, ring finger and middle finger. / None (purely motor)	None / None
Finger flexion	Flexor digitorum superficialis and profundus	**C8** / *Median* / *Ulnar*	Little finger, ulnar ½ of ring finger and ulnar aspect of hand / Palmar aspect of lateral side of hand, thumb, index finger, middle finger and lateral (radial) border of ring finger / Palmar aspect of medial side of hand, little finger and medial (ulnar) border of ring finger	Finger flexion / None / None
Index (first) finger abduction	First dorsal interosseous	C8, **T1** / *Ulnar*	Little finger, ulnar ½ of ring finger, ulnar aspect of palm, medial **aspect of forearm to elbow** / Palmar aspect of medial side of hand, little finger and medial (ulnar) border of ring finger	None / None
Little finger abduction	Abductor digiti minimi	C8, **T1** / *Ulnar*	Little finger, ulnar ½ of ring finger, ulnar aspect of palm, ulnar aspect of forearm to elbow / Palmar aspect of medial side of hand, little finger and medial (ulnar) border of ring finger	None / None

(Continued)

Table 6.1 (Contd.)

Movement	Muscle(s)	Root (top line; main innervated root in **bold**)/Nerve (bottom line)[b]	Area of sensory loss corresponding to root/nerve lesion[b]	Reflex (if impaired)
Thumb abduction	Abductor pollicis brevis	C8, **T1**	Little finger, ulnar ½ of ring finger, ulnar aspect of palm, ulnar aspect of forearm to elbow	None
		Median	Palmar aspect of lateral side of hand, thumb, index finger, middle finger and lateral (radial) border of ring finger	None
Thumb opposition	Opponens pollicis	C8, **T1**	Little finger, ulnar ½ of ring finger, ulnar aspect of palm, ulnar aspect of forearm to elbow	None
		Median	Palmar aspect of lateral side of hand, thumb, index finger, middle finger and lateral (radial) border of ring finger	None
Thumb flexion	Flexor pollicis brevis	C8, **T1**	Little finger, ulnar ½ of ring finger, ulnar aspect of palm, ulnar aspect of forearm to elbow	None
		Median	Palmar aspect of lateral side of hand, thumb, index finger, middle finger and lateral (radial) border of ring finger	None
Finger adduction	Palmar interossei	C8, **T1**	Little finger, ulnar ½ of ring finger, medial forearm	None
		Ulnar	Palmar aspect of medial side of hand, little finger and medial (ulnar) border of ring finger	None

[a] Information in Tables 6.1 and 6.2 is presented in the order of the clinical examination.

[b] For dermatomal loss of sensation in association with a root lesion, see Fig. 6.1.

Remember that most muscles are often innervated by >1 nerve root. The lesion of a single nerve root does not produce well-defined sensory loss due to overlapping of the branches of dorsal root terminals from different segments. Therefore an isolated root lesion often results in a significantly smaller area of sensory impairment than indicated in the dermatomal diagrams (Fig. 6.1).

Specific examinations such as those of the cerebellar or extrapyramidal systems are described later in this chapter. It is recommended that, in PACES, where clear instructions are given, pointing towards a particular disorder, e.g. 'examine this patient's gait', the tailored examination should be commenced. Where the instructions are less clear, e.g. 'examine this patient's limbs and proceed', the general examination should be started, but as soon as abnormal signs become apparent, the examination should then become focused.

To emphasize, practice of the general and more focused examinations is crucial in this station. The process of examination should be automatic, to permit concentration on eliciting and interpreting the signs as you go along. Ensure that you have read a text on the standard neurological examination early in your preparation for PACES.

📖 **Further reading**

Fuller G. *Neurological Examination Made Easy*. Edinburgh: Churchill Livingstone, 2008.
O'Brien M. *Aids to the Examination of the Peripheral Nervous System*. London: Saunders Ltd, 2010.

Approach to gait disorders

Gait is a poorly examined feature of the neurological examination, and is frequently omitted altogether. However, a multitude of neurological conditions result in gait disorders, and abnormal gait may be the only obvious sign. Proper assessment of gait will quickly provide important clues to the underlying diagnosis and is an excellent discriminator of candidates.

You will be asked to examine the patient by the following likely commands: 'This patient has difficulty walking. Please examine gait and proceed', or 'This patient has had frequent falls. Please examine the gait and proceed'.

Candidates may be required to assess gait disorders in Station 5 as well as in the neurology station.

Initial examination

- Prior to asking the patient to walk, look for clues at the bedside. These may include walking aids, a wheelchair, ankle–foot orthoses (AFOs) indicating foot drop, blood sugar monitoring devices suggesting diabetic neuropathy or medication for Parkinson's disease.
- Ask the patient to remove trousers and shoes/slippers.
- Look for wasting, pes cavus or foot drop.
- Carefully observe the patient for vital clues as they stand up from the chair e.g. use of arms in proximal myopathy.
- Ask the patient to walk a few metres. Initially you should stand in close proximity to the patient, remembering to accompany them should he/she be unbalanced. Once you have established the stability of the patient, stand back to observe the gait pattern.
- Ask the patient to walk on tip-toes and then on their heels. This helps to assess distal lower limb power very quickly.
- Perform Romberg's test.
- Attempt to classify the gait early by considering the key features:
  - Gait asymmetry points towards hemiparesis, Parkinson's disease, or a unilateral cerebellar hemisphere lesion. Additional features such as the upper limb being held in flexion and lower limb held in

Table 6.2 Correlation between muscle weakness and potential nerve or root lesions in the lower limbs[a]

Movement	Muscle	Root (top line; main innervated root in bold)/Nerve (bottom line)	Area of sensory loss corresponding to root/nerve lesion[b]	Reflex (if impaired)
Hip flexion	Iliopsoas	**L1, L2**, L3 Lumbar sacral plexus	Anteromedial thigh and inner leg distally to mid-calf	None
		Femoral	Groin and upper thigh anteriorly (lateral cutaneous nerve of thigh)	Knee
Hip extension	Gluteus maximus	L5, S1 Inferior gluteal	Lateral lower leg, dorsum and sole of foot None (purely motor)	None None
Knee flexion	Hamstrings	L5, S1 Sciatic	Lateral lower leg, dorsum and sole of foot Outer aspect of leg, dorsum of foot, sole and inner aspect of foot	Ankle Ankle
Knee extension	Quadriceps femoris	L3, L4 Femoral	Anteromedial mid thigh and anteromedial lower leg Anteromedial thigh and inner leg as far down as ankle	Knee Knee
Ankle dorsiflexion	Tibialis anterior	L4, L5 Deep peroneal	Across knee, medial and lateral lower leg 1st interosseous web space (between big and 2nd toe)	None None

	Muscle / Nerve	Root	Sensory distribution	Reflex
Ankle plantar flexion	Gastrocnemius	S1	Anterolateral aspect of lower leg, dorsum of lateral border of foot, most of sole	Ankle[c]
	Tibial		Anterolateral aspect of lower leg, dorsum of lateral border of foot, most of sole	Ankle[c]
Ankle inversion	Tibialis posterior	**L4**, L5, S1	Across knee, medial and lateral lower leg[d]	None
	Tibial		Anterolateral aspect of lower leg, dorsum of lateral border of foot, most of sole	Ankle[c]
Ankle eversion	Peroneus longus and brevis	L5	Lateral aspect of lower leg, lateral border of foot, most of sole[d]	None
	Superficial peroneal branch of common peroneal		Lateral distal portion of lower leg, dorsum of foot	None

[a] Information in Tables 6.1 and 6.2 is presented in the order of the clinical examination.

[b] For dermatomal loss of sensation in association with a root lesion, see Fig. 6.1.

Remember that most muscles are often innervated by >1 nerve root. The lesion of a single nerve root does not produce well-defined sensory loss due to overlapping of the branches of dorsal root terminals from different segments. Therefore an isolated root lesion often results in a significantly smaller area of sensory impairment than indicated in the dermatomal diagrams (Fig. 6.1).

[c] The ankle jerk is conveyed through the S1 root via the tibial branch of the sciatic nerve and is therefore spared in a peroneal nerve lesion (See Top Tips box, p. 374).

[d] Sensory impairment is often minimal.

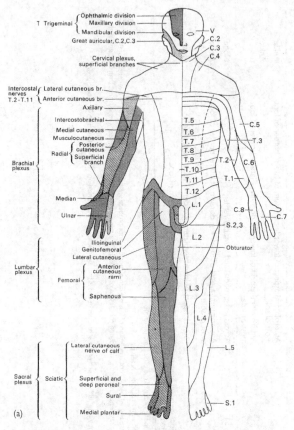

Fig. 6.1 a) Distribution of dermatomes: anterior. b) Distribution of dermatomes: posterior. c) Cutaneous innervation of the foot.
Reproduced from Murray Longmore, Ian Wilkinson, Tom Turmezei, Chee Kay Cheung, *Oxford Handbook of Clinical Medicine*, 2007, with permission from Oxford University Press.

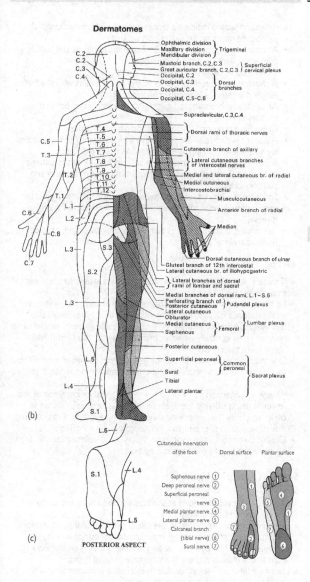

Dermatomes

Ophthalmic division ⎫
Maxillary division ⎬ Trigeminal
Mandibular division ⎭

Mastoid branch, C.2, C.3 ⎫ Superficial
Great auricular branch, C.2, C.3 ⎬ cervical plexus

Occipital, C.2 ⎫
Occipital, C.3 ⎬ Dorsal
Occipital, C.4 ⎪ branches
Occipital, C.5–C.8 ⎭

Supraclavicular, C.3, C.4

Dorsal rami of thoracic nerves

Cutaneous branch of axillary

Lateral cutaneous branches of intercostal nerves

Medial and lateral cutaneous br. of radial

Medial cutaneous
Intercostobrachial

Musculocutaneous

Anterior branch of radial

Median

Dorsal cutaneous branch of ulnar
Gluteal branch of 12th intercostal
Lateral cutaneous br. of iliohypogastric

Lateral branches of dorsal rami of lumbar and sacral

Medial branches of dorsal rami, L.1–S.6
Perforating branch of ⎫ Pudendal plexus
Posterior cutaneous ⎭

Lateral cutaneous
Obturator ⎫
Medial cutaneous ⎬ Femoral ⎫ Lumbar plexus
Saphenous ⎭

Posterior cutaneous

Superficial peroneal ⎫ Common
Sural ⎬ peroneal ⎫ Sacral plexus
Tibial ⎭
Lateral plantar ⎭

(b)

POSTERIOR ASPECT

(c)

Cutaneous innervation
of the foot   Dorsal surface   Plantar surface

Saphenous nerve ①
Deep peroneal nerve ②
Superficial peroneal
nerve ③
Medial plantar nerve ④
Lateral plantar nerve ⑤
Calcaneal branch
(tibial nerve) ⑥
Sural nerve ⑦

extension would indicate a stroke patient. Circumduction of the paretic leg may also be evident on walking.

- A scissoring gait, presenting with extended knees or stiff legs, is consistent with a spastic paraparesis.
- Contractures suggest longstanding spasticity.
- A shortened, wasted leg points to old poliomyelitis with the limb length discrepancy indicating childhood disease.
- An unsteady, broad-based gait points towards a cerebellar or sensory ataxia.
- Consider a proximal myopathy if the patient waddles.
- A patient with a foot drop will have a high stepping of the affected leg with the foot slapping down hard as it hits the floor.
- A stamping gait in proprioceptive sensory loss helps the patient to localize the position of their feet from resulting sensory and auditory clues.
- Small steps with reduced arm swing and poor turning suggest an extrapyramidal disorder, which will be asymmetric in Parkinson's disease.
- Remember that not all gaits have a neurological origin: consider musculoskeletal disorders.

❶ Top Tips

- If there is a wheelchair ask the patient if they are able to stand even if they cannot walk.
- Be ready to assist (quickly!) a poorly mobile patient. If they fall over this is almost a fail sign, not to mention any injury they may sustain!
- It is inappropriate to tandem walk very unstable patients for the same reason. Think carefully whether this test may do you (and them) more harm than good.
- Use the right word when describing gait as this can often commit you to a particular diagnosis. If in doubt use terms like 'small steps' or 'unsteady'.
- Always volunteer to carry out a full neurological examination of the lower limbs, specifying the likely findings (e.g. cerebellar signs), in order to clarify the underlying diagnosis – the examiners may or may not allow you to proceed to a full neurological examination.
- Do not be put off if the examiners stop you completing the examination before the time has elapsed.

Spastic (scissoring) gait
Signs
- Legs stiff and held extended at the hips and the knees and partially plantar flexed at the ankles.
- Legs are functionally longer as a result of postural changes, therefore toes may drag on floor, or legs may circumduct during walking to accommodate this apparent leg lengthening. Shoes may therefore be worn at the toes, and there is an increased risk of falling.
- Hips may be drawn together due to increased adductor tone when the patient walks – hence the term 'scissoring'.
- Hyper-reflexia, ankle clonus, upgoing plantar responses.

- Ascertain the presence of a sensory level.
- Determine if there are UMN signs in arms (localizes the lesion to C4 or above, producing a spastic quadriparesis).
- Pseudobulbar signs such as brisk jaw jerk or dysarthria indicate brainstem or bilateral cerebral lesions.
- Extra-ocular eye movement disorders, especially internuclear ophthalmoplegia (INO), or a relative afferent pupillary defect (RAPD) and poor visual acuity indicative of optic atrophy suggests multiple sclerosis (MS), particularly in a young patient.
- Surgical scars, either of a craniotomy or a spinal procedure.
- Note the presence of a urinary catheter. In its absence, offer to palpate the abdomen to rule out a distended bladder.
- Wasting or fasciculations are suggestive of LMN pathology – LMN signs at one level imply a lesion at that level causing anterior horn cell damage (e.g. cervical spondylosis), while more diffuse LMN signs are consistent with MND. Dysarthria with tongue fasciculations may also be present in MND.

❶ Top Tips

- Once a spastic gait has been identified, attempt to localize the lesion e.g. sensory level or signs pointing to brainstem or cerebrum.
- Look for any additional features suggestive of a diagnosis e.g. INO of MS, wasting and fasciculations of MND.

Causes

- Demyelination/MS: young patient, particularly in the presence of cerebellar signs, dysarthria, eye movement disorders or poor visual acuity (think of neuromyelitis optica in someone with very poor vision), urinary catheter (➋ p. 337).
- Cerebral palsy: longstanding weakness often associated with contractures.
- Transverse myelitis: infective, post-infective or inflammatory (e.g. sarcoid or lupus). Paraparesis may be asymmetric (dependent on location of lesion(s)), and may occur with sensory level and bladder involvement.
- Motor neuron disease: mixed UMN and LMN signs, but spasticity may dominate (➋ p. 355).
- Spinal cord compression e.g. cervical myelopathy secondary to cervical spondylosis (elderly patient), trauma, compressive tumour.
- Syringomyelia: Horner's syndrome, cape-like distribution of dissociated sensory loss (i.e. pain and temperature impairment), wasting of the small muscles of the hands, loss of upper limb reflexes (➋ p.356).
- Anterior spinal artery infarction: sensory level with sparing of posterior column sensory modalities (➋ p.329).
- Hereditary spastic paraparesis: legs usually much more stiff than weak, bladder involvement is a late feature.
- Tropical spastic paraparesis: HTLV-1 is endemic in the West Indies.
- Parasagittal (falx) meningioma: compression on both sensorimotor cortices can cause a spastic paraparesis with proprioception and two-point discrimination impairment (which are features of parietal lobe cortical damage), but without a sensory level.

- Bilateral cerebral infarcts – may be cortical or subcortical (➔ p. 323).
- If there is evidence of a significant peripheral neuropathy and cerebellar signs, Friedreich's ataxia and vitamin B1 or B12 deficiency should be considered (➔ p. 346).

❶ Top Tips

- A sensory level may be caused by a lesion at that level or above.
- In a young patient, check for cerebellar and eye signs suggesting demyelination. In an older patient, consider a vascular cause.
- Ask about bladder, bowel and visual disturbance.
- In an elderly patient with brisk upper limb reflexes, wasting of the small muscles of the hands and a sensory neuropathy may suggest dual pathology e.g. compressive cervical myelopathy with diabetes.

Parkinsonian gait

Signs

- Expressionless face (hypomimia) and asymmetrical pill-rolling tremor.
- Cogwheel rigidity and tremor (both accentuated by movement of contralateral arm [synkinesis]).
- Bradykinesia (a reduction in both amplitude and speed of movement). Ask the patient to rapidly tap the thumb and index finger of both hands together as quickly as possible. Demonstrate micrographia by asking the patient to write.
- Low volume, monotonous voice (dysphonia).
- Small stepping, shuffling (festinant) gait.
- Reduced arm swing (asymmetry suggests idiopathic Parkinson's disease).
- Stooped posture with flexed hips.
- Difficulties with initiation of gait, turning (wide turning circle) or avoiding obstacles (do not test!).
- Impaired postural reflexes. If testing, candidate must ensure that they are able to protect the patient from falling (place one arm in front and one arm behind the patient).
- Parkinson's plus syndrome:
  • Progressive supranuclear palsy (PSP) is suggested by frontalis overactivity, axial rigidity and vertical gaze palsy (overcome by the vestibulo-ocular (doll's eye) reflex).
  • Early autonomic features such as postural hypotension or impotence suggest multisystem atrophy (MSA).
- A prominent parkinsonian gait in the absence of signs in the face and upper limbs is consistent with vascular parkinsonism.

Causes

(➔ Movement disorders, p. 342.)
- Idiopathic Parkinson's disease.
- Parkinson's plus syndromes:
  • MSA: autonomic, pyramidal and cerebellar signs.
  • Progressive supranuclear palsy: vertical gaze palsy.
  • Corticobasal degeneration: asymmetrical, dystonic posturing, myoclonus, 'alien limb' phenomenon.
  • Dementia with Lewy bodies: early cognitive impairment, visual hallucinations.

- Vascular parkinsonism due to multiple lacunar infarcts or extensive small-vessel disease.
- Drug-induced e.g. neuroleptics and anti-emetics (prochlorperazine, metoclopramide).
- Toxic e.g. MPTP (1-methyl-4-phenyl-1,2,3,6-tetrahydropyridine), manganese toxicity (occupational exposure in welders).
- Genetic disorders:
  - Huntington's disease (juvenile form more likely to present with an akinetic-rigid syndrome).
  - Wilson's disease.
- Dementia pugilistica: repetitive head trauma, esp. boxers.
- Normal pressure hydrocephalus: classical triad of apraxic gait (→ Ataxic gait, see below), cognitive impairment and urinary incontinence.
- Encephalitis lethargica.

❶ Top Tips

- Ask about day-to-day function: How far can the patient walk? Can they climb stairs? Can they dress and feed themselves? Can they get into a bath? Can they get out of a chair?
- Remember the carers.
- Remember that postural hypotension is a feature of Parkinson's disease itself as well as being a side effect of the anti-parkinsonion medication used. It also occurs in multisystem atrophy.

Ataxic gait

Signs

- Unsteady broad-based stamping gait often requiring support. May weave from side to side. Subtle gait ataxia may only be detected on heel-toe walking. The patient may veer towards side of the lesion.
- Romberg's test: ask the patient to stand with feet close together. The test is positive if the patient becomes unsteady on closing their eyes, not if unsteady with eyes open. A positive Romberg's test indicates sensory ataxia; proceed to test joint position sense.
- Other features of a cerebellar syndrome – dysarthria, nystagmus, intention tremor, past-pointing, dysdiadochokinesis, hypotonia, and pendular reflexes (→ p. 346).

Causes

(→ Cerebellar disorders, p. 346.)

Ataxic gait or truncal ataxia results from damage to the cerebellar vermis – alcoholic degeneration particularly affects this region.

❶ Top Tips

- Gait ataxia may be due to cerebellar, vestibular or sensory disturbance. Romberg's test and joint position sense testing is necessary to identify the cause.
- Remember to stand close to the patient in order to ensure patient safety when performing this test.

Apraxic gait (synonyms: magnetic gait disorder, 'marche à petit pas')

The apraxic gait may be confused for a parkinsonian gait, but in contrast, the patient can move their legs at will, despite a severe gait disorder.

Signs
- Difficulty initiating gait.
- Inability to lift feet = 'magnetic gait'.
- When pushed forward, the heels will rise, but the toes may 'grab' the floor.
- Turning is broken into many small steps and may precipitate the feet becoming glued to the floor.
- Distal volitional movements such as the heel–shin manoeuvre or cycling movements are normal.
- In contrast to parkinsonian gait, arm swing will be normal.
- Falls are common.

Causes
- Bilateral ischaemic white matter lesions: 'vascular parkinsonism'.
- Normal pressure hydrocephalus: classical triad of gait apraxia, urinary incontinence and cognitive impairment.

Neuropathic gait

Signs
- Ankle–foot orthoses (AFOs) may be present at the bedside.
- Feet do not dorsiflex and are raised high off the ground with each step to avoid catching toes.
- Feet slap down on the ground.
- May be unilateral, suggesting foot drop due to a common peroneal nerve palsy or L5 radiculopathy, or bilateral, consistent with a more diffuse disease.
- Foot inversion is preserved in a common peroneal nerve palsy, but is weak in an L5 radiculopathy; eversion is weak in both these conditions. Distinguishing these may be difficult on sensory testing, but L5 does not mediate sensation from the lateral aspect of the dorsum of the foot.
- Distal wasting, particularly with pes cavus, suggests Charcot–Marie– Tooth disease – look for muscle wasting in the hands (◑ p. 375).
- Reflexes:
  • Absent or diminished in a peripheral neuropathy.
  • May be brisk in association with wasting and fasciculations in MND.
- In the absence of motor signs, loss of joint position sense may also result in a stamping gait, as the patient relies on auditory and additional sensory clues to know when their feet contact the ground. Look for Charcot's joints.
- Look at the hands for wasting of the small muscles.

Causes
(◑ Neuropathies, p. 376.)
- Peripheral motor neuropathy with peroneal muscle involvement:
  • Hereditary: Charcot–Marie–Tooth disease, hereditary neuropathy with liability to pressure palsies (HNPP).
  • Diabetes.

- • Vasculitis.
- • Sarcoidosis.
- • Paraproteinaemia.
- • Amyloidosis.
- • Guillain–Barré syndrome.
- • Critical care neuropathies.
- Unilateral/bilateral common peroneal palsy e.g. trauma, compression by plaster cast, prolonged bed rest.
- Unilateral/bilateral L5 radiculopathies.
- MND.
- Causes of loss of joint position sense include tabes dorsalis, subacute combined degeneration of the cord, diabetes, neuropathies associated HIV, Sjögren's syndrome and paraneoplastic syndromes.

Myopathic gait

Signs

- Difficulty or inability to stand up from chair with arms folded, or to climb stairs.
- Difficulty sitting up from the lying position.
- Evidence of respiratory muscle weakness: forced vital capacity (spirometer may be present by the bedside), paradoxical indrawing of the abdomen on inspiration.
- Weak neck flexors and extensors.
- Waddling gait, unstable pelvis due to marked proximal weakness.
- Normal sensation and reflexes, excluding a radiculoneuropathy.
- Evidence of systemic disease (◆ Myopathies, p.383), e.g. thin hair of hypothyroidism, purple striae of Cushing's syndrome, myotonia of myotonic dystrophy, Gottron's papules and heliotropic rash of dermatomyositis.
- Other features of specific myopathies, e.g. frontal balding and percussion myotonia of myotonic dystrophy, pseudohypertrophy of calf muscles in some muscular dystrophies (e.g. Becker's), prominent scapular winging of facioscapulohumeral dystrophy, wasting of the quadriceps and forearm flexors in inclusion body myositis (◆ p.387).
- Fatiguability or diurnal variation in symptoms – suggestive of myasthenia gravis.
- Muscle biopsy scars (classically overlying triceps, lateral quadriceps).

Causes

◆ Myopathies, p.383.

Approach to limb weakness

Limb weakness may result from a wide range of neurological lesions. Therefore rapid localization is crucial to determining the likely underlying diagnosis.

Initial examination

- Look for bedside clues:
  - AFOs may point towards foot drop.
  - A catheter bag may imply a spastic paraparesis.
  - Crutches suggest that upper limbs are strong.
  - Look around the bedside for a wheelchair, or walking aids.
- Inspect the limbs carefully:
  - General muscle bulk – look for wasting, fasciculations, and particularly at the intrinsic muscles of the hand. If wasting is present, consider the distribution e.g. symmetrical and distal or localized to a specific nerve. Pseudohypertrophy of the calf suggests a dystrophy.
  - Check for deformities such as contractures, pes cavus (suggesting a hereditary sensorimotor neuropathy or polio) or Charcot's joints (consistent with a sensory neuropathy).
  - Look at limb posture e.g. wrist drop of a radial nerve palsy, clawing of the hand due to ulnar nerve palsy.
  - Look for muscle biopsy scars (often deltoid, triceps, or lateral quadriceps) or spinal procedure.
- During the general neurological examination, decide on the pattern of weakness:
  - UMN weakness is suggested by hypertonia, hyper-reflexia and a pyramidal pattern of weakness (flexors stronger than extensors in the arm, with hand held pronated with wrist and fingers flexed, extensors stronger than flexors in the leg, with foot plantarflexed).
  - Significant wasting is almost always a feature of LMN pathology.
  - Proximal weakness is most likely due to a myopathy or neuromuscular junction disorder (check for fatiguability), but can occasionally be caused by a polyradiculopathy.
  - Determine if this is a hemiparesis, a paraparesis, isolated limb weakness (monoparesis), or a generalized process.
  - Look for weakness above the neck – head drop suggests weakness of neck extensors, found in myasthenia gravis and MND.

❶ Top Tips

- If asked to examine the upper limbs neurologically, start by asking the patient to hold their hands outstretched and then to close their eyes. This simple procedure will quickly screen for a wrist drop, a pronator drift and will allow you to look for rebound by tapping firmly on the arms. Any deformities and muscle wasting will also become apparent.
- If symmetrical signs are found in the limbs you have been asked to examine always question whether the same process is occurring in all four limbs, e.g. if peripheral wasting is present in the lower limbs, is there also wasting of the small muscles of the hands?
- Do not expect always to find all the textbook signs in an UMN lesion – a pyramidal pattern of weakness, increased tone and hyper-reflexia are not invariably all present

Hemiparesis

Signs

- Unilateral pyramidal weakness, hypertonia, hyper-reflexia, upgoing plantar response, hemi-sensory disturbance.
- Look for UMN facial weakness with sparing of the frontalis.
- Assess visual fields for homonymous hemianopia.
- Check speech for dysarthria and cerebellar signs (suggestive of demyelination), and offer to assess bulbar function.
- Attempt to find a sensory level.
- Examine the scalp, neck and back for surgical scars, and enquire about bladder and bowel function.

Causes

- *Intracranial*:
  - Cerebral infarction: middle cerebral artery (arm weaker than leg), anterior cerebral artery (leg weaker than arm), lacunar infarct (usually affects face, arm and leg equally), small cortical infarct (may produce isolated limb weakness).
  - Space-occupying lesion: tumour, haemorrhage, abscess.
  - Demyelination/inflammation.
- *Brainstem* – look for crossed signs (⊙ p.328):
  - Posterior circulation vascular event.
  - Demyelination/inflammation (esp. internuclear ophthalmoplegia).
- *Spinal cord* – identify sensory level, wasting and fasciculations at level of lesion (due to anterior horn cell damage), and ipsilateral loss of vibration sense and joint position sense with contralateral loss of temperature and pinprick:
  - Trauma
  - Tumour e.g. neurofibroma, schwannoma or meningioma (skin changes of NF1, and bilateral deafness of NF2)
  - Abscess
  - Arteriovenous malformation (AVM) or haemorrhage

❶ Top Tips

- Remember: the spinal cord ends at T12/L1, and therefore lumbar lesions do not cause UMN signs.
- Paresis means weakness, plegia signifies paralysis.

Para/quadraparesis

Symmetrical weakness of limbs may be due to an UMN lesion (spastic para/quadraparesis), or due to a generalized process affecting LMNs (flaccid para/quadraparesis).

Spastic paraparesis

Signs

- Hypertonia bilaterally, hyper-reflexia, ankle clonus, upgoing plantar responses (NB in MND, the plantar response is sometimes downgoing), sensory disturbance.
- Symmetry suggests an intrinsic or complete lesion, asymmetry may suggest lateral compression or a myelitis.
- Localize the lesion by determining a sensory level.

- UMN signs in arms must be caused by a cervical cord lesion or above.
- Look for surgical scars over the cervical and thoracic spine.
- Examine cranial nerves for evidence of multiple sclerosis (oculomotor abnormalities, esp. INO, and dysarthria) or MND (dysarthria, bilateral facial weakness, tongue fasciculations).
- LMN signs at one level imply a lesion causing damage to the anterior horn cells at that level.
- If LMN signs are widespread, consider MND.

Causes ➔ Spastic gait, p. 302.

Flaccid paraparesis

Signs

- Wasting of the lower limbs, fasciculations, hypotonia, diminished or absent reflexes, downgoing or mute plantars.
- Wasting of the upper limbs, esp. in the intrinsic muscles of the hands (Charcot–Marie–Tooth or other neuropathy – ➔ p.375).
- Deformity such a pes cavus suggests onset of a peripheral nerve problem during development.
- Action tremor may be seen in demyelinating neuropathies.
- Absence of sensory signs suggests Guillain–Barré syndrome, chronic inflammatory demyelinating polyradiculoneuropathy (CIDP), motor neuropathy, or MND.

Causes ➔ High steppage gait, p.302.

Wasted hand

Signs

- Hand position: look for ulnar clawing, or wrist drop associated with a radial nerve palsy.
- Wasting:
  - Localize the wasting, paying special attention to thenar eminence (median nerve) and dorsal interossei (esp. first dorsal interosseous) and hypothenar eminence (ulnar nerve).
  - A smaller wasted, areflexic limb suggests polio.
  - Brachial plexopathy produces a wasted shoulder with winging of the scapula.
- Assess tone and reflexes:
  - Hypotonia or hyporeflexia will confirm a LMN lesion.
  - Hypertonia or hyper-reflexia may suggest MND (upper or lower limbs) or syringomyelia (lower limbs only).
- Look for weakness in the intrinsic hand muscles but also in the rest of the arm.
- Clarify if any sensory deficit is in a dermatomal or nerve distribution (see Figs. 6.1 & 6.2), and look for dissociated sensory loss.
- Look for the scars of carpal tunnel decompression or ulnar nerve transposition.
- Finger pulp pin pricks may be present, confirming diabetes.

Causes

(➔ Peripheral nerve, p.367.)
- Median or ulnar nerve palsies.

- Generalized neuropathy.
- C8/T1 radiculopathy: look for T1 dermatomal sensory loss. Check for lymphadenopathy and Horner's syndrome (Pancoast tumour).
- MND: focal or generalized wasting with UMN signs and absence of sensory signs.
- Polio: wasting (may follow myotomal distribution), shortened limb (if onset in childhood), areflexia, absence of sensory and UMN signs.
- Plexopathy: more generalized wasting, winging of scapula, with diminished or absent reflexes, ± multiple dermatomal sensory loss.
- Syringomyelia.

Proximal weakness

Signs

- Look for signs of underlying systemic conditions e.g. habitus and purple striae of Cushing's syndrome, heliotropic rash and Gottron's papules of dermatomyositis and dry skin, coarse hair and loss of outer third of eyebrow in hypothyroidism.
- Weakness around shoulders and pelvic girdle. Neck flexors and extensors may also be weak.
- Difficulty raising hands above head, getting out of chair, or sitting up from lying.
- In a myopathy or NMJ disorder, the tone, reflexes and sensation will be normal.
- Check for fatiguability of proximal and ocular muscles (myasthenia gravis); the voice may also fatigue (can be checked simultaneously e.g. by asking the patient to count loudly).
- Look for evidence of a ptosis or ophthalmoparesis (myasthenia gravis or mitochondrial myopathy).
- Examine for:
  - Facial weakness, wasting of the shoulder girdle and upper arm or winging of the scapula (FSHD).
  - Myotonia, temporalis wasting, cataracts (myotonic dystrophy).
  - Calf pseudohypertrophy (Becker's or other dystrophies).
  - Respiratory muscle weakness – look for paradoxical respiration, i.e. inhalation causing indrawing of abdomen, as seen in diaphragmatic weakness.
  - Scoliosis or lordotic gait, suggesting a longstanding muscle weakness.
- Rarely, a diffuse peripheral disorder such as Guillain–Barré syndrome may cause isolated proximal weakness, but will be accompanied by diminished reflexes and/or sensory signs.

Causes

(Myopathies, p.383 and Neuromuscular junction, p.379.)
- Metabolic/endocrine myopathies e.g. hypothyroidism.
- Inflammatory myopathies e.g. polymyositis, dermatomyositis.
- Dystrophies.
- Congenital metabolic myopathies e.g. McArdle's, late onset acid maltase deficiency.
- Toxic/drug-induced myopathies e.g. alcohol, statins.
- Myasthenia gravis – fatiguability, ocular and bulbar involvement, thymectomy scar, Cushing's syndrome due to steroid treatment.

- Lambert–Eaton syndrome – predominantly lower limb, reflexes facilitated by repetitive stimulation, dry mouth (suggesting autonomic dysfunction).
- Polyradiculopathy – may be largely motor, but reflexes will be diminished or absent e.g. Guillain-Barré syndrome or CIDP.
- Cord lesion – rarely may present with isolated proximal muscle weakness.
- Idiopathic.

Approach to sensory disturbance

When performed both skilfully and rapidly, the sensory component of the neurological examination will demonstrate to the examiners both experience and clinical competence at the neurology station. Done well, it provides valuable information regarding the patient's underlying pathology, allowing confident localization of the underlying lesion.

Examination

- Look for bedside clues:
    - AFOs point towards foot drop and either distal sensory loss in keeping with a sensorimotor peripheral neuropathy or loss of sensation over the lateral aspect of the foot due to common peroneal nerve palsy.
    - A catheter bag may imply a sensory level in the context of a spastic paraparesis.
- Examine the limbs carefully: look for clues from tone, power, reflexes and coordination as to cause of sensory impairment:
    - Patterns of wasting or fasciculations suggesting peripheral neuropathy, mononeuropathy or radiculopathy.
    - Generalized hyporeflexia of a sensorimotor neuropathy, or absent reflex of a mononeuropathy or radiculopathy.
    - Increased tone and hyper-reflexia of a brain and spinal cord lesion.
    - Look for the scar of a spinal procedure.
- Romberg's test: ask the patient to stand (if able) with feet together and eyes closed. If the patient is stable with eyes open, but is unsteady with eyes closed, this is a positive test, demonstrating a sensory ataxia due to impaired proprioception.
- Pseudoathetosis: ask the patient to hold both arms up, with fingers spread. If the fingers start to drift when the eyes are closed, this also suggests impaired proprioception.
- Test each sensory modality systematically:
    - Remember to provide a reference for normal sensation by touching the forehead or chest first, asking 'Does this feel normal?'.
    - Start proximally and work distally, testing each dermatome along the way for light touch and pinprick.
    - If any sensory impairment is detected, focus on trying to delineate the deficit.
    - For vibration sense, only use bony points e.g. big toe, 1st metatarsophalangeal joint, medial malleolus, tibial tuberosity,

anterior superior iliac spine, sternum. If present distally, do not test proximally. Use the 128Hz tuning fork (the *long* tuning fork for the *long* limbs!).

- Assess gait for the stamping gait of a sensory neuropathy.

❶ Top Tips

- Sensory loss is rarely an isolated finding – look for accompanying motor signs.
- If the pattern of weakness suggests a specific nerve lesion look carefully for sensory deficit in the distribution of the nerve e.g. regimental badge sensory loss in a patient with a weak deltoid.
- Do not forget to assess the dermatomes at the back of the leg – an L4 and L5 radiculopathy may look like a stocking distribution impairment if this is not done.
- Do not forget to examine the back and offer to examine the saddle area.
- Check for a sensory level and dissociated sensory loss.

The dermatomal distribution of sensory loss is illustrated in ➔ Fig. 6.1.

Distribution of sensory impairment

The differing patterns of sensory loss are illustrated in Fig. 6.2.

Peripheral causes

- *Radiculopathy:* dermatomal sensory impairment.
- *Peripheral nerve:*
  - *Asymmetrical:* due to mononeuropathy or rarely plexus lesion. Expect to find associated weakness and wasting in the corresponding muscle groups. Remember – diabetes and other diseases can cause a mononeuritis multiplex (➔ Mononeuritis multiplex, p.376).
  - *Symmetrical:* results from a diffuse length-dependent neuropathy, causing a stocking, or glove-and-stocking, distribution sensory impairment. Predominant pin-prick and temperature impairment suggests a small-fibre neuropathy, especially with pain and skin changes reflecting autonomic involvement. ➔ Polyneuropathies, p.375 for more details.

Central causes

- *Spinal cord:*
  - Total transection: impairment of all sensory modalities below the level of the transection.
  - Hemisection of the cord (Brown–Séquard syndrome): impairment of all modalities at the site of the dorsal root; impaired light touch, 2-point discrimination, vibration sense and proprioception below the level of the lesion ipsilaterally; impaired pain and temperature sensation on the contralateral side.
  - Central cord syndrome: bilateral impairment of pain and temperature in the segments affected by the lesion; dorsal column modalities spared (➔ Syringomyelia, p.356).

- Anterior spinal artery syndrome: impairment of pain and temperature sensation below the level of the lesion; dorsal column modalities preserved (➲ Stroke, p.323).
- Posterior column syndrome: impaired light touch, two-point discrimination, vibration and proprioception below the level of the lesion; pain and temperature sensation preserved (➲ B12 deficiency, p.352).

- *Brain:*
  - Parietal cortex: impairment of 2-point discrimination, astereognosis (object recognition by touch), agraphaesthesia (discriminating letters or numbers traced on the palm of the hand), and proprioception contralateral to the side of the lesion.
  - Thalamic: impairment of all sensory modalities contralateral to the lesion; often associated with a thalamic pain syndrome – pain often has a strong emotional component.
  - Brain stem (above medullary decussation): impairment of all sensory modalities contralateral to the side of the lesion.
  - Medial medulla: impaired 2-point discrimination, proprioception and vibration sense on the contralateral side of the lesion; sensation to the face is preserved.
  - Lateral medulla: ipsilateral impaired pain and temperature sensation over the face; impaired pain and temperature sensation in the contralateral body (➲ Lateral medullary syndrome, p.328).

❶ Top Tips

- Pin prick and light touch are usually the best discriminators in the examination.
- Remember, when testing light touch, not to stroke or tickle the skin, as this will stimulate the spinothalamic tracts.
- Romberg's test is unreliable in patients with cerebellar disorders or moderate to severe weakness from any cause as the patient will be unsteady anyway, irrespective of whether there is sensory ataxia.

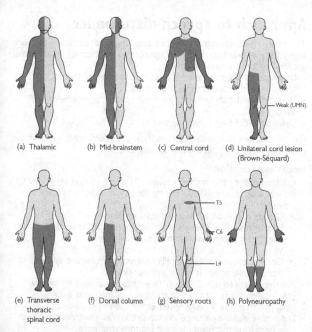

Fig. 6.2 Patterns of sensory loss. a) Thalamic lesion: sensory loss throughout opposite side. b) Brainstem lesion (rare): contralateral sensory loss below face and ipsilateral loss on face. c) Central cord lesion, e.g. syrinx: 'suspended' areas of loss often asymmetrical and 'dissociated', i.e. pain and temperature loss but light touch remaining intact. d) 'Hemisection' of cord or unilateral cord lesion = Brown–Séquard syndrome: contralateral spinothalamic (pain and temperature) loss with ipsilateral weakness and dorsal column loss below lesion. e) Transverse cord lesion: loss of all modalities below lesion. f) Isolated dorsal column lesion, e.g. demyelination: loss of proprioception vibration and light touch. g) Individual sensory root lesions, e.g. C6 (cervical root compression), T5 (shingles), L4 (lumbar root compression). h) Polyneuropathy: distal sensory loss.
Reproduced from Charles Clarke, Robin Howard, Martin Rosor, and Simon D. Shorvon, *Neurology: A Queen Square Textbook*, 2009, with permission from Wiley-Blackwell.

Approach to speech disturbance

The patient with speech disturbance provides an opportunity to score highly for the examinee, but rests upon early classification of abnormal speech into 1 of 3 major categories:

- Dysphasia (difficulty generating or comprehending content of speech) – expressive, receptive, or mixed.
- Dysarthria (difficulty articulating words) – bulbar, pseudobulbar, or mixed.
- Dysphonia (difficulty producing sound).

Once the nature of speech disturbance has been confirmed, a few simple steps may easily ascertain the correct diagnosis.

Initial examination

- Ask the patient a few simple questions: 'How did you get here?', 'What did you have for breakfast?', 'Tell me about your speech difficulties.' Listen for:
  - Quality of speech: is it slurred, nasal, or hoarse?
  - Rate of speech: is it slow and deliberate? Is it explosive or telegraphic (abnormal rhythm of speech)?
  - Volume of speech: is it quiet or monotonous? Does it fatigue?
  - Content of speech: does it utilize correct grammar and syntax, and does it make sense? Is it fluent or non-fluent?
- Ask the patient to repeat 'la la la' (lingual consonants), 'mm mm mm' (labial consonants), 'ga ga ga' (guttural consonants), and 'baby hippopotamus' and 'West Register Street' (cerebellar speech).
- Determine that the patient understands complex commands e.g. 'with your right hand touch your left ear and then your nose'.
- Ask the patient to repeat a phrase or sentence.
- Ask the patient to cough, and say 'Aaaah'.
- Determine if the patient can read and write a sentence.
- Ascertain whether the patient is right- or left-hand dominant.

> **❶ Top Tips**
>
> - Remember: all right-handed people are left-hemisphere dominant, while only 75% of left-handers are right-hemisphere dominant.

Dysphasias

Signs

- Loss of production of spoken language = expressive dysphasia. The patient will understand you but will generate broken or meaningless speech. Patients are aware of this disability and may find it frustrating.
- Loss of comprehension of speech = receptive dysphasia. The patient will speak normal complete sentences but will often reply inappropriately due to a lack of understanding.
- Problems with repetition of phrase or sentence = conduction aphasia.
- Assess for further evidence of dominant hemisphere damage:
  - Visual agnosia (inability to name or describe function of an object shown = lesion of posterior occipital/temporal lobe) and

prosopagnosia (inability to recognize faces = fusiform gyrus lesion in temporal lobe).
- Gerstmann's syndrome (dyscalculia, finger agnosia, dyslexia, left–right discrimination problems), from lesion in dominant parietal lobe.
- Limb apraxias – ask the patient to copy hand gestures and mime brushing teeth, drinking tea and combing hair = contralateral parietal lobe lesion.
- Suggest that a full neurological examination is appropriate, to look for other UMN signs.

Causes

Any lesion of Broca's (expressive dysphasia) or Wernicke's (receptive dysphasia) areas, or the arcuate fasciculus (conduction dysphasia) connecting the 2 areas:
- Middle cerebral artery branch occlusion due to embolus.
- Space-occupying lesion: tumour, abscess, intra- or extra-parenchymal haemorrhage.
- Neurodegenerative disorder e.g. Alzheimer's, frontotemporal lobar degeneration (esp. semantic or progressive non-fluent aphasia variants).
- Thalamic stroke is a rare cause of dysphasia.

Dysarthrias

Pseudobulbar (UMN or spastic) dysarthria

Signs
- Speech is slow, effortful, and harsh.
- Associated UMN facial weakness – forehead-sparing.
- 'Donald Duck' speech due to spastic tongue held in back of mouth – labial consonants especially affected.
- Tongue movements are slow and protrusion is difficult.
- Tongue fasciculations or wasting point to LMN pathology of MND.
- Associated dysphagia (bulbar).
- Exaggerated facial reflexes – glabellar tap, pout, snout, jaw jerk, palmomental.
- Apparent emotional lability may be a feature – the patient may laugh or cry inappropriately.

Causes

Bilateral damage to the corticobulbar tracts:
- Bilateral internal capsule infarcts or small-vessel disease
- Demyelination
- MND
- Neurodegenerative disorders
- Neurosyphilis
- Traumatic brain injury
- High brainstem tumours.

Bulbar (LMN) dysarthria

Signs
- Speech is indistinct, due to lack of tone in tongue and lips, and may be nasal if soft palate weak.
- May have LMN facial weakness.
- Tongue may be wasted and fasciculating.

- Poor or absent palatal movements.
- Associated nasal regurgitation, dysphonia and dysphagia.
- The jaw jerk may be absent.
- Fatiguability suggests a neuromuscular junction defect i.e. myasthenia gravis.
- Cough may be poor, with associated risk of aspiration.

Causes

- Myasthenia gravis
- Guillain–Barré syndrome or other neuropathies
- MND
- Poliomyelitis
- Brainstem infarction damaging bulbar nuclei or fascicles
- Brainstem tumour
- Syringobulbia.

Ataxic dysarthria

Signs

- Slurred speech.
- May be 'explosive' due to increased effort and variability of volume.
- Tendency to place equal and excessive stress on each syllable ('scanning' speech).
- Other features of cerebellar syndrome:
  • Nystagmus
  • Finger-nose ataxia
  • Intention tremor
  • Dysdidochokinesis
  • Hypotonia/hyporeflexia
  • Gait ataxia.

Causes

(➔ Cerebellar disorders, p.346.)
- Posterior circulation infarction
- Cerebellar haemorrhage, tumour or abscess
- Demyelination
- Cerebellar degeneration

Parkinsonian dysarthria

Signs

- Soft and monotonous speech, with little inflection.
- Slow rate of speech that may get quieter in the middle of the sentence.
- Difficult speech initiation.
- Associated lack of facial expression (hypomimia).
- Glabellar tap.
- Sialorrhoea.
- Other extrapyramidal signs – bradykinesia, tremor, cogwheel rigidity, postural hypotension and instability.

Causes ➔ Movement disorders section, p.342.

Dysphonia

Signs

- Deficient sound production.

- Patient may speak in whispers and sound hoarse, suggesting a LMN lesion.
- Voice may sound strangulated in a spastic dysphonia (laryngeal dystonia).

Causes
- Laryngitis.
- Local pathology e.g. neoplasm, trauma.
- Inhaled steroids.
- Syringobulbia or other medullary damage causing lesions to the vagal nuclei.
- Recurrent laryngeal nerve palsy, due to thyroid surgery, bronchial tumour or aortic aneurysm.
- Laryngeal dystonia (can be a feature of MSA ➲ p.342).

Approach to the eye

Neurological examination of the eye is a source of significant anxiety for many candidates. However, with a systematic approach, most neurological diagnoses can be easily teased out.

The following aspects of eye examination, which have been covered in the Ophthalmology section in Chapter 8 (➲ p.532–546), should be read in conjunction with this chapter:
- Initial examination
- Visual acuity
- Fundoscopy
- Visual fields
- Eye movements
- Pupils
- Ptosis, eye movement disorders, and nystagmus are also important components of eye examination and are discussed next.

Ptosis

Examination
- Check carefully for ptosis in the contralateral eye.
- Observe for eyelid fatiguability on upgaze, suggesting myasthenia gravis.
- Assess pupil:
  - Dilated – IIIrd nerve palsy.
  - Constricted – Horner's syndrome.
  - Normal – consider myasthenia gravis or a myopathy.
- Assess eye movements:
  - Look for confirmation of a IIIrd nerve palsy, with limitation of up- and down-gaze and adduction only (abduction normal).
  - If there is limitation in abduction, or any limitation of movement in the contralateral eye, consider this a 'complex ophthalmoplegia' – almost always suggests myasthenia gravis or a muscular disorder.
- Check visual fields for constriction due to retinitis pigmentosa, suggesting a mitochondrial disorder.
- Volunteer further appropriate neurological signs e.g. bulbar, respiratory or limb weakness or fatiguability.
- Ask about worsening of symptoms towards the end of the day in myasthenia gravis.

- Ask for old portrait photographs of the patient to check if the ptosis is longstanding.

Causes

- IIIrd nerve palsy.
- Horner's syndrome.
- Myasthenia gravis (➔ p. 379).
- Myotonic dystrophy.
- Oculopharyngeal muscular dystrophy (OPMD) – autosomal dominant.
- Chronic progressive external ophthalmoplegia or other mitochondrial disorders (look for pacemaker associated with cardiac conduction block, white stick).
- If no other signs except for ptosis, consider senile or congenital ptosis, or a structural lesion of the eyelid – these are the commonest causes of ptosis outside PACES!

❶ Top Tips

- Always describe the ptosis to be unilateral or bilateral, partial or complete and, if partial, whether or not it is fatiguable.
- If you find evidence of weakness of eye movements in more than one nerve distribution, refer to this as a 'complex ophthalmoplegia' – this is usually due to myasthenia gravis, but can be seen in thyroid eye disease or more rarely in myopathies affecting the eye or multiple cranial nerve lesions.
- If myasthenia is considered, check for facial, bulbar, limb and respiratory weakness and for a thymectomy scar.

Eye movement disorders

Ophthalmoplegia

Examination

- Look for disconjugate gaze. The position of the eye will often reveal the diagnosis – with a IIIrd nerve palsy, the eye will be down and out, and with a VIth nerve palsy the eye will be held in adduction.
- If disconjugate gaze is present, check if the difference between the 2 eyes changes with different directions of gaze, to confirm a nerve or muscle cause. If the difference is consistent in all directions of gaze, and there is a vertical component, this is termed 'skew deviation' and likely represents a brainstem lesion.
- If disconjugate gaze is inconsistent, this points towards an external ocular muscle, nerve lesion or an INO. Perform a formal eye movement examination (utilize finger or pen and move in an H-shape), asking the patient to report any double vision. In an INO, the eye on the side of the lesion will fail to adduct, and the contralateral eye will demonstrate nystagmus in abduction.
- Characterize diplopia or limitation of eye movement in terms of a lesion of the IIIrd, IVth or VIth nerve. Look for additional features to confirm your diagnosis e.g. partial or complete ptosis. If unable to localize to one nerve, consider this a complex ophthalmoplegia

(→ Ptosis pp.319, 541, 575) and look for evidence of myasthenia gravis, thyroid eye disease or a myopathy.
- Look for further evidence of ocular myasthenia by maintaining upgaze – the patient may complain of diplopia after a few seconds.
- Limitation of vertical eye movements without disconjugate gaze is consistent with a supranuclear gaze palsy. Limitation of lateral gaze without disconjugate gaze suggests a lateral gaze palsy due to a pontine lesion.

❶ Top Tips

- In the presence of a IIIrd nerve lesion a IVth nerve lesion can be identified by failure of intorsion of the eye on attempted inward and downward gaze. Whilst the oculomotor nerve lesion would prevent the eye from adducting, intorsion would occur if the trochlear nerve was intact.

Causes
- Muscle/neuromuscular junction:
  - Myasthenia gravis.
  - Myopathies – thyroid eye disease, OPMD, mitochondrial.
- Nerve (Peripheral nerve → p.367):
  - IIIrd.
  - IVth.
  - VIth.
  - Mononeuritis multiplex or lesion in the cavernous sinus or superior orbital fissure e.g. Wegener's granulomatosis.
  - Miller–Fisher syndrome (ophthalmoplegia, cerebellar signs and areflexia).
- Brainstem – causing skew deviation or INO (→ p.359).

Nystagmus → Fig. 6.3
- Examine the eyes in the primary position of gaze first: lateral nystagmus in one direction suggests a unilateral vestibular lesion, downbeat nystagmus points to a craniocervical junction lesion, and upbeat nystagmus implies a cerebellar or brainstem lesion.
- Then look for nystagmus in lateral, up- and downgaze. This may bring out nystagmus not seen in the primary position. Do not bring the eyes out >30° as this may produce physiological nystagmus.
- Horizontal gaze-evoked nystagmus suggests a cerebellar lesion. The fast phase will always be in the direction of gaze.
- Assess saccadic eye movements by asking patient to look from one object to another e.g. hand and examiner's nose. This may bring out a subtle INO – the adducting eye on the side of the lesion will be slow and left behind (as opposed to failure of adduction in a more severe INO).
- Offer to perform a full neurological examination.

❶ Top Tips

- Nystagmus is described as being in the direction of the fast phase, despite the slow phase being the pathological element.
- Check horizontal saccades to bring out an INO.
- The term 'supranuclear' refers to the lesion being above (more central to) the ocular motor nuclei, not to the direction of gaze paresis.
- Differentiate a supranuclear gaze palsy from a ophthalmoparesis due to nerve involvement by checking the vestibulo-ocular (doll's eye) reflex – the eyes will move up and down in a supranuclear gaze palsy with neck extension and flexion (ask the patient to fixate on a distant object as they flex and extend their neck).

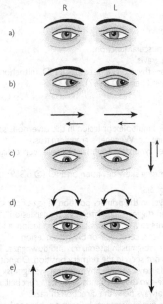

Fig. 6.3 Illustration of directions of nystagmus. a) Primary position. b) Horizontal nystagmus (demonstrated on left gaze). In nystagmus there is difficulty maintaining conjugate deviation. Both eyes drift slowly back to the central position (slow, pathological phase, smaller arrow), followed by a fast (saccadic) phase towards the target and the correct position of the eyes (larger arrow). Nystagmus is maximal on looking towards the lesion. c) Vertical nystagmus (downbeat nystagmus illustrated). Often seen in brainstem disease, but also with drug toxicity (e.g. from phenytoin). d) Congenital (pendular) nystagmus. Horizontal nystagmus is evident at rest (primary position) and is worsened by gaze in any direction. Pendular nystagmus has no fast phase. Often familial. Not associated with vertigo or oscillopsia (oscillation of the image). e) See-saw nystagmus. There is rapid see-saw movement of the eyes. One eye rises whilst the other falls (i.e. dysconjugate). May be seen in optic chiasm lesions.

Causes
- Cerebellar lesions: upbeat or gaze-evoked, either uni- or bi-directional nystagmus, always in the direction of gaze.
- Brainstem lesions: causing upbeat or downbeat nystagmus, or an INO (medial longitudinal fasciculus):
  - Downbeat nystagmus almost always results from lesions at the craniospinal junction, including Arnold–Chiari malformation, syringobulbia and demyelination.
  - Upbeat nystagmus suggests upper brainstem disease; causes include demyelination, stroke and Wernicke's encephalopathy.
- Vestibular lesions: nystagmus beating away from the side of lesion, worsened by gaze in the direction of the nystagmus.
- Optic chiasmal lesion.
- Congenital nystagmus.

Stroke

The term 'stroke' describes a group of heterogeneous disorders, in terms of anatomy, mechanism and cause. Figs. 6.4 and 6.5 illustrate the cerebral anatomy and its vascular supply.

Types of stroke
- Ischaemic:
  - Embolic
  - Atherosclerotic
- Haemorrhagic:
  - Intracerebral
  - Sub-arachnoid
  - Subdural
  - Extradural
- Venous.

Precise classification of the underlying mechanism causing stroke permits a more guided approach to defining the underlying aetiology, and thus modification of risk factors. Aetiology of the stroke also determines the treatment e.g. thrombolysis for thromboembolic stroke.

In the PACES setting, acute stroke will not be encountered, but its diagnosis and management is likely to feature as a subject in the discussion. However, chronic stroke patients with their associated neurological deficits and the long-term sequelae, such as spasticity, contractures and urinary dysfunction, are commonly encountered, particularly in view of the extremely high prevalence of the condition.

A basic understanding of the anatomical basis of stroke syndromes is crucial, since the candidate will be expected to look for additional neurological signs that aid localization of the lesion.

Cerebral arterial infarction

Cerebral infarctions can be categorized as large- and small-vessel occlusion. This can be helpful in determining likely pathophysiological mechanisms. Small vessel perforator occlusion (lacunar infarction) is more commonly related to local atheromatous disease due to hypertension or smoking, while large vessel occlusion is frequently associated with emboli from the carotid arteries or heart.

Risk factors for ischaemic stroke

- Smoking
- Hypertension
- Diabetes mellitus
- Atrial fibrillation – embolic stroke
- Transient ischaemic attacks
- Carotid artery stenosis
- Family history of stroke, cardiac or other vascular disease
- Alcohol abuse
- Oral contraceptive pill
- Obesity
- Coagulopathies
- Patent foramen ovale/atrial septal defect.

Lacunar infarct

- Due to occlusion of small perforator vessels through atheromatous change.
- Rarely due to embolic disease.
- Results in infarctions up to 1.5cm in diameter.
- Affects the deep white matter, usually in the corona radiata or internal capsule (the bundle of fibres containing ascending and descending tracts from the cortex to the brainstem and beyond), basal ganglia, thalamus and pons.
- Due to density of fibres, often results in significant loss of function.
- Does not affect cortex, and so does not result in deficits of higher cortical function.
- Common lacunar syndromes:
  - Pure motor hemiparesis: weakness of face, arm, and leg.
  - Sensorimotor: weakness and sensory loss in face, arm and leg.
  - Pure sensory: isolated hemisensory loss, involving face, arm, leg and hemi-trunk, usually due to thalamic infarction.
  - Ataxia-hemiparesis: hemiparesis with ataxia disproportionate with the degree of weakness caused by damage to cerebellar projections. Often, but not invariably, due to brainstem lacunar events.
  - Dysarthria – clumsy hand: facial weakness, dysarthria, dysphagia, with mild hand weakness or clumsiness.
  - Other syndromes e.g. hemiballismus, dystonias, eye movement disorders.
- Main risk factors are age, hypertension, diabetes, smoking and hyperlipidaemia.

Large vessel arterial occlusion

An ischaemic stroke, thought to be caused by occlusion of a large vessel, necessitates a thorough examination and investigation of likely causes of embolism, including the carotid or vertebral arteries (atherosclerosis or dissection), cardiac structure and rhythm, and prothrombotic tendencies.

Anterior circulation infarction

The anterior circulation comprises the anterior and middle cerebral arteries, both supplied by the internal carotid.

Anterior cerebral artery (ACA) supplies parasagittal cortex, including the motor and sensory cortices for the lower limb.

Clinical features of occlusion
- Contralateral leg weakness and sensory impairment. There may be similar but milder upper limb signs and symptoms. The face is spared.
- Loss of voluntary micturition, resulting in urinary incontinence.

Middle cerebral artery (MCA) supplies almost whole lateral surface of the frontal, parietal and temporal lobes, auditory cortex and insula, as well as lenticulostriate perforating vessels.

Clinical features of occlusion
- Contralateral weakness and sensory impairment, face and arm more than leg – inability to detect sensory stimuli, rather than due to a lack of attention.
- Homonymous quadrant- or hemi-anopia due to damage to optic radiations in the parietal (inferior quadrantanopia) or temporal (superior quandrantanopia) lobes.
- Expressive and/or receptive dysphasia if the dominant hemisphere is involved.
- Cortical symptoms and signs:
  - Sensory cortical impairment: 2-point discrimination, astereoagnosis (inability to recognize objects by touch), localization of pain and touch, texture recognition, sensory inattention (e.g. when touched on both hands simultaneously, will only notice the touch on the right, despite being able to detect touch on the left and right independently), agraphaesthesia (impaired recognition of numbers drawn on the palm of the hand).
  - Dominant parietal lobe: in addition to sensory cortical features, visual agnosia (inability to recognize a familiar object), prosopagnosia (inability to recognize familiar faces), auditory agnosia (inability to recognize familiar sounds), autotopagnosia (inability to identify parts of the body), anosagnosia (unaware of any disability), Gerstmann syndrome (inability to calculate, read or write [acalculia, alexia, agraphia], finger agnosia [unable to correctly identify the finger touched], and loss of left–right discrimination).
  - Non-dominant parietal lobe: hemi-neglect (multi-modality), apraxias (inability to execute or carry out skilled or coordinated movements and gestures, despite having the desire and the physical ability to perform them) e.g. dressing apraxia, gait apraxia, constructional apraxia (inability to draw intersecting pentagons).

ⓘ Top Tips

- Hemi-neglect or hemi-inattention usually affects the left side of the body (i.e. non-dominant side). There is redundant processing of the right hemispace by both parietal lobes, whereas the left hemispace is only processed by the right parietal lobe. Therefore damage to the left parietal lobe does not usually result in a significant attentional deficit.

Cerebral blood supply

ACA supplies the frontal and medial areas of the cortex. MCA supplies most of the cortex. The superior division supplies the cortex above the Sylvian fissure. The inferior division supplies the cortex below the Sylvian fissure, including the lateral temporal lobe and a variable portion of the parietal lobe. PCA supplies the inferior, medial temporal and occipital cortex.

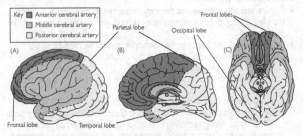

Fig. 6.4 Regions of the cortex supplied by the anterior cerebral artery (ACA), middle cerebral artery (MCA), and posterior cerebral arteries (PCA). a) Lateral view; b) medial view; c) Inferior view.
From Blumenfeld: *Neuroanatomy Through Clinical Cases*, Second Edition, Sinauer Associates, Inc., 2010, Figure 10.5 A, B, and C, page 396.

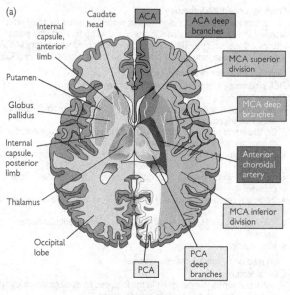

(a)

Caudate head — ACA

Internal capsule, anterior limb

ACA deep branches

MCA superior division

Putamen

MCA deep branches

Globus pallidus

Internal capsule, posterior limb

Anterior choroidal artery

Thalamus

MCA inferior division

Occipital lobe

PCA deep branches

PCA

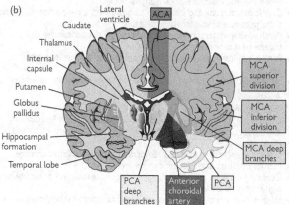

(b)

Lateral ventricle — ACA

Caudate

Thalamus

Internal capsule

MCA superior division

Putamen

MCA inferior division

Globus pallidus

Hippocampal formation

MCA deep branches

Temporal lobe

PCA deep branches

Anterior choroidal artery

PCA

Fig. 6.5 a) Axial blood supply. b) Coronal figure.
From Blumenfeld: *Neuroanatomy Through Clinical Cases*, Second Edition, Sinauer Associates, Inc., 2010, Figure 10.9 A, and B page 399.

Posterior circulation infarction

The posterior circulation refers to the vessels supplied by the vertebral arteries, and comprises the basilar artery and its perforators, the posterior inferior cerebellar artery (PICA), anterior inferior cerebellar artery (AICA), superior cerebellar artery (SCA), and the posterior cerebral artery (PCA).

Common posterior circulation syndromes

PICA syndrome (lateral medullary or Wallenberg's syndrome)
Clinical features:
- Ipsilateral pain and pinprick impairment in the face, due to damage to the spinal trigeminal nucleus.
- Contralateral trunk and extremity pain and pinprick impairment, due to damage to lateral spinothalamic tract.
- Dysphagia, hoarseness and loss of gag reflex, due to nucleus ambiguus damage.
- Ipsilateral Horner's syndrome, due to descending sympathetic fibre damage.
- Ipsilateral cerebellar signs, due to involvement of the inferior cerebellar peduncle.
- Vertigo, nystagmus, vomiting and diplopia due to vestibular nuclei damage.
- Hiccupping.

AICA syndrome (lateral pontine syndrome)
Clinical features:
- Ipsilateral sensory impairment in the face, due to damage to the spinal trigeminal and main sensory trigeminal nuclei.
- Contralateral trunk and extremity pain and pinprick impairment, due to damage to lateral spinothalamic tract.
- Paralysis of ipsilateral muscles of mastication, due to damage to trigeminal motor nucleus.
- Paralysis of ipsilateral face (LMN lesion), due to damage to facial nucleus.
- Ipsilateral hemi-ataxia due to damage to middle cerebellar peduncle.

PCA occlusion
Clinical features:
- Contralateral homonymous hemianopia, frequently with macular sparing (occipital pole at site of rich anastomosis between MCA and PCA).
- Contralateral loss of pain and temperature due to thalamic damage.
- Memory deficits due to hippocampal involvement.
- Cortical blindness, visual hemineglect, prosopagnosia and other visual higher cortical deficits.
- Weber's syndrome: third nerve palsy and contralateral hemiplegia due to infarction of the medial midbrain.
- Dominant hemisphere infarction may cause aphasia ± alexia without agraphia.
- Larger PCA infarcts involving the thalamus and internal capsule may cause contralateral hemisensory loss and hemiparesis.

Top of the basilar syndrome
Emboli may lodge at the top of the basilar artery, causing infarction of the midbrain:
- Loss of vertical eye movements
- Pupillary abnormalities
- Coma
- Locked-in syndrome.

Spinal cord infarction

The most common territory for spinal cord infarction is the anterior spinal artery, which supplies the anterior 2/3 of the spinal cord. The anterior spinal artery is supplied by 8–10 unpaired anterior medullary arteries, which are branches of the aorta, vertebral and iliac arteries. The largest anterior medullary artery, the artery of Adamkiewicz, usually located at T9–T11, is susceptible to occlusion with neurological deficit. The commonest level for spinal cord infarction is the upper thoracic cord as this is a watershed area. Occasionally the cervical cord may be affected. Figs. 6.6a and 6.6b illustrate the arterial supply to the spinal cord.

Signs
- Acute flaccid paraparesis, becoming more spastic later on.
- Loss of sphincter control.
- Anaesthesia to pain and temperature due to involvement of spinothalamic tracts, but relative preservation of dorsal column-mediated joint position and vibration sense.

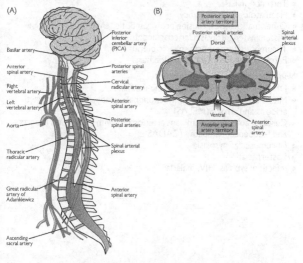

Fig. 6.6 Spinal cord arterial supply. a) Vertebral and radicular arteries give rise to anterior and posterior spinal arteries forming the spinal arterial plexus. b) Spinal cord cross-section showing regions supplied by the anterior and posterior arteries. From Blumenfeld: *Neuroanatomy Through Clinical Cases*, Second Edition, Sinauer Associates, Inc., 2010, Figure 6.5 A and B, page 229.

Causes of ischaemic stroke

Cardiac causes

- Atrial fibrillation
- Valvular heart disease
- Prosthetic heart valves
- Bacterial or marantic endocarditis
- Cardiac surgery
- Myocardial infarction
- Intracardiac aneurysm
- Cardiomyopathy
- Septal abnormality e.g. patent foramen ovale
- Intracardiac lesions e.g. myxoma.

Pathology of the arterial tree

- Carotid or aortic atherosclerosis.
- Dissection of the aorta, carotids or vertebrals – may be related to trauma, drugs or collagen disease.
- Vasculitides – giant cell arteritis, Wegener's granulomatosis, SLE, polyarteritis nodosa, syphilitic aortitis.

Haematological causes

- Sickle cell disease
- Polycythaemia
- Thrombocythaemia
- Antiphospholipid antibody syndrome
- Thrombophilias
- Haematological malignancy
- Other malignancies, causing prothrombotic tendency
- Disseminated intravascular coagulopathy
- Thrombotic thrombocytopaenic purpura
- Paroxysmal nocturnal haemoglobinuria.

Non-atherosclerotic vasculopathies

- Drug misuse: heroin, cocaine, amphetamine
- Mitochondrial disease e.g. mitochondrial encephalomyopathy, lactic acidosis and stroke (MELAS)
- Cerebral autosomal dominant arteriopathy with subcortical infarcts and leucoencephalopathy (CADASIL)
- Fibromuscular dysplasia
- Post-irradiation
- Infection: syphilis, HIV, malaria.

Intracerebral haemorrhage

- Major differential for cerebral infarction – comprises 10% of patients with stroke.
- Consider if evidence of raised intracranial pressure, >1 vascular territory or prominent headache.
- Focal signs depend on haemorrhage location.
- Deep haemorrhages centred on the basal ganglia are more likely to be related to hypertension.
- Lobar haemorrhages more likely to be associated with structural abnormalities (such as tumours or AVMs), trauma or other abnormalities of the vasculature e.g. amyloid angiopathy or vasculitis.
- Intraventricular extension increases the likelihood of acute obstructive hydrocephalus.

Causes

- Hypertension
- Anticoagulation or bleeding tendency
- Trauma
- Tumour – primary or secondary
- Aneurysm
- AVM or cavernoma
- Infective endocarditis, due to haemorrhagic transformation of a septic embolus, or mycotic aneurysm
- Venous thrombosis (◆ p.332)
- Vasculitides
- Amyloid angiopathy

Subarachnoid haemorrhage

The main cause of non-traumatic subarachnoid haemorrhage (SAH) is rupture of an intracranial aneurysm, accounting for 85% of cases. The most common location is the circle of Willis. 10% are due to non-aneurysmal perimesencephalic haemorrhage, while 5% are due to rare causes such as AVMs, tumours, vasculitides and arterial dissection.

Risk factors

- Genetic: family history, polycystic kidney disease, Ehlers–Danlos, Marfan's, pseudoxanthoma elasticum
- Smoking
- Hypertension
- Illicit drugs: cocaine, methamphetamine
- Infective endocarditis with mycotic aneurysm formation

Clinical features

- 'Thunderclap' headache
- Confusion and lethargy
- Transient loss of consciousness or coma
- Meningeal irritation
- Focal signs related to intraparenchymal extension of blood, or later vasospasm
- Retinal or subhyaloid haemorrhage

Complications
- Vasospasm – 46%. Most common 4–10 days after haemorrhage. Nimodipine reduces risk of cerebral infarction by 34%.
- Hydrocephalus – 20%. Consider this as a cause in any patient who exhibits a deterioration in consciousness or confusion, new onset of a VIth nerve palsy (false-localizing sign), or a rise in BP, widened pulse pressure and bradycardia (Cushing's triad – a late feature, suggestive of impending coning).
- Rebleeding – 7%, most commonly in first 48 hours.
- Seizures.
- Pulmonary oedema – cardiogenic or neurogenic (mechanisms poorly understood).
- Cardiac arrhythmias (probably due to autonomic changes or deranged electrolytes).
- Hyponatraemia, due to SIADH or cerebral salt-wasting.

Venous infarction
Venous infarction is usually caused by thrombosis within the deep veins, venous sinuses or the cortical veins. Secondary haemorrhage may result, due to forced local arterial hypertension.

Signs
- Features of raised intracranial pressure:
  - Headache
  - Papilloedema
  - VIth nerve palsy
  - Focal signs related to herniation
- Seizures
- Focal signs related to location of the infarction
- Altered consciousness.

Causes
- Raised oestrogen levels related to pregnancy, puerperium or oral contraceptive pill
- Dehydration
- Sepsis
- Thrombophilias e.g. anti-phospholipid antibodies, Factor V Leiden
- Behçet's disease
- Local infection – facial cellulitis, purulent otitis media, mastoiditis
- Direct trauma
- Tumour infiltration of dural sinuses.

Differential diagnosis of stroke
- Space-occupying lesions:
  - Cerebral tumour
  - Abscess
  - Parasitic e.g. neurocystercercosis, echinococcus (hydatid disease)
- Viral encephalitis
- Neuroinflammatory
  - Demyelinating plaque in MS
  - Neurosarcoid
  - Behçet's

- Metabolic: hypoglycaemia.
- Migraine: may present with aphasia and hemiparesis.
- Epilepsy: Todd's paresis following a focal seizure.
- Neuropsychiatric: may present with functional hemiparesis; weakness unlikely to be of pyramidal pattern.
- Hemi-Parkinson's disease: in the initial phase of the disease, there may be unilateral increased tone with apparent mild weakness.

In the acute setting, the major differential diagnoses for stroke include migraine, CNS infection, Todd's paresis and functional weakness. There are some important diagnostic clues:

- Positive motor phenomena before onset of neurological deficit are very rare in stroke, although are occasionally seen in TIA, and suggest focal epilepsy.
- Neurological deficit in stroke usually develops over a few seconds or minutes. Instantaneous onset is more in keeping with epilepsy.
- A neurological deficit such as numbness or weakness spreading down the body over minutes e.g. from the hand, up the arm, to the face, then the shoulder, is known as a 'migrainous march', and is thought to represent spreading cortical depression in migraine. Similarly, visual aura slowly spreads across the visual field. Positive sensory or visual phenomena, such as paraesthesiae or shimmering lights and zig-zag lines respectively, are also much more consistent with migraine than stroke. Sensory, aphasic or motor aura is rare without visual aura.
- Pyrexia, or a preceding history of lethargy or fever, raise the possibility of encephalitis, or stroke in the context of bacterial endocarditis.
- Fluctuating or inconsistent signs, especially if they disappear on distraction, suggest non-organic illness.

Investigation of stroke

- *Immediate:*
  - Oxygen saturations, glucose, BP, 12-lead ECG, blood tests (FBC, clotting, ESR, TFTs, LFTs, ANA, blood cultures).
  - CT brain (often normal in the acute phase in embolic stroke) – may see thrombus (e.g. in proximal middle cerebral artery) or the hyperdense signal of blood in haemorrhagic stroke.
  - If CT scan is normal within 3 hours, some centres proceed to CT perfusion scan, which correlates blood flow with tissue perfusion.
- *Urgent:*
  - Speech and language therapy (patient nil by mouth till then).
  - CXR (to rule out aspiration).
  - Fasting glucose and lipids.
  - Thrombophilia screen in young patients or if history of recurrent thromboembolism or miscarriage. Sickle cell screen in Afro-Caribbean patients.
  - MRI brain (± neck and cerebral angiography to rule out AVM or aneurysm).
  - 24-hour ECG, TTE, transcranial Doppler and, if appropriate, TOE (young patients with few or no risk factors).

Treatment

- Rule out hypoglycaemia, hyperglycaemia, Todd's paresis, TIA, functional hemiparesis.
- If presentation within 3 hours of symptom onset, and no contraindications, then consider thrombolysis with tissue plasminogen activator (tPA).
  - Given intravenously peripherally.
  - Transfer to monitored bed in Specialist Stroke Unit.
  - Regular (15-min) neurological observations. Watch for drop in GCS, which may indicate haemorrhagic transformation, or oedema (or hydrocephalus in the case of haemorrhage) causing raised intracranial pressure.
- Currently, thrombolysis beyond 3 hours is outside the licence, but there is evidence that thrombolysis within a 4.5-hour window may be appropriate. The IST-3 trial is currently ongoing to study the effectiveness of thrombolysis in patients outside the terms of the licence, e.g. minimal or severe neurological deficit, up to 6 hours after onset, age >80.
- Contraindications to thrombolysis:
  - Any previous intracranial haemorrhage, AVM or aneurysm.
  - History of stroke or head injury in the last 3 months.
  - Evidence of active internal bleeding.
  - History of gastrointestinal bleeding, liver disease or varices.
  - Major surgery or trauma in the last 14 days.
  - Pancreatitis or pericarditis.
  - Recent lumbar puncture or arterial puncture at a non-compressible site.
  - Systolic BP >185mmHg; diastolic BP >110mmHg.
- Bleeding risk:
  - 1% natural risk in ischaemic stroke.
  - 6% with active treatment within 3 hours.
  - Increases with delay from time of onset.
  - 11–12% between 3–6 hours.
- Perform post-thrombolysis CT brain (within 24 hours, or sooner if GCS drops).
- Avoid catheterization, venepuncture or other invasive procedures for 24 hours.

Complications of stroke

- Acute:
  - Raised intracranial pressure and herniation
  - Haemorrhagic transformation
  - Aspiration and pneumonia
- Complications due to immobility:
  - Pneumonia
  - Contractures
  - Deep vein thrombosis
  - Pressure sores
  - Urinary tract infections

- Constipation
- Disuse atrophy from immobility
- Later complications:
  - Depression and reduced social interaction
  - Seizures
  - Thalamic pain syndrome.

Viva questions

What is the effectiveness of thrombolysis?

The NINDS trial demonstrated that thrombolysis within a 3-hour window increased the proportion of patients with minimal or no disability at 3 months from 38% to 50%.[1] The number needed to treat for 1 more patient to have a normal or near outcome was 8, and the number needed to treat (NNT) for 1 more patient to have an improved outcome was 3.1. Brain haemorrhage related to tPA caused severe worsened final outcome in 1% of patients.

The ECASS3 trial analysed the effect of thrombolysis between 3 and 4.5 hours.[2] This trial found that major symptomatic haemorrhage occurred in 2.4% of thrombolysed patients, compared with 0.2% in the placebo group. The proportion of patients with minimal or no disability increased from 45% to 52%. The NNT for a normal or near normal outcome was 14, and the NNT for an improved outcome was 8.

Discuss the treatments for secondary prevention of ischaemic stroke

- Aspirin 300 mg stat, for 2 weeks then 75mg daily.
- Dipyridamole MR 200 mg BD.
- Consider changing anti-platelet therapy to clopidogrel if ischaemic stroke occurred on aspirin ± dipyridamole.
- Consider warfarin for AF-induced embolic stroke.
- Statin.
- ACE inhibitor.
- Consider carotid endarterectomy if symptomatic stenosis >70%.

What is the significance of the NIH stroke scale in the decision to thrombolyse?

The NIH stroke score (NIHSS) is used to assess the severity of stroke. It is scored out of 42, and is based upon clinical findings such as level of consciousness, gaze, visual field deficit, motor and sensory deficit, dysarthria and ataxia. Patients with an NIHSS of between 5–20 are eligible for thrombolysis. For patients with an NIHSS <5 or >20, the IST-3 trial is currently ongoing to assess the safety and effectiveness of thrombolysis.

How would you investigate and manage a patient with possible subarachnoid haemorrhage?

Investigations include:

- A mandatory CT brain:
  - Demonstrates blood in 95% if done within 48 hours.
  - Sensitivity drops to 80% at 3 days, 50% at one week, 30% at 2 weeks.
- If CT normal, lumbar puncture must be performed:
  - Should be delayed by 12 hours to permit xanthochromia to develop.
  - Xanthochromia should be determined by spectrophotometry.
  - Negative CSF, if performed properly, excludes a SAH.

- Arterial imaging:
  - CT or MR angiography
  - Digital subtraction angiography is the gold standard.

Management:
- Supportive care – stabilize BP, ventilation, oxygenation and circulating volume.
- Avoid hyperglycaemia and hyperthermia.
- Stop aspirin or warfarin.
- Commence nimodipine 60 mg 4-hourly to reduce risk of vasospasm.
- Liaise with neurosurgery urgently for clipping or endovascular coiling – early intervention is generally favoured to reduce the risk of rebleeding.

References

1. The National Institute of Neurological Disorders and Stroke rt-PA Stroke Study Group. Tissue plasminogen activator for acute ischemic stroke. *NEJM* 1995; **333**(24):1581–7.

2. Hacke W, et al. Thrombolysis with alteplase 3 to 4.5 hours after acute ischemic stroke. *NEJM* 2008; **359**(13):1317–29.

📖 Further reading

NICE. *Guidance for management of Stroke and TIA.* London: NICE, 2010. Available at: http://guidance.nice.org.uk/CG68/Guidance.

🔗 Useful websites

IST-3 Trial Website: http://www.dcn.ed.ac.uk/ist3/.
NIH stroke scale: http://www.strokecenter.org/trials/scales/nihss.html.

Multiple sclerosis and other CNS inflammatory disorders

Multiple sclerosis

MS is a recurrent multifocal inflammatory disorder of the central nervous system, and is frequently described as 'CNS inflammation disseminated in time and space'.

Due to the variety of signs, and the chronicity of the disease, patients with MS frequently appear in the PACES examination, and due to the recent introduction of novel therapies, MS and its treatment is often discussed in the viva section.

Epidemiology
- MS is the commonest cause of neurological disability in young adults, with significant healthcare costs.
- Prevalence is 100–150/100,000 population, with 85,000 patients in the UK.
- Incidence increases with increasing latitude, with a few exceptions, and even small distances demonstrate variation, e.g. commoner in Scotland than in South-East England.
- Migration studies suggest that risk is acquired before adolescence, although not all studies are consistent.
- Typically presents at 20–40 years of age, with females twice as frequently affected.

Aetiology
- Complex aetiology, which cannot be ascribed to a single genetic or environmental factor.
- Genetic susceptibility – higher concordance in monozygotic twins, with an increased risk in those with 1st-degree relatives with MS. Associations with HLA class II alleles, and a polymorphism of the interleukin-7 receptor alpha (*IL7RA*) gene have been described.
- Environmental factors – transmissible agents such as EBV, HHV-6, *Chlamydia pneumoniae* and other viruses have all been hypothesized to play a role. Vitamin D deficiency has also been proposed as a contributing factor.

Clinical features
- MS can affect any part of the CNS, and as such, the clinical features mirror this.
- Optic neuritis is frequently the presenting feature – pain behind the eye on movement, followed by a reduction in visual acuity, colour desaturation and the development of a relative afferent pupillary defect. Visual acuity reaches a nadir within 2 weeks. Optic atrophy usually takes 6–8 weeks to develop.
- Diplopia is usually symptomatic of a VIth nerve palsy or an INO (→ p. 359).
- A spinal cord syndrome may present with sensory disturbance or paraparesis, with or without urinary or bowel dysfunction.
- Motor involvement tends to occur later in the disease, with weakness and spasticity.

- Cerebellar signs at presentation are unusual, but become common during the course of the disease, due to cerebellar or brainstem disease.
- Cognitive impairment is common, but tends to be a later feature.
- Other features include dysarthria, dysphagia, vertigo, pain, Lhermitte's symptom (electrical sensation radiating from neck to arms or legs on flexion of the neck), Uthhoff's phenomenon (worsening of symptoms with a rise in body temperature e.g. during a hot shower or on exercise), trigeminal neuralgia, depression.
- Systemic infections may trigger a relapse or exacerbate existing symptoms.
- Pregnancy appears to reduce the likelihood of relapse, but this is balanced by a slightly increased relapse rate in the first 3 months post-partum.

Common Pitfalls

- MS is frequently mentioned by candidates as a differential diagnosis for a peripheral nerve lesion. MS is a disease of the CNS, and therefore only rarely causes cranial neuropathies through demyelination of the nucleus or fasciculus. MS does not affect other peripheral nerves.

Clinical course

- 85% present with relapses and remissions, with an average frequency of 1 relapse per year – relapsing-remitting MS (RRMS).
- RRMS may evolve into a gradually progressive decline, called secondary progressive MS (SPMS). After 20 years of RRMS, ~80% go on to develop SPMS, without clear relapses but accumulating neurological deficits.
- ~10–15% of patients present with a gradually progressive disorder – primary progressive MS (PPMS).
- By definition, MS requires 2 or more discrete episodes. The first acute episode is referred to as a clinically isolated syndrome (CIS). The risk of developing MS after a CIS has been quoted as 30–70%, depending on length of follow-up, but an abnormal MRI on presentation increases the risk from 8–22% to 56–88%.

Diagnosis

- The diagnosis of MS is a clinical one, based upon the exclusion of other conditions and the provision of dissemination in time and space. Basic blood tests will help exclude common mimics – ESR, ANA, ANCA, dsDNA, extractable nuclear antigen (ENA), and anti-phospholipid antibodies for autoimmune causes, B12 level, treponemal serology; further investigations should be guided by clinical presentation to exclude other diagnoses.
- Investigations may help to provide further evidence of dissemination in time and space, and immunological disturbance confined to the CNS.
- The MRI characteristically shows periventricular white matter lesions, and involvement of the corpus callosum (the large white matter tract joining the 2 hemispheres). Other common sites for lesions are the juxtacortical white matter (lesions are visible just under the grey matter of the cortex), brainstem, cerebellar white matter and spinal cord.
- Visual and auditory evoked potentials may be useful in demonstrating lesions in the optic pathway or brainstem respectively.

- CSF is usually normal, but occasionally a mildly raised CSF white cell count may be found (<50 mononuclear cells/mm^3). In 90% of clinically definite MS patients, unmatched oligoclonal bands (OCB) are present in the CSF. If bands are matched in CSF and serum, this suggests OCB spill-over into the CSF indicating a systemic disorder, not just limited to the central nervous system.
- Diagnostic criteria for MS have taken on new significance, since disease-modifying therapy is increasingly being commenced after a CIS. The development of new criteria for proving dissemination in time on the basis of a new T2 lesion 30 days after clinical onset (revised McDonald criteria[1]), now permits the diagnosis of MS after a CIS, without the need for a second clinical episode.

Management
- Management of acute relapses:
  - Steroid therapy is the only recommended drug treatment. It hastens recovery, but does not appear to affect long-term outcome.
  - Screen for systemic infection (commonly a urinary tract infection) that might trigger relapse or exacerbate existing symptoms.
- Symptomatic management:
  - Physiotherapy, occupational therapy, speech and language therapy.
  - Anti-spastic agents such as baclofen, tizanidine or intramuscular botulinum toxin.
  - Intermittent self-catheter or indwelling catheter, oxybutynin, tolterodine or solifenacin for bladder symptoms.
  - Laxatives for constipation.
  - Treatment of pain, respiratory dysfunction, swallowing difficulties, depression, sexual dysfunction.
- Disease-modifying therapy (DMT):
  - At present, beta-interferon and glatiramer acetate are prescribed according to guidelines from the Association of British Neurologists (ABN). Patients must be ambulant and have a diagnosis of MS established by McDonald criteria with relapsing onset. Patients with RRMS must have active disease, as defined by 2 significant relapses in last 2 years, 1 disabling relapse in last year, or active MRI scan with new or gadolinium-enhancing lesions that have developed in the last year. These drugs are not recommended in SPMS or PPMS, unless SPMS has superimposed relapses that are felt to be the predominant causes of increasing disability.
  - Beta-interferon and glatiramer acetate are given by subcutaneous or intramuscular injection, on a daily to weekly basis, depending on the drug.
  - Both drugs reduce the relapse rate by ~1/3.
  - Natalizumab is a monoclonal antibody, directed against an adhesion molecule expressed on T-cells. It blocks the migration of activated T-cells across the blood–brain barrier. It is given once a month by infusion, and reduces relapse rate by ~2/3. However, as well as hypersensitivity reactions, progressive multifocal leucoencephalopathy (PML) as a result of JC virus has been reported in individuals on natalizumab, with some fatalities. Natalizumab is therefore currently restricted for patients with severe active disease and evidence of active disease on MRI.

- Other DMTs currently being used include alemtuzumab, an anti-CD52 antibody that causes prolonged T cell depletion (may cause life-threatening immune-mediated thrombocytopaenia), and mitoxantrone (a cytotoxic agent which is reserved for very aggressive disease as it can cause cardiac failure, bone marrow suppression and leukaemia).
- Oral therapies. Fingolimod has now been approved in the UK as the first oral treatment for RRMS. Cladribine, another oral DMT is approved for use in Russia and Australia, but concerns about the increased risk of cancer associated with its use have delayed its licensing for use in the US and Europe.
- All DMTs should be withdrawn during pregnancy or if the patient plans to become pregnant.

MS mimics

The list of conditions that can present in a similar manner to MS is extremely long, but the main differential diagnosis includes:

- Vasculitides/auto-immune: SLE, Sjögren's, Behçet's, sarcoid, primary CNS angiitis, neuromyelitis optica.
- Vascular: recurrent TIAs/stroke, CADASIL, Fabry's disease, antiphospholipid syndrome.
- Mitochondrial disease: MELAS.
- Infection: Lyme, HIV encephalitis, syphilis, brucellosis, progressive multifocal leucoencephalopathy (PML).
- Metabolic: B12 deficiency.
- Leucodystrophies.

Differentiation of MS from other mimics can be extremely problematic, but is usually based upon atypical clinical features such as systemic symptoms, raised inflammatory markers, matched OCB in CSF and serum, or unusual radiological findings.

Neuromyelitis optica (NMO)/Devic's disease

This disease causes demyelination of the spinal cord and optic nerves:

- Typically, optic neuritis in NMO is more severe and recovers less well.
- Spinal cord lesions are usually more extensive than in MS, and on imaging tend to be central and extend over 3 vertebral segments.
- NMO is mediated by an antibody directed against aquaporin-4, a water channel. This antibody can be detected in blood serum.
- NMO is responsive to intravenous immunoglobulin and plasma exchange in the acute setting, and steroids and immunosuppressants in the long term.

Viva questions

Do you know of any rating scales for disability in MS?

The widest utilized scale is called the Expanded Disability Status Scale (EDSS), and ranges from 0 to 10. 0 represents normal neurological examination, 5 is ambulatory without aid or rest for about 200m, with disability enough to impair full daily activity, 10 is death due to MS. The ABN guidelines for initiating beta-interferon or glatiramer acetate state that the patient should have a maximum EDSS of 6.5 (constant bilateral assistance (canes, crutches, braces) to walk about 20 m with or without resting).

Why would beta-interferon or glatiramer acetate be stopped?

These 1st-line DMTs are stopped either due to adverse side effects such as injection site reactions, flu-like symptoms, autoimmune hepatitis and depression, or due to lack of efficacy. Beta-interferon treatment is associated with the development of neutralizing antibodies, which may reduce efficacy after some time. These antibodies do not interfere with glatiramer acetate, so patients can be switched to this treatment.

Reference

1. Polman CH *et al.* Diagnostic Criteria for Multiple Sclerosis: 2005 Revisions to the 'McDonald' Criteria. *Ann Neurol* 2005; **58**:840–6.

🖰 Useful website

Multiple Sclerosis Society: http://www.mssociety.org.uk [Information for doctors and patients, including downloadable PDF information sheets.]

Movement disorders

Parkinsonism

Idiopathic Parkinson's disease (IPD) is the commonest form of hypokinetic movement disorder but, should be distinguished from other syndromes with parkinsonian features. These include the Parkinson's-plus syndromes, a group of degenerative disorders with additional features, described as follows.

Signs
- Walking aids, or anti-parkinsonian medication.
- Hypomimic facies (lack of expression), reduced blink rate, sialorrhoea (drooling due to reduced swallowing frequency and facial bradykinesia).
- Festinant gait (→ p.304), reduction of armswing, camptocormia (marked flexion of the thoracolumbar spine), difficulties with turning or initiation of gait, postural instability.
- Asymmetrical 4–6Hz resting tremor, often pill-rolling, made worse by distraction (e.g. asking patient to count backwards from 100) or repetitive movements of the contralateral hand. A symmetrical tremor should alert the candidate to question the diagnosis of IPD.
- Bradykinesia (reduced speed and amplitude of movement) – ask the patient to make repetitive pincer grip motions or pronate and supinate the hands.
- Lead-pipe rigidity (+ superimposed tremor = 'cogwheel rigidity').
- Quiet, monotonous speech.
- Micrographia.
- Impaired sense of smell (can be a very early feature).

Causes
- Idiopathic Parkinson's disease
- Drug-induced: mainly neuroleptics, anti-emetics, or valproate
- Parkinson's plus syndromes: progressive supranuclear palsy (PSP), multisystem atrophy (MSA), corticobasal degeneration (CBD)
- Dementia with Lewy bodies
- Toxins: MPTP, manganese, carbon monoxide
- Wilson's disease (→ pp.120–122)
- Juvenile form of Huntington's disease (Westphal variant)
- Normal pressure hydrocephalus (triad of gait apraxia, urinary incontinence and cognitive decline)
- Post-traumatic e.g. dementia pugilistica in boxers
- Post-encephalitic
- Vascular parkinsonism
- Vasculitis (SLE, Sjögren's)

Additional signs that point away from a diagnosis of IPD
- Symmetry of signs: IPD almost always starts on one side, and throughout the disease that side is more affected than the other.
- Tardive dyskinesias: peri-oral or tongue involuntary movements (drug-induced).

- Early falls, especially backward, supranuclear gaze palsy (limitation of up- or down-gaze or slow vertical saccades), frontalis overactivation and axial rigidity point to progressive supranuclear palsy (PSP).
- Early autonomic disturbance such as impotence, urinary incontinence or postural hypotension, and cerebellar signs suggest MSA.
- Early dementia and visual hallucinations suggest dementia with Lewy bodies (DLB).
- Unilateral apraxia or pyramidal signs, 'alien limb', myoclonus, dystonic posturing suggest CBD, which results in degeneration of the cortex (predominantly parietal lobe) and the basal ganglia.
- Lower limb involvement only suggests vascular parkinsonism due to diffuse small-vessel disease.

❶ Top Tips

- Having demonstrated the characteristic signs (e.g. festinant gait, bradykinesia) in a patient with Parkinson's disease, always look for features associated with Parkinson's plus syndromes including supranuclear gaze palsy, postural hypotension, axial rigidity etc.

Chorea

Chorea is characterized by unpredictable jerky movements affecting different body parts in a random fashion – in subtle cases, the patient may look very fidgety.

Causes

- Sydenham's chorea (St Vitus' Dance): rheumatic fever
- Drug-induced: anti-convulsants, oral contraceptive pill
- Pregnancy
- Polycythaemia rubra vera
- Cerebral infarction
- Wilson's disease
- Huntington's disease
- Other hereditary neurological disorders: autosomal dominant spinocerebellar ataxias (SCAs), neuroacanthocytosis (a group of hereditary conditions characterized by the presence of acanthocytes on the blood film), ataxia telangiectasia
- Vasculitides
- Prion disease

Other hyperkinetic disorders

- Hemi-ballismus (ballistic movements of the limb, usually arm), which is usually related to a vascular lesion of the subthalamic nucleus.
- Athetosis: writhing movements of the limbs, more obvious distally (often coexists with chorea). In contrast to pseudoathetosis, this is present both with eyes open and closed.
- Dystonia: sustained involuntary contractions causing abnormal posture or twisting, repetitive movements. May be caused by drugs (e.g. neuroleptics, tricyclics, metoclopramide), a primary genetic syndrome, Parkinson's

disease (or L-dopa), an inherited neurodegenerative or metabolic syndrome (e.g. Wilson's or leucodystrophies), trauma, tumours and toxins.

Tremor

Tremor is defined as an involuntary rhythmic movement. Key to determination of the cause is to define the nature of the tremor.

Clinical examination

- Assess the hands, resting on the patient's lap. Look for the slow rhythmic tremor of Parkinsonism, with pill-rolling. Assess if the tremor is asymmetrical, suggesting IPD, or symmetrical, suggesting some other cause. Examine the rate and rhythmicity of the tremor. A jerky tremor suggests a dystonic component.
- If no tremor is present, attempt distraction by asking the patient to count backward.
- Ask the patient to hold the hands up, to see if there is a postural component, or if a resting tremor disappears on movement, as in Parkinson's disease.
- Perform finger–nose testing to examine for an intention tremor (tremor increases as the finger approaches the target) or past-pointing.
- Look at the head. Isolated head tremor is not a feature of Parkinson's disease. A 'yes-yes' tremor suggests essential tremor, a 'no-no' tremor, especially associated with torticollis, suggests a dystonic tremor.
- If the tremor is suggestive of Parkinsonism, examine for other features such as cogwheeling, lead-pipe rigidity, bradykinesia and gait.
- If there is evidence of past-pointing and intention tremor, go on to examine for other cerebellar signs, including dysdiadochokinesis, nystagmus, dysarthric speech and gait ataxia.
- If the tremor is present on maintaining a posture and also on performing an action, consider a peripheral neuropathy, and check for sensory disturbance, especially joint position sense, and reflexes.
- If the tremor only occurs with a particular task, ask the patient to reproduce that task – some dystonic tremors are task specific e.g. writing tremor.
- Ask for a drug history.

Types of tremor

- Parkinsonian tremor: present at rest, worsened by distraction or synkinesis, alleviated by movement, low-frequency, rhythmic.
- Essential tremor: predominantly postural or on action, may have a family history, is alleviated by alcohol or beta-blockers.
- Drug-induced tremor: often seen with inhaled beta-agonists, theophylline, caffeine, ciclosporin, sodium valproate and lithium.
- Cerebellar tremor: low frequency, absent at rest, present with movement, exacerbated towards end of goal-directed motion, may be unilateral or asymmetrical if related to a focal lesion (➲ see p. 346).
- Demyelinating tremor: seen in demyelinating neuropathies, present in posture (e.g. holding arms outstretched) and action, but not at rest.

- Task-specific tremor: often has a jerky component, and may only be produced by a particular activity like writing.
- Midbrain (Holmes) tremor (previously called a rubral tremor): present at rest, worsened significantly by posture and action, coarse. It is caused by damage to the cerebellorubrothalamic and nigrostriatal pathways, and is usually associated with MS or vascular insult.
- Nutritional: coeliac disease.

Further reading

Clarke H et al. (eds) Neurology: A Queen Square Textbook. Chapter 5: Movement disorders. Chichester: Wiley-Blackwell, 2009.

Cerebellar disorders

The cerebellar syndrome is caused by a heterogeneous group of disorders, and can occur in isolation or as part of range of neurological or systemic features. The candidate will often be directed towards a cerebellar examination by instructions referring to imbalance, incoordination or the patient having difficulties performing certain tasks.

Cerebellar disorders

Signs
- Gaze-evoked nystagmus and hypo- or hypermetric saccadic eye movements: on looking to either side, the fast phase of nystagmus will be in the direction of gaze, and on generation of saccadic eye movements, the patient may under- or overshoot, with resultant small corrective saccades.
- Cerebellar 'staccato' speech (in music, staccato refers to unconnected or detached notes; ⊃ p.318).
- Hypotonia of arms and legs.
- Upper limb signs of intention tremor, past-pointing, dysmetria and dysdiadochokinesis.
- Rebound phenomenon: the patient is asked to maintain his arms in the outstretched position with eyes closed. Downward pressure is applied to the arms and is released suddenly. In a cerebellar syndrome, the arms will shoot upward when pressure is released and will oscillate before returning to the original position. The cerebellum functions as a calibrator of forces, and dysfunction results in inappropriate muscle forces being generated to fix the limb in a particular position.
- Look for evidence of a sensory rather than cerebellar ataxia: positive Romberg's test or pseudoathetosis (apparent writhing of fingers of outstretched hands when eyes are closed, due to proprioceptive impairment). If sensory ataxia is suspected, look for sensory impairment (especially joint position sense) and distal weakness associated with a peripheral sensory or sensorimotor neuropathy.
- Ataxic gait (⊃ p.305).
- Heel–shin ataxia.
- Truncal ataxia.
- Pendular reflexes: the movement elicited by percussion is not dampened, resulting in swinging back and forth of the limb. Once again, this is due to a failure of calibration of muscle forces, resulting in abnormal 'dampening'.

Causes
- Demyelination: look for evidence of an RAPD (⊃ p.544), INO (⊃ p.359) or UMN signs, especially in a young woman.
- Vascular: infarction or haemorrhage.
- Space-occupying lesion (especially if unilateral or markedly asymmetrical signs).
- Alcoholic degeneration.
- Drugs esp. carbamazepine, phenytoin and barbiturates.
- Metabolic: B12, copper or vitamin E deficiency (may also cause sensory ataxia).
- Hypothyroidism.
- Nutritional: coeliac disease.

- Genetic:
  - Spinocerebellar ataxias: may have a variety of additional signs including UMN and extrapyramidal signs, peripheral neuropathy and ophthalmoplegia; autosomal dominance inheritance.
  - Friedreich's ataxia: ataxia with peripheral neuropathy, spasticity, optic atrophy, diabetes mellitus, hypertrophic cardiomyopathy and deafness. Typical onset is between 8–15 years of age; autosomal recessive inheritance. Patients frequently wheelchair-bound.
  - Ataxia telangiectasia: skin and eye telangiectasiae, dystonia and chorea; autosomal recessive inheritance.
  - Von Hippel–Lindau syndrome with cerebellar haemangioblastomas (associated with renal cell carcinoma).
- Multiple system atrophy with predominant cerebellar features (often referred to as MSA-C).
- Paraneoplastic: associated with small cell lung, breast, gynaecological and testicular tumours, and Hodgkin's lymphoma.

> **❶ Top Tips**
>
> - Consider the nature of the cerebellar dysfunction and order your list of causes according to the pattern of cerebellar signs elicited:
>   - Global dysfunction, i.e. symmetrical signs, suggests a degenerative, nutritional or toxic cause.
>   - Unilateral or asymmetrical signs suggest demyelination, a vascular lesion or space-occupying lesion.
>   - A cerebellar gait in isolation suggests damage to the cerebellar vermis, which is usually caused by chronic alcohol toxicity. If gait abnormality found, look for truncal ataxia.
> - Do not forget to examine gait, as this may be the only cerebellar sign elicited, especially in cerebellar degeneration related to alcohol.

Viva questions

What do you know about the genetics of the spinocerebellar ataxias?
The SCAs are a heterogeneous group of autosomal dominant genetic conditions causing a degenerative cerebellar syndrome. Over 25 have now been described. A majority of known mutations are trinucleotide CAG repeats, similar to those seen in Huntington's disease. These diseases show an inverse correlation between repeat length and age of onset, and demonstrate anticipation, the phenomenon of earlier onset and more severe disease in subsequent generations.

What do you know of Miller–Fisher syndrome?
Miller–Fisher syndrome is an autoimmune, usually post-infectious, disorder of acute or subacute onset, which causes ophthalmoplegia, ataxia and loss of lower limb reflexes, associated with the anti-GQ1b ganglioside antibody. It may overlap with Guillain–Barré syndrome.

With which cancers is a paraneoplastic cerebellar syndrome most frequently associated?
Paraneoplastic cerebellar degeneration is generally subacute in onset and aggressive in time course, with most people losing mobility within a year to 18 months. It is usually associated with small cell lung, breast, gynaecological and testicular tumours, and Hodgkin's lymphoma.

Spinal cord disorders

The basic spinal cord anatomy is illustrated in Fig. 6.7.

Spinal cord lesions may result from a variety of pathologies:

- Compressive – either extra- or intradural
- Vascular
- Inflammatory
- Nutritional/toxic
- Infective
- Degenerative/hereditary.

Differentiating these causes can be difficult on a clinical basis, but certain clinical features may be helpful.

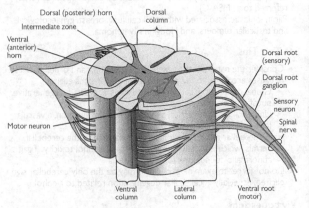

Fig. 6.7 Basic spinal cord anatomy. Grey matter, white matter and dorsal and ventral roots.
From Blumenfeld: *Neuroanatomy Through Clinical Cases*, Second Edition, Sinauer Associates, Inc., 2010, Figure 6.3 A only, page 227.

Spinal cord disorders

Signs

- Paraparetic spastic gait
- Spasticity in the lower limbs
- Pyramidal weakness (extensors weaker than flexors in the arm, flexors weaker than extensors in the leg)
- Hyper-reflexia with upgoing plantar responses
- Sensory level above L1
- Catheter *in situ*
- Spinal surgery scars.

Helpful differentiating clinical features

- Rapidity of onset:
  - Seconds to minutes: vascular or trauma.
  - Hours: inflammatory, compressive, infective.
  - Days: nutritional, inflammatory, compressive.
  - Weeks to months: degenerative/hereditary, infective, nutritional.
- Very predominant sensory features point toward an inflammatory myelitis, while predominant motor features suggest cord compression.
- Sparing of posterior column sensory modalities suggests an anterior cord infarction or a syrinx, whilst predominant loss of posterior column sensory modalities suggests B12 deficiency, neurosyphilis or HIV-associated vacuolar myelopathy.
- Asymmetry suggests a myelitis or compressive lesion rather than a degenerative or nutritional process.
- Marked spasticity out of keeping with degree of weakness suggests MND, hereditary spastic paraparesis or tropical spastic paraparesis.
- Early bladder involvement in a motor syndrome would be highly unusual in MND, and would suggest a compressive myelopathy.
- Additional associated neurological signs:
  - LMN signs such as wasting, fasciculations or hyporeflexia: e.g. MND, syringomyelia, B12 deficiency, conus lesion (➲ Mixed upper and lower motor neuron signs, p.354).
  - Cerebellar signs: B12 deficiency, demyelination or other inflammatory disorders (➲ Mimics of multiple sclerosis, p.340), spinocerebellar ataxias (some SCAs have myelopathy as a feature).
  - Dysarthria: demyelination, MND.
  - Eye movement abnormalities: demyelination, spinocerebellar ataxias.
  - Reduced visual acuity: demyelination (especially neuromyelitis optica – Devic's syndrome), spinocerebellar ataxias.

Compressive lesions

Cord compression may result from a variety of pathologies. Classically, cord compression presents clinically as a predominantly motor syndrome, with bilateral spasticity and pyramidal weakness with a sensory level, but variations may occur depending on the degree and cause of compression, e.g. lateral compression causing Brown–Séquard syndrome, anterior compression causing sparing of posterior column modalities. Lesions above T1 may give rise to arm signs and high anterior cervical lesions can also result in respiratory compromise. A sensory level may result from a lesion at that level or at any site in the cord rostrally. Sacral sparing (preservation of pinprick in the saddle area) suggests an intrinsic cause since the sacral fibres are arranged most laterally in the spinothalamic tracts.

Causes
- Degenerative disease:
  - Central disc herniation – especially in cervical spine.
  - Atlanto-axial instability (e.g. rheumatoid arthritis).
  - Osteophytic compression.
- Tumours – benign and malignant:
  - Most commonly metastatic: myeloma, lung, breast, colon, thyroid, prostate, kidney.
  - Primary intramedullary: ependymoma, astrocytoma, glioblastoma, haemangioblastomas (25% have von Hippel–Lindau syndrome).
  - Primary extramedullary: meningioma, neurofibroma (associated with NF1), schwannoma (associated with NF2), arachnoid cysts, epidermoid.
- Trauma.
- Infection:
  - Epidural abscess: *S. aureus, E. coli*, often seen in IV drug users.
  - Spinal TB (Pott's disease): results from vertebral collapse.
  - Vertebral osteomyelitis.
- Congenital:
  - Klippel–Feil syndrome results from failure of normal segmentation of the cervical vertebrae during the early weeks of fetal development, leading to a decreased number of cervical vertebrae and fusion of 2 or more vertebrae (C2–C7). Patients typically have a short (webbed) neck, low hairline at the back of the head, restricted mobility of the head and upper spine. Patients with Klippel–Feil syndrome may have cranial nerve abnormalities (particularly cranial nerves VI, VII and VIII, which may result in facial asymmetry or hearing loss, respectively) and a combination of spasticity and cerebellar signs in the limbs, the latter resulting from Arnold–Chiari malformations (downward displacement of the cerebellar tonsils through the foramen magnum). Associated abnormalities may include cleft palate, scoliosis, spina bifida, anomalies of the kidneys, genitourinary organs and the ribs, respiratory problems and cardiovascular malformations. High cervical abnormalities can cause acute spinal cord compression following comparatively minor trauma.
- Haematoma.

Vascular cord lesions

Causes
- Spinal artery infarction: almost always anterior spinal artery (Ͻ p.329).
- Neoplastic vascular lesions e.g. cavernous angiomas, haemangioblastomas (von Hippel–Lindau): may cause focal intraparenchymal haemorrhage.
- AVMs: usually present subacutely with progressive sensory, motor and sphincter loss, occasionally with radiculopathy and LMN signs. A dural fistula may produce an audible bruit over the spine.

Inflammatory cord lesions

Inflammatory transverse myelitis may occur in isolation or be part of a multifocal inflammatory process, either confined to the CNS or with multi-systemic involvement. As with compressive myelopathies, the clinical hallmark is that of a sensory level, but in contrast, a predominant sensory syndrome is sometimes seen.

Causes
- MS (→ p.337): by far the commonest cause of transverse myelitis in the young. May be a clinically isolated episode of demyelination or a relapse.
- Post-infectious acute disseminated encephalomyelitis (ADEM) e.g. measles, rubella, varicella, mumps, or less commonly, post-vaccination (esp. rabies vaccine).
- Sarcoidosis.
- Auto-immune disorders:
  - SLE, Sjögren's, scleroderma.
  - Vasculitides.
  - Antiphospholipid syndrome.
  - Ulcerative colitis.
- Devic's disease (neuromyelitis optica) (→ p.340): longer segments of myelitis associated with optic neuritis.
- Paraneoplastic disorders, esp. small-cell lung and lymphoma.

Infections of the spinal cord

The majority of infections infecting the spinal cord result in involvement of the vertebra or intervertebral disc, with subsequent extradural abscess formation. This causes cord compression but may also result in intradural involvement or local vasculitis with resulting infarction.

Causes
- Bacterial:
  - *Staphylococcus**
  - *Mycoplasma*
  - TB*
  - Lyme disease
  - Syphilis
- Viral:
  - Enteroviruses: esp. poliomyelitis**, coxsackie
  - Herpes viruses*: esp. VZV, HSV1 and 2
  - CMV and EBV*
  - Influenza
  - HIV-associated vacuolar myelopathy: slowly progressive spastic paraparesis with posterior column involvement
  - HTLV1-associated myelopathy (tropical spastic paraparesis). HTLV-1 is endemic in the Caribbean. 5% of carriers of the virus develop a slowly progressive myelopathy.
- Parasitic:
  - Schistosomiasis
  - Cysticercosis
  - Toxoplasma
  - Malaria

(*Common causes; ** frequently leads to permanent neurological deficit and therefore more commonly encountered in PACES; causes a flaccid weakness, both acutely and chronically.)

Nutritional/toxic cord disorders

Subacute combined degeneration (SCD) of the cord manifests as symmetrical dysaesthesiae, loss of posterior column sensory modalities and a spastic para- or quadraparesis, and results from B12 deficiency. It is usually seen in patients with pernicious anaemia (look for associated vitiligo), but may also be seen in severe malnutrition, or in nitrous oxide abuse (nitrous oxide interrupts normal B12 metabolism). Look for other features of B12 deficiency such as anaemia and beefsteak tongue.

SCD may rarely be caused by copper deficiency (associated with high zinc intake, which competes with copper for absorption) or vitamin E deficiencies.

Toxic causes of myelitis:

- Heroin (other drugs may cause spinal infarction)
- Snake and spider bite.

Degenerative/hereditary cord disorders

A variety of degenerative or hereditary disorders may present with a slowly progressive myelopathic picture. MND (➔ p.355) may present with a spastic paraparesis and is common in the PACES exam.

Hereditary spastic paraparesis (HSP), a heterogenous group of disorders, can be autosomal dominant, recessive or X-linked. The pure form presents with a slowly progressive gait disturbance, spasticity and hyperreflexia with upgoing plantars. Weakness is not a prominent feature, nor is sphincter disturbance. The complicated form is associated with features such as cerebellar, extrapyramidal and cognitive signs, neuropathy, optic atrophy and retinopathy.

Other hereditary or degenerative disorders with a prominent myelopathic component include:

- Friedreich's ataxia (➔ p. 346)
- Spinocerebellar ataxias (➔ p. 346)
- Leucodystrophies.

Viva questions

What is the definition of spasticity, and how is it differentiated from other types of hypertonia?

Spasticity is the increased tone due to an upper motor lesion, which is velocity-dependent, i.e. resistance increases with the rate the muscle is stretched. It is usually described as 'clasp-knife'; initial resistance to a passive movement suddenly disappears, much like a pen-knife when it is opened. In contrast, in extrapyramidal syndromes, the rigidity is constant throughout the range of movement and is not velocity-dependent. It may have superimposed tremor, resulting in 'cogwheel' rigidity. Paratonia, or Gegenhalten, is a feature of diffuse bilateral frontal lobe dysfunction – the patient appears to actively resist movement, and the tone increases in proportion to the strength used by the examiner moving the joint.

How are spinal tumours classified according to their anatomical location?

- Spinal tumours are usually classified into intra- or extradural tumours. Intradural tumours may be intramedullary (within the substance of the spinal cord), or extramedullary (compressing the spinal cord). Classification according to these groupings is helpful with respect to forming a differential diagnosis based upon imaging findings.
- Intramedullary tumours usually enlarge the cord, focally or diffusely. The majority are ependymomas, but include atrocytomas, glioblastomas, haemangioblastomas, and more rarely, other glial tumours, metastases and cavernomas.
- Intradural extramedullary tumours include meningiomas, neurofibromas, schwannomas, metastases, arachnoid cysts or epidermoid tumours.
- Extradural tumours are more likely to be metastases, as the vertebral bodies are the most frequent site of metastatic disease to the spine. Common cancers associated with spinal metastasis include breast, prostate, lung and kidney.

Do you know of any other neurological and non-neurological features of HTLV-1 infection?

In addition to causing tropical spastic paraparesis and T-cell leukaemia/lymphoma, HTLV-1 can cause a peripheral sensorimotor neuropathy and low-grade myositis. Other features include arthritis, sicca syndrome, uveitis and alveolitis.

What is the treatment for tropical spastic paraparesis?

To date, both the use of anti-retroviral drugs, to prevent viral replication, and immunosuppressants, to reduce the secondary inflammatory response, have not demonstrated either improved clinical outcome or a reduction in disease progression.

What do you know about stiff-person syndrome?

Stiff-person syndrome is a rare auto-immune or even rarer paraneoplastic syndrome driven by anti-glutamic acid decarboxylase (GAD) antibodies. It is characterized by rigidity of the axial and sometimes lower limb muscles, and can sometimes be mistaken for a spastic paraparesis, as the reflexes are frequently brisk. Treatment usually consists of immunosuppression or plasma exchange. Diagnosis is based upon continuous activity on EMG of the paraspinal musculature and anti-GAD testing.

Mixed upper and lower motor neuron signs

Candidates may encounter patients with various combinations of mixed upper and LMN signs in the PACES examination.

Remember that some patients may have dual (or even triple) pathology and do not easily fit into a single disease or syndrome. The candidate should be ready to recognize this and be able to discuss the findings in a clear and succinct way.

This section will review some of the typical clinical features and causes of lesions affecting both the upper and lower motor neurons.

Examination

- Look for bedside clues in the scenario given by the examiners. An elderly patient might suggest cervical spondylosis with a myelopathy, MND or a dual pathology such as neuropathy with cervical myelopathy.
- Listen to speech for dysarthria. Is there bulbar or pseudobulbar dysarthria?
- Offer to test for a jaw jerk (should be brisk in MND and other causes of a pseudobulbar palsy).
- Examine the gait and limbs – are there mixed upper and lower motor neuron signs (e.g. wasting and fasciculation with preserved or brisk reflexes and extensor plantars).
- Ask about swallowing, bladder and bowel function.

Bulbar and pseudobulbar palsy

Bulbar palsy is due to LMN lesion of the lower cranial nerves:

- Characterized by nasal speech
- Nasal regurgitation
- Tongue wasting and fasciculations.

Pseudobulbar palsy is due to UMN lesion affecting the supply to the tongue and oropharynx:

- Spastic, hoarse voice
- Slow tongue movements
- Associated with brisk facial reflexes, jaw jerk and emotional lability (spontaneous laughter or crying).

Both may cause dysphagia and drooling.

Causes of bulbar palsy include:

- Myasthenia gravis
- MND
- Neuropathy (particularly Guillain–Barré syndrome)
- Myopathy.

Causes of pseudobulbar palsy include:

- MS
- Brainstem stroke
- MND.

Advanced PD and other extrapyramidal syndromes also cause poverty of movement of the bulbar muscles.

Conditions characterized by the presence of upper and LMN signs include:

Dual pathology
In the PACES setting, the most common cause of mixed UMN and LMN signs is the presence of 2 pathologies, usually cervical myelopathy with a peripheral neuropathy:

* Look for a surgical scar over the posterior or anterior neck.
* There will be no signs above the neck.
* Verify the presence of a stocking (± glove) sensory impairment.
* Reflexes may be brisk despite the neuropathy if the myelopathy is severe and the neuropathy is mild.
* Examine for evidence of what is causing the neuropathy, e.g. pinpricks in the fingertips, suggesting diabetes.

Cervical radiculomyelopathy
Multilevel degenerative disease of the cervical spine leads to compression of the exiting nerve roots (radiculopathy) and the spinal cord (myelopathy). Features include:

* Wasting and weakness:
  * C5–C6 nerve root compression leads to flaccid weakness of biceps and supinators with loss of the biceps and supinator reflex.
  * Involvement of C7–T1 leads to wasting of the triceps, forearm or intrinsic hand muscles.
* Brisk reflexes and spasticity, below the level of cord compression. The biceps or supinator jerks may be 'inverted' i.e. percussion does not elicit the reflex itself, but due to hyper-reflexia at lower levels, finger jerks will be present.
* Pain localized to the neck or in a radicular pattern.
* Sensory disturbance in a radicular distribution.

Motor neuron disease
MND is a progressive neuronal degenerative disease affecting the motor neurons (anterior horn cells) of the spinal cord and the motor cranial nuclei. It leads to severe disability and death. There is considerable variability in presentation, clinical course and prognosis. The condition is divided into several different clinical subtypes:

* *Amyotrophic lateral sclerosis (ALS)*: the most common and characterized by upper and lower motor neuron involvement of the bulbar system and upper and lower limbs; If it presents with predominantly (or exclusive) bulbar weakness, it is referred to as progressive bulbar palsy (PBP).
* *Primary lateral sclerosis (PLS)*: exclusively UMN involvement.
* *Progressive muscular atrophy (PMA)*: involves only LMNs.

Diagnosis is made through demonstration of widespread upper and LMN signs, with active denervation on EMG. Other causes, such as cervical myelopathy, need to be excluded.

The majority of cases are sporadic, but 5–10% are familial (20% of these are due to a mutation in the *SOD1* gene).

Management
- Mainly supportive:
  - Respiratory management with early use of antibiotics and consideration of non-invasive ventilation.
  - Management of bulbar weakness – swallowing assessment, nutritional assessment, treatment of sialorrhoea with anticholinergic agents. Speech and language therapists may be able to advise regarding communication aids.
  - Psychological support.
  - Riluzole has been shown to prolong survival in MND by 3 months after 18 months' administration. However, it can cause nausea and deranged liver function.

Syringomyelia

Arises due to a fluid filled cyst within the central canal of the spinal cord. Similar signs may occur with an intrinsic spinal cord tumour. When the brain stem is affected it is referred to as syringobulbia. A syrinx may be associated with an intrinsic cord tumour or a Chiari malformation, so adequate imaging is crucial.

Signs include:
- 'Dissociated' sensory loss – loss of pain and temperature sensation with preservation of light touch, vibration, and position sense. Due to interruption of decussating spinothalamic fibres in the central grey matter with preservation of the dorsal columns. May be described as 'suspended' or 'cape-like' – a patch of dissociated sensory loss that does not extend to the lower limbs and is thus 'hanging', usually on the arms and thorax or abdomen.
- Sensory loss may also be unrecognized by the patient. Look for scars from painless burns or painless minor injuries.
- Wasting and weakness of the small muscle of the hand.
- Lower limb reflexes are brisk and plantars are extensor.
- Examine for Horner's syndrome (due to involvement of sympathetic neurons at C8/T1).
- There may be associated kyphoscoliosis.
- Look also for loss of sensation to pin prick on the posterior scalp (C2).

Lesions of the conus medullaris and cauda equina

The spinal cord tapers and ends in a distal bulbous swelling (conus medullaris) at the L1–L2 vertebral level. The nerve roots emerge at the cauda equina and are arranged according to the spinal segments from which they originate. They extend within a CSF-containing dural sac to the S2 vertebral level.

Conus and cauda equina lesions can be difficult to differentiate, especially in the acute setting. The conus medullaris contains UMNs, so acutely, a conus lesion may cause loss of lower limb reflexes, but upgoing plantars later emerge.

Lesions of the conus result in:
- Early and prominent sphincter disturbance (neurogenic bladder, faecal incontinence)
- Impotence
- Saddle anaesthesia (L5–S5)

- Inconsistent and mild leg weakness
- Upgoing plantars.

They are usually due to demyelination, central disc herniation, intrinsic spinal cord tumours or infection (herpes zoster, human herpes simplex virus 1 and 2).

Lesions of the cauda result in:
- Prominent low back and radicular pain
- Asymmetrical LMN signs including atrophy, flaccid weakness and areflexia
- Sphincter disturbance and diminished anal tone
- Radicular sensory loss.

Common causes of lesions of the cauda equina include extrinsic compression (prolapsed intervertebral disc, epidural abscess or tumour), inflammation (chronic inflammatory demyelinating neuropathy, sarcoidosis), carcinomatous meningitis or infection (herpes zoster, cytomegalovirus).

Subacute combined degeneration of the cord
Due to vitamin B12 deficiency. There may be:
- Brisk knee jerks, absent ankle jerks and extensor plantars.
- Symmetrical, distal (often painful, burning) sensory neuropathy (loss of light touch, vibration and joint position sense).
- Lower limb weakness.
- Positive Romberg's sign.
- Lhermette's phenomenon – tingling or electric shock-type feeling that passes down the spine and often the lower limbs when the neck is flexed or extended.
- Look for signs of anaemia (pale conjunctival membranes, tongue for glossitis, skin for yellow lemon tinge).
- There may be optic atrophy and/or dementia.
- Offer to check the abdomen for splenomegaly, laparotomy scar from previous surgery.
- Ask about pernicious anaemia and other autoimmune conditions, and consider nitrous oxide abuse as a cause.

Treatment is parenteral B12 replacement. If pernicious anaemia is the cause, this necessitates lifelong treatment. The neuropathy generally recovers better than the myelopathy.

Viva questions
What is your differential for absent ankle jerks and extensor plantar responses?
- MND
- Friedrich's ataxia
- Subacute combined degeneration of the cord
- Syringomyelia
- Tumours involving conus and cauda
- Neurosyphilis.

Approach to cranial nerves

Cranial nerve lesions may appear either in the Neurology station or Station 5, or indeed in both these stations of the PACES examination. The candidate should examine the cranial nerves both skilfully and rapidly. Remember, the cranial nerve findings may be part of a wider spectrum of neurological disease, involving the peripheral nervous system. Look for clues in the scenario given.

This section reviews typical features of lesions of individual cranial nerves and conditions affecting them, and combinations of cranial nerve lesions, which may occur together in the PACES exam. The relevant anatomy of the cranial nerves, their nuclei and central connections are also highlighted in this section. Conditions affecting the optic nerves and cranial nerves III, IV and VI are discussed in ➲ Eye movement disorders, p.541.

Olfactory nerve (I)

Examination

Ask the patient whether they have noticed a change in their sense of smell. A simple and quick assessment of olfaction at the bedside can be carried out with the peel of an orange, scented soap or coffee, if available. Check whether the patient can distinguish between, rather than recognize, odours. Test one nostril at a time.

Causes

- Unilateral anosmia:
  - Usually diseases of the nasal cavity.
  - Rarely, pressure on one olfactory tract by a space-occupying lesion such as a frontal lobe meningioma.
- Bilateral anosmia:
  - Post-head injury (may be associated with rhinorrhoea due to CSF leak caused by fracture of the cribriform plate).
  - Following viral infections such as the common cold.
  - Space-occupying lesion.
  - Early sign of Parkinson's disease.

Please see the ➲ Ophthalmology section in Chapter 8 (pp.532–546), for examination of vision and pupillary reflexes.

Third, fourth and sixth nerves (III, IV, VI) – eye movements

Check each extraocular muscle individually by asking the patient to track movements in the shape of an 'H'. Lateral movements are assessed, followed by elevation and depression to about 30° of lateral gaze.

In order to determine which muscle is weak, the following points should be considered:

- The false image is usually the less distinct.
- Diplopia occurs in positions that depend upon contraction of a weak eye muscle.
- A false image is projected in the direction of action of a weak muscle.
- Image separation increases in the direction of action of a weak muscle.

Remember that extraocular muscle palsies can be caused by the relevant cranial nerve lesion (e.g. abducens nerve in lateral rectus palsy), a disorder of the muscle or neuromuscular junction, or a structural intraorbital lesion.

(For complex ophthalmoplegia, ➔ Eye movements, p.541, and ➔ Myasthenia gravis, p.379.)

III. Oculomotor nerve palsy

Oculomotor nerve palsy is presented as a case in the Ophthalmology section (➔ p.572–574).

A complete, e.g. compressive, IIIrd nerve palsy typically causes:
* Complete ptosis.
* A dilated pupil that is unreactive to direct or consensual light (the contralateral pupil constricts normally when light is shown in either eye).
* An eye pointing down and out.

The term partial IIIrd nerve palsy usually implies sparing of the pupillary and lid parasympathetic fibres; these lie on the outer rim of the IIIrd nerve and have a separate blood supply:
* The pupil is not dilated and responds to light (direct and indirect).
* Partial or complete ptosis.
* Eye faces down and out.

IV. Trochlear nerve palsy

A distinct rarity compared with IIIrd and VIth nerve palsies, a IVth nerve palsy causes:
* A complaint of double vision on looking down e.g. descending stairs.
* 'Twisted' images i.e. one at an angle to the other.
* A head tilt away from the side of the superior oblique muscle weakness.
* No obvious squint.

VI. Abducens nerve palsy

This causes:
* A convergent squint.
* Diplopia with 2 images side by side (i.e. diplopia with horizontal separation). The double vision is maximal on attempted abduction (i.e. direction of action of lateral rectus) of the effected eye (and disappears on adduction).
* No abnormality of pupillary light reaction.

Internuclear ophthalmoplegia

INO results from damage to the medial longitudinal fasciculus in the brainstem and causes:
* Disconjugate horizontal eye movements i.e. movements not yoked together – the eyes move horizontally at different velocities.
* Incomplete adduction of the ipsilateral eye.
* Coarse jerky nystagmus of the opposite abducting eye.

❶ Top Tips

- The lesion of the medial longitudinal fasciculus is on the side of failure of adduction
- Observe conjugate gaze by fixing your own gaze on the patient's forehead – otherwise there a tendency for the examiner to fixate on the movement of one eye and miss what is happening to the other.

Trigeminal nerve (V)

The *sensory* territory includes the face and head anterior to the vertex, the eyes, the mucous membranes of the oral, nasal cavities and paranasal sinuses, and the teeth. The angle of the jaw is supplied by C2, not the trigeminal nerve. There are 3 divisions of the trigeminal nerve: ophthalmic (V_1), maxillary (V_2) and mandibular (V_3) – see ❸ Fig. 6.1a.

The *motor* root supplies the muscles of mastication.

Examination

- Sensory examination should include examination of all 3 divisions of the nerve and comparison made with the other side. Cutaneous sensation is best done by examining pin-prick sensation.
- Central lesions (brainstem) can cause circumoral, 'onion-skin' sensory loss.
- Ask the patient to bite, and palpate over the masseters and temporalis muscles. Opening the jaw against resistance tests pterygoid muscles. Motor lesions of V are unusual – but easy to miss unless jaw deviation (to the side of weakness) is assessed carefully.
- The corneal reflex tests the trigeminal and facial nerve but should not be performed in PACES, although you should state that you would normally do it; loss of the corneal reflex is usually the first sensory deficit in V1 lesion.
- The jaw jerk should be assessed – brisk in pseudobulbar palsy.

Facial nerve (VII)

- Motor branches supply muscles of facial expression. A small motor branch supplies the stapedius (hence a Bell's palsy causing hyperacuisis).
- Sensory: taste fibres from the anterior 2/3 of the tongue carried by the chorda tympani.
- Part of the VIIth nucleus on each side supplying the upper face (principally frontalis) receives supranuclear fibres from both hemispheres and, therefore, an UMN lesion of VII has sparing of the 'upper muscles' of the face.

Facial weakness

Weakness of the face should be characterized as unilateral or bilateral. It may be UMN (affecting lower parts of the face, sparing blinking and the wrinkling of the forehead, due to bilateral innervation of the parts of the VIIth nuclei supplying upper facial muscles) or LMN (affecting all facial muscles on the same side). Bell's phenomenon – the eyeball rolling upwards when the patient tries to blink – is a hallmark of a LMN lesion, since the eye is unable to close properly.

Causes of unilateral LMN facial weakness

- Bell's palsy: idiopathic, possibly secondary to a viral cause.
- Ramsay Hunt syndrome: this is the result of herpes zoster reactivation in the geniculate ganglion. Ask the patient if their taste has been affected. Look for vesicles over the external auditory meatus or in the canal. Offer to also look in the ear canal itself – an occasional site for vesicles.
- Stroke: brainstem lesion within the VIIth cranial nerve nucleus.
- Demyelination: plaques may present within the brainstem nuclei.
- Space-occupying lesion: cerebellar pontine angle (CPA) lesion, e.g. acoustic neuroma (frequently bilateral in neurofibromatosis type 2), cholesteatoma, neurofibroma. Ask to assess the corneal reflex, facial sensation and hearing. With cerebellar compression, there may also be nystagmus and other ipsilateral cerebellar signs. Check for a surgical scar.
- Infection e.g. Lyme disease, TB.
- Nerve infiltration e.g. sarcoid, lymphoma.
- Vasculitides.

Causes of bilateral LMN facial weakness

- Bilateral Bell's palsies.
- Sarcoidosis.
- Autoimmune causes: myasthenia gravis, vasculitides.
- Inflammatory: Guillain–Barré syndrome (prodromal illness – gastrointestinal upset with diarrhoea, chest infection, ascending weakness). Assess for other signs of motor neuropathy.
- Dystrophies e.g. facioscapulohumeral dystrophy, myotonic dystrophy- look for associated signs of MD e.g. myotonic facies, delayed relaxation, percussion myotonia, pacemaker (**◆** p.385 Myotonic dystrophy).
- Amyloidosis.
- Congenital e.g. Mobius syndrome (congenital facial weakness associated with bilateral VIth nerve palsies).

Vestibulocochlear (acoustic, VIII) nerve

You are unlikely to be asked to formally assess hearing in the PACES examination. If there is a degree of deafness, record the distance at which a whisper (or speech) is heard. Perform Rinne's and Weber's tests to assess the VIIIth nerve formally.

Rinne's test verifies that air conduction is better than bone conduction. Place a vibrating 512Hz tuning fork over the mastoid process, and ask the patient to tell you when they stop hearing it. At this point, hold the tuning fork in front of the ear – they should be able to hear it.

For Weber's test, hold the vibrating tuning fork on the forehead in the midline. If hearing is normal, the patient will hear the tuning fork equally in both ears. If Rinne's test is normal, demonstrating that air conduction is normal bilaterally, then a Weber's test producing a louder noise on the left suggests a lesion of the right cochlear nerve.

In practice, any suspicion of a CPA lesion should be followed by careful examination of the Vth, VIth, VIIth, and VIIIth cranial nerves and the demonstration of any associated cerebellar signs.

Patients with impaired vestibular nerve function complain of dizziness, vertigo and may have nystagmus. Remember Station 5 may include patients with benign paroxysmal positional vertigo (BPPV), so candidates should be aware of how to perform Hallpike's manoeuvre. This test is performed by moving the patient from the seated to the supine position, with the head turned to the side by 45° and the neck extended by 20°. The eyes are observed for nystagmus, which in BBPV characteristically has a latent period and a rotatory component. The test is repeated with the head turned to the other side.

Glossopharyngeal and vagus nerves (IX and X)

Examine these nerves together:

- Illuminate the uvula and fauces with a pen torch and ask the patient to say 'Aaah.' Check for symmetrical elevation of the soft palate, and that the uvula remains in the midline (will be pulled away from the side of the lesion).
- Ask the patient to cough – a Xth nerve palsy may result in laryngeal paralysis and a 'bovine' cough.
- The voice will sound 'wet' in the early stages of bulbar muscle weakness.

The gag reflex should not be elicited in the PACES examination – it is extremely unpleasant for the patient. However, it should be mentioned if there is any indication of a XIth or X^{th} nerve lesion.

Accessory nerve (XI)

Palpate the sternomastoid when the patient is turning his head away to the opposite side against resistance. To test shoulder elevation ask the patient to shrug the shoulders against resistance. While examining trapezii and sternomastoids, look for winging of the scapula and at the neck muscles. Winging is best seen if the patient extends his arms and pushes against resistance, e.g. leaning forwards with arms outstretched onto a wall.

Hypoglossal nerve (XII)

- Inspect the tongue at rest on the floor of the mouth. Fasciculations may be seen in MND. Remember, when the tongue is protruded, twitching is commonly found in normal individuals.
- Look for wasting of the tongue and deviation to the weak side (and of the lesion) when protruded.
- Power of the tongue can be assessed by asking the patient to push against the inside of the cheek. Compare the strength by feeling the cheek on each side in turn.
- Examine tongue movements generally. The speed and amplitude of tongue movements are diminished in bilateral pyramidal lesions and often early in Parkinson's disease.

Multiple cranial nerve syndromes

Since the nuclei and the courses of the cranial nerves often lie in close proximity, multiple cranial neuropathies may result from focal lesions.

Table 6.3 describes the commonly occurring multiple cranial neuropathies that might be encountered in the PACES examination.

Table 6.3 Multiple cranial nerve syndromes

Syndrome	Nerves affected	Common signs and symptoms
Cavernous sinus syndrome	Ipsilateral III, IV, VI, V_1	Painful ophthalmoplegia, usually with fixed dilated pupil
		Orbital congestion, chemosis, periorbital oedema, proptosis, sensory loss over V_1 ($\pm V_2$). Possible Horner's syndrome (from involvement of sympathetic fibres)
Orbital apex syndrome	II, III, IV, VI, V_1	Same deficits as cavernous sinus syndrome, plus more likely to involve cranial nerve II, causing visual loss
Jugular foramen syndrome (Vernet's syndrome)	Ipsilateral paralysis of IX, X and XI	Dysphagia, dysphonia
		Sensory loss over posterior 1/3 of the tongue, soft palate, pharynx, and larynx (IXth and X^{th}) and ipsilateral sternocleidomastoid/trapezius atrophy and weakness (XIth)
Cerebellopontine angle syndrome	Ipsilateral V	Facial sensory loss
	Ipsilateral VII	LMN facial weakness without hyperacusis
	Ipsilateral VIII	Progressive sensorineural hearing loss, tinnitus
	VI, IX, X less commonly involved	If the lesion continues to grow, pressure on cerebellum or its peduncles results in ipsilateral ataxia
		Nystagmus and gaze palsies may result from pontine compression

Orbital apex syndrome/superior orbital fissure syndrome
Involves the ophthalmic division (V_1) through the superior orbital fissure (SOF) together with the IIIrd, IVth and VIth cranial nerves. May be involved in various combinations by pathological processes at this site.

Clinical features
- Ophthalmoplegia.
- Sensory disturbance and often pain in V_1 distribution.
- Proptosis with large orbital lesions.
- Horner's syndrome.
- Visual loss may occur if the optic nerve becomes involved, suggesting extension to the orbital apex, which is more serious and called orbital apex syndrome (involves II, III, IV, VI and V_1, and occasionally V_2).

Causes

- Inflammatory/vasculitic disorders e.g. sarcoidosis, Wegener's granulomatosis, Churg–Strauss syndrome, giant cell arteritis.
- Fracture of the superior orbital fissure.
- Infections (bacterial, epidural abscesses, fungal mucomycosis spreading from a paranasal sinus, herpes zoster).
- Nasopharyngeal tumours.

❶ Top Tips

- Remember, if you isolate a single cranial nerve lesion, then look 'above' and 'below' that nerve in order to localize the likely anatomy of the lesion.
- If you find an unusual collection of cranial nerve signs suggesting disparate multiple cranial nerve lesions, then suspect traumatic causes (e.g. a IInd, IIIrd and XIIth nerve lesion).
- Learn the anatomical locations for the most common visual defects.
- Remember the divisions of the sensory branches of the trigeminal nerve.

Cavernous sinus syndrome

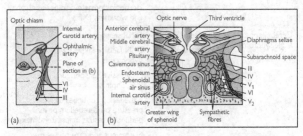

Fig. 6.8 Relations of III, IV, VI, V$_1$ and V$_2$ within the cavernous sinus. a) Right middle cranial fossa from above (cavernous sinus removed). b) Coronal section through pituitary.
Reproduced from Charles Clarke, Robin Howard, Martin Rosor, and Simon D. Shorvon, *Neurology: A Queen Square Textbook*, 2009, with permission from Wiley-Blackwell.

Affects cranial nerves III, IV, VI and V$_1$ (ophthalmic) and possibly V$_2$ (maxillary) division. The anatomical localization of these cranial nerves within the cavernous sinus is illustrated in Fig. 6.8.

Clinical features

- Ipsilateral complete/incomplete ophthalmoplegia (often painful).
- Chemosis.
- Proptosis.
- Horner's syndrome.
- Trigeminal V$_1$ sensory loss (absent corneal reflex) ± V$_2$.
- Can be indistinguishable from superior orbital fissure syndrome, except that V$_2$ as well as V$_1$ may be involved in cavernous sinus syndrome.

Causes
- Tumours: metastatic or direct extension of nasopharyngeal tumours, meningiomas.
- Pituitary apoplexy.
- Vascular: aneurysms of the intracavernous carotid, cavernous sinus arteriovenous fistula, aseptic thrombosis.
- Infections: bacterial infection causing cavernous sinus thrombosis, fungal infections (aspergillosis or mucormucosis).
- Granulomatous disease e.g. sarcoid, Wegener's granulomatosis, polyarteritis nodosa, idiopathic (Tolosa–Hunt syndrome).

Differential diagnosis
- Aneurysms of the posterior communicating artery with painful ophthalmoplegia
- Thyroid eye disease
- Basilar artery aneurysm
- Basilar meningitis
- Ophthalmoplegic migraine
- Lesions involving the orbital apex.

Cerebellopontine angle (CPA) lesion
Affects cranial nerves V, VI, VII and VIII and is often associated with ipsilateral cerebellar signs.

Clinical features
- Corneal reflex (V_1) may be absent (mention that this reflex should ideally be assessed in clinical practice, but do not perform this test in the PACES examination).
- Nystagmus.
- VIth and LMN VIIth nerve palsies.
- VIIIth nerve palsy (usually present with sensorineural deafness).
- Tremor ± other cerebellar features.
- Look for scar(s) behind ear over petrous bone.
- Headache, hydrocephalus and elevated intracranial pressure may be produced by obstruction to CSF flow.

Common Pitfalls

- Candidates may miss a unilateral hearing deficit if:
  - They whisper too loudly in the affected ear (as the words will be heard by the opposite ear).
  - They do not mask the noise input into the opposite ear (by rubbing the opposite tragus or their own fingers just outside the opposite ear).

Causes
- Tumours of the middle cranial fossa: acoustic neuroma (consider neurofibromatosis type 2 if bilateral), meningioma, cholesteatoma, glioma of the pons, cerebellar astrocytoma, medulloblastoma, nasopharyngeal carcinoma.
- Vascular: vertebrobasilar dolichoectasia (elongation and dilatation of the vertebrobasilar artery).
- Meningeal infection from syphilis or TB.

Jugular foramen syndrome
Lesion of cranial nerves IX, X and XI.

Clinical features
- Absent gag reflex (do not test in the examination).
- Ipsilateral impaired taste over the posterior 2/3 of the tongue.
- Ipsilateral decreased palatal movements.
- Uvula drawn to the opposite side.
- Ipsilateral wasted/weak sternocleidomastoid muscle.
- Headache, hydrocephalus, raised intracranial pressure.
- Look for scar over petrous bone, suggesting patient has had resective surgery.

Causes
- Neurofibroma or schwannoma of IXth, Xth or XIth cranial nerves.
- Meningioma.
- Glomus or carotid body tumours (may complain of pulsatile tinnitus).
- Cholesteatoma.
- Carcinoma (primary or metastatic).
- Granulomatous disease.
- Lymphoma.

Differential diagnosis
A brainstem lesion involving the lower cranial nerve nuclei may produce a similar clinical picture, but would be associated with contralateral spinothalamic sensory involvement.

Approach to peripheral nerve problems

Patients with neuropathies are commonly encountered in the PACES examination. A peripheral nerve disorder may occur by itself or with other conditions, leading to dual or even triple pathology. The consideration of the combination of any motor deficit in relation to the sensory involvement will provide valuable information to localize the underlying lesion.

Terminology

'Neuropathy' is a general term meaning disorder of the peripheral nerves. Diseases of the peripheral nerve can be genetic or acquired (either primary or secondary), symmetrical or asymmetrical, and predominantly sensory, motor or, more commonly, mixed sensorimotor. Peripheral neuropathies may be divided into axonal forms, in which degeneration of the nerve body develops distal to nerve damage, and demyelination, when the myelin sheath is denuded and conduction velocity is slowed.

- Polyneuropathy usually refers to diffuse involvement of the peripheral nerves, and is usually first noted distally in the feet and later in the lower legs and hands.
- Mononeuropathy refers to involvement of a single nerve e.g. ulnar, median, radial, common peroneal nerve palsy.
- Mononeuritis multiplex signifies focal involvement of 2 or more nerves.
- Radiculopathy describes involvement of a single spinal nerve root.
- Neuronopathy refers to primary involvement of the nerve cell body, rather than its axon.
- Plexopathy or plexitis refers to involvement of brachial or lumbosacral plexus.
- Neuropraxia refers to the mild mechanical disruption of a nerve which causes temporary impairment of nerve conduction, usually resolving within hours to weeks.

Radiculopathies

- Involvement of nerve root causing symptoms and signs in the corresponding dermatome and myotome.
- Often associated with burning, tingling or lancinating pain that radiates or shoots down a limb and is exacerbated by coughing, straining or sneezing.
- Weakness and sensory loss may be incomplete because of overlap of innervation.
- Loss of reflexes and motor strength in a myotomal distribution.
- Chronic radiculopathy can result in atrophy and fasciculations.
- A T1 radiculopathy can interrupt the sympathetic pathway to the cervical sympathetic ganglia, resulting in Horner's syndrome.
- Involvement of multiple nerve roots below L1 can result in cauda equina syndrome.

❶ Top Tips

- Testing sensation with pin prick is more sensitive than light touch for detailing radicular sensory impairment.
- Remember, relatively mild or recent-onset radiculopathy can cause sensory changes without motor deficits.

Common causes of radiculopathy
- Disc herniation: most frequently at L5 and S1 ('sciatica'), but also C6 and C7.
- Cervical/lumbar spondylosis with osteophyte formation.
- Spinal stenosis.
- Compression: nerve sheath tumours (schwannomas and neurofibromas), epidural abscess, epidural metastases.
- Inflammation: acute inflammatory demyelinating polyradiculoneuropathy (Guillain–Barré syndrome).
- Infection: herpes zoster, *Borrelia*, CMV (particularly in AIDS).

❶ Top Tips
- Upper limbs:
  - The 3 most clinically useful nerve roots to differentiate lesions in the upper limb are C5, C6 and C7. Memorize the reflexes, motor, and sensory function of these roots.*
  - About 20% of all cervical radiculopathies involve 2 or more cervical levels.
- Lower limbs:
  - The 3 most clinically useful nerve roots to differentiate lesions in the lower limb are L4, L5 and S1. Once again, memorize the reflexes, motor and sensory function of these roots.*

(*Summarized in Tables 6.1 and 6.2, Fig. 6.1)

Plexopathies
Plexopathies can result from traumatic injury, infiltrative or compressive tumors, infections, haematomas, autoimmune reactions, or following radiotherapy.

Brachial plexopathy
The brachial plexus is formed by the nerve roots arising from cervical enlargement at C5, C6, C7, C8 and T1. These nerve roots provide the major sensory and motor innervation for the upper extremities. Fig. 6.9 provides an overview of the brachial plexus with its roots (C5–T1), trunks (upper, middle and lower), divisions (anterior and posterior) and cords (medial, lateral and posterior).

Clinical features
- Muscle weakness and atrophy.
- Tendon reflexes may be reduced in weak muscles.
- Sensory loss which commonly involves the axillary nerve distribution, but may be diffuse or reflect the distribution of other involved nerves or cords.

Causes
- Neuralgic amyotrophy (brachial neuritis): inflammatory disorder of the brachial plexus characterized by severe pain at onset, followed by patchy weakness in the distribution of the upper and/or middle brachial plexus, usually involving winging of the scapula.

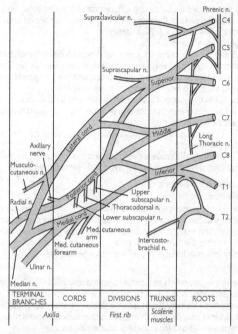

Fig. 6.9 Brachial plexus.
Reproduced from Graeme McLeod, Colin McCartney, and Tony Wildsmith (2012, forthcoming) *Principles and Practice of Regional Anaesthesia* fourth edition, figure 17.1, with permission from Oxford University Press.

- Neoplastic:
  - Breast and lung cancers most frequently cause an infiltrative brachial plexopathy.
  - Commonly leads to pain in the shoulder and axilla.
  - Invasion of the lower plexus (inferior trunk and medial cord) occurs more frequently than the upper trunk.
  - Pancoast syndrome is most commonly due to non-small cell lung cancer. Horner's syndrome occurs in 3/4 of patients. Weakness usually occurs in a lower plexus distribution, but may also be more widespread and patchy in distribution.
- Paraesthesias and weakness are more prominent symptoms in radiation-induced brachial plexopathy than in neoplastic cases.
- Thoracic outlet syndrome: slowly progressive unilateral atrophic weakness of intrinsic hand muscles and numbness in the distribution of the ulnar nerve, due to chronic traction injury to the lower plexus from rudimentary cervical rib or other structural abnormality.
- Iatrogenic plexopathies following traction or pressure during surgery – usually results in painless weakness in the distribution of the upper brachial plexus, sometimes accompanied by paraesthesiae.

- A C8 motor root lesion can be differentiated from an ulnar nerve lesion by weakness of flexor pollicis longus (median nerve) and extensor pollicis brevis (radial nerve).
- Congenital brachial plexus palsy:
  - C5 and C6 injury (Erb's palsy) – weakness involves the deltoid and infraspinatus muscles (mainly C5) and biceps (mainly C6). The upper arm is adducted and internally rotated, and the forearm is extended, while hand and wrist movement are preserved.
  - C5–C7 injury – arm is internally rotated and held in adduction with the forearm in extension and pronation, and the wrists and fingers flexed (the 'waiter's tip' posture).
  - C5–T1 injury usually presents with arm paralysis and some sparing of finger flexion.
  - C8–T1 injury (Klumpke's palsy) is the most infrequent pattern and manifests as isolated hand paralysis and Horner's syndrome.

Lumbosacral plexopathies
Clinical features
- These usually present with diffuse weakness of the affected lower extremity, although a patchy distribution of weakness may occur.
- Weakness can involve the femoral and sciatic territories depending upon whether the lumbar and/ or sacral plexi are involved.
- Sensory loss may involve any of the nerve territories.

Causes
- Diabetic amyotrophy: high lumbar radiculopathy involving L2, L3 and L4 roots, associated with subacute onset of severe proximal leg and hip pain and weakness. Sensory symptoms are fleeting or nonexistent, although most patients already have an established sensory peripheral neuropathy.
- Compressive lesions (haematoma, abscess or tumour).
- Radiation-induced injury: slowly progressive weakness and sensory loss affecting the entire leg. May occur at the time of radiotherapy or decades after.

Mononeuropathies (may also appear in Station 5)
These are easy to recognize once seen! Ulnar, median, radial and common peroneal nerve palsies are the most likely to be encountered in the examination. Most are caused by traumatic entrapment, but there are other causes such as diabetes, nerve tumours and vasculitis.

Upper limb mononeuropathies
Median nerve palsy
The median nerve supplies:
- The 'LOAF' muscles, i.e. only four muscles of the hand, including the thenar eminence – all T1:
  - Lateral 2 lumbricals (supplying the index finger and middle finger).
  - Opponens pollicus – opposition of the thumb to the finger tips ('make an 'O' sign').
  - Abductor pollicis brevis (APB) – abduction of the thumb at right angles to the palm. APB is the only intrinsic muscle in the hand that is invariably supplied by the median nerve. The opponens pollicis is supplied by the median nerve in about 90% of the population.
  - Flexor pollicis brevis – flexion of the thumb.

- The pronators of the forearm (C6).
- The lateral wrist flexors – flexor carpi radialis (C7).
- The long finger flexors via the anterior interosseous branch of the median nerve, including flexors digitorum profundus and superficialis to index and middle fingers and flexor pollicis longus (C8).
- Sensation to the lateral 2/3 of the palm, and the palmar aspect and distal dorsal aspect of the lateral three and a half fingers.

Sites of damage:
- Carpal tunnel syndrome due to median nerve entrapment at the wrist.
- More proximal upper limb compression is rare:
  - In the upper arm, trauma may result in an isolated median nerve lesion.
  - Numerous injuries can occur at the elbow.
- Median nerve compression in the axilla usually occurs in combination with radial and ulnar nerve involvement. Causes include trauma or surgical injury, or unusual compressive forces (e.g. crutches or heavy sleep through intoxication).

Carpal tunnel syndrome (CTS)
- Caused by median nerve compression between the flexor retinaculum of the wrist and the bones of the carpus and is the most common of the median compression palsies (prevalence estimated at >6% of the population).
- More common in females (F:M, up to 8:1).
- Commonly bilateral with dominant hand typically affected first.
- There are many recognized causes of CTS.

Symptoms:
- Numbness, paraesthesiae and pain in the hand, with occasional extension to the forearm. Symptoms most frequently nocturnal.
- Intermittent symptoms relieved by shaking the hand or wrist (this action is a relatively reliable sign of compression at the wrist).
- Left untreated, sensory symptoms and muscle weakness and wasting of the thenar eminence may become permanent.

Signs:
- Typically wasting of the outer aspect of the thenar eminence and APB.
- Weakness APB, opponens pollicis, the 1st and 2nd lumbricals and sometimes flexor pollicis brevis.
- Sensory disturbance on the palmar skin of the thumb, 2nd, 3rd and 1/2 of the 4th digit.
- Many anatomical variations exist.
- Sensory loss typically over the palmar aspect of thumb, index, middle and radial side of ring finger, as well as the tips of corresponding fingers on dorsum of hand. A lesion of the median nerve in the forearm affects the lateral 2/3 of the whole palm, not just of the fingers.
- The sensory symptoms may be more extensive in CTS.
- Provocative tests include:
  - Tinel's test – percussion over the flexor retinaculum causes tingling along the course of the median nerve in the hand and can also induce tingling in the forearm.
  - Phalen's test: ask the patient to keep both hands with wrists in complete palmar flexion for 1 minute; in CTS this may reproduce the symptoms of numbness or tingling in the distribution of the median nerve.

🖣 Common Pitfalls

- Weakness of flexor pollicis longus results in inability to make, or to maintain (against resistance), an 'O' sign. This does not indicate a carpal tunnel syndrome, but a more proximal median nerve lesion, as this muscle is supplied by the anterior interosseous branch of the median nerve, which enters the hand superficial to the carpal tunnel.

Causes:
- Idiopathic
- Work-related repetitive strain
- Pregnancy
- Hypothyroidism
- Diabetes
- Acromegaly
- Rheumatoid arthritis
- Bony osteophytes, degenerative wrist disease, wrist fractures
- Gouty tophi
- Chronic renal failure, uraemia and dialysis
- Congenitally narrow tunnel
- Multiple myeloma
- Hereditary neuropathy with liability to pressure palsies
- Inflammatory neuropathies (e.g. CIDP, MMNCB [multifocal motor neuropathy with conduction block])
- Amyloidosis
- Vasculitides.

Ulnar nerve palsy
The ulnar nerve supplies all small muscles of the hand except the 'LOAF' muscles (which are supplied by the median nerve). The most important ones are:
- Hypothenar muscles.
- Medial 2 lumbricals (which flex the metacarpophalangeal [MCP] joints of the fingers when the proximal interphalangeal [PIP] and interphalangeal [IP] joints of the fingers are held in extension).
- Interossei (palmar adduct and dorsal abduct the fingers – PAD, DAB).
- Adductor pollicis (T1).
- The medial wrist flexors (C8).

Signs:
- Wasting of the dorsal interossei ('dorsal guttering').
- Wasting of hypothenar eminence.

Clawing of the 4th and 5th fingers (i.e. hyperextension at the MCP joints and flexion of the IP joints of these fingers).
- Generalized weakness of the hand, sparing the thenar eminence.
- Sensory impairment most appreciated to pin prick over the palmar and dorsal aspects of the little finger and ulnar aspect of the ring finger ('splitting of the ring finger') and corresponding area of the hand.
- Sensory loss does not extend proximal to the wrist.
  - The ulnar nerve can be damaged anywhere along its course from the brachial plexus to the hand. Most common site of damage is

at the elbow where the nerve is exposed to trauma, pressure and stretching as it passes the medial epicondyle, through the ulnar groove and then deep to the flexor aponeurosis under flexor carpi ulnaris.

Causes:
- Compression at the elbow:
  - Bony
  - Prolonged elbow flexion e.g. prolonged use of elbow crutches
  - Perioperative/ITU compression
  - Soft tissue/neural/bony masses
- Bony deformity at elbow:
  - Fractures (including childhood supracondylar fracture of the humerus 'tardy' ulnar nerve palsy)
  - Rheumatoid arthritis, osteophytes, Paget's disease
- Idiopathic
- Variable anatomy (muscles/fibrous bands)
- Diabetes
- Hereditary neuropathy with liability to pressure palsies
- Inflammatory neuropathies (e.g. CIDP, MMNCB)
- Vasculitides
- Leprosy.

> ## ❶ Top Tips
>
> - Assessing abductor pollicis brevis (APB) and first dorsal interosseous (FDIO) differentiates between median, ulnar and T1 radiculopathy:
>   - APB weak and FDIO normal suggests a median nerve lesion.
>   - APB normal and FDIO weak suggests an ulnar nerve lesion.
>   - Weakness of *both* APB and FDIO suggest a T1 radiculopathy.

Radial nerve palsy
Muscles supplied:
- Wrist extensors – extensor digitorum, extensor indicis and extensor carpi ulnaris (C8).
- Posterior interosseous branch of the radial nerve (branches out in the forearm) supplies the extensors of the fingers, so the weakness invariably accompanies a wrist drop.
- Brachioradialis, supinator (both C6) and the triceps (C7). Examine for weakness of these muscles to find the site of the lesion which is often located in the spiral groove in the posterior part of the middle of the humerus.

Signs:
- Weakness of wrist and elbow extension (elbow flexion is normal).
- Finger drop – the patient is unable to straighten the fingers.
- If the wrist is passively extended, the patient can straighten the fingers at the IP joints (due to the action of interossei and lumbricals supplied by the ulnar nerve). No extension is possible at the MCP joints.
- Apparent weakness of finger abduction and adduction. This can, however, be overcome by placing the hand on a flat surface as this allows the interossei to use their attachments to the long extensor tendon to abduct and adduct the fingers.

Sites of neuropathy:
- At the elbow: fractures, dislocations, ganglions.
- At the humeral shaft (fractures).
- At the axilla (traumatic compression from using crutches, or from sleeping with the arm slumped over the back of a chair ('Saturday night palsy').

❶ Top Tips

- Remember to test elbow extension and the triceps reflex. An intact triceps reflex suggests a lesion below the spiral groove.
- Wasting of the triceps, weakness of elbow extension and absent/diminished triceps reflex is suggestive of a high radial nerve lesion at the axilla or C7 radiculopathy.
- A C7 radiculopathy results in weakness of shoulder adduction (C7), but not abduction (C5), elbow extension (C7), wrist flexion and wrist extension (also C7). Thus a root lesion at C7 can significantly affect both the median and radial nerves.

A radial nerve injury spares shoulder abduction (C5, axillary nerve) and wrist flexion (C7 and C8 (mostly C7), median and ulnar nerves).

Lower limb mononeuropathies

Common peroneal nerve palsy (L4, L5)
Signs:
- A high-steppage gait, indicating footdrop.
- Wasting of the muscles on lateral aspect of the lower leg (peronei and tibialis anterior).
- Weakness of ankle dorsiflexion and eversion of the foot.
- There may be slight sensory impairment over the anterolateral aspect of the lower leg and dorsum of the foot.

Causes:
- Compression (from a plaster cast or tourniquet) at the fibula head – the CPN lies superficially here and is therefore vulnerable to trauma.
- Direct trauma to the nerve.
- Diabetes mellitus.
- As part of a mononeuritis multiplex – diabetes, Wegener's granulomatosis, amyloidosis, rheumatoid arthritis, systemic lupus erthromatosis, polyarteritis nodosa, Churg–Strauss syndrome.
- Leprosy (commonest cause worldwide) – look for palpable thickening of this and other peripheral nerves e.g. the greater auricular nerve.

❶ Top Tips

- The ankle jerk is conveyed through the S1 root via the tibial branch of the sciatic nerve and is therefore spared in a peroneal nerve lesion.
- An absent ankle jerk indicates 1 of 3 possibilities:
  - A lesion of the tibial nerve (far less common than lesions of common peroneal nerve (CPN) or its deep/superficial braches).
  - A complete lesion of the sciatic nerve.
  - An S1 radiculopathy (the most common cause).
- If possible, patient with a suspected sciatic nerve lesion or S1 radiculopathy should be asked about history related to trauma, back pain, sciatica and 'red flag' features.

Polyneuropathies

- The clinical manifestations of neuropathy depend on the type and distribution of affected nerve and the degree of nerve or myelin damage, and the course of the disease.
- When *motor nerves* are damaged, cramps, fasiculations, weakness and muscle atrophy occur.
- Damage to *sensory nerves* can cause loss of sensation, paraesthesia and dysaesthesia, pain and sensory ataxia.
- Autonomic dysfunction can result in postural hypotension, impotence, gastrointestinal (diarrhoea or constipation) and genitourinary dysfunction (urinary retention), abnormal sweating and hair loss.
- Involvement of small myelinated and unmyelinated sensory fibres typically results in impaired pin prick and temperature sensation, numbness and painful burning, cold, stinging or tingling paraesthesia. Large diameter sensory fibre involvement manifests as loss of vibration and position sensation, sensory ataxia, numbness or tingling and paraesthesia.
- Deep tendon reflexes are frequently diminished or absent, particularly in the demyelinating neuropathies.
- Because most nerve trunks have a mixture of fibre types, damage to the peripheral nerves often affects more than one of these functions.

Examination

- Ensure that you are dealing with a polyneuropathy by checking for the typical glove and stocking distribution of sensory impairment:
  - First establish the presence of a peripheral sensory loss by asking the patient whether they perceive a difference in sensation when examined at a proximal and then a distal point of the same limb.
  - When suspecting a peripheral neuropathy, start distally and work proximally. Ask the patient to mention when sensation becomes normal. If sensation is absent at the extremity, establish when sensation first returns and then, when it becomes normal.
- Be suspicious of a mononeuritis multiplex if there is asymmetry or if the hands are affected in the absence of sensory disturbance to above the knees (in a length-dependent neuropathy, the hands usually remain unaffected until the impairment has risen above the knees).
- Exclude the presence of any UMN signs.
- Characterize the polyneuropathy as sensorimotor, predominantly sensory, or predominantly motor, as this will point to a different list of possible causes. The pattern and rate of development often provide important clues to the aetiology with inflammatory, vasculitic and infective neuropathies developing over days or weeks.

✿ Common Pitfalls

- Candidates frequently check the distal sensation only on the medial and lateral aspects of the legs.
- Be careful not to omit sensation on the back of the leg to verify that you are dealing with a true 'stocking' rather than an L4 and L5 radiculopathy.

Causes: peripheral neuropathies (glove and stocking)

Axonal sensori-motor neuropathy

- Diabetes mellitus (2nd commonest worldwide after leprosy – classically predominantly sensory, but also affects motor fibres)
- Nutritional (B12/folate) deficiency
- Alcohol
- Drugs and toxins:
  - Anti-tuberculosis drugs (isoniazid, ethambutol)
  - Antibiotics (metronidazole, nitrofurantoin)
  - Anti-cancer (chemotherapeutic agents e.g. cisplatin, vincristine)
  - Anti-arrhythmics (amiodarone)
  - Anti-convulsants (phenytoin)
- Endocrine and metabolic:
  - Hypothyroidism
  - Renal failure
  - Hepatic failure
- Infections: herpes zoster, HIV, leprosy, syphilis
- Vasculitis
- Inherited: hereditary motor and sensory neuropathy (Charcot–Marie–Tooth disease).

Predominantly motor neuropathies

- Inflammatory:
  - Acute inflammatory demyelinating polyradiculoneuropathy (Guillain–Barré syndrome)
  - Chronic inflammatory demyelinating polyradiculopathy
  - Multifocal motor neuropathy with conduction block
  - Paraprotein-associated – e.g. monoclonal gammopathy of unknown significance (MGUS)
- Toxins: heavy metals
- Diabetic amyotrophy
- Inherited:
  - Inherited distal motor neuropathy
  - Spinal muscular atrophy.

Sensory neuronopathies

- Characterized by dysasthesiae, disabling, asymmetrical sensory loss and ataxia, absent reflexes but no motor loss:
  - Paraneoplastic
  - Sjögrens syndrome
  - Friedreich's ataxia
  - Drugs e.g. chemotherapy.

Mononeuritis multiplex

- Vasculitis:
  - Primary: Churg–Strauss, Wegener's granulomatosis, PAN, microscopic polyangiitis
  - Secondary: RhA, SLE, vasculitis secondary to hepatitis B or C, cryoglobinaemias
  - Other autoimmune disorders
- Sjögren's syndrome

- Sarcoidosis
- Hepatitis C

Causes of thickened nerves
- Hypertrophic Charcot–Marie–Tooth diseases
- CIDP
- Neurofibromatosis
- Refsum's disease
- Leprosy
- Infiltration (lymphoma/secondary deposits)
- Amyloidosis
- Acromegaly.

Viva questions

How would you investigate the causes of a sensorimotor peripheral neuropathy?

Stage 1 investigations
- The commonest causes of neuropathy can be identified from the history, examination, and simple stage 1 investigations:
  - Urine: glucose, protein.
  - Haematology: FBC, ESR, vitamin B12 and folate levels.
  - Biochemistry: fasting blood glucose level, renal function, liver function, TFTs.
- If the patient has a clear cause for their neuropathy and a typical clinical picture, treatment for instance, of diabetes mellitus or alcohol misuse can be started without further investigation.
- If the cause of the neuropathy is not clear from the stage 1 investigations or is atypical, the patient should be referred to a neurologist.

Stage 2 investigations
- The most important stage 2 investigation is neurophysiological investigation. About 80% of symmetrical peripheral neuropathies are axonal.
- Electrophysiological investigation (electromyography [EMG] and nerve conduction study [NCS]): assessment of distal and proximal nerve stimulation.
- Biochemistry: serum protein electrophoresis, serum angiotensin converting enzyme.
- Immunology: antinuclear factor, antiextractable nuclear antigen antibodies (anti-Ro, anti-La), ANCAs.
- Other: CXR.

Stage 3 investigations
This will depend on whether neurophysiological testing has shown the neuropathy to be demyelinating or axonal.
- Urine: Bence Jones protein.
- Biochemistry: oral glucose tolerance test.
- Cerebrospinal fluid: cells, protein, immunoglobulin oligoclonal bands.
- Immunology: anti-HIV antibodies, antineuronal antibodies (Hu, Yo), antigliadin antibodies, serum angiotensin converting enzyme,

antiganglioside antibodies, antimyelin associated glycoprotein antibodies.

- Tests for Sjögren's syndrome: Schirmer's test, Rose Bengal test, salivary flow rate, labial gland biopsy.
- Search for carcinoma, lymphoma, or solitary myeloma: skeletal survey, pelvic ultrasonography, abdominal and chest CT, mammography or PET.
- Molecular genetic tests: peripheral nerve myelin protein 22 gene duplication (the commonest cause of Charcot–Marie–Tooth disease type 1) or deletion (hereditary neuropathy with liability to pressure palsies), connexin 32 mutation (X-linked Charcot–Marie–Tooth disease), PO gene mutation (another cause of Charcot–Marie–Tooth disease type 1).

What is the differential diagnosis of a predominantly motor neuropathy?
These would include:

- Neuromuscular junction disorders:
  - Myasthenia gravis (look for complex ophthalmoplegia, ptosis, fatiguability).
  - Lambert–Eaton myasthenic syndrome (associated with SCLC – chachexia, post titanic potentiation).
- Distal myopathies:
  - Myotonic dystrophy (frontal balding, facial muscle wasting, cataracts, learning disability, cardiac pacemaker, percussion myotonia).
  - Inclusion body myositis (wasting and weakness of finger and wrist flexors (scalloping), knee extensors and ankle dorsiflexors. Weakness of the wrist and finger flexors is often disproportionate to that of their extensor counterparts. Hence, loss of finger dexterity and grip strength may be a presenting or prominent symptom.

📖 **Further reading**

Clarke H et al. (eds) *Neurology: A Queen Square Textbook*. Chapter 5: Movement disorders. Chichester: Wiley-Blackwell, 2009.
Hughes RAC. Peripheral neuropathy. *BMJ* 2002; **24**:466–9.

Myasthenia gravis and other neuromuscular junction disorders

Disorders of the neuromuscular junction (NMJ) arise from functional or structural abnormalities interfering with the transmission of neural impulses from motor nerves to muscles. Myasthenia gravis (MG) is by far the commonest of the NMJ disorders.

Myasthenia gravis

MG is an autoimmune disorder caused by antibodies directed against the acetylcholine receptor (AChR) in the muscle membrane.

- Bimodal pattern of onset: most commonly women in 2nd and 3rd decade, with second peak in 6th and 7th decade, the latter more frequently affecting men.
- Associated with IgG AChR antibodies (Ab) in 75%, and anti-muscle-specific kinase (MuSK) antibodies in >50% of patients with anti-AChR seronegative ocular/generalized MG. MuSK antibodies predominantly seen with facial, bulbar and respiratory weakness in young women (positive in ~5% of patients with generalized myasthenia).
- May affect ocular, bulbar, respiratory or limb muscles; 15% have pure ocular MG.
- Often coexists with other autoimmune diseases such as pernicious anaemia, SLE, vitiligo, RA and thyroiditis.
- 15% of patients with MG have a thymoma.

Clinical features

- Inspect the patient for Cushingoid appearance related to steroid treatment, a thymectomy scar, or a vital capacity meter (if you suspect MG, always offer to check the FVC).
- Ptosis (usually bilateral and asymmetrical, but may affect only one eye) and diplopia, which are fatiguable – often worse towards the end of the day, or visibly worsen when the eyes are held in a particular position of gaze. Extraocular muscle weakness that cannot be explained by a single cranial nerve palsy ('complex ophthalmoplegia') is most frequently due to MG.
- Pupillary reflexes are normal, in contrast to botulism and Guillain–Barré syndrome.
- Weakness of the jaw, face, speech, or swallowing musculature. Speech may be bulbar in quality (⊃ p. 317).
- Respiratory muscle weakness, as demonstrated by limited chest wall movement or excessive use of accessory muscles of respiration.
- Proximal limb weakness (the patient may have their arm propped up on an armrest or a bedside table).
- Fatiguability is a hallmark – repetitive or sustained activity exacerbates weakness.
- Reflexes will be initially normal but may diminish with repeated percussion.

❶ Top Tips

- The patient may complain of diplopia before any ophthalmoparesis is evident on examination. If this is the case, ask in which directions the diplopia is worse, and if the images get further apart on prolonged gaze, as this suggests fatiguability.
- On examination of eye movements, hold upgaze for several seconds to see if a ptosis develops or worsens.

Diagnostic testing

- Tensilon (edrophonium) test involves the injection of a short-acting acetylcholinesterase inhibitor to see if symptoms or signs improve. However, the high incidence of false positives and false negatives, and possibility of precipitating heart block, has resulted in this test falling out of favour, and it is now rarely performed.
- Serological testing for AChR Ab (75% in generalized and 50% in ocular), striated muscle Ab (seen in 90% with associated thymoma) and MuSK Ab.
- Electrophysiological studies – repetitive stimulation, and single-fibre EMG (most sensitive).

Medical management

- Supportive care:
  - Assess respiratory function. Can the patient speak complete sentences? Is there evidence of diaphragmatic weakness (look for paradoxical breathing)? Check the FVC as saturations drop late in respiratory failure – if FVC <1.5L, patient should be in HDU; if <1.2L, in ITU.
  - Speech therapy assessment to ensure that swallowing is safe – if not, make nil by mouth and arrange nasogastric feeding.
- Avoid drugs likely to exacerbate MG – aminoglycosides, quinine, beta-blockers, phenytoin, D-penicillamine, neuromuscular blockade anaesthetic agents. Iatrogenic worsening of MG is a common cause of inpatient referrals to neurology.
- Anticholinesterases e.g. pyridostigmine, are useful in the early symptomatic stages or as an adjunct to immunotherapy. However, at high doses, they may precipitate myasthenic crisis – a worsening of secretions and weakness which may lead to respiratory failure.
- Corticosteroids may establish remission, but can cause a paradoxical worsening of MG in the first 2 weeks of therapy, so should be initiated in hospital. Patients on long-term steroids should all be placed on bone-protecting agents to avoid osteopenia.
- Immunomodulatory therapies act as steroid sparing agents and include azathioprine, methotrexate, mycophenolate and ciclosporin. MuSK Ab-positive MG may respond less well to immunosuppressive therapy.
- IV Ig or plasma exchange can be helpful in the acute setting (do not cause a paradoxical worsening), but occasionally IV Ig may also have a role in long-term maintenance therapy.

Differential diagnosis for myasthenia gravis

Ophthalmoplegia

- Isolated cranial nerve palsies
- Thyroid eye disease

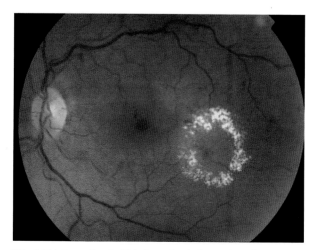

Plate 1 Diabetic maculopathy. Diabetic maculopathy frequently manifests as rings of exudate around areas of oedema (circinate exudates).
With permission from Moorfields Eye Hospital. See also Figure 8.12, page 551.

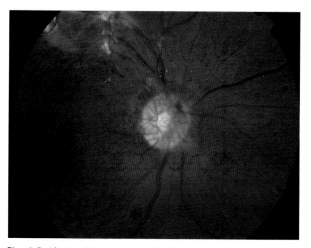

Plate 2 Proliferative diabetic retinopathy. This fundus photograph shows florid new vessels on the optic disc (NVD). Frequently neovascularization is more subtle and may also be seen arising from vessels elsewhere (NVE), typically from one of the four major veins that run from the disc to each quadrant of the retina.
With permission from Moorfields Eye Hospital. See also Figure 8.13, page 552.

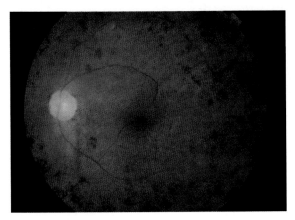

Plate 3 Retinitis pigmentosa. This fundus photograph shows retinal pigmentation, attenuation of retinal vessels and pallor of the optic disc.
With permission from Moorfields Eye Hospital. See also Figure 8.14, page 558.

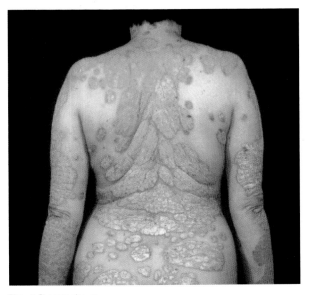

Plate 4 Psoriatic plaques.
With permission from St John's Institute of Dermatology. See also Figure 8.15, page 614.

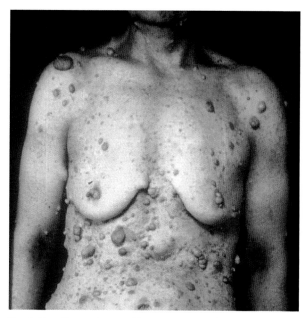

Plate 5 Neurofibromatosis – neurofibromas.
With permission from St John's Institute of Dermatology. See also Figure 8.16, page 618.

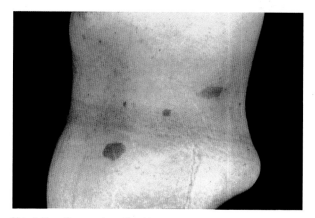

Plate 6 Neurofibromatosis – café-au-lait spots.
With permission from St John's Institute of Dermatology. See also Figure 8.17, page 618.

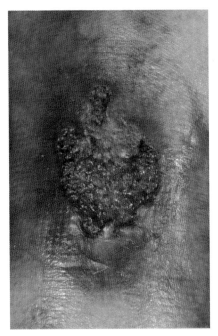

Plate 7 Pyoderma gangrenosum.
With permission from St John's Institute of Dermatology. See also Figure 8.18, page 624.

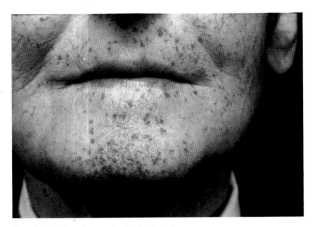

Plate 8 Hereditary haemorrhagic telangiectasia.
With permission from St John's Institute of Dermatology. See also Figure 8.19, page 629.

- Guillain–Barré syndrome
- Mitochondrial disease
- Oculopharyngeal muscular dystrophy
- Central causes such as aneurysm, MS
- Botulism.

Bulbar and respiratory weakness
- MND
- Acid maltase deficiency
- Botulism.

Proximal limb weakness
- Myopathies
- Inflammatory myositis
- Congenital myasthenia – a group of inherited disorders of the NMJ
- Lambert–Eaton myasthenic syndrome.

Lambert–Eaton myasthenic syndrome

Lambert–Eaton myasthenic syndrome (LEMS) is a rare autoimmune disorder caused by impaired release of ACh from the pre-synaptic terminal, and is characterized by weakness and fatigue. It is frequently associated with malignancy (50%) or autoimmune disease (50%). It is driven by antibodies to the voltage gated calcium channel (VGCC Ab), present in 90% of patients.

Clinical features
- Can occur at any age but usually >40 years.
- Insidious onset of fatigue and progressive weakness.
- Weakness affects the proximal limb muscles, usually legs, often associated with stiffness or aching. There may be some fatiguability.
- Autonomic features – dry mouth, constipation, impotence.
- Ophthalmoplegia, bulbar and respiratory involvement are much rarer than in MG.
- Reflexes are reduced or absent, but become brisker with sustained effort ('post-tetanic potentiation'). If LEMS is suspected, test reflexes before power, as power testing can make the reflexes brisker.

Investigations
- Serological testing for VGCC Ab.
- Electrophysiological studies.
- A search for underlying malignancy or autoimmune disorder.

Treatment
- If found, treatment of an underlying malignancy will often lead to improvement.
- Pyridostigmine may have a mild effect.
- 3,4-diaminopyridine increases pre-synaptic ACh release.
- Immunomodulatory therapy with steroids, azathioprine and ciclosporin may be useful, but plasma exchange and IV immunoglobulin are generally less helpful than in MG.

Viva questions

What are the neurophysiological findings in MG and LEMS?

Nerve conduction studies in these 2 neuromuscular conditions demonstrate normal nerve conduction velocities, since there is no demyelination or axonal damage to the nerves themselves.

One of the hallmarks of MG on neurophysiology is a decrement in response on repetitive stimulation:

- With normal NMJ function, there is a natural decrement in the total amount of ACh released with each nerve depolarization, but even after long-term high frequency stimulation, the amount of ACh released is far more than is required for adequate NMJ signal transmission.
- In MG, a reduction in effective post-synaptic receptor density results in failure of NMJ transmission at lower levels of ACh release, resulting in a sequential reduction in amplitude of the muscle response.
- In contrast, in LEMS, where the problem is related to pre-synaptic transmitter release, repetitive stimulation at a fast rate can facilitate neurotransmitter release, resulting in an increment in response.

Single-fibre EMG is a technique primarily limited to academic centres, and is a time-consuming test. It measures the difference in firing times between 2 fibres that are part of the same motor unit. Increased variability of the interval, or 'jitter', suggests that neuromuscular transmission is abnormal. 'Jitter' on SFEMG is the investigation of choice for MG, with >95% sensitivity, but is not specific for MG, and may also be seen in MND, myositis and LEMS.

What is the role of thymectomy in MG?

CT or MR imaging of the mediastinum should be performed in all patients with MG, since 15% of patients have a thymoma (50% of patients with thymoma will develop MG). Most are benign, but in 10% the thymoma shows malignant features, so all patients with thymoma should undergo a resection. Those patients with thymomas with malignant features should receive post-resection radiotherapy.

For those patients without thymoma, the role of thymectomy is still under debate, although there is some evidence that thymectomy increases the probability of remission or improvement. At present, thymectomy is recommended for seropositive patients with generalized disease under the age of 60, particularly if there is thymic hyperplasia. Its role in ocular myasthenia is less certain.

MuSK Ab-positve MG does not respond to thymectomy.

What underlying malignancies is LEMS associated with?

LEMS is most commonly associated with small-cell lung cancer, but has been described to be associated with lymphoproliferative disorders, thymoma, and more rarely carcinomas of the stomach, breast, colon, prostate, kidney and bladder.

All patients with LEMS without a clear autoimmune cause should have an FDG-PET scan if routine imaging does not demonstrate a tumour. If no malignancy is found, patients should be closely followed, as LEMS may precede a demonstrable malignancy by many years.

🖰 **Useful websites**
Myasthenia Gravis Association: http://www.mgauk.org.
Neuromuscular Disease Centre, Washington University, St Louis: http://www.neuromuscular. wustl.edu.

Muscle disorders

The muscle disorders comprise a mixed group of disorders, some limited to muscle pathology, others being associated with more systemic disease, with cardiac, endocrine and other system involvement.

Major categories of muscle disorders are:
- Inflammatory: relating to an auto-immune process, which may be systemic or limited to muscle.
- Dystrophies: due to genetic defect in the components of the muscle fibre.
- Metabolic: due to hereditary disorders of metabolism.
- Inflammatory: relating to an autoimmune process, which may be systemic or limited to muscle.
- Secondary causes:
  - Endocrine abnormalities e.g. hypo/hyperthyroidism
  - Systemic disease e.g. critical illness myopathy
  - Drugs e.g. statins, steroids.

Muscle disorders

Signs
- Muscle wasting – classify as predominantly proximal or distal, or identify any particular muscle groups that are spared.
- Weakness in the absence of sensory signs.
- No UMN signs.
- Reflexes are normal, unless the degree of muscle wasting is very severe.
- No fatiguability (cf. MG).
- Muscle biopsy scar over the deltoid or quadriceps.

Additional helpful features
The majority of diagnostic information comes from the history, such as age of onset, exercise tolerance, myoglobinuria after exercise, and family history, but there are some signs that are extremely helpful in determining the underlying diagnosis.
- Estimate the age of the patient. In the young, a genetic cause is more likely.
- Examine for signs of an endocrine disturbance or another systemic disorder, e.g. loss of the outer 1/3 of the eyebrow and sallow dry skin of hypothyroidism, spade-like hands and macroglossia of acromegaly, Gottron's papules and heliotrope rash of dermatomyositis, Cushingoid appearance of steroids (may be a cause of the myopathy, or may be as a result of treatment of an inflammatory myopathy).
- Look for evidence of contractures or deformity, which suggest a chronic process.
- Facial or ocular involvement point toward myotonic dystrophy, facioscapulohumeral dystrophy or another genetic myopathy.

- Search for additional features of the hereditary dystrophies such as percussion myotonia or typical facies of myotonic dystrophy, retinitis pigmentosa, hearing aid and ophthalmoplegia of a mitochondrial disorder, scapular winging and sparing of deltoid in facioscapulohumeral dystrophy. There may be apparent hypertophy of the trapezii on shoulder abduction because the scapulae are pulled up.
- Examine the calves for evidence of pseudohypertrophy, features of Duchenne's or Becker's dystrophy.
- Look for a pacemaker, suggesting cardiac involvement, seen mainly in the genetic dystrophies or myopathies, but also occasionally seen in dermatomyositis.

> **❶ Top Tips**
>
> - If there is a urine sample present, look for reddish discoloration or a positive dipstick for blood, as this is likely to represent myoglobinuria. In the context of the PACES examination, this will point towards a metabolic myopathy such as McArdle's disease.

Helpful patterns of involvement
- Distal >proximal:
  - Inclusion body myositis – flexors of forearm and quadriceps.
  - Facioscapulohumeral dystrophy – involvement of anterior tibial compartment may cause foot drop.
  - Myotonic dystrophy.
- Face with external ocular muscle involvement:
  - Myopathy due to Grave's disease.
  - Mitochondrial disorders – look for ptosis, deafness, retinitis pigmentosa.
  - Oculomusculopharyngeal dystrophy.
  - Consider MG.
- Face without external ocular muscle involvement:
  - Myotonic dystrophy – with ptosis and typical 'hatchet' facies.
  - Facioscapulohumeral dystrophy – winging, wasting of upper arm, foot drop.
- Calf pseudohypertrophy:
  - Duchenne's muscular dystrophy.
  - Becker's muscular dystrophy.

Muscular dystrophies

This is a group of disorders characterized by the degeneration of muscle, hereditary in nature, usually occurring after a period of normal muscle development and function:
- There is often a family history (remember that non-penetrance, non-paternity and genetic anticipation means that this is not always the case with autosomal dominant conditions).
- Weakness often precedes wasting as degenerating muscle is frequently replaced by fat, resulting in pseudohypertrophy.
- The pattern of wasting and weakness usually reflects the underlying type of dystrophy.

Myotonic dystrophy

Myotonic dystrophy is the most common adult muscular dystrophy with onset usually in early adult life.

Clinical features

- Myotonia: failure of relaxation of voluntary contraction may become evident on shaking the patient's hand or prolonged contraction after percussion can be elicited with a tendon hammer by gently percussing the thenar eminence.
- Frontal balding.
- Early partial ptosis and wasting of the masseters, with narrowing of lower half of face ('hatchet face').
- Wasting of sternocleidomastoid.
- Weakness tends to be distal >proximal with initial weakness and wasting of the intrinsic hand muscles and extensors of forearm.
- Wasting of the pretibial muscles, with foot drop.
- The voice may be weak, monotonous and nasal due to pharyngeal and laryngeal weakness.
- Dysphagia – often progressive and patient may have a percutaneous endoscopic gastrostomy (PEG) *in situ*.
- Frequent low IQ.
- Cataracts.
- Diabetes mellitus and testicular atrophy.
- Cardiac involvement, with bradycardia, AV block, or heart failure – this is a frequent cause of death.
- Hypersomnolence (cause unknown).
- Diaphragmatic weakness and respiratory failure.
- Usually wheelchair-dependent within 15–20 years of onset.

Myotonic dystrophy is an autosomal dominant condition, caused by expansion of an unstable trinucleotide repeat on chromosome 19q, and is therefore prone to genetic anticipation. A second gene on chromosome 3q has been identified, causing a milder phenotype, proximal myotonic myopathy (PROMM). Facial involvement, cognitive impairment and cardiac pathology are rare in this variant, and the myopathy tends to be more proximal. As with classical myotonic dystrophy, age of onset depends on repeat length of the causative mutation.

Duchenne's/Becker's muscular dystrophy

These disorders are caused by mutations in the dystrophin gene, on the X chromosome. In Duchenne's the mutation results in an absence of dystrophin, whilst in Becker's, dystrophin is present but structurally abnormal. Since the diseases are X-linked, patients are almost always male (occasional females, nearly always have Turner's syndrome, i.e. only one X chromosome, but note that carriers can be symptomatic).

Due to the natural history of Duchenne's, patients with this condition are unlikely to present in PACES, and Becker's is much more likely to be encountered.

Duchenne's muscular dystrophy

- Onset between ages 3–10.
- Most die by age 25, but a few survive much longer.
- Usually wheelchair-dependent by early in the 2nd decade.

- Onset in proximal muscles of legs and lower trunk, with later involvement of shoulder girdle and distal musculature.
- Other features: low IQ, macroglossia, calf pseudohypertrophy, cardiomyopathy, respiratory failure, osteoporosis due to immobility, scoliosis.
- Creatine kinase (CK) very high initially, falling with severe muscle atrophy.

Becker's muscular dystrophy
- Later onset – 5–45 years of age.
- Weakness and hypertrophy in same distribution as Duchenne's.
- Much milder, with many walking in adulthood.
- IQ usually normal, cardiac involvement less frequent, but rarely patients may present with cardiac abnormalities.

Diagnosis is based upon a raised CK, EMG consistent with myopathy, muscle biopsy and dystrophin gene testing.

Facioscapulohumeral dystrophy
- Usually autosomal dominant.
- Onset 6–20 years of age.
- Slowly progressive disease, affecting facial musculature and shoulder girdle.
- Facial weakness, with difficulty closing eyes tightly, pursing lips and whistling.
- Difficulty raising arms above head, winging of scapulae – the scapulae are pushed off the back due to weakness of serratus anterior. They may also rise up on shoulder abduction, giving the appearance of hypertrophy of the trapezeii.
- Triceps is usually more wasted than the biceps, with relative preservation of deltoid.
- Pectoralis major weakness leading to reversal of the anterior axillary fold.
- Later in the disease, the pelvic girdle and pretibial muscles may also become affected, causing a waddling gait and foot drop.
- Cardiac and respiratory involvement is rare. IQ is normal.
- Non-muscular features uncommonly associated with FSHD include scoliosis, sensorineural hearing loss and retinal telangectasias.

Other dystrophies
- Limb-girdle muscular dystrophies – a group of genetic conditions, usually autosomal recessive, affecting shoulder and pelvic girdles, with variable age of onset.
- Emery–Dreifuss muscular dystrophy – an X-linked disorder, usually affecting the upper limbs first, with early contractures of the flexors of the elbow and neck extensors.
- Oculopharyngeal dystrophy – autosomal dominant, late onset, causing bilateral ptosis and dysphagia. MG (→ p.379) is an important differential for this condition

Metabolic muscle disorders
Myopathies can result from disorders of energy metabolism and can be grouped into 3 main classes:

Disorders of the mitochondrial respiratory chain

- May be maternally inherited due to mitochondrial DNA mutations, but may also be autosomal dominant or recessive, as some mitochondrial proteins are produced by nuclear DNA.
- Can cause exercise intolerance, isolated proximal myopathy, or less frequently, distal myopathy.
- Associated features include:
  - Progressive external ophthalmoplegia (leading to complex ophthalmoplegia), retinitis pigmentosa and cardiac conduction defects (Kearns–Sayre).
  - Encephalopathy (MERRF and MELAS).
  - Stroke (MELAS).
  - Optic atrophy.
  - Sensorineural deafness.
  - Diabetes mellitus.

Disorders of glycogen storage

- Almost all are autosomal recessive.
- Characterized by cramping on exercise, with 'second-wind' phenomenon (prolonged exercise results in an improvement due to switching over to metabolism of free fatty acids and blood glucose), myoglobinuria with resulting renal failure, but may present with progressive limb weakness in late life (McArdle's disease).
- Acid maltase deficiency may present in infancy or childhood, but in the adult-onset form, usually presents with slowly progressive truncal or proximal myopathy, with severe diaphragmatic involvement, resulting in respiratory failure.

Disorders of lipid metabolism

- Autosomal recessive inheritance.
- Usually presents with a progressive proximal myopathy, with or without cardiac involvement, but may present with myoglobinuria or rhabdomyolysis, often provoked by sustained exercise or fasting.

Inflammatory myopathies

The inflammatory myopathies are a group of acquired disorders whose primary pathology is of inflammation within the muscle. They may be idiopathic (e.g. isolated dermatomyositis, polymyositis or inclusion body myositis), associated with systemic inflammatory diseases, or infective/post-infective.

Idiopathic

- Patients with dermatomyositis and polymyositis may have overlap with other connective tissue diseases e.g. SLE and systemic sclerosis:
  - The patient may have a butterfly rash or sclerodactyly suggesting SLE or systemic sclerosis respectively.
  - Periungual erythema.
- Dermatomyositis:
  - More common in women and non-Caucasians, may affect any age.
  - Humorally-mediated autoimmune disorder.
  - Subacute, progressive, proximal, affecting legs more than the arms, associated with myalgia.

- Severe cases may affect the oesophagus, heart, respiratory musculature, and may be associated with interstitial lung disease.
- Skin manifestations usually precede the myopathy: 'heliotrope' rash affecting the face and upper trunk, Gottron's papules (thickening over the surface of the knuckles), periorbital oedema.
- 20% associated with underlying malignancy, most commonly adenocarcinoma and gynaecological tumours.
- Polymyositis:
  - Progressive proximal and symmetric weakness, without skin lesions.
  - Typically a disease of middle or later life.
  - Respiratory musculature, heart and lungs may be affected, as with dermatomyositis.
  - Cell-mediated (CD8+ T lymphocytes).
- Inclusion body myositis:
  - Most commonly a disease of Caucasian males, occurring late in life.
  - Insidious onset, with classic pattern of weakness involving the quadriceps and deep finger flexors. Patients may demonstrate the 'tear drop' sign when asked to make a pincer grip with their thumb and index finger. As the thumb and index remain in a relative extended position due to weakness of the finger flexors a tear shape is formed between the thumb and index finger instead of an 'O'.
  - Occasional dysphagia and foot drop.
  - Pulmonary and cardiac complications are rare.
  - Uncertain aetiology, but not thought to be associated with malignancy.
  - IBM can look similar to inflammatory motor neuropathies or a predominantly LMN form of MND. It is important to clarify the diagnosis with nerve conduction studies and EMG, and ideally perform a muscle biopsy.

Associated with systemic disorders

Dermatomyositis and myositis can be associated with other immune disorders:

- SLE and systemic sclerosis (mixed connective tissue disease refers to the overlap syndromes of myositis, SLE and systemic sclerosis), Sjögren's, RA.
- Vasculitides.
- Sarcoidosis.
- Eosinophilic syndromes.

Look for additional features of these conditions:

- Butterfly rash of SLE
- Sclerodactyly of systemic sclerosis
- Lupus pernio and lymphadenopathy of sarcoidosis
- Vasculitic skin rash/erythema nodosum.

Infective/post-infective

- Viral: HIV, CMV, EBV, HTLV-1
- Bacterial: staphylococcal, Lyme, TB
- Parasitic: nematodes, cestodes, protozoa.

HTLV-1 and parasitic infections tend to cause a more chronic myopathic picture, whilst CMV and EBV may produce an acute post-infectious myopathy.

Endocrine myopathies

Muscle disorders are associated with a wide range of endocrinopathies:

- Thyroid disease: hypothyroidism can cause myalgia, cramps and a proximal myopathy, and hyperthyroidism may also cause a proximal, or occasionally a distal, myopathy. Hyperthyroidism may also be associated with periodic paralysis. Hypothyroidism may result in a mildly raised CK.
- Adrenal disorders: Cushing's syndrome may cause a proximal myopathy, while Addison's typically causes myalgia, cramps and fatigue.
- Parathyroid under- or overactivity may lead to a mild proximal myopathy, although unlikely to have wasting.
- Acromegaly may cause proximal weakness, sometimes with muscle hypertrophy.

Toxic myopathies

- Lipid-lowering agents: statins, fibrates, nicotinic acid, ezetimibe
- Steroids
- Cardiac drugs, esp. amiodarone
- Rheumatological treatments: colchicines, chloroquine, hydroxychloroquine
- Drugs of abuse: alcohol, heroin, cocaine
- Others: zidovudine, alpha-interferon, d-penicillamine, ipecac.

Viva questions

How would you investigate a possible myopathy?

In the first instance, a family history and drug history should be carefully elicited. Blood tests to confirm a raised CK and to look for potential causes should be performed. These should include an ESR, FBC, U&E, liver profile, bone profile, blood glucose, thyroid function, ANA, ANCA and RF. An EMG should be obtained to determine the presence of myopathic changes. If an inflammatory myopathy is being queried, a muscle biopsy is important for histological diagnosis as the patient may be embarking on chronic immunosuppressive treatment. A CXR and an ECG should be requested. Further investigations may include a high resolution CT of the chest, 24-hour ECG and an echocardiogram. In dermatomyositis and, to a lesser extent, polymyositis, unless an alternative cause has been found, the patient should be screened for underlying malignancy, with CT of the chest, abdomen and pelvis, and if negative, possibly with PET.

What features of the EMG suggest a myopathy?

Myopathies produce damage to the muscle fibre membrane, resulting in influx of sodium that can occasionally cause the muscle fibre to depolarize, resulting in fibrillation potentials and positive sharp waves. These changes are also seen in denervation, but the nature of motor unit potentials differs. In denervation, reinnervation of muscle fibres by remaining neurons results in many more fibres being innervated by a single motor axon, resulting in giant potentials. New nerve connections are not as fast or as consistent as the original connections, resulting in polyphasic potentials. In contrast, in myopathies, each motor unit supplies fewer muscle fibres with normal function, resulting in smaller potentials. Conduction in abnormal muscle fibres is dispersed, and so the motor potentials are also polyphasic, but these are of short duration and are of small amplitude.

What treatments are there for inflammatory myopathies?

The mainstays of treatment are steroids, initially at a dose of 1mg/kg/day, but steroid-sparing agents are almost always required. Options include azathioprine, methotrexate, or for refractory cases, ciclosporin, cyclophosphamide or IV immunoglobulin. Although evidence for the latter is limited, resistant cases can show significant clinical response to this treatment.

Which patients are at increased risk of a statin-induced myopathy?

There is an eightfold increase in myopathy in patients taking statins, increasing to a 42-fold risk if a fibrate is co-administered. The risk is dose-related, but is higher in the elderly, diabetics, hypothyroidism, or concurrent renal or liver disease. Drugs such as ciclosporin, proton pump inhibitors, calcium-channel blockers, selective serotonin reuptake inhibitors (SSRIs), and grapefruit juice all increase the risk.

Current recommendations are that in asymptomatic patients with a raised CK, the CK should be rechecked after 1 month, and the statin should be discontinued if the CK rises or if symptoms develop. For patients with symptoms, stop the statin, and if the CK returns to normal, consider restarting at the lowest possible dose. If symptoms persist or the CK remains elevated following withdrawal of the statin, proceed to muscle biopsy to rule out another cause.[1]

Reference

1. Sathasivam S, Lecky B. Statin-induced myopathy. *BMJ* 2008; **337**:a2286.

Communication skills and ethics

Michael Nandakumar
Rupa Bessant

Introduction

The communication skills and ethics station aims to assess your ability to guide and organize an interview with a patient, relative or surrogate (such as a healthcare worker). The skills specifically tested in this station include:

- Clinical communication skills
- Managing patients' concerns
- Clinical judgement (including knowledge of ethics and law)
- Managing patient welfare.

Station format

Written instructions are provided for the scenario during the 5-minute interval before the station starts. 14 minutes are allowed for the patient interaction, followed by 1 minute for the candidate to reflect their thoughts. A 5-minute discussion with the 2 examiners will then take place after the patient has left the station. Each examiner has a structured mark-sheet for the case (➔ Useful websites, p.395).

Station strategy

Revision

- Approach the station as a 2-way discussion rather than a rigid 'tick-box task'.
- Set aside time each week to practise scenarios with colleagues under timed conditions.
- Familiarize yourself with recent NICE guidance (especially with new or controversial or rationed treatments) and DVLA advice.
- Remember that skills needed in this station are also particularly applicable to those required in station 2 (history taking) and station 5 (brief clinical consultations), and it is therefore essential that you spend adequate time practising these skills to maximize your performance in the examination.

5-minute preparation time

- Identify key issues that need to be addressed during the consultation (e.g. breaking bad news) as well as 'hidden clues' (e.g. a single parent may have concerns regarding childcare if she herself is admitted to hospital).
- Make notes during this time, but avoid the temptation to make notes during the consultation itself, as it distracts from the flow of the discussion.

15-minute consultation

- Start with open-ended questions and establish the patient's understanding, knowledge and concerns at an early stage – these are all specifically mentioned in the clinical marksheet.
- Use '2-way acting' where appropriate – you can improvise within reason to aid the flow and realism of the consultation (e.g. 'Are you feeling better since I saw you on the ward last week?').
- Facilitate the consultation by demonstrating empathy, providing words of reassurance and offering realistic optimism where possible.

1-minute reflection time

- Anticipate questions regarding your management plan and any relevant ethical principles.
- Consider how you might proceed differently if the consultation did not go as well as you had expected.

5-minute discussion with examiners

- Show confidence and aim to lead the discussion with the examiners.
- Demonstrate that you can deal effectively with the clinical problem presented to you with due regard to good clinical and ethical practice.

The key to successful communication

- *A clear greeting is important:* e.g. 'Hello, my name is Dr Chatterjee, I am one of the junior doctors in the chest clinic today'.
- *Remember non-verbal communication:* smiling, eye-contact nodding, open body posture.
- *Agree the purpose of the consultation:* surprisingly this is often missed out by candidates.
- *The 'golden minute':* the patient's agenda will often become evident in the first minute if they are allowed to speak without early interruption from the doctor.
- *Elicit the patient's Ideas, Concerns, and Expectations* (ICE) regarding the problem.
- *Reflect and respond:* to verbal and non-verbal cues (e.g. 'You seem disappointed' or 'I can see that you're angry').
- *Allow regular pauses:* for clarification and questions.
- *Consider the patient's agenda:*
  - Weaker candidates tend to focus only on the doctor's agenda.
  - Ask yourself – who does most of the talking during the consultation? (Weaker candidates tend to dominate the discussion.)
- *Provide written information:* including follow-up and access to support groups and appropriate members of the multidisciplinary team.
- *Negotiate a management plan.*
- *Summarize:* the key features of the consultation and check understanding.

---

❶ Top Tips

- *Familiarize yourself with the clinical marksheet:* ➲ Useful websites, p.395.
- *Appear confident:* the examiners want to see that as a registrar you can communicate well with patients, relatives and colleagues, and can confidently manage and problem-solve challenging situations with ease.
- *Adopt a holistic approach:* e.g. if faced with a patient with a terminal illness, consider spiritual care in addition to the physical symptoms of their condition.
- *Demonstrate knowledge of multidisciplinary team working:* involve agencies such as occupational therapy, meals-on-wheels, Macmillan nurses etc. where appropriate.

(Top Tips continued)

- *Consider the potential psycho-social impact:* on activities of daily living, family life, relationships, employment and any relevant hobbies.
- *Consider how you might 'rescue' a consultation that is going badly:* e.g. 'I can see that you're very angry about what has happened, how do you see that we can move forward from here?' or 'I appreciate that this is a difficult subject for you to talk about, can you tell me what thoughts are going through your mind right now?'.
- *Be prepared for real patients as well as actors in the examination:* e.g. counselling a non-compliant diabetic patient.

✪ Common Pitfalls

- *Revising only for the clinical stations:* candidates often underestimate the amount of preparation required for stations 2 and 4.
- *Taking too long to break bad news:* check understanding, give a warning shot and impart the bad news within the first 2–3 minutes of the consultation.
- *Overloading the patient with too much information:* be clear what can and cannot be covered during the consultation, and use pauses as an opportunity to check understanding and clarify information. You can always offer a further consultation at a later date.
- *Tick-box approach to the consultation:* the best candidates stand-out because their consultation looks like a natural discussion rather than a forced routine for the examination.
- *Spending too long summarizing and checking understanding:* do not spend any more than 1 minute on this at the end of the consultation.
- *Finishing too early:* it is essential to practice with colleagues under timed conditions.

Scenarios

The communication skills and ethics scenarios that follow allow you to practise the most common types of scenario that you would be expected to face in the PACES examination. They are grouped according to the main themes that are represented in the examination:

- Breaking bad news (scenarios 1–3)
- Explaining a new diagnosis (scenarios 4–5)
- Counselling (scenarios 6–9)
- Chronic disease management (scenarios 10–12)
- Speaking to relatives and colleagues (scenarios 13–16).

Each scenario begins with 'Information for the candidate,' which is similar to the written instructions that candidates would expect to receive in the examination. Also included is 'Information for the actor,' and although this is not provided to candidates during the examination, it will be useful when practising scenarios with colleagues. In addition, it serves as an insight in to the background information, prompts and questions that the actors are supplied with in the examination itself. Each scenario includes a suggested approach to tackling the clinical case. All of the main ethical and legal frameworks that you would be expected to be familiar with are discussed where appropriate in each scenario. Finally, there are 2 viva-style example questions at the end of each themed section, specifically to help prepare you for the 5-minute discussion with the examiner at the end of the station.

✍ Useful websites

Driver and Vehicle Licensing Agency (DVLA): http://www.dft.gov.uk/dvla.
MRCP(UK): http://www.mrcpuk.org.
MRCP(UK) PACES Marksheets: http://www.mrcpuk.org/PACES/Pages/PacesMarkSheets.aspx
National Institute for Health and Clinical Excellence (NICE): http://www.nice.org.uk.

Scenario 1

Information for the candidate

Your role

You are the specialty registrar on the acute medical ward.

Problem

Explaining the diagnosis of cerebral metastases in a patient with known thyroid carcinoma.

Patient

Mrs Debbie Jacks, a 38-year-old woman.

Please read the scenario which follows. When the bell sounds, enter the examination room to begin the consultation.

Background to Scenario

Mrs Jacks was admitted to the acute medical unit 3 days ago following a seizure at work.

She was diagnosed with papillary adenocarcinoma of the thyroid 2 years ago, and subsequently underwent thyroidectomy and radioiodine treatment. She has been well for the last 18 months.

A CT head scan performed on admission has been reported as showing appearances highly suggestive of cerebral metastases.

Mrs Jacks is now feeling back to her normal self and is expecting to go home later today.

Your task is to speak to the patient and explain the results of the CT head scan.

Information for the actor

You are a primary school teacher, and married with 2 children.

You were diagnosed with cancer of the thyroid 2 years ago, and at that time had an operation to remove your thyroid gland. This was followed by treatment with radioactive iodine tablets. You have been feeling well for the last 18 months.

You were feeling well yesterday until lunchtime when you suddenly developed a sickness feeling followed by jerking of your arms and legs. You were taken to hospital for further tests. You are now feeling better, and anxious to get home to your children. You have no idea that this may be related to your previous thyroid cancer.

Questions you might ask
- 'Why wasn't this picked-up at my last outpatient review?'
- 'Can this be cured with chemotherapy?'
- 'Am I going to die?'

Breaking bad news

- Preparation: ask whether they would like a relative to be present, and consider the use of '2-way acting':
  - *'I have asked a nurse to sit in with us today if that is okay?'*
- Set the scene:
  - *'I have come to talk to you about the results of your tests.'*
- Check understanding:
  - *'Can you tell me what you understand by what has been happening so far?'*
  - *'Do you know why we did the CT scan and what we were looking for?'*
- Ask about specific concerns (including psychosocial worries e.g. childcare).
- Gauge how much information she wants to know.
- Warning shot:
  - *'The results are not normal . . . I'm afraid I've got some bad news . . .'*
- Give small amounts of information and use pauses and silence.
- Acknowledge her distress and be prepared to deal with anger and denial. Facilitate expression of emotion:
  - *'I can see that was a shock for you . . . What's going through your mind at the moment?'*
- Allow questions and check understanding as you go:
  - *'Does that make sense so far?'*
- Briefly explain details of immediate management plan. It is important to offer realistic hope. Mrs. Jacks may ask directly how long she has left to live. In this situation it is important to give some idea, without committing to a specific time,
  - *'We are probably talking about a few months rather than a few years.'*
- Arrange follow-up, including use of allied health professionals. Suggest bringing a friend or relative to the next visit
  - *'Is there anyone you would like to have with you when we next meet in 2 weeks?'*

- Re-check understanding:
  - *'What do you think you will say to your husband when you get home?'*

❶ Top Tips

- Use non-verbal empathy to build a rapport: voice, tone, facial expression, posture and eye contact are all important.
- Be guided by the patient when pacing the consultation – remember that you cannot possibly cover everything in 14 minutes.
- Be mindful of the balance between the patient's or relative's agenda (what the patient or relative wants to discuss) and the doctor's agenda (what the doctor wants to discuss) throughout the consultation.
- Ask about family and work, and consider how these will be affected by the news.
- Consider the use of touch if this feels appropriate during the consultation.
- Although you may feel unable to answer difficult questions regarding prognosis and survival, try not to evade the questions completely – attempt to provide a response however vague this may seem to you.
- Consider use of diagrams to aid explanation.
- Provide written information at the end of the consultation.
- Remember multidisciplinary professional support (e.g. specialist nurses, palliative care team, hospital chaplain, GP).
- Offer a further meeting to speak to family members.
- Encourage questions.
- Ensure patient is not left alone at the end of the consultation and think about whom they have at home with them for further support.

⟐ Common Pitfalls

- Taking too long to break the bad news, leaving the patient frustrated and second-guessing the diagnosis.
- Use of medical jargon without adequate explanation.
- Focusing only on the doctor's agenda – trying to impart detailed and complex information regarding treatment and prognosis.
- Doing too much of the talking during the consultation.
- Missing important verbal and non-verbal cues (e.g. when patient starts crying or looking down at the floor).
- Rushing the consultation and missing out on valuable pauses and periods of silence.
- Focusing only on the physical aspects of the case, and ignoring psychosocial factors.
- Dodging questions when asked about prognosis and survival times.

♫ Useful websites

Breaking Bad News: http://www.patient.co.uk/showdoc/40002053
Breaking Bad News Regional Guidelines: http://www.dhsspsni.gov.uk
Guidelines for Breaking Bad News: http://www.lnrcancernetwork.nhs.uk/healthcareprofessionals

Scenario 2

Information for the candidate

Your role

You are the specialty registrar in the haematology clinic.

Problem

Explaining the diagnosis of HIV.

Patient

Mr Abdi Mohamed, a 36-year-old man.

Please read the scenario which follows. When the bell sounds, enter the examination room to begin the consultation.

Background to Scenario

Mr Mohamed was referred urgently to the haematology clinic following a 6-week history of painless cervical lymphadenopathy, weight loss and malaise.

He moved to the UK from Turkey 4 years ago, and only registered with a GP last month, as he had been well up until that time.

Your consultant saw him in clinic last week and arranged further investigations including blood and urine tests, a lymph node biopsy and a CXR.

Unfortunately, the HIV test has come back as positive. The results of the remaining tests are all normal.

Mr Mohamed has returned to clinic today to discuss the results of his tests.

Your task is to speak to the patient and explain the diagnosis of HIV.

Information for the actor

You moved to the UK from Turkey 4 years ago. You live with your wife and 3 young children, and work in a sandwich factory. You have been having an affair with a colleague from work for the last 18 months, and your wife is unaware of this.

You are normally healthy, and only registered with a GP for the first time last month. You noticed a painless swelling on the right side of your neck 6 weeks ago, which has persisted despite a course of antibiotics from your GP. You have also lost weight and felt generally very tired since first noticing the neck swelling.

Your main concern is that this may be diabetes, as your father was diagnosed with this in his late 30s. You are also anxious that you are able to continue to work, as you need to be able to support your wife and children. You are completely shocked to learn that this is HIV, as you thought that this only affected gay men.

Questions you might ask
- 'How did I get HIV?'
- 'Can my children catch HIV from me?'
- 'You won't tell my wife about this, will you?'

Explaining the diagnosis of HIV
- Explain the diagnosis, utilizing the principles of breaking bad news as discussed in ➔ Scenario 1, p.396.
- Acknowledge the shock of an unexpected diagnosis:
  - *'I can see that this news has come as a big shock to you . . . had the thought of HIV ever crossed your mind?'*
- Explain the difference between HIV and AIDS.
- Remember sources of support such as the Terence Higgins Trust.
- Explain the need for his wife to be informed so that she has an opportunity to be tested to determine her HIV status.
- If he refuses to tell his wife, consider whether you would breach his confidentiality and disclose his HIV status to her.
- There is no right or wrong answer, since there is no absolute indication to breach confidentiality here.
  - Arguments *for* breaching confidentiality include concern for the wife's health, given that she may actually have HIV herself and therefore could potentially benefit from treatment.
  - Arguments *against* breaching confidentiality include the desirability not to compromise the doctor-patient relationship in a patient with a new diagnosis of HIV who is likely to require frequent contact with health professionals in the future.
- Be mindful of the underlying ethical principles of good medical practice:
  - **Autonomy**: respect for the individual patient and their ability to make decisions regarding their own health.
  - **Beneficence**: acting in the best interest of the patient.
  - **Non-maleficence**: 'first do no harm'.
  - **Justice**: fairness and equality in the wider community.

- Before disclosing confidential information, seek advice from sources such as senior colleagues, the General Medical Council (GMC), Medical Defence Union (MDU), Royal College of Physicians (RCP) or British Medical Association (BMA).

Confidentiality

- Confidentiality is a patient's right and must be respected by the entire healthcare team (Human Rights Act 1998).
- The Data Protection Act 1998 regulates the processing of information about individuals, which includes paper and computer records.
- The duty of confidentiality continues after a patient has died (Access to Health Records Act 1990).

Disclosure of confidential information

- Information may be disclosed in the *public interest*, without the patient's consent, where the benefits to an individual or to society of the disclosure outweigh the public and the patient's interest in keeping the information confidential.
- Disclosure may also be justified to *protect the patient or others*, where failure to disclose may expose the patient or others to risk of death or serious harm.
- The information disclosed must be *proportionate and limited* to the relevant details only.
- Seek consent to disclosure where practicable.
- Inform the patient in writing as soon as the disclosure has been made.

Consent requirements

- *Implied consent sufficient:*
  - Sharing information within the healthcare team.
  - Using information for clinical audit.
- *Express consent required:*
  - Disclosure of identifiable information to third parties (e.g. insurance companies).
  - Medical research.
- *No consent required:*
  - Reporting terrorist activity under the Terrorism Act 2000.
  - Notification of communicable diseases.
  - Reporting serious crime (e.g. murder).
  - If ordered by a judge.

🕭 Useful websites

British HIV Association: http://www.bhiva.org
GMC Confidentiality: Protecting and Providing Information: http://www.gmc-uk.org/guidance
The Medical Defence Union: http://www.the-mdu.com
The NHS Confidentiality Code of Practice: http://www.dh.gov.uk
Terence Higgins Trust: http://www.tht.org.uk

Scenario 3

Information for the candidate

Your role
You are the specialty registrar on the intensive care unit (ICU).

Problem
Explaining to a mother the death of her teenage daughter.

Patient's mother
Ms Sandra Curtis, a 43-year-old woman.

Patient
Carla Curtis, a 19-year-old woman.

Please read the scenario which follows. When the bell sounds, enter the examination room to begin the consultation.

Background to Scenario

Carla Curtis was admitted to the acute medical unit 4 days ago following a co-codamol overdose.

She was diagnosed with opiate drug dependence 4 years ago, and had subsequently been under the care of the drug and alcohol team. She had been admitted to hospital 12 times over the last year due to acts of deliberate self-harm including drug overdoses. This recent overdose was precipitated by an argument with her boyfriend.

Carla's condition deteriorated 48 hours after admission, and she was transferred to ICU where she was ventilated and treated for sepsis and renal failure.

Unfortunately, Carla died earlier this morning following a cardiac arrest from which she could not be resuscitated.

Ms Curtis has just arrived on the unit to visit Carla, as she has done for the last 2 days.

Your task is to speak to Ms Curtis and explain that Carla has died.

Information for the actor

You are the mother of Carla, who is your only child. You separated from Carla's father 12 years ago. Carla has not had a job since leaving school 3 years ago.

She was diagnosed with heroin addiction 4 years ago, and since then has had repeated admissions to hospital following drug overdoses. On each occasion you have pleaded with the doctors for her to be sectioned as you believed that this would have enabled her to get the help that she needed.

On the day of Carla's overdose you came home from work to find her surrounded by empty co-codamol packets. You called an ambulance immediately and she was taken to hospital. You are shocked to see how poorly Carla has been in the last few days following this overdose, as she has never been on the ICU or required the use of a ventilator before.

Questions you might ask

- 'Why wasn't she moved straight to the ICU from the emergency department?'
- 'Why wasn't she sectioned after the last overdose?'
- 'Could she have been saved if I had found her earlier?'

Bereavement

- Ask Carla's mother whether she would like anyone else in the room with her – in reality a nurse would be present.
- Confirm that Carla has been very poorly over the last 2 days.
- Give the warning shot, and allow silence for the news to sink in:
  - *'I'm afraid that I have some very bad news to tell you . . .'*
- Explain clearly that Carla has died, and avoid euphemisms.
- Be ready to deal with immediate feelings of anger and guilt.
- Consider the Kübler-Ross model of grief to understand the emotions that may be expected over the following days, weeks and months:
  - **Shock**
  - **Denial**
  - **Bargaining:** begging for their loved one to be returned to life in exchange for whatever price such a bargain would demand
  - **Depression**
  - **Acceptance**.
- The first 3 phases may feature during the consultation itself, whilst the last 2 phases tend to arise at a later stage, and are probably best discussed with the examiners after the consultation.
- Gently discuss why Carla may not have been 'sectioned' previously.
- Ask about family support and consider what further support may be available to Ms Curtis after the consultation (e.g. GP can offer support in the community, professional bereavement counselling services such as CRUSE may be helpful).

Mental Health Act (MHA) 2007

- Gives health professionals the power, in certain circumstances, to detain, assess and treat people with mental illness.

- Excludes:
  - Alcohol and drug dependence (as in Carla's case).
  - Learning disability (unless associated with abnormal aggression).
- *For assessment* to occur under the MHA, the patient:
  - Must be suffering from a mental disorder of a degree that warrants the detention of the patient in hospital for assessment.
  - Ought to be detained in the interests of their own health and safety or for the protection of others.
- *For treatment* to occur under the MHA, appropriate medical treatment must be available – the *purpose* of which is to alleviate or prevent deterioration *even if this is unlikely to occur in reality* (e.g. in borderline personality disorder a short in-patient stay may result in a temporary improvement, even if the long-term prognosis is not necessarily altered).

Summary of sections: MHA 2007

Section 2: Admission for assessment
- Requires application by a relative or an approved mental health practitioner (AMHP) and authorization by a responsible clinician (RC) and an approved clinician (AC).
- Lasts 28 days.

Section 3: Admission for treatment
- Requires application and approval as in section 2.
- Is valid for 6 months.

Section 4: Admission for assessment in cases of emergency
- Requires application by a relative or AMHP and one clinician.
- Is valid for 72 hours.

Section 5: Application in respect of patient already in hospital
- Is used when there is difficulty in finding an approved clinician (e.g. due to time constraints).
- Section 5(2) allows a doctor to detain any in-patient for 72 hours.
- Section 5(4) allows a nurse to detain a patient (who is already receiving treatment for mental illness) for 6 hours.

The roles of AMHP, RC, and AC (which were previously only held by doctors and approved social workers) have been widened to include occupational therapists, psychologists and nurses.

♫ Useful websites
Bereaved Parents' Network: http://www.careforthefamily.org.uk/bpn
Cruse Bereavement Care: http://www.cruse.org.uk
Implementing the amended Mental Health Act: http://www.mhact.csip.org.uk
Mental Health Act 2007: http://www.dh.gov.uk
Mind (National Association for Mental Health): http://www.mind.org.uk

Viva questions: Breaking bad news (scenarios 1–3)

Do you know what a 'DS 1500 form' is?
- A DS 1500 form is completed by a GP, consultant, hospital doctor or specialist nurse.
- It enables a patient who is terminally ill to claim the higher rates of disability living allowance (DLA) or attendance allowance (AA) under what are called 'special rules'.

- It is designed to 'fast-track' claims to be processed within a few weeks.
- Forms can be completed if the patient's death can 'reasonably be expected' within the next 6 months.
- The DS 1500 form is not a claim form itself, and the appropriate claim form needs to be submitted with the 'special rules' box ticked.

Tell me some situations in which HIV testing is undertaken in the community

- When HIV is clinically suspected (e.g. in a patient presenting with an opportunistic infection).
- Screening (e.g. at a walk-in sexual health clinic).
- Contact-tracing in patients who have had sexual contact with an affected individual.
- Pregnancy (all pregnant women in the UK are routinely offered an HIV test).
- Blood donors (this is part of a series of tests undertaken on all donated blood in the UK).
- Children of affected individuals (vertical transmission).
- Organ donors and recipients.
- High-risk jobs (e.g. sex workers).

Useful websites

Department for Work and Pensions: http://www.dwp.gov.uk/directgov

The National Blood Service (includes information for both donors and recipients): http://www.blood.co.uk

Scenario 4

Information for the candidate

Your role
You are the specialty registrar on the acute medical unit.

Problem
Explaining the diagnosis of type 1 diabetes mellitus.

Patient
Mr Kieran De Silva, a 21-year-old man.

Please read the scenario which follows. When the bell sounds, enter the examination room to begin the consultation.

Background to Scenario

Mr De Silva was admitted to the acute medical unit 2 days ago following a 5-day history of diarrhoea and vomiting.

He has been a soldier in the army for the last 4 years, and has recently returned from overseas for a period of home leave. He had been out with friends celebrating his 21st birthday the day before becoming unwell. The diarrhoea quickly settled, but he continued vomiting until the day of his admission.

Upon arrival to the ward, he was lethargic and dehydrated. His blood glucose on admission was 38.6mmol/L. He was diagnosed with type 1 diabetes mellitus and diabetic ketoacidosis secondary to viral gastroenteritis.

Your task is to speak to Mr De Silva and explain the diagnosis of type 1 diabetes mellitus.

Information for the actor

You are a soldier in the army, and have recently returned home from a period of service overseas. You have previously worked as a trainee electrician.

You celebrated your 21st birthday with friends last week, which resulted in you drinking a lot of alcohol. The following day you started to feel unwell with vomiting and diarrhoea. The diarrhoea stopped after 1 day, and you thought that it was probably caused by the alcohol and kebab that you had had on your birthday. However, the vomiting continued for a further 4 days until your admission to hospital, at which point you were feeling lethargic and generally unwell.

You are feeling better today and looking forward to going back home to relax and prepare for your next deployment abroad in 2 weeks' time.

Questions you might ask
- 'How did I get diabetes?'
- 'Can't I just have some strong tablets instead of insulin?'
- 'Can diabetes be cured?'

Explaining the diagnosis of diabetes mellitus
- Check his understanding of events preceding his admission.
- Explain that he was feeling so unwell because he has diabetes.
- Explore his knowledge of diabetes (including any family or friends who may have diabetes) and any specific concerns that he may have.
- Provide information in small pieces, allowing time throughout for questions and to re-check understanding:
  - *'The pancreas produces insulin hormone to control sugar levels in the blood . . . in diabetes the insulin-producing cells are destroyed, and so your body can no longer control sugar properly.'*
  - *'This recent gastroenteritis tummy bug has unmasked this diabetes problem which has probably been building up for a while.'*
  - *'Your body still needs insulin hormone to keep control of the sugar levels in the blood . . . insulin doesn't come in tablet form, and therefore it has to be given as a small injection just underneath the skin.'*
- Gently explore his understanding of how diabetes and insulin treatment may affect his current job.
- Explain that insulin treatment would prohibit him continuing in the army.
- Suggest careers advice agencies to offer guidance regarding alternative employment and/or training courses.
- Acknowledge feelings of shock, anger and denial – refer to principles of breaking bad news in ➲ Scenario 1, p.396.
- Offer realistic hope:
  - *'Most people with diabetes are well and live normal lives.'*
- Explain that he will need long-term multidisciplinary care which will be provided at both his GP surgery and by a hospital diabetology service.
- Arrange a follow-up appointment and provide him with contact details of the diabetic specialist nurse.

❶ Top Tips

- Ask about hobbies and recreational activities and consider how diabetes may affect these.
- Adopt a multidisciplinary team approach, involving attention to nutrition, exercise and psychological well-being.
- Smoking, alcohol and recreational drugs are important issues to be mindful of, particularly in young patients.
- Consider the use of a medic-alert bracelet or similar.
- Explain the use of support groups, including those specifically for younger patients.

Prohibited jobs in patients taking insulin

- Driving heavy goods vehicles (HGVs), buses and taxis.
- Armed forces.
- Airline pilots.

Blanket bans have now been lifted in the emergency services for insulin-treated diabetics – patients are now assessed on an individual basis.

Disability Discrimination Act (DDA) 2005

- Defines a disabled person as someone who has a physical or mental impairment that has a substantial and long-term (has lasted or is likely to last >12 months) adverse effect on his or her ability to carry out normal day-to-day activities.
- Gives disabled people rights in the areas of:
  - Employment (i.e. entitlement to workplace adjustments).
  - Access to goods, facilities and services.
  - Buying or renting land or property.
- Applies to all employers and everyone who provides a public service, *except* the Armed Forces.
- Whilst the Armed Forces are exempt from the DDA 2005, any other employer in this situation would be obliged to make reasonable workplace adjustments if he was unable to continue in his current role for health reasons.
- Patients with HIV, cancer and MS are covered by the act effectively from the point of their diagnosis, rather than from the point when the condition has some adverse effect on their ability to carry out normal day-to-day activities.

⌘ Useful websites

Department for Work and Pensions: http://www.dwp.gov.uk/employers/dda
Diabetes UK: http://www.diabetes.co.uk
Directgov [The official government website for citizens]: http://www.direct.gov.uk/en/disabledpeople
NICE. *Type 1 diabetes: diagnosis and management in adults: Quick reference guide.* London: NICE, 2004. Available at: http://www.nice.org.uk/guidance .

Scenario 5

Information for the candidate

Your role

You are the specialty registrar in the cardiology clinic.

Problem

Explaining the diagnosis of hypertrophic obstructive cardiomyopathy (HOCM).

Patient

Mr Jason Grainger, a 29-year-old man.

Please read the scenario which follows. When the bell sounds, enter the examination room to begin the consultation.

Background to Scenario

Mr Grainger is attending cardiology clinic today following episodes of palpitations and dizziness over the preceding 3 months.

He finds that he particularly develops symptoms during or after exercise. His GP diagnosed an anxiety disorder and has prescribed a beta-blocker, which he thinks may have slightly improved his symptoms.

An echocardiogram performed today has confirmed a diagnosis of HOCM.

Mr Grainger is keen to be seen in clinic promptly today, as he is playing in an important football match later this evening.

Your task is to speak to Mr Grainger and explain the diagnosis of HOCM.

Information for the actor

You work as a bus driver, and live with your partner and 2-year-old son. Your father died suddenly aged 22, although you do not know any further details regarding the cause of death. You enjoy playing football with your old school friends most weekends.

You have been experiencing intermittent episodes of palpitations and light-headedness over the last 3 months. You have noticed that these episodes mostly occur during or shortly after playing football. Your GP diagnosed an anxiety disorder and has been treating you with beta-blockers, which you feel may have slightly improved your symptoms.

You are keen to be seen promptly in clinic today, as you are playing in an important football match later this evening.

You have been particularly stressed recently as you have doing a lot of overtime work to earn extra money. You are very shocked to learn that this is actually a heart problem. Driving is your livelihood, so you are angry at being told that you must stop.

Questions you might ask
- 'Why wasn't this heart problem detected earlier?'
- 'Can this heart problem be cured?'
- 'Will my son have the same heart problem as well?'

Explaining the diagnosis of HOCM
- Establish prior knowledge including specific concerns and expectations from today's discussion.
  - *'Has anything in particular been going through your mind about what might be causing your dizziness and palpitations?'*
- Explain the diagnosis and the possible familial nature of HOCM in a clear manner, avoiding medical terms. Diagrams to aid can be useful.
- Acknowledge the shock of this diagnosis, and deal with any anger.
  - *'I can see that this news has come as a big shock for you today . . .'*
- Explain the risk of further episodes and the need for definitive treatment, including medical and surgical options and the use of an implantable defibrillator.
- Explain the legal requirement to cease driving and inform the DVLA.
- Acknowledge the financial and social difficulties to his family that may arise from him being unable to drive (ask if there are any alternative office-based roles available at his current employment).
- Ask about his family, and consider the potential psychosocial impact of this diagnosis.
- Aim to reach a shared understanding of his current situation and help to offer potential solutions to some of the problems.
- Advise him to contact his company occupational health department for specific employment advice.

DVLA guidelines
- The DVLA is legally responsible for deciding if a person is medically unfit to drive.

- Make sure that the patient understands that the condition may impair their ability to drive. If a patient is incapable of understanding this advice, for example because of dementia, you should inform the DVLA immediately.
- Explain to patients that they have a legal duty to inform the DVLA about the condition and make clear that documentation to this effect will be recorded in their medical notes.
- If the patient refuses to accept the diagnosis or the effect of the condition on their ability to drive, you can suggest that the patient seeks a second medical opinion. Advise patients not to drive until the second opinion has been obtained.
- If patient continues to drive when they are not fit to do so, you should make every reasonable effort to persuade them to stop.
- If you do not manage to persuade patients to stop driving, or you are given or find evidence that a patient is continuing to drive contrary to advice, you should disclose relevant medical information immediately, in confidence, to the medical adviser at the DVLA.
- Before giving information to the DVLA you should inform the patient of your decision to do so. Once the DVLA has been informed, you should also write to the patient, to confirm that a disclosure has been made.

Licence groups

Group 1
- Motor cars, motor cycles.
- Issued until age 70 years, and renewed every 3 years thereafter.

Group 2
- Large lorries, buses and taxis.
- Issued from age 21–45 years, and renewable every 5 years to age 65, and annually thereafter.
- The medical standards are significantly more stringent than those for group 1 because of the size and weight of the vehicle, the higher risk caused by the length of time the driver may spend at the wheel, and in cases of public service vehicles, the responsibility to public passengers being transported (Table 7.1).

Useful websites
DVLA: At a Glance Guide to the Current Medical Standards of Fitness to Drive: http://www.dft. gov.uk/dvla/medical/ataglance.aspx
GMC: Good Medical Practice: http://www.gmc-uk.org/guidance

Viva questions: Explaining a new diagnosis (scenarios 4-5)
How would you respond to a patient asking about genetic testing for his children for a disease where there is no clear inheritance pattern (e.g. diabetes mellitus)?
- Many diseases and conditions do run in families.
- Some diseases are passed on to children with a 'clear pattern of inheritance' (e.g. neurofibromatosis).
  As these diseases are caused by a faulty chromosome, they can be detected by a simple blood test.
- Other conditions have a 'multifactorial inheritance' (e.g. diabetes), and there are no simple tests which will accurately predict those children that will become affected.

Table 7.1 DVLA standards

	Type 1 licence	Type 2 licence
Epilepsy	6-month ban	Needs to remain seizure-free for 5–10 years, depending on specialist neurological assessment
Stroke and transient ischaemic attack (TIA)	At least 1-month ban	At least 1-year ban
Acute coronary syndrome (ACS)	1-week ban (if treated successfully by angioplasty) or 4-week ban (if not successfully treated by angioplasty)	At least 6-week ban
Implantable cardioverter-defibrillator (ICD)	Various lengths of ban depending on exact circumstances of ICD insertion	Permanently banned
Hypertrophic obstructive cardiomyopathy (HOCM)	Can continue	Permanently banned
Diabetes mellitus (on insulin)	1-, 2- or 3-year licence as long as signs of hypoglycaemia are recognized and visual standards are met	Licence can be renewed on an annual basis if: Free of hypoglycaemic episodes during past 12 months. Full awareness of hypoglycaemia. 3-month record of glucose monitoring carried out on at least a twice daily basis.

- Whilst we know that diabetes does run in families, and therefore there is an increased chance of your child developing this condition (compared to the background population), there is no clear or predictable pattern to the condition.
- We do know that certain lifestyle measures can reduce the chance of your child developing the condition (such as maintaining a normal healthy body weight, taking regular exercise and enjoying a healthy low fat diet).

What would you say to a patient who has just been diagnosed with type 1 diabetes and tells you that he has a phobia of needles?

- Elicit their specific concerns – is it the sight of the needle, or the thought of the pain of the needle, or is it based on a previous 'bad experience'?

- Reassure them that a degree of initial needle phobia is quite normal.
- However, most patients will overcome this fear and quickly become accustomed to the routine of insulin injections.
- Patient education and reassurance are the key factors – offer to make an appointment for them to see a specialist nurse or to attend a patient support group.
- Note: NICE[1] *only* recommends continuous subcutaneous insulin infusion as an option in adults and children >12 years with type 1 diabetes in certain situations including inadequate glycaemic control or unpredictable hypoglycaemia.

Reference

1. NICE. *Appraisal Technology Guidance 151 – insulin pump therapy: guidance*. London: NICE, 2008. Available at: http://guidance.nice.org.uk/TA151/Guidance/pdf/English.

Scenario 6

Information for the candidate

Your role

You are the specialty registrar in the clinical genetics clinic.

Problem

Counselling for genetic testing for Huntington's disease (HD).

Patient

Miss Lisa Dempsey, a 22-year-old woman.

Please read the scenario which follows. When the bell sounds, enter the examination room to begin the consultation.

Background to Scenario

Miss Dempsey has been referred to the clinical genetics clinic following a recent diagnosis of HD in her father.

Her 48-year-old father was diagnosed with HD 6 weeks ago following an 8-month history of abnormal arm movements and increasing clumsiness. He has since had to take early retirement from his job as a building site manager due to a deterioration in his symptoms.

Miss Dempsey is currently asymptomatic. She is attending clinic today asking to be tested for the HD gene in view of her father's recent diagnosis.

Your task is to speak to Miss Dempsey and counsel her regarding genetic testing for HD.

Information for the actor

You work as an occupational therapist at the local hospital, and live with your fiancé. You are hoping to start a family after you get married later this year.

Your father has recently been diagnosed with Huntington's disease following a 4-month episode of clumsiness and abnormal movements of his arms. You had suspected that this might have been the beginnings of multiple sclerosis, and are shocked to hear that this is actually HD, which you know very little about. You and your 2 younger brothers have all been referred to see a clinical geneticist to discuss testing for the HD gene.

Questions you might ask
- 'What treatment is available?'
- 'Will this affect me being able to get a mortgage and life insurance?'
- 'What about any children I have – will they be affected?'

Genetic counselling for Huntington's disease
- Explain that you are sorry to hear about her father's recent diagnosis.
- Enquire if anyone else in the family has had similar symptoms.
- Elicit her understanding of HD and specific concerns (which may relate to her father's current symptoms).
- Explain that HD is usually transmitted in an autosomal dominant manner, and there is therefore a 50% chance of herself and her brothers carrying the HD gene.
- Details regarding the specific mutation (in this case, the short arm of chromosome 4) are not appropriate at this stage.
- Explain that although there is no current preventative or curative treatment for HD, medication is available which may help control specific symptoms (e.g. tetrabenazine for chorea).
- Offer her predictive genetic testing, and explain that this is *different* to diagnostic testing which her father had and involves a blood test.
- Discuss the small possibility of a false positive or false negative test result.
- Phrases 'predicted to be affected' or 'predicted not to be affected' are less ambiguous than 'positive' and 'negative' – explore how she would feel if she was given each of these results.
- Consider how testing may affect her personally:
  - *Financial* (including career and life insurance).
  - *Psychological* (including anxiety due to uncertainty).
  - *Social* (including family, friends and any potential children).
- Remember the principles of informed consent before proceeding to testing – ➔ Scenario 8, p.420.
- Explain that a lot of patients decide not to actually go ahead with testing in the end.
- How would she feel if she proceeded to be tested, but one of her siblings declined the test (or vice versa)?
- If following the test she is 'predicted to be affected', it will not show at what *age* she will be affected or *how* she will be affected (e.g. symptoms, severity, rate of progression).

- If following the test she is 'predicted not to be affected', she would not pass on the gene to any children, due to autosomal dominant inheritance.
- Reassure her that she can take time to consider her decision, and offer her a follow-up appointment – there should be at least a few weeks between the initial consultation and any subsequent testing.
- Finally, ask if she would like to bring a friend or relative to the next appointment, although this should not be a relative who could be potentially affected (e.g. brother) as there is potential for a conflict of interest.

Principles of genetic counselling

- Provision of specialized non-directive genetic counselling.
- Use of simple printed information that can be consulted after counselling.
- Aim is to help individuals or families understand or cope with genetic disease, *not* to decrease the incidence of genetic disease.
- History and pedigree construction.
- Examination.
- Diagnosis (including clinical presentation, treatment, natural history, prognosis, complications and clear explanation of the genetics).
- Counselling.
- Follow-up (including communication of test results).

Ethical considerations

- Respect for the patient's *autonomy* – the individual has both the right to know and not to know.
- *Confidentiality* must be respected – including access to a patient's personal information and tissue samples.

Association of British Insurers (ABI) genetic testing code of conduct

- No insurer can request that an applicant undertake a genetic test in order to obtain insurance.
- Individuals can apply for £500,000 of life insurance and £300,000 of critical illness insurance, without having to tell the insurer the results of any predictive genetic tests.
- For life insurance applications worth more than £500,000, the results of any genetic test will *not* be used in the assessment of an application, unless they are in the applicant's favour, or the test has been approved by the Genetics and Insurance Committee (GAIC) – *HD* is currently the only test that has been approved.

Pre-implantation genetic diagnosis

- Available for couples who have had a 'predicted to be affected' pre-symptomatic HD result.
- Involves *in vitro* fertilization (IVF) treatment, even if they are a normal fertile couple.
- Embryos are then tested for HD before they are implanted.

✆ Useful websites

Association of British Insurers (ABI) Genetic Testing Code of Conduct: http://www.abi.org.uk

Huntington's Disease Association: http://www.hda.org.uk

Recommendations on the ethical, legal and social implications of genetic testing: http://ec.europa. eu/research

Scenario 7

Information for the candidate

Your role

You are the specialty registrar on the gastroenterology ward.

Problem

Counselling a patient regarding the use of intravenous steroids in acute ulcerative colitis.

Patient

Mrs Jasmine Gupta, a 27-year-old woman.

Please read the scenario which follows. When the bell sounds, enter the examination room to begin the consultation.

Background to Scenario

You have been called by the gastroenterology ward sister to speak to Mrs Gupta.

Mrs Gupta was admitted yesterday following an exacerbation of ulcerative colitis. She presented with a 6-day history of acute bloody diarrhoea, fever and abdominal pain which had deteriorated despite mesalazine enemas. She was seen by the consultant gastroenterologist, and commenced on intravenous steroid therapy.

However, Mrs Gupta refused the intravenous steroid on the drugs round this morning, and is now asking to speak to a doctor as she would like to discuss this further.

Your task is to speak to Mrs Gupta and discuss with her the use of intra-venous steroids for her acute exacerbation of ulcerative colitis.

Information for the actor

You are married with 2 young children, and work part-time in a crèche. You smoke 5 cigarettes per day.

You were diagnosed with ulcerative colitis 3 years ago, and have since been well-controlled on medication. You have not required any previous hospital admissions. You became unwell 1 week ago with a flare-up of ulcerative colitis. Your GP prescribed mesalazine enemas, but you deteriorated despite this, and were admitted to hospital yesterday morning.

You saw the consultant on the ward round, who explained that he wanted to start a course of intravenous steroids. At the time, you did not get the chance to explain your concerns regarding this, and you are worried about the side effects of the steroids. In particular, you and your husband are trying for another baby, and you are concerned that steroids may reduce your chance of becoming pregnant.

Questions you might ask
- 'Will steroids stop me getting pregnant?'
- 'What has caused this flare-up?'
- 'Will I need surgery?'

Intravenous steroid therapy in ulcerative colitis
- Explore Mrs Gupta's understanding of this admission and of UC in general.
- Ask about any pervious episodes of acute exacerbations.
- Ask about concerns and more specifically about her anxieties regarding the use of intravenous steroids:
  - *'Lots of patients actually worry when we mention steroid medication – is there anything in particular that concerns you about steroids?'*
- Explain the difference between short- and long-term use of steroids:
  - *'The steroid side effects that most people worry about usually occur after long-term use of steroids for weeks or months, and not after a few days or a one week course.'*
- Mrs Gupta may then want reassurance that she will only be on steroids for a few days, although you would be unable to guarantee this.
- Ascertain her understanding of the potential complications of untreated acute UC:
  - *'Sometimes, if the flare-up gets out of control, then the colon can become very inflamed and swollen, and can actually burst if left untreated . . . this would be a serious problem and would need an emergency operation, and possibly the use of a special pouch called a stoma . . .'*
  - *'Fortunately however, the steroids are very good at controlling flare-ups and preventing these more serious problems.'*
- Acknowledge her concerns regarding the use of steroids and pregnancy:
  - *'A short course of steroids would not prevent you getting pregnant in the future . . . Steroids can be used in pregnancy, although we would*

weigh up the risks and benefits at the time, and discuss this with you if we were considering using them whilst you were pregnant.'

- Explain that by maintaining good control of her UC, she would optimize the chances of her falling pregnant and enjoying a healthy pregnancy:
  - *'With steroid treatment we find that patients tend to improve quite quickly . . . the better your general health is, including your UC, then the less likely you are to encounter problems either conceiving or during an actual pregnancy itself.'*
- Emphasize the desirability to start intravenous steroid therapy as soon as possible.
- Direct her to support groups (e.g. National Association for Colitis and Crohn's Disease [NACC]), and explain how many patients find these useful.
- Offer further discussion with other family members present and the opportunity to speak to the consultant.
- Summarize and check understanding before finishing:
  - *'What are your feelings about having the steroids now, after having this chat?'*
  - *'Do you think that you would feel able to explain some of these things that we have talked about today to your husband?'*

❶ Top Tips

- Asking about previous episodes is important as this has a significant impact on any further explanation offered. If a patient has had a previous episode and is now refusing treatment, then it is essential to elicit the reasons behind this (including previous adverse effects). However if this is a first episode, the patient may accept treatment following a simple explanation.
- Written information and diagrams are often helpful (e.g. in explaining what a stoma is).
- Remember to explain fully in simple language any jargon words which she may have heard (e.g. 'intravenous', 'stoma' and 'exacerbation').
- Involve the inflammatory bowel disease nurse specialist.
- 'Normalize' her emotions – most other patients in her situation would have exactly the same concerns.
- Offer to return in a couple of hours to answer any further questions and allow time for her to re-consider her decision.

✂ Useful website

National Association for Colitis and Crohn's Disease: http://www.nacc.org.uk

Scenario 8

Information for the candidate

Your role
You are the specialty registrar on the acute medical unit.

Problem
Counselling a patient who is refusing a blood transfusion.

Patient
Mr Neil Keenan, a 53-year-old man.

Please read the scenario which follows. When the bell sounds, enter the examination room to begin the consultation.

Background to Scenario

Mr Keenan was admitted to the acute medical unit yesterday following a massive haematemesis.

Upon arrival to the emergency department (ED) he was tachycardic, hypotensive and drowsy. He was given an immediate 2U blood transfusion and then transferred to the acute medical unit once his condition had stabilized.

He has a history of depression and alcoholism, and is known to have oesophageal varices. He was admitted to hospital a year ago following a paracetamol overdose.

An FBC taken earlier this morning has revealed an Hb of 4.7g/dL, and your consultant has asked you to arrange a further transfusion.

However, Mr Keenan has made it clear that he does not wish to receive any further blood transfusions, as he feels that he doesn't have anything to live for, and 'wouldn't mind dying now'.

Your task is to speak to Mr Keenan and discuss the blood transfusion with him.

Information for the actor

You are currently living in a hostel, after losing your bedsit 3 months ago. You are unemployed, and have not worked for the last 5 years. Your family have disowned you because of your continual alcohol and debt problems.

You were admitted to hospital a year ago following a paracetamol overdose, and at that time you were told that you had developed liver problems due to an excessive alcohol intake.

In the last few weeks you have been feeling depressed, and have been drinking more heavily, although you have not done anything to try to harm yourself.

You started to feel unwell yesterday whilst in the off licence, and subsequently vomited a large amount of blood. The shopkeeper called an ambulance, and you were taken to hospital.

Your life seems to be full of despair and you cannot see any hope for the future. You have therefore decided to decline all medical treatment whilst in hospital, including blood transfusions, as you feel that it would be best for everybody if you were to die now.

Questions you might ask

- 'I didn't want a blood transfusion – so why was I given blood in the ED?'
- 'You can't force treatment on me, can you?'
- 'What will happen if I do not have the transfusion?'

Consent for blood transfusion

- Explore his understanding of his current admission.
- Ask about events leading up to his admission:
  - 'You are obviously feeling quite low at the moment – can I ask you about some of the things that have been happening recently that might be making you feel like this?'
- Essentially, the key question is whether he has *capacity* to make a decision to refuse a blood transfusion.
- Inform him of the consequences of both receiving a blood transfusion, and not receiving a blood transfusion:
  - 'Your blood count is extremely low, and although you have mentioned dying, it is more likely that you will actually just become very tired, breathless and distressed over the next few days and weeks as your body struggles to cope with the very low blood count.'
- Explain to him why he was given blood in the ED:
  - 'We were unable to obtain your consent for the blood transfusion, as you were extremely unwell, and not in a position to be able to weigh-up all of your options . . . we gave you blood in the ED because this was deemed to be in your best interests at the time.'
- Suggest to him that by improving his current medical condition, he would hopefully feel much better. He would then be more likely to be in a position to be able to benefit from further sources of support.
- Allow time for reflection before exploring psycho-social factors further:
  - 'Do you think that we might be able to help you with some of the problems that you've been having recently with your depression and alcohol drinking?'

- Consider how referral to other agencies may help support him after the acute situation has been managed (e.g. citizen's advice bureau, social services, alcohol team, GP, Samaritans).
- Ask how he feels about the blood transfusion now following your discussion.

Valid consent

For consent to be valid, it must be given *voluntarily* (i.e. not coerced). The patient must be appropriately *informed* of the intervention, and have *capacity* to make the decision.

Capacity

To have capacity, the patient must be able to *comprehend*, *retain* and *weigh* the information, and *understand the consequences* of having or not having the intervention. The Mental Capacity Act 2005 provides a framework to protect vulnerable people who are not able to make their own decisions.

Mental Capacity Act 2005: key principles

- Every adult has the right to make his or her own decision, and must be *assumed to have capacity* unless proved otherwise.
- Individuals have the right to be *supported to make their own decisions*.
- Individuals have the right to make what might be seen as unwise or 'eccentric' decisions (including refusing life-sustaining treatment).
- Anything done for or on behalf of people without capacity must be in their *best interests*.
- Anything done for or on behalf of people without capacity must be the *least restrictive* of their basic rights and freedoms.

Assessing lack of capacity

- Assessment of capacity (competence) is *decision-specific*.
- No one can be labelled incompetent as a result of a particular medical condition or diagnosis.
- Age, appearance or any aspect of a person's behaviour cannot be used to establish a lack of capacity.
- No one can consent for an incompetent adult – an assessment is made of what decision would be in the *best interests* of the patient.

Self-harm and consent

- If the patient is able to communicate, an urgent assessment of their mental capacity should be made.
- If they are judged to be incompetent, they are treated on the basis of temporary incapacity – and the principle of best interests applies. In such cases, assessment of competence is reviewed on a continual basis.
- If the patient is unconscious, they should be given emergency treatment – again applying the principle of best interests, unless an advance directive is in place and contradicts this.
- If they are judged to be competent, and they refuse treatment, then a psychiatric assessment should be made to decide whether the use of the MHA is appropriate (i.e. are they suffering from a psychiatric illness that requires further assessment and/or treatment?)
- If use of the MHA is *not* appropriate, then their *refusal must be respected*.

- If there is good reason to believe that a patient was competent when they took the decision to end their life with a genuine intention, and use of the MHA is not applicable, then treatment must not be forced upon the patient, although clearly attempts should be made to encourage them to accept help.
- In reality, it is very difficult to know whether a patient was indeed competent at the time of the act of self-harm.
- As with all complex decisions, senior colleagues and medical defence organizations can provide further support and advice.

Lasting power of attorney (LPA)

Individuals can appoint an LPA to act on their behalf if they should lose capacity in the future (e.g. a patient in the early stages of dementia). LPAs can make decisions regarding health, welfare, finance and property.

Independent mental capacity advocate (IMCA)

This is a new role created by the Mental Capacity Act 2005. IMCAs are appointed to support a person who lacks capacity, but has no one to speak for them. Patients who are 16 years or older and who lack capacity to make decisions regarding serious medical treatment or a major change of accommodation are eligible for an IMCA. Every health authority will have a local IMCA service to which patients can be referred.

Advance refusals

Advance refusals and advance directives should be respected and are *legally-binding*.

℘ Useful websites

Consent: Patients and Doctors Making Decisions Together: www.gmc-uk.org
Mental Capacity Act 2005: http://www.opsi.gov.uk/acts
Reference Guide to Consent for Examination or Treatment: http://www.dh.gov.uk

Scenario 9

Information for the candidate

Your role
You are the specialty registrar on the coronary care unit.

Problem
Dealing with an angry patient who has been admitted with a myocardial infarction (MI).

Patient
Mr Ian Spokes, a 56-year-old man.

Please read the scenario which follows. When the bell sounds, enter the examination room to begin the consultation.

Background to Scenario

Mr Spokes was admitted to the coronary care unit 4 days ago following a myocardial infarction.

He has a history of hypertension, and smokes 30 cigarettes per day. He started to develop epigastric pain last week. His GP diagnosed acid reflux and prescribed lansoprazole.

Unfortunately, 2 days later he developed worsening pain during a business meeting. Colleagues called an ambulance, and he was subsequently transferred to hospital where he was diagnosed with an anterior MI.

Mr Spokes is now angry as he feels that his GP was negligent in not diagnosing his MI, and he would like to speak to you further regarding this.

Your task is to speak to Mr Spokes and discuss his concerns regarding his medical management.

Information for the actor

You are a managing director for a computer company and married with 2 grown-up children and a 5-month-old granddaughter. You smoke 30 cigarettes per day.

You have been particularly stressed recently, as there have been financial problems within your company.

You were diagnosed with high blood pressure 8 years ago, and have been on medication for this ever since. You have continued to smoke despite repeated advice against this. You saw your GP last week because of abdominal pain and were prescribed a tablet for acid reflux.

You were subsequently admitted to hospital 2 days later with worsening abdominal pain, where you were diagnosed with a heart attack. You are now angry as you have been told that you cannot drive for the next 4 weeks. You feel that this is all your GP's fault, and want something to be done.

Inwardly, you feel guilty for having continued to smoke, despite previous medical advice. You suddenly now realize that you may not see your granddaughter grow up if you continue to smoke.

Questions you might ask
- 'Can you tell me how I make a complaint against my GP?'
- 'Could this have been prevented if my GP had done a blood test?'
- 'The GP didn't even listen to my heart – I must be able to sue her?'

Dealing with an angry patient
- A relaxed, open posture, gentle calming voice and giving the patient time to talk can all go a long way in defusing a tense situation.
- Acknowledge the patient's anger and invite him to talk:
  - *'I can see that you are very angry – do you want to tell me what happened at your last appointment with the GP . . .?'*
- Explore what has upset him and the contributory reasons for his anger, and be mindful of potential escalation of anger:
  - Triggering events → Escalation → Crisis → Resolution.
- Recognize and consider common triggering events e.g.:
  - Fear (for his own health).
  - Guilt (of continuing to smoke despite medical advice).
  - Poor communication skills (missing cues, dismissive attitude of the GP or hospital staff).
  - Problems at home (financial, psychological and social issues).
- Take his concerns seriously.
- Answer any questions you can – remembering that you are only hearing one side of the story, and do not have all of the facts.
- Discuss how you can help – present the patient with realistic, achievable options and come to a shared agreed plan.
  - *'The issues that you have raised are important, and we would need to get in touch with your GP to get their thoughts regarding this . . .'*

Dealing with complaints

'**A soft answer turneth away wrath**' – each of us will never know how many times we have escaped the misery of a complaint thanks to the calming influence of another colleague.

NHS and social care complaints procedure

- A complaint must be made within 12 months from the date on which the matter occurred.
- Patients can seek further advice from the Patient Advisory Liaison Service (PALS) or Independent Complaints and Advocacy Service (ICAS) – both of which are accessible in primary and secondary care.

Local resolution

- Initially aim to resolve verbally with the consultant or ward manager (GP or practice manager if relates to a complaint in primary care).
- If unresolved, the complaint should be made to the ward manager, consultant or practice manager in writing.
- If still unresolved, the complaint should be referred to the complaints manager at the hospital or primary care trust.

Parliamentary and Health Service Ombudsman

- If the matter remains unsettled, the patient can complain to the Health Service Ombudsman.

Medical negligence

To bring a claim for medical negligence, a patient must prove:

- That the treatment fell below a minimum standard of competence.
- *And* that he or she has suffered an injury.
- *And* that it is more likely than not that the injury would have been avoided or have been less severe with proper treatment.
- The claim must be made within 3 years of the date of injury (exceptions exist – e.g. when the patient is a child or has a mental illness that makes them incapable of managing their own affairs).

Proving negligence: the Bolam test

- The standard of care in medical litigation is determined by the Bolam test.
- In law, a practitioner does not breach the standard if a responsible body of similar medical peers supports the practice in question.
- The principle criticism of the Bolam test is that it allows the standard in law to be set subjectively by doctors.

Proving negligence: the Bolitho test

- Following the Bolitho case, the court will now enquire more closely in to the justification of a defendant's practice, and must be satisfied that the body of opinion relied upon has a logical basis.
- In the *Bolitho v. City & Hackney Health Authority* [1997] case, a 2-year-old boy was admitted to hospital with croup and the next day developed 2 episodes of respiratory distress, followed by a fatal respiratory arrest.
- It was established that only intubation before the final episode would have averted the tragedy, and therefore the case hinged on whether a

competent doctor would have intubated the child after the 1st or 2nd episodes of respiratory distress.
- One expert's professional opinion suggested the child's symptoms did not indicate a progressive respiratory collapse, and there was only a small risk of total respiratory failure which did not justify the invasive procedure of intubation.
- The judge accepted that this expert opinion withstood logical analysis, and consequently the defending doctor was acquitted.
- However, if it can be demonstrated that the defendant's professional opinion was illogical, then the judge can hold that opinion unreasonable, thus supporting the claim for negligence.

Clinical Negligence Scheme for Trusts (CNST)
- Administered by the NHS Litigation Authority (NHSLA).
- Provides an indemnity to members and their employees in respect of clinical negligence claims arising from events that occurred on or after 1 April 1995.

✍ Useful websites
Bolitho v. City & Hackney Health Authority [1997]. Available at:
http://www.publications.parliament.uk.
The NHS Litigation Authority: http://www.nhsla.com
Understanding Anger: http://www.ltscotland.org.uk/Images/DB05_tcm4-341611.pdf

Viva questions: Counselling (scenarios 6–9)
Suppose the gentleman admitted with a myocardial infarction asks you for your opinion about the GP's initial diagnosis of acid reflux – what would you say to him?
- It is important not to be drawn in to colluding with the patient, and equally not to be seen to defend the appropriateness of the GP's diagnosis.
- Be careful with verbal (choice of words) and non-verbal communication (e.g. such as raised eyebrows).
- After acknowledging and dealing with his initial anger, explain the reasons for which you are not in a position to comment on the GPs diagnosis:
  - You do not have all the 'facts' elicited by the GP.
  - Clinical findings (including investigations) may change over time. Even if it was obvious that he was having a heart attack on admission to hospital, this may not necessarily have been the case at the time of the initial consultation with his GP.
  - Many conditions can present in an unusual manner, such as a heart attack presenting with non-specific abdominal pain.
- Explain that you are sure that his GP will be upset to learn that he has had a heart attack. Encourage him to speak to his GP following his discharge home.
- If this appointment with his GP fails to alleviate misunderstandings, suggest that he should contact the practice manager in the first instance.

At what age are teenagers or adolescents presumed to be competent to give their own consent for medical treatment?

- Once children reach the age of 16, they may be admitted to an adult medical ward.
- The Mental Capacity Act applies to people aged 16 and over; at this age they are presumed in law to be competent.
- As with any adult, a child over the age of 16 may not necessarily be competent. In this situation, consent would need to be obtained from someone with parental responsibility.
- The Department of Health recommends that it is nevertheless good practice to encourage children of this age to involve their families in decisions about their care.
- If a competent child requests that confidentiality is maintained, this should be respected unless the doctor considers that failing to disclose information would result in significant harm to the child.
- A child aged 16–18 cannot refuse treatment if it has been agreed by a person with parental responsibility or the Court, and it is in their best interests.

Further reading

GMC. *0 to 18 years: Guidance for All Doctors.* London: GMC, 2007. Available at: http://www.gmc-uk.org/guidance/ethical_guidance/children_guidance_index.asp.

Scenario 10

Information for the candidate

Your role

You are the specialty registrar on the respiratory ward.

Problem

Discussing recurrent hospital admissions with a patient with poorly-controlled asthma.

Patient

Miss Vicky Ollerton, an 18-year-old woman.

Please read the scenario which follows. When the bell sounds, enter the examination room to begin the consultation.

Background to Scenario

You have been asked by your consultant on the respiratory ward to speak to Miss Ollerton before she is discharged home later today.

Miss Olletton was admitted to the ICU 9 days ago with acute asthma. She was transferred to the respiratory ward 5 days ago, and is now ready to be discharged home.

She was diagnosed with asthma at the age of 5, and this has been particularly poorly-controlled over the last few years. She has had 8 admissions with acute asthma over the last year – 4 of which have required admission to ICU. She was ventilated on 2 of these occasions.

Your task is to speak to Miss Ollerton and discuss her recurrent hospital admissions for acute asthma.

Information for the actor

You currently work part-time as a carer in a residential home, and are hoping to start a beautician course at college later on in the year. You live with your mother and younger brother. You smoke 10 cigarettes per day, as well as smoking cannabis occasionally. You go out with friends and drink alcohol most evenings.

You were diagnosed with asthma as a child, and have been prescribed blue and brown inhalers ever since, although have not been shown how to correctly use them. As a result, you rarely use your inhalers, as they do not seem to make you feel any different.

You have been admitted to hospital 8 times over the last year, and have been put on a ventilator on 2 of those occasions. You feel that your asthma would improve if you were given a nebulizer to use at home, as you grandfather has a nebulizer which helps with his breathing problems.

Questions you might ask
• 'Why do I keep getting these asthma attacks?'
• 'Could I just have some stronger inhalers?'
• 'Could I not just have a nebulizer at home?'

Recurrent admissions for acute asthma
• Explore her understanding of asthma and the severity of this current admission.
• Check her knowledge of the use of her inhalers and any difficulties using them:
  • *'I just wanted to check what you've been told about when to use your inhalers ... How do you think you are getting on with actually using your inhalers?'*
• Consider potential precipitating factors (e.g. pets, occupation):
  • *'Is there anything in particular that you have noticed that sets off your asthma?'*
• Outline the specific problems caused by acute admissions including the risk of death, radiation risks associated with repeated chest x-rays and the adverse effects associated with frequent use of antibiotics and systemic steroids (e.g. antibiotic resistance and steroid side effects).
• Emphasize the need for regular inhaler use, and check technique: consider the use of a spacer device or changing to an alternative inhaler.
  • *'Can you show me or describe to me how you use your inhaler ...?'*
• The use of a peak-flow meter and diary may aid understanding, motivation and adherence with medication.
• Consider prescribing 2 of each inhaler – allowing her to keep one at home and one in her handbag.
• Explore her ideas regarding smoking (➔ Smoking cessation, p.429).
• Involve the specialist asthma nurse.

Supporting medicines adherence
• Adopt an open no-blame approach, encouraging the patient to discuss any doubts or concerns.

- If the patient is non-adherent, discuss whether this is because of ideas and concerns (intentional) or practical problems (unintentional – e.g. if the patient has difficulty using the inhaler).
- Involve patient in decisions about medicines and explain the likely consequences of not taking the medication.
- Discuss how medicines fit in with their daily routine (e.g. keeps forgetting to take the salbutamol inhaler to work).
- Enquire about any medication side effects (e.g. oral thrush from inhaled corticosteroids).
- Ask if prescription costs are a problem, and consider options for reducing costs (e.g. prescribing 2 inhalers on 1 prescription or using a prescription prepayment certificate).
- Provide clear information, re-inforced with regular agreed intervals (e.g. with the asthma nurse specialist).
- Accept that a patient has the right to decide not to take a medicine, even if you do not agree with the decision, as long as the patient has the capacity to make an informed decision.

Smoking cessation

- Explore health beliefs and establish readiness to change when consulting with patients who smoke (see 'cycle of change' model in Fig. 7.1).
- When consulting, give brief advice on stopping tobacco use.
- If patient wants to stop using tobacco, refer to the local NHS stop smoking service.
- In addition, in patients with pre-existing respiratory and cardiovascular disease, consider the use of nicotine replacement therapy, varenicline or bupropion.

'Cycle of Change' Model (Prochaska and DiClemente)

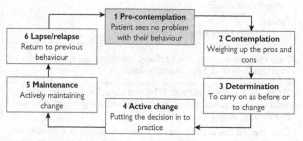

Fig. 7.1 'Cycle of change' model (Prochaska and DiClemente).

- Identify where the patient currently fits in on the 'cycle of change' – if they do not perceive smoking as a problem, then they are unlikely to be successful in trying to stop smoking.
- Explore the patient's view of the problem:
  - *'What problems do you see with smoking?'*
- Discuss motivation:
  - *'What do you enjoy about smoking?'* or
  - *'Why do you want to stop smoking now?'*
- Give practical advice on stopping smoking:
  - *'Plan a quit day, and stick to it.'*
  - *'Prepare for vulnerable times (e.g. times of increased stress).'*
  - *'Plan a daily routine that includes activities to keep occupied.'*
  - *'Spend time with non-smokers.'*
- Facilitate the patient around the cycle – providing information, supportive advice and reassurance as appropriate.

Useful websites

British Thoracic Society: http://www.brit-thoracic.org.uk
Medicines Adherence: http://www.nice.org.uk/CG76
Smoking Cessation Services: http://www.nice.org.uk/PH010
The Cycle of Change and Drugs and Alcohol Treatment: http://www.alcohol-drugs.co.uk

Scenario 11

Information for the candidate

Your role
You are the specialty registrar (ST2) in the renal clinic.

Problem
Discussing end stage renal failure in a patient with systemic lupus erythematosus (SLE).

Patient
Ms Anita Socchi, a 43-year-old woman.

Please read the scenario which follows. When the bell sounds, enter the examination room to begin the consultation.

Ms Socchi was diagnosed with SLE 8 years ago. She is currently taking hydroxychloroquine and mycophenolate mofetil and is under the care of a rheumatologist.

Over the last few months she has been complaining of increasing lethargy, and investigations have unfortunately revealed a progressive deterioration in her renal function. Her estimated glomerular filtration rate (eGFR) is 13mL/min, and a recent ultrasound scan has revealed 2 small kidneys. Consequently she has been referred to the renal clinic for consideration of renal replacement therapy, and specifically the option of renal transplantation.

Your task is to speak to Ms Socchi regarding her deteriorating renal function and discuss with her the option of renal transplantation.

Information for the actor

You are a single parent with 5-year-old twin boys. You work part-time as a ward clerk at the local hospital.

You were diagnosed with systemic lupus erythematosus (SLE) 8 years ago after complaining of painful wrists and hands, and have been under the care of a rheumatologist since that time. Until 6 months ago, your disease had been well-controlled with hydroxychloroquine tablets. You had always attended for regular blood test monitoring and an eye examination annually with your optician as part of your treatment.

6 months ago you began to feel more tired, and initially attributed this to doing extra hours at work to cover staff sickness. Over the past few months you have needed more frequent blood tests as your rheumatologist has informed you that some of the kidney tests were abnormal. You have been treated with oral steroids and had a new medication mycophenolate mofetil.

Your father died suddenly of a heart attack 4 months ago. You have also recently found out that one of your sons is being bullied at school and this has been causing additional stress within the family.

You feel that your tiredness is probably due to recent stressful events. You do not realize how serious the problem is with your kidneys, and are completely shocked to hear the mention of a kidney transplant. You are reluctant to be admitted to hospital for any period of time, as you do not trust your ex-partner looking after your sons. You had previously refused intravenous steroids for this reason.

Questions you might ask
- 'Surely I can just increase some of my tablets again?'
- 'Where would the donated kidney come from?'
- 'How long would I have to wait for a transplant?'
- 'What would happen if I do not have a kidney transplant?'

Discussing end-stage renal disease
Check understanding
Establish the patient's knowledge of her disease, especially regarding the deterioration in her condition 6 months ago.

Explain end-stage renal disease
- Give her information a little bit at a time, check understanding frequently and acknowledge and respond to verbal and non-verbal cues and emotions along the way.
- Explain how the kidneys have an important role in removing waste products from the body, helping make new blood cells (erythropoiesis) and regulating essential salts in the body (potassium, phosphate and calcium).
- Inform her that her kidney function has continued to deteriorate. Make it clear that, unfortunately, her kidneys are now failing and that this is a life threatening problem.
- Explain that increasing the dose of the medication which she had been taking has not controlled her disease sufficiently, and that further

medication (either tablets or intravenously) will not be able to improve her kidney function.

Renal replacement therapy

Outline the possible options:

- *Haemodialysis* (hospital-based or home-based): haemodialysis requires the formation of an arteriovenous fistula or the insertion of a permanent dialysis line
- *Peritoneal dialysis:* this requires the insertion of a peritoneal dialysis catheter into the abdomen.
- *Transplantation:*
  - There are 2 types of transplants: cadaveric and living (related or unrelated).
  - Transplantation is possible pre-emptively (i.e. before dialysis is started) or after dialysis has started.

Additional considerations

Depending on the results of blood tests, she may need to start treatment with:

- Erythropoietin subcutaneously to help her anaemia.
- Intravenous iron (oral iron not absorbed well in renal failure).
- 1α-calcidol to help replace calcium.

Multidisciplinary team working will include the dietician (as she may need to reduce dietary potassium and phosphate, and if phosphate levels are very high she may need to start a phosphate binder).

Dialysis should be viewed as a temporary measure. In the longer term she would be a potential candidate for a renal transplant which is the gold standard of treatment for most patients, and this should result in returning to an almost normal lifestyle.

Ethical issues relating to renal transplantation

- Donor organs may become available from a cadaver or from a living donor. In general, transplants from a living donor function better and for longer.
- Living organ donation is always *non-conditional* (i.e. if a potential donor states that they would be willing to donate one of their kidneys on the condition that Ms Socchi agrees to marry them, then this is clearly *not* ethically acceptable).
- Careful screening of a living donor for suitability is essential. The health of the donor is paramount, and it must be ensured that the donor's health is not compromised by the donation (e.g. the perioperative risk in a donor with COPD or the risk of developing end-stage renal failure in a donor with hypertension).
- The 'work-up' of a living donor can potentially reveal conditions or problems which were not known about before (e.g. previously undiagnosed HIV or awkward questions regarding paternity).
- Blood group or HLA incompatible transplants may be possible in more specialist centres, but would require a higher degree of immunosuppression.

- Post transplantation, she will need long-term care from the renal team. Compliance with medication and clinic appointments is essential to ensure optimal benefit of a transplant without risking rejection or complications from over-immunosuppression.

Human Tissue Act 2004

- Regulates removal, storage and use of human tissue.
- Makes consent the fundamental principle underpinning the lawful removal and use of body parts, organs and tissue.
- Establishes a Human Tissue Authority to advise on and oversee compliance with the act.
- Provides a number of exceptions to the general rule that appropriate consent is always required in order to store human tissue (e.g. consent is not needed for the use of surplus or 'residual' tissue taken from a living patient which is left over from a diagnostic or surgical procedure.
- Any commercial dealings in organs for transplantation are prohibited.
- Before organ donation, the donor must be interviewed by an independent assessor who is fully familiar with the Human Tissue Act and is not a member of the renal or transplant team.

Useful websites

British Kidney Patient Association: http://www.britishkidney-pa.co.uk
Human Tissue Authority: http://www.hta.gov.uk
Kidney research UK: http://www.kidneyresearchuk.org/home.php
Mykidney website: http://www.mykidney.org.uk

Scenario 12

Information for the candidate

Your role

You are the specialty registrar in the rheumatology clinic.

Problem

Discussing the use of monoclonal antibody therapy with a patient who has rheumatoid arthritis.

Patient

Miss Kelly Chamberlain, a 34-year-old woman.

Please read the scenario which follows. When the bell sounds, enter the examination room to begin the consultation.

Background to Scenario

Miss Chamberlain was diagnosed with rheumatoid arthritis 4 years ago. She is currently under the care of a rheumatologist, although often fails to attend her outpatient clinic appointments.

She was started on methotrexate 3 years ago, and has been taking this intermittently since. She repeatedly fails to attend for blood tests for methotrexate monitoring and consequently her methotrexate prescriptions have often been withheld by her GP. Her joints have remained active and symptomatic.

Her GP has referred her back to the rheumatology clinic as she is demanding to try a new monoclonal antibody treatment that she has read about on an Internet website.

Your task is to speak to Miss Chamberlain regarding her suitability for monoclonal antibody therapy.

Information for the actor

You are married and have 3 young children aged under 5 years old. You work in a call centre for a bank in the evenings.

You were diagnosed with rheumatoid arthritis 4 years ago and there is a family history of this condition in your mother. Following your diagnosis, you were initially started on sulphasalazine but became intolerant of this medication due to gastrointestinal side effects. Shortly afterwards, you were switched onto methotrexate tablets, although you have had long periods off this treatment. You have repeatedly missed blood tests and outpatient clinic appointments, and consequently your GP has withheld repeat prescriptions for methotrexate.

You are annoyed that your prescriptions keep getting stopped, and do not understand why you should need to have blood tests so frequently when you are feeling otherwise well. Your youngest child has cerebral palsy and has been particularly unwell over the last year with recurrent hospital admissions.

Your mother has been receiving a new injection treatment for her rheumatoid arthritis and you have researched this further on the Internet. You are very keen to try this new treatment, as it appears to be a much easier option and has really helped your mother. You have asked your GP to refer you back to a rheumatologist to discuss this further.

Questions you might ask

- 'My Mum is getting this treatment which has made her a real difference to her, so why can't I have it as well?'
- 'Are you refusing the treatment because it's expensive?'
- 'My Dad is willing to pay for a private consultation – would I be able to get the treatment then?'

Use of monoclonal antibody treatment in rheumatoid arthritis

The benefits and risks of biologic treatment in the management of rheumatoid arthritis need to be considered carefully (➔ p. 495 and Useful websites, p. 438).

There are several issues highlighted in this case

- Establish why she is unable to comply with the recommended disease-modifying antirheumatic drug (DMARD) treatment.
- Explain that methotrexate has potential side effects that have to be monitored by regular blood tests.
- Establish why she wants to have a biologic treatment.
- It will be important to establish how severely affected her mother is as this may help to explain her wish to commence biologic treatment. Miss Chamberlain may have accompanied her mother to hospital appointments and seen other patients with rheumatoid arthritis being wheelchair bound, which is much less common in today's arthritis clinics.
- Clarify to her that more aggressive treatment, which includes DMARDs, is currently commenced immediately following diagnosis, and that this has had a significant impact on disease progression.

- Explain that when taken regularly, DMARD therapy can lead to good control of rheumatoid arthritis, avoiding the need to consider anti-TNF therapy.
- Explain that under existing NICE and British Society for Rheumatology (BSR) guidelines she is not currently eligible for anti-TNF therapy, although this does not imply that this treatment would not be offered to her should she fulfil the criteria in the future:
  - Biologic therapies have potential serious side effects including life-threatening infections, malignancy and induction of SLE or demyelinating disease.
  - If eligible for anti-TNF therapy this patient will still require monitoring.
  - Most patients are also prescribed a DMARD, which will necessitate more frequent monitoring.
  - Each of the biologics have a different regimen (most are subcutaneously administered; others such as infliximab require repeated venepuncture, usually every 2 months). Infliximab therefore has an advantage if compliance is felt to be an issue.
- The patient should be encouraged to give methotrexate a fair trial.
- Candidates should recognize the importance of a multidisciplinary team approach:
  - She will need to agree to make a special effort with monitoring. Explore ways in which monitoring can be made easier for her (for example attending the GP surgery).
  - Offer an early follow-up out-patient appointment with the rheumatology clinical nurse specialist as she may value the opportunity to discuss any difficulty with medication, fears etc.

The NICE Guidelines recommend a TNFα inhibitor (adalimumab, etanercept and infliximab, and more recently certolizumab pegol and golimumab) as possible treatments for people with rheumatoid arthritis who:
- have already tried methotrexate and another DMARD, and
- have 'active' rheumatoid arthritis, as assessed by a rheumatologist on 2 separate occasions.

People who are given anti-TNF treatment should normally also be given methotrexate.

UK guidelines outlined by NICE and BSR have been developed to take account of cost effectiveness of biologic agents. Current NICE guidelines recommend biological therapies as options for the treatment of adults who have the following characteristics:
- active RA (as measured by DAS-28 >5.1) with at least 3 or more tender and 3 or more swollen joints; and
- have undergone trials of 2 DMARDs, including methotrexate (unless contraindicated). A trial of DMARDs is defined as at least 2 DMARDs usually given concurrently over a 6-month period, with 2 months at standard doses, unless significant toxicity has limited the dose or duration of treatment.

Rationing expensive treatments: ethical principles

In the context of healthcare, rationing implies that resources will be denied or redistributed to certain patients. The Society of Critical Care Medicine defined rationing as: 'the allocation of healthcare resources in the face of limited availability, which necessarily means that beneficial interventions are withheld from some individuals'.

Across the NHS, there are various examples of rationing on a daily basis. Allocating our time to certain patients, triaging of critical care or high dependency beds, withholding diagnostic procedures in patients who are unlikely to benefit, and deciding how aggressively to treat certain patients with end of life diseases are all examples. Rationing, in a sense, might be the ethical thing to do. The ethical principle of justice would support this: 'the greater good for everyone concerned'.

The other key ethical principles highlighted in this case include:

Autonomy: as a competent adult, Miss Chamberlain has the right to control decision-making over own health needs. However, no one has the right to demand treatments which are considered futile.

Beneficence: 'Doing good for the sick'. Miss Chamberlain has active rheumatoid arthritis and biological drugs are available which can potentially improve her quality of life. The principle of beneficence argues that she should be entitled to receive these treatments.

Maleficence: 'To cause no harm'. This principle considers that Miss Chamberlain may not actually derive further benefit from treatment escalation. In fact, such treatment may do more harm than good – either by causing side effects or by prolonging suffering by prolonging the quantity but not quality of life.

The following model summarizes the key principles underpinning rationing of healthcare, and may be useful when justifying or explaining difficult decisions to patients, such as in this scenario:

- Resources are limited.
- Help patients understand the consequences of limits and the need to be fair.
- Change to thinking as the 'most benefit per pound'.
- Focus on populations rather than individuals.
- Ineffective treatments given to one individual limit the resources available for other patients.

National Institute for Health and Clinical Excellence (NICE)

NICE is an NHS organization based in London and Manchester set up on 1 April 1999. It has a role in rationing and streamlining healthcare. It aims to ensure that everyone has equal access to medical treatments and high-quality care from the NHS – regardless of where they live in England and Wales.

NICE makes recommendations to the NHS on:

- New and existing medicines, treatments and procedures.
- Treating and caring for people with specific diseases and conditions.
- How to improve people's health and prevent illness and disease.

NICE guidelines are frequently followed in Scotland. The equivalent body is NHS Quality Improvement Scotland.

ℬ Useful websites

Eligibility criteria for BSR and BHPR rheumatoid arthritis guidelines on eligibility criteria for the first biological therapy: http:// www.rheumatology.org.uk/resources/guidelines/bsr_guidelines.aspx

NHS Quality Improvement Scotland: http://www.nhshealthquality.org

NICE. *Adalimumab, etanercept and infliximab for the treatment of rheumatoid arthritis.* London: NICE, 2007. Available at: http://www.nice.org.uk/TA130.

NRAS National Rheumatoid Arthritis Society (provides support and information for people with Rheumatoid Arthritis): http://www.nras.org.uk

📖 Further reading

Bloomfield EL. The ethics of rationing of critical care services: Should technology assessment play a role? *Anesthesiol Res Pract* 2009; **pii:** 915–197.

Deighton C et al. BSR and BHPR rheumatoid arthritis guidelines on eligibility criteria for the first biological therapy. *Rheumatology (Oxford)* 2010; **49**(6):1197–9.

Eddy DM. Oregon's methods: did cost-effectiveness analysis fail?' *JAMA* 1991; **266**(15): 2135–41.

Levy MM. Rationing in the ICU. In: *Proceedings of the Society of Critical Care Medicine: 34th Critical Care Congress.* Phoenix, AZ, January 2005.

Viva questions: Chronic disease management (scenarios 10–12)

What is your feeling about patients with asthma having a supply of antibiotics and oral steroids at home to use in case of acute exacerbations?

- This strategy may be beneficial to asthmatic patients who:
  - Experience recurrent acute exacerbations.
  - Are able to identify the early signs of an acute exacerbation.
  - Have a good understanding of their condition, knowing exactly how and when to use the medication.
- Patient education is key to this 'self-escalation' strategy. Careful selection should include those:
  - Who realize that they still need to see a health professional for early review (and to obtain further supplies of stand-by medication).
  - Who understand when it is *not* appropriate to use this approach (e.g. in severe acute asthma).

Regular review should identify those who escalate their treatment inappropriately (e.g. excessive oral steroid use).

How would you respond if a patient with end-stage renal disease told you that they didn't want to receive a kidney from a donor with a specific ethnic background?

- As doctors, some of our patients will express prejudicial views from time to time, but we must remain professional and be mindful of our reactions – however much we may disagree with their views.
- Explore their thoughts and ask them gently what has prompted them to express this wish.
- Do they have any specific concerns? If they are hesitant in elaborating further, be explicit:
  - *'Some patients are concerned about catching infections such as HIV – is this something that you were worried about . . .?'*
- Briefly explain the general shortage of suitable organs, being mindful of the potential to evoke feelings of guilt in the patient.
- Explaining the donation process may help – all blood and organ donors are screened before they are allowed to donate, and donated organs and blood products are rigorously tested for infections such as hepatitis and HIV.

- The organs (or blood) are then matched very closely to a particular patient according to genetic make-up, to minimize the risk of any problems to the recipient.
- Applying the principle of blood donation may help to rationalize their thoughts:
  - Blood donors come from all ethnicities.
  - This increases the diversity of the pool of donors.
  - Thereby optimizing the donor–recipient match.
- Tell them clearly that it is not possible to specify any restrictions with regard to the donor. In addition, it is important to emphasize that the demand for organs far outweighs donor availability.
- Offer them an appointment with one of the transplant liaison team to discuss any issues further.
- Addressing specific concerns, education and reassurance is the key to successfully managing a potentially awkward situation.

Scenario 13

Information for the candidate

Your role

You are the specialty registrar on the stroke ward.

Problem

Discussing the prognosis and resuscitation status of a patient with her son.

Patient's son

Mr John Kershaw, a 47-year-old man.

Patient

Mrs Brenda Kershaw, a 79-year-old woman.

Please read the scenario which follows. When the bell sounds, enter the examination room to begin the consultation.

Background to Scenario

Mrs Kershaw was admitted to the surgical admission unit 3 days ago with acute cholecystitis. She was commenced on intravenous fluids and antibiotics. Unfortunately she was found unresponsive by nursing staff later that afternoon, and a subsequent CT head scan confirmed an extensive haemorrhagic stroke.

She has a past medical history of hypertension, diabetes mellitus and vascular dementia.

She remains poorly responsive, and has now been transferred to the stroke ward, where she is continuing to receive intravenous fluids and antibiotics. The stroke consultant has since made the decision that Mrs Kerhshaw should not be resuscitated in the event of a cardiorespiratory arrest.

Mrs Kershaw's son, who is also her next of kin has arrived this morning to visit her. He has asked to speak to you today regarding his mother.

Your task is to speak to Mr Kershaw regarding his mother's current condition, including discussion of her resuscitation status.

Information for the actor

You live over 200 miles away from your mother. She has no other living relatives and you are her next of kin. You work as a headteacher at a secondary school and are divorced with a young daughter.

Your mother was diagnosed with dementia 3 years ago, and has since gradually deteriorated. She has lived in a residential home for the past year. You last saw her 6 months ago on her birthday and generally find it difficult to visit because of work commitments and the time involved in travelling.

You received a telephone call from a staff nurse yesterday evening explaining that your mother had been admitted to hospital with a severe gallbladder infection. You have arrived at the hospital today to see her and are alarmed to find out that she has been transferred to the stroke ward.

You have asked to speak to one of the doctors on the stroke ward to find out more about her condition.

Questions you might ask
- 'Why did she have a stroke?'
- 'Is she in any pain?'
- 'Why are you asking me about resuscitating her – is she about to die?'

Discussing cardiopulmonary resuscitation (CPR) with relatives

- Confirm his relationship to the patient, and ascertain the presence of any other relatives, to avoid repeated discussions with different family members.
- If the patient has capacity to give consent, then ask permission to discuss their care with their relatives.
- As Mrs Kershaw does not have capacity to give consent, then it would be considered to be in her best interests for relevant aspects of her medical care to be discussed with her son.
- Check his understanding of his mother's health prior to her admission.
- Explain that she is now very unwell following a stroke and discuss her likely prognosis and current treatment.
- Explain the importance for advance planning of her ongoing care:
  - *'Your mother is very poorly, and we need to make sure that we make the right decisions for her, should her condition deteriorate . . .'*
- Approach the subject of CPR, checking his understanding at each stage:
  - *'Although this is a difficult subject to talk about, if your mother's heart was to stop beating, or if she was to stop breathing, we need to consider what we would actually do at that stage, and whether we would try to restart her heart and breathing with emergency treatment called CPR . . . this would involve repeatedly pushing down very firmly on the chest and using electric shocks to the heart . . .'*
- Ask whether his mother had ever expressed any views or wishes regarding CPR.
- Enquire to his views regarding CPR.

- Explain the medical team's view regarding CPR for Mrs Kershaw, and that accordingly a 'Do Not Attempt Resuscitation' decision has been made, as this is considered to be in her best interests.
- Make clear that this decision relates to CPR only, and that this is not an 'all-or-none' decision about her care – she will continue to receive active treatment that is appropriate for her (e.g. intravenous fluids and antibiotics).
- Shock and possibly guilt, which are common feelings experienced by relatives in this situation may result in unusually aggressive behaviour or irrational thoughts – it is important to consider and acknowledge these emotions as appropriate.

Cardiopulmonary resuscitation (CPR)

- Has a low success rate, especially for patients who are in poor general health.
- May do more harm than good by prolonging the dying process and the pain and suffering of a seriously ill patient.
- If used inappropriately, may be seen as degrading and undignified.
- Decisions regarding CPR should ideally be made in advance as part of the care plan for the patient, following discussion with the patient and or relatives.
- There is no obligation however, to provide treatment that is considered futile. The final decision about the merits of attempting resuscitation rests with the most senior clinician in charge of the patient's care.

Withholding life-prolonging treatment

- Withholding or withdrawing treatment is regarded in law as an 'omission', rather than an 'act'.
- Life-prolonging treatment (e.g. intravenous fluids) may lawfully be withheld or withdrawn from an incompetent patient when continuing or commencing treatment is not in their best interests.
- Where an adult patient has become incompetent, a refusal of treatment made when the patient was competent (advance decision to refuse treatment) must be respected.
- 'The right to life' and 'the prohibition to inhuman or degrading treatment' as outlined in **The Human Rights Act 1998** are important in informing medical decision-making in this area.

✍ Useful websites

Cardiopulmonary Resuscitation Standards for Clinical Practice and Training: http://www.resus. org.uk

The Human Rights Act 1998: http://www.opsi.gov.uk/acts/acts1998

Withholding and Withdrawing Life-Prolonging Treatments: http://www.gmc-uk.org/guidance

Scenario 14

Information for the candidate

Your role
You are the specialty registrar on the oncology ward.

Problem
Discussing the management of a terminally ill patient, with her daughter.

Patient's daughter
Mrs Denise Harrison, a 59-year-old woman.

Patient
Mrs Elizabeth Williams, an 85-year-old woman.

Please read the scenario which follows. When the bell sounds, enter the examination room to begin the consultation.

Background to Scenario

Mrs Williams was diagnosed with endometrial cancer 4 years ago, for which she had a total abdominal hysterectomy. Unfortunately she developed recurrent disease 3 months ago, and currently has hepatic and bony metastases.

A palliative approach has been agreed between Mrs Williams and her consultants, and no further active treatment is planned.

Unfortunately, she was admitted to the oncology ward at the weekend with poorly controlled back pain.

Mrs Williams' daughter, Mrs Harrison has expressed concern at the continuing pain that her mother is experiencing. She has asked to speak to you today to see if anything else can be done to relieve her mother's distress and help her to die in peace.

Your task is to speak to Mrs Harrison regarding her mother's current condition, and management.

Information for the actor

You live and work on a farm with your husband. You have a daughter and grandson who both live abroad.

Your mother had a hysterectomy for cancer of the womb 4 years ago, but has recently learned that the cancer has returned and now spread to her liver and bones. It has since been decided that she will not receive any further active treatment for her cancer, which you are unhappy with, as you felt that this decision was based purely on her age.

Unfortunately she was admitted to hospital at the weekend with severe back pain. She is currently quite drowsy as a result of the strong pain-killers that she is being given. You feel that your mother has been through a lot in the last few years, and now deserves to rest in peace and be free of pain and distress. If she cannot be cured of her cancer, then you believe that she should not have to suffer any longer.

You have asked to speak to the doctor today to see if your mother can be given a strong injection to help her die peacefully.

Questions you might ask
- 'Why has she suddenly developed this back pain?'
- 'She didn't want to die in hospital – can she come back home with us?'
- 'Can't you just give her something to put her out of her misery? Animals get better treatment than this.'

Discussing end of life care with relatives
- Acknowledge the daughter's sadness of seeing her mother in the terminal stages of her illness.
- Listen to her specific concerns.
- Explain that the aim of palliative care is to minimize pain and other distressing symptoms at the end of life, and so adequate analgesia will be administered to control her mother's pain.
- Establish her mother's prior wishes (if known), and explain that these will be integrated into the planning and delivery of her end of life care where possible.
- As the daughter gains understanding of aspects of palliative care, she may well move away from her initial thoughts of assisted dying. In the event that these thoughts remain, explain that assisted dying (e.g. giving a lethal injection with the intent of ending life) is currently illegal in the UK.
- Advise her that community palliative care services can be arranged in her mother's own home in keeping with her prior wishes.
- Remember the role of the multidisciplinary palliative care team, including spiritual carers (e.g. chaplain) for both the patient and relatives.

Advanced care planning
- Involves discussion between a patient, their care providers and relatives (or those close to them).

- An Advance Statement details patients' wishes and preferences.
- An Advance Decision to Refuse Treatment:
  - Only applies to medical treatment.
  - Can only be made by a patient whilst they still have capacity.
  - Only becomes active when they lose capacity.
  - Must be specific about the treatment that is being refused and the circumstances in which the refusal will apply.

Liverpool care pathway

- Used in the final phase of terminal illness – the last few days and weeks.
- Transfers the hospice model of care into other care settings.
- Multiprofessional document which provides an evidence-based framework for end of life care.
- Designed to deliver high-quality proactive care to dying patients and their relatives, regardless of diagnosis or place of death (diagnosis does not have to be cancer e.g. can include end-stage heart failure).
- Includes attention to psychological and spiritual care and family support.

Assisted dying

- Is currently illegal in the UK.
- Is legally and morally different to the withholding or withdrawal of treatment.
- Raises issues regarding *autonomy* (i.e. the right to decide to end one's life) and *non-maleficence* (the duty of the doctor to do no harm)
- Encompasses:
  - *Euthanasia:* where someone other than the patient administers a fatal injection.
  - *Assisted suicide:* where patients are assisted to end their own lives.
- Consider whether there has been adequate provision of quality palliative care services in patients requesting assisted dying.

Doctrine of double effect

- Administration of large doses of medication to reduce pain or suffering may consequently hasten a patient's death.
- This is legal providing that the *intention* was to relieve pain or suffering (rather than to cause or hasten death).

◌ Useful websites

Advance Care Planning: http://www.rcplondon.ac.uk
End-of-Life Decisions: http://www.bma.org.uk
Liverpool Care Pathway: http://www.mcpcil.org.uk

Scenario 15

Information for the candidate

Your role

You are the specialty registrar on the rheumatology ward.

Problem

Discussion with a foundation year 1 (FY1) colleague regarding their professional behaviour.

Colleague

Dr Anil Desai, a 24-year-old man.

Please read the scenario which follows. When the bell sounds, enter the examination room to begin the consultation.

Background to Scenario

Dr Desai is currently an FY1 doctor with whom you work on the rheumatology ward.

There have been various concerns raised regarding Dr Desai's behaviour over the past few weeks. Nursing staff have complained that he has been rude and shouted at them in front of patients on several occasions. More seriously, the ward manager claims that she could smell alcohol on his breath on a ward round last week.

You have noticed that recently he is late for ward rounds and outpatient clinics, and is often uncontactable for large periods of the day, without explanation. Last week a verbal complaint was received from a patient regarding his inappropriate and casual dress on the ward.

Your consultant is currently on annual leave, and the ward manager has therefore asked you to speak to Dr Desai urgently in relation to these events, as she is concerned that his attitude and behaviour is affecting patient care.

Your task is to speak to Dr Desai regarding his recent professional behaviour.

Information for the actor

You are a foundation year doctor (FY1) in rheumatology. You have been revising for postgraduate exams for the last 5 months as you had been planning to emigrate to Canada with your fiancée.

Unfortunately, you found out last month that your fiancée was having an affair. You have since separated and left the family home, and are now living in hospital accommodation.

In the last 3 weeks you have become increasingly withdrawn and have started drinking alcohol heavily. As a result, you have often overslept and arrived for morning ward rounds late and with a hangover. You have become more irritable, and often find yourself shouting at the nursing staff. Last week you reduced one of the student nurses to tears.

Your life seems to have been turned upside-down in a matter of a few weeks, and you cannot see a solution to your current problems.

Your specialty registrar colleague (who is 3 years your senior) has asked to speak to you urgently before today's ward round. You expect this to be a quick question regarding an audit presentation tomorrow, and are shocked to be confronted regarding your recent behaviour.

Questions you might ask
- 'What right have you got to speak to me like this? – This is none of your business.'
- 'You won't tell the consultant, will you?'
- 'What do you think I should do next?'

Discussing inappropriate behaviour with a colleague
- Aspects of life outside work will impact in the working environment.
- The aim of the discussion is to encourage the doctor to accept that his outside life has changed his work behaviour.
- Explain the purpose of the discussion, and give a warning shot:
  - *'There's something serious that I need to talk to you about.'*
  - *'I need to speak to you about certain concerns that have been raised by some of the medical and nursing staff on the ward.'*
- Give him time to reflect on this and allow him to respond:
  - *'Actually, we have been genuinely worried about you over the last few weeks, as your behaviour seems to have changed.'*
- Acknowledge the difficulty of this discussion for both of you, given that you actually work together as colleagues.
- Discussion with a fellow health professional requires skill – avoid being patronizing, but at the same time do not assume knowledge (even if they are a doctor) as the stress of the situation can cause chaotic thinking, even in the most measured individuals.
- Enquire about any current stressors that may be responsible for his behaviour change.
  - *'Is there anything that has been troubling you recently?'*
- Use gentle prompts to encourage him to reflect on his own behaviour – this is less likely to result in confrontation than an interrogatory approach.

- Show empathy towards his current difficult circumstances, and acknowledge that these events would cause stress and some degree of behaviour change in most people in the same situation.
- Enquire to his psychological well-being:
  - *'I know that this may seem like a difficult question, but do you think that you might actually be depressed?'*
- Ask about his alcohol use, and then explain the most serious concern that has been raised regarding the allegation of him smelling of alcohol.
- Explain that you both have a duty to act – as together you must make the care of patients your first concern.
- Suggest that in the first instance he may benefit from some time off work.
- Explain that people at work can help him to change his work behaviour by signposting to sources of support regarding his problems outside of work (e.g. relationship counselling).
- Advise that he arranges to see the occupational health department and his GP for further confidential advice and support.
- Mention other sources of self-help (Ⓢ Supporting doctors in difficulty, see below).
- Remind him of the need for him to speak to his consultant, and suggest booking an appointment with protected time for discussion:
  - *'The consultant will obviously need to be aware of your current situation and what has been happening – this will be better coming from you, rather than him hearing it secondhand from anybody else.'*

Good medical practice[1]

- You should support colleagues who have problems with performance or health.
- You must protect patients from risk of harm posed by another colleague's conduct, performance or health.
- You must raise any concerns with an appropriate person from your employing or contracting body.
- If unsure how to proceed, discuss your concerns with an impartial colleague, defence body, professional organization or GMC for advice.
- All doctors should be registered with a GP to ensure access to independent and objective medical care.

Supporting doctors in difficulty

- Encourage colleagues to seek advice from the occupational health department or their GP at an early stage as mental illness is common amongst health professionals, and may require treatment.
- Signpost to self-help groups, e.g. Doctors' Support Network, which can advise on issues such as accommodation, addiction, bereavements, relationships and stress.
- Suggest that they speak with their educational supervisor and possibly the postgraduate deanery – modification of their training programme (e.g. less than full-time training) may be helpful in some circumstances.
- Consider what the concerns are e.g. do they relate to clinical competence or probity?
- Concerns about a doctor should be dealt with at a local level where possible (e.g. consultant, medical director or chief executive).

National Clinical Assessment Service (NCAS)

- Provides an advisory role to healthcare organizations regarding doctors, dentists and pharmacists in difficulty.
- Can advise on the handling of concerns.
- Have effective local systems for handling poor performance.
- Will carry out assessments of professionals if there are concerns about poor performance.

General Medical Council (GMC)

- Is made up of doctors and lay members.
- Can take action if a doctor's fitness to practice is impaired, and resolution at a local level has failed.

Reference

1. GMC. *Good Medical Practice*, 2006. Available at: http://www.gmc-uk.org/guidance/good_medical_practice.asp.

Useful websites

Doctors' Support Network: http://www.dsn.org.uk
National Clinical Assessment Service: http://www.ncas.npsa.nhs.uk
Resources for Doctors in Difficulty: http://www.bma.org.uk/doctors_health

Scenario 16

Information for the candidate

Your role
You are the specialty registrar on the diabetes ward.

Problem
Discussion with a foundation year 2 (FY2) doctor regarding a clinical incident.

Colleague
Dr Hannah Somerby, a 25-year-old woman.

Please read the scenario which follows. When the bell sounds, enter the examination room to begin the consultation.

Background to Scenario

Dr Somerby is currently a foundation year 2 (FY2) doctor with whom you work on the diabetes ward.

You have just discovered that a patient who was discharged from your ward 2 weeks ago has been re-admitted under the care of your team with neutropenic sepsis.

The clinical notes from 2 weeks ago show that the patient was taking carbamazepine 100mg daily for trigeminal neuralgia. Unfortunately however, he was discharged with carbimazole 100mg instead of carbamazepine, as Dr Somerby entered the drug information incorrectly on to the computerized discharge letter.

The patient is clinically stable and not expected to experience any permanent adverse effects. He is unaware of the medication error, although his family is enquiring as to the nature of his admission.

Dr Somerby is currently unaware that the patient has been re-admitted to hospital.

Your task is to speak to Dr Somerby regarding this clinical incident.

Information for the actor

You are a foundation year 2 (FY2) doctor working on the diabetes ward. You started this post 3 weeks ago after rotating from another hospital in the region. Unfortunately you missed the trust induction last week as you had just finished working a night shift at your previous hospital.

Consequently, you are still familiarizing yourself with completing computerized rather than handwritten discharge letters, which you have not done before. Your specialty registrar has asked to speak to you regarding a medication error on a patient who was discharged from your ward 2 weeks ago, and has now been re-admitted to the acute medical unit.

Initially you are shocked and embarrassed to learn of this incident, as this is the first time that you have made such a serious clinical error. However, you soon become angry and frustrated as you feel that you should have received a proper induction, including training on how to complete computerized discharge letters.

Questions you might ask
- 'Do we have to tell the patient about this?'
- 'Will I face disciplinary action because of this?'
- 'Will this affect my application to enter specialist training?'

Discussing clinical errors with a colleague
- Make sure that you have read the necessary documentation regarding the incident (the copy of the discharge prescription in this case).
- Explain the reason for the discussion, and give a warning shot:
  - *'There's something serious I need to speak to you about.'*
  - *'I wanted to talk to you about a clinical incident on one of our patients who was unfortunately discharged with the wrong medication . . .'*
- Allow her time to respond – is she already aware of this incident?
- Have the clinical notes available (including a hard copy of the computerized prescription), and adopt a non-threatening and non-judgemental manner to encourage openness and honesty.
- Confirm the error and other possible parties involved (e.g. pharmacist checking or dispensing the medication).
- Consider 'system errors' (e.g. limitations or faults with the computerized discharge procedure).
- Listen to her ideas and concerns regarding the cause(s) of the error.
- Remember common causes of clinical error, and discuss these where appropriate: poor communication, personal ill health, poor clinical knowledge, unfamiliar systems, repetitive tasks and high workload.
- Advise her that it is good clinical practice to discuss the event openly and honestly with the patient (and family), and to document the discussion in the clinical notes.
- Depending on the exact circumstances, it may be sensible to seek medico-legal advice from a medical defence union.
- Outline the importance of incident reporting and significant event analysis – particularly in identifying and preventing systematic errors (e.g. inadequate induction/training).

Reporting clinical incidents

- Allows NHS organizations to analyse the type, frequency and severity of incidents in an effort to make changes to improve patient care.
- Incidents that have occurred, incidents that have been prevented ('near-misses') and incidents that might happen (e.g. due to faulty equipment) should all be reported.
- Local incident-reporting systems exist in each hospital trust.
- For incidents and injuries to staff, patients and the public, completion of an Incident Record 1 (IR1) form is required.
- The IR1 form prompts as to whether the incident requires reporting to the Health and Safety Executive (HSE) as part of the Reporting of Injuries, Disease and Dangerous Occurrences Regulations 1995 (RIDDOR).
- The National Patient Safety Agency (NPSA) set up in 2001 acts as a single, confidential, national collection point for the reporting and analysis of adverse events and 'near misses' within the NHS.

Significant event analysis

- Aims to identify events in individual cases that have been critical and to improve the quality of patient care from the lessons learnt.
- Encourages a culture of openness and reflective learning.
- Can be used as important evidence of learning in annual appraisal.
- Includes 7 stages:
  1. Identify significant event.
  2. Collate information.
  3. Facilitated team-based meeting.
  4. Analysis of the significant event.
  5. Agree, implement and monitor change.
  6. Write it up.
  7. Report, share and review findings.

℘ Useful websites

Learning from Prescribing Errors: eprints.pharmacy.ac.uk/358/1/Deanpreserrorsqshc.pdf
National Patient Safety Agency: http://www.npsa.nhs.uk
Management for Doctors: http://www.gmc-uk.org/guidance
Significant Event Analysis: http://www.nes.scot.nhs.uk/sea

Viva questions: Speaking to relatives and colleagues (scenarios 13–16)

At the end of your morning post-take ward round your foundation year 1 (FY1) tells you that she has tonsillitis, and asks if you could prescribe her some amoxicillin. What would you say to her?

- Explain that you are sorry to hear that she is feeling unwell, however it is inappropriate for you to prescribe her antibiotics for several reasons:
  - A proper assessment of her condition should be carried out by an independent practitioner (occupational health department or her GP).
  - There are a number of other possible diagnoses (e.g. glandular fever, quinsy).
  - Consequently, the requested antibiotic may not be the appropriate management for her condition.
  - She may be reluctant to disclose certain aspects of her medical history (e.g. potential interaction of antibiotics with any co-prescribed oral contraceptive).

- Ask her whether she feels too unwell to be at work; if you have significant concerns regarding her health or potential risk to patients, you may need to inform your consultant.
- Further issues which make it inappropriate to prescribe antibiotics in this case include:
  - No access to her past medical record.
  - Inability to pursue further follow-up and correspondence with other healthcare professionals (e.g. GP).
- The GMC advises that wherever possible, doctors should avoid providing medical care to anyone with whom they have a close personal relationship (➔ Useful Websites).

The daughter of one your elderly patients approaches you explaining that her father is struggling to cope at home since his wife has been admitted to hospital. What would you say to her?

- If possible, arrange to meet together with the nurse in charge to enable the daughter to raise any specific concerns. If appropriate, include her mother (your patient) in this discussion.
- Explain that as her father is not your patient:
  - you can offer her some general advice on this matter, as this will not involve breaching any confidential medical information.
  - the responsibility for coordinating the services required would lie with her father's GP.
- Check a background social history and establish her views regarding her father's difficulties:
  - Are they physical (e.g. is he visually impaired?)
  - Are they psychological (e.g. does he forget to take his tablets)
  - Are they social? (e.g. is he self-caring?)
- Social services, who may be contacted by the family directly, can arrange a home assessment to determine any further social support required.
- Additional specific services can be instated on either a temporary or long-term basis, depending on the principal identified problems:
  - A 'Meals-on-Wheels' service can provide a hot meal every day if nutrition is a concern.
  - Citizens Advice Bureau can give advice regarding any further benefits or allowances that he may be entitled to claim.
  - Charities such as Age UK (previously called Age Concern) can offer support and advice regarding local services and useful products for older people (e.g. bath appliances).
- Day centres and locally-organized luncheon clubs can improve well-being and mood by facilitating social interaction.
- Respite care in a residential home may be a useful temporary solution if the support of community services has not been sufficient to meet his needs.

Useful websites

Age UK: http://www.ageuk.org.uk

GMC. *Good Medical Practice*, 2006. Available at: http://www.gmc-uk.org/guidance/good_medical_practice.asp.

Brief clinical consultation

Edited by
Rupa Bessant
Jonathan Birns

* Joint first authors
* Joint senior authors

Introduction

The brief clinical consultation station, which was introduced in the 3rd diet of the PACES examination in 2009, aims to assess the way in which the candidate approaches a clinical problem in an integrated manner, using history taking, examination and communication with a patient or a surrogate patient. The objective of this station is to reflect the way in which clinical problems are considered in the ward, emergency medical admissions unit, or medical outpatient clinic in normal clinical practice. During this station the candidate will be assessed on their ability to focus on the most important parts of history and examination when posed with a clinical problem. In addition, the candidate will be expected to explain their management plan succinctly to the patient and answer any questions they might have. Careful preparation for this station is vital, particularly as it carries a third of the overall marks of the PACES examination.

Procedure

There are 2 cases in this 20-minute station – each lasting 10 minutes. Candidates will be given written instructions for each of the 2 cases, usually in the form of short notes or referral letters, during the 5-minute interval before this station. During this time candidates ought to draw up a list of differential diagnoses based on the presenting complaint. They should plan the questions that they will need to ask and the most important aspects of the clinical examination that they will be required to perform in order to enable them to differentiate between these diagnoses. The timekeeper will sound a bell to signal the start of the station and 1 examiner will take the candidate into the first of the 2 cases.

Candidates will have 8 minutes to take a focused history, carry out a relevant examination, and respond to the patient's concerns. After 6 minutes have elapsed, candidates will be alerted that they have 2 minutes left with the patient. During the remaining 2 minutes, an examiner will ask the candidate to describe the positive physical findings and discuss the preferred diagnosis and any differential diagnosis as well as the management plan. If the physical findings and diagnosis have already been conveyed to the patient during the consultation, the examiners are likely to concentrate on issues related to patient management. In contrast, if the candidate has not covered appropriate aspects of the history and examination in the first 8 minutes, then the examiner may well ask questions regarding the areas omitted.

After 10 minutes, the candidate will be moved on to the second case and the same procedure will be repeated. As information related to both scenarios is given simultaneously and prior to starting the first of the two Station 5 cases, if needed, candidates are advised to ask the examiners for a few moments during which they re-read the next scenario. This will help to recall the planned approach or help to remember what differential diagnoses had been considered, although it is important to note that the 8 minute stopwatch will have already started!

History taking and clinical examination

8 minutes is a relatively short time for history taking, clinical examination, and a discussion of management and concerns with the patient. Therefore, the way in which candidates approach this station is very different to the formal examination of systems at Stations 1 and 3, and very different to the structured and comprehensive history taking and communication exercise at Stations 2 and 4.

An initial careful inspection for a few seconds may provide vital clues which may, for example, guide further questioning and examination. For example, if the scenario states that a patient has difficulty using their hands it may be quickly apparent that they have deformities suggesting rheumatoid arthritis and that the candidate should focus on this presumptive diagnosis rather than looking for a neurological cause for the patient's disability.

A brief history should confirm the initial findings on inspection or, if an underlying diagnosis is not immediately apparent, the early questions should establish the most likely diagnosis or differential diagnoses. Subsequently, candidates may examine the patient and take further aspects of the history in any order, or concurrently. For example, if a patient complains of a physical abnormality, the candidate may wish to examine the affected area whilst simultaneously asking the patient about relevant history.

The history must be adapted to focus on a specific symptom or disability. In most scenarios it is important to ascertain:

- Date of onset of symptoms (including any precipitating factors e.g. history of trauma if appropriate).
- Rate of progression (e.g. sudden onset strongly suggests a vascular aetiology, whereas gradual onset might indicate a compressive lesion).
- The presence and severity of any associated symptoms.
- Whether symptoms are constant or intermittent during the day.
- Investigations/treatment to date.
- Monitoring of disease and treatment.
- What effect the symptom/disability is having on the patient's activities of daily living.

There will also be a number of questions that are specific to a particular scenario and these should be prepared in the 5 minutes prior to commencing the Station 5 assessment. These will be highlighted as we deal with specific Station 5 scenarios.

Candidates should also be prepared to tailor their examination to specific cases and show the examiner that they are looking for associated clinical signs. For example, if the candidate assesses the patient to have a homonymous hemianopia on examination of their visual fields, it would be appropriate to examine for sensory and/or motor neurological deficits on the same side as well as feel the pulse and auscultate the heart for any cardioembolic source.

Marking

Each examiner has a structured marksheet for the cases and Station 5 is the only station in the PACES examination to cover all 7 of the clinical skills that are assessed:

- Clinical communication skills (C)
- Physical examination (A)
- Clinical judgement (E)
- Managing patients' concerns (F)
- Identifying physical signs (B)
- Differential diagnosis (D)
- Maintaining patient welfare (G).

As a result, **the marks awarded at Station 5 are proportionately greater than for Stations 1–4**. The maximum marks available for Station 5 equal 56 out of a possible total of 172 for the entire PACES examination. It is therefore crucial to practise for Station 5 by carrying out timed consultations with patients prior to the actual PACES examination.

The authors' of this chapter have all been involved in preparing PACES candidates for the Station 5 examination which has included simulated mock examination scenarios. Collectively, they have observed that candidates' time management is frequently poor and that they fail to focus adequately on the salient aspects of the scenarios. This highlights the need for candidates to practise undertaking as many Station 5 cases as possible prior to their examination in order to optimize their chances of demonstrating their ability to address the key history questions, undertake the relevant and important aspects of examination and discuss the key management issues with the patient, as well as incorporating the patient's concerns within the allocated 8 minutes.

Cases

The cases presented to candidates will all offer a clinical problem relevant to general or acute medicine that can be addressed in an 8-minute consultation and **may comprise any clinical problem encountered by trainee physicians in routine hospital medical practice**. The spectrum of conditions used in the examination is determined by a variety of factors including the availability of patients with demonstrable physical signs, the prejudice of the doctors choosing the cases and occasionally the specialty bias of the examination centre. In order to provide a representative sample of the types of cases likely to be encountered in Station 5, the authors have undertaken a survey of Station 5 cases experienced by candidates' during their PACES examination.[*] Of the 250 cases in this survey, 6 scenarios were demonstrated to occur frequently and together made up 46% of all cases encountered. Indeed, other cases never occurred >5% of the time. The 6 most commonly encountered cases were:

- Rheumatoid hands (29 cases)
- Thyroid status – hypothyroidism or hyperthyroidism (23 cases)
- Breathlessness (19 cases)
- Diabetic retinopathy (17 cases)
- Acromegaly (16 cases)
- Systemic sclerosis (12 cases).

[*]The authors would like to thank the candidates who attended the PassPACES course and participated in this survey.)

All cases surveyed to occur >5% of the time are described in this chapter or elsewhere to provide the candidate with the information required to succeed at this station.

The following cases, featured in the Station 5 survey, have been dealt with in other chapters:

• Neurology: carpal tunnel syndrome, peripheral neuropathy, stroke.
• Abdomen: inflammatory bowel disease, polycystic kidneys, alcoholic liver disease.

Although they have been covered in the chapters specified, the candidate needs to be aware of the symptomatic perspective in which they may be presented and the subsequent problem-based approach expected.

We have subdivided the chapter into sections pertaining to different relevant clinical subspecialities:

• Acute medicine
• Rheumatology
• Ophthalmology
• Endocrinology
• Dermatology.

Whilst any case may potentially be examined in this station, we aim to demonstrate the systematic approach to this station that may be adapted to other scenarios. In particular, we provide advice to enable the candidate to be the lateral quick thinking individual that the examiner is seeking to find. We have also included a more fully dialogued case (➜ Sudden loss of vision: diabetic vitreous haemorrhage, p.547) providing instructions for the candidate, patient, and examiner respectively, as would occur in the examination itself.

Acute medicine: **Shortness of breath**

Shortness of breath is one of the, if not the, most common presenting acute medical complaint.

> ### Scenario
>
> A multitude of scenarios exist involving patients complaining of shortness of breath, either alone or in conjunction with other symptoms. Sometimes, information about the time course or recently measured O_2 saturation may be given.
>
> E.g. Mrs Edna Thomas, aged 40 years.
>
> This lady with a history of Raynaud's phenomenon has been complaining of increasing shortness of breath.
>
> Please take a focused history and examine her appropriately.

History

Shortness of breath has an enormous differential diagnosis and a focused history is important to making the correct diagnosis. Key features relate to:
- Mode of presentation:
  - Acute
  - Episodic (± diurnal variation)
  - Exertional
  - Progressive
- Precipitating factors:
  - Recent long-haul travel – ask regarding calf tenderness
  - Exposure to dust/smoke/asbestos/cold
  - Position – ask about orthopnoea and paroxysmal nocturnal dyspnoea
  - Sleep
  - Trauma (may lead to pneumothorax/haemothorax, although unlikely in PACES)
- Rate of progression (see Table 8.1)
  - Sudden; rapid; gradual
- Associated symptoms:
  - Fever ± rigors/sweats
  - Cough ± sputum; haemoptysis
  - Pain e.g. crushing (IHD) or pleuritic (PE)
  - Wheeze
  - Change in weight:
    - Gain: hypothyroidism, cardiac failure
    - Loss: neoplasia, cardiac cachexia, COPD
  - Rash e.g. vasculitic
  - Generalized weakness; fatiguability (muscular dystrophies; myasthenia gravis)
- Previous respiratory history/investigations/treatment
- Comorbidities with respiratory associations e.g. rheumatological disease
- Smoking history

- Occupational history
- Travel abroad (particularly if associated symptoms of infection)
- Effect on the patient's activities of daily living.

Table 8.1 Onset of breathlessness

Sudden (within minutes)	Rapid (hours–days)	Gradual (days–weeks–months)
Pneumothorax	Haemothorax	Pleural effusion
Severe acute asthma	Acute asthma	COPD
Pulmonary oedema	Pulmonary oedema	Fibrosing alveolitis
Pulmonary embolism	Pneumonia	Tuberculosis
Laryngeal oedema	Acute bronchitis	Neuromuscular disease
Foreign body inhalation	Allergic alveolitis	Lung neoplasia

It is also important for the candidate to ascertain the severity of the breathlessness and this can be assessed using the MRC Breathlessness Scale (Table 8.2):

Table 8.2 MRC Breathlessness Scale

Grade	Degree of breathlessness
0	No breathlessness except with strenuous exercise
1	Breathless when walking up an incline or hurrying on the level
2	Walks slower than most on the level or stops after 15 minutes of walking on the level
3	Stops after a few minutes of walking on the level
4	Breathless with minimal activity such as getting dressed; too breathless to leave the house

Examination

The patient with shortness of breath will require a focused respiratory examination that may be adapted to that undertaken in Station 1 (→ p.21) but that should be comprehensive in order to elicit all appropriate signs. The candidate would also be expected to demonstrate the presence of any associated signs. For example, in a patient with pulmonary oedema, examination for arrhythmia, valvular abnormalities and peripheral/sacral oedema would be expected.

Investigations

These will depend on the differential diagnoses of each case but the candidate needs to start with basic tests before moving on to more specialized investigations:

- Pulse oximetry.

- Blood tests:
  - FBC to assess for infection, anaemia; U&E/LFT as a baseline for management; CRP for infection/inflammation.
  - Specialized blood tests, e.g. autoantibodies; avian precipitins.
- Arterial blood gas analysis.
- Pulmonary function tests:
  - Bedside spirometry.
  - Formal respiratory function tests including transfer factor.
- Chest imaging: CXR, CT, HRCT, PET.
- Bronchoscopy.
- Echocardiography (myocardial function and valvular lesions).
- Pulmonary angiography/right heart catheter studies.

Treatment/patient concerns

Treatment will depend entirely on the specific case but the candidate will always be expected to address the patient's concerns. In some cases this may require dealing with sensitive issues such as, 'Have I got cancer, doctor?', 'Is it HIV, doctor?', 'Am I going to die, doctor?'. The candidate needs to show sympathy and empathy and explain clearly the management plan with appropriate reasoning. In other scenarios, the candidate will be expected to discuss with the patient why they need to be admitted to hospital, or in contrast, why it is safe for them to be managed as an outpatient.

Viva questions

The survey undertaken by the authors demonstrated that in this case the viva questions will always focus on the differential diagnosis and appropriate investigation and management of the individual case.

E.g. Should this 28-year-old man with asthma be discharged from A&E?

The candidate needs to be aware of national guidelines[1] outlining criteria for admission and discharge:
Admit patients with any feature of life-threatening or near fatal attack:
- PEFR <33% best of predicted
- O_2 saturation <92%
- PO_2 <8kPa
- Normal or raised PCO_2
- Silent chest
- Cyanosis
- Poor respiratory effort
- Arrhythmia
- Exhaustion/altered consciousness.

Admit patients with any feature of a severe attack persisting after initial treatment:
- PEFR 33–50% best of predicted
- Respiratory rate ≥25/min
- Heart rate ≥110/min
- Inability to complete sentences on 1 breath
- Patients whose PEFR >75% best of predicted 1 hour after initial treatment may be discharged (unless there are other reasons for admission).

Reference

1. The British Thoracic Society and Scottish Intercollegiate Guidelines Network. *British Guideline on the Management of Asthma*. Edinburgh: SIGN, 2009.

Transient ischaemic attack

A transient ischaemic attack (TIA) is defined as a rapid onset of focal neurological deficit lasting <24 hours, with no apparent cause other than disruption of blood supply to the brain. The majority resolve within 1 hour and episodes of amaurosis fugax commonly last <5 minutes.

> **Scenario**
>
> 1. Mr Ted Hughes, aged 67 years.
> Earlier today, this man had right arm weakness and difficulty with speech that lasted for 45 minutes. Please take a focused history and examine him appropriately.
>
> 2. Mrs Gill Smith, aged 79 years.
> This lady had transient monocular loss of vision lasting 2 minutes. Please take a focused history and examine her appropriately.

History

- The history needs to focus on 4 key questions about the presenting complaint:
  1. Were the neurological symptoms *focal* rather than *non-focal*?
  2. Were the symptoms *negative* rather than *positive*?
  3. Was the *onset* of the symptoms *sudden*?
  4. Were the symptoms *maximal at onset* rather than progressing over a period?
- If the answer is 'Yes' to each of the 4 questions, then the symptoms were almost certainly caused by a vascular pathology.
- In addition if the symptoms have fully resolved then the diagnosis is a TIA.

The candidate should start by asking about the presenting symptoms but should then inquire about other potential focal neurological symptoms. The symptoms of a TIA are anatomically determined by the insult to the neurological structures that are supplied by the vasculature affected:

- TIA affecting the anterior cerebral artery territory may result in emotional changes, dysphasia and contralateral weakness.
- TIA affecting the middle cerebral artery territory may result in dysphasia and contralateral weakness, sensory loss, visual field loss and neglect.
- TIA affecting the posterior cerebral artery territory may result in contralateral visual field loss, neglect, weakness and sensory loss.
- TIA affecting the posterior brain structures supplied by the vertebrobasilar arterial system may cause nausea, vomiting, vertigo, visual disturbance, dysarthria, ataxia, weakness and/or sensory disturbance.

TIAs that involve only a small blood vessel (<400µm in diameter) supplying deep brain structures lack cortical features (e.g. dysphasia, visual field loss, neglect, perceptual abnormalities) and present as pure hemiparesis, pure hemisensory loss, combined hemiparesis and hemisensory loss or unilateral ataxic hemiparesis.

Temporary reduction in retinal blood flow causes transient monocular blindness (amaurosis fugax) with the symptoms classically described as 'a curtain coming down vertically' into the field of vision in one eye. Other descriptions of this experience include a dimming or fogging.

The history should also focus on:
- Risk factors for TIA
- Current anti-thrombotic medication e.g. aspirin, warfarin
- Current medications to reduce vascular risk e.g. anti-hypertensives, statins.

Risk factors for TIA

- Age
- Previous TIA or stroke
- Hypertension
- Diabetes mellitus
- Dyslipidaemia
- Cardiac disease
- Obesity
- Cigarette smoking
- Alcohol excess
- Recreational drug misuse.

Examination

- A focused neurological examination should commence with the symptomatic deficit encountered by the patient. There should be no residual neurological deficit in a patient with a TIA.
- The candidate should then examine the pulse, particularly for AF, ask for the BP, and auscultate for any cardiac murmurs or carotid bruits.

Differential diagnosis/TIA mimics

- Migraine
- Focal epilepsy
- Metabolic disturbance e.g. hyper/hypoglycaemia
- Transient global amnesia
- MS.

Investigations

- Blood tests:
  - FBC for underlying thrombophilic tendencies such as polycythaemia and thrombocythaemia.
  - Glucose to exclude hyper/hypoglycaemia.
  - HbA$_1$c for glycaemic control.
  - Lipid profile.
- ECG and 24-hour ECG (Holter monitoring) particularly to assess for paroxysmal AF.

- Echocardiography to assess for left ventricular dyskinesia or other structural cause of cardioembolism.
- Carotid arterial imaging (for anterior circulation TIAs).
- Duplex ultrasound.
- CT angiography.
- MR angiography.
- Brain imaging.
- MRI, including diffusion weighted imaging (that will highlight any areas of infarction) and gradient echo imaging (that will highlight any areas of haemorrhage), in patients seen acutely after TIA in whom there is uncertainty about the diagnosis, vascular territory or underlying cause.

Treatment

Lifestyle advice

- Optimize diet to include:
  - ≥5 portions of fruit and vegetables/day
  - 2 portions of fish/week
  - Reduced saturated fat
  - Reduced salt
- Weight loss if overweight (BMI >25)
- Increase physical activity
- Cessation of cigarette smoking/recreational drug use
- Reduction of alcohol intake to <3 units/day for men and <2 units/day for women.

Control of vascular risk factors

- BP to be ≤130/80mmHg (or ≤150/80 if >70% carotid stenosis bilaterally)
- Cholesterol to be <3.5mmol/L
- HbA₁c to be <7.5%.

Anti-thrombotic medication

- Commence aspirin and dipyridamole as dual anti-platelet therapy; if patients are aspirin-intolerant then clopidogrel should be used as monotherapy.
- If a TIA is found to cardioembolic then the patient should be anticoagulated in the absence of contraindications.

Carotid endarterectomy

This should be offered within a maximum of 2 weeks of symptoms (although ideally within 2 days) to those patients with TIA who have symptomatic carotid stenosis of 50–99% according to the North American Symptomatic Carotid Endarterctomy Trial criteria or 70–99% according to the European Carotid Surgery Trialists' Collaborative Group criteria.

Patient concerns

Suspecting a 'mini-stroke', the patient is likely to ask regarding the likely cause of their symptoms, the consequences of a TIA and will want to know what to do if the symptoms recur. The differential diagnosis and management plan should be explained, focussing on the importance of stroke prevention.

❶ Top Tips

- Candidates should emphasize to the patient that they are at increased risk of stroke and must act **FAST** should there be any sudden:
  - **F**acial weakness
  - **A**rm weakness
  - And/or **S**peech problems
  - With that being the **T**ime to call 999.

Viva questions

Can you tell me about how you would manage a TIA?

- Patients with TIA should be assessed for their risk of subsequent stroke using the ABCD² scoring system (Table 8.3).
- TIAs with an ABCD² score ≥4 are classified as high risk and guidelines advise specialist assessment and investigation (as described above) within 24 hours.
- TIAs with an ABCD² score <4 are classified as low risk and should have specialist assessment and investigation (as described above) within 1 week.

Table 8.3 ABCD² scoring system

Age	≥60 years	1 point
	<60 years	0 points
Blood pressure	≥140/90mmHg	1 point
	<140/90mmHg	0 points
Clinical features	Speech impairment without weakness	1 point
	Unilateral weakness	2 points
Duration	10–59min	1 point
	≥60min	2 points
Diabetes mellitus	Yes	1 point

What is this patient's risk of suffering a stroke?

- Overall, patients who have suffered a TIA have a:
  - 2-day stroke risk of ~4%
  - 7-day stroke risk of ~5.5%
  - 30-day stroke risk of ~7.5%
  - 90-day stroke risk of ~9%
- However, the risk may be stratified using the ABCD score with 2-day stroke risk being:
  - 1% for ABCD² score 0–3
  - 4% for ABCD² score 4–5
  - 8% for ABCD² score 6–7

📖 **Further reading**

Clairborne Johnston S, et al. Validation and refinement of scores to predict very early stroke risk after transient ischaemic attack. Lancet 2007; **369**:283–92.

Department of Health. National Stroke Strategy. London: Department of Health, 2007.

NICE. Stroke: Diagnosis and initial management of acute stroke and transient ischaemic attack (TIA). London: NICE, 2008.

Royal College of Physicians Intercollegiate Stroke Working Party. National Clinical Guidelines on the Management of people of Stroke, 3rd edn. London: RCP, 2008.

Headache

Headache has a lifetime prevalence of 90% and has >200 causes, ranging from harmless to life threatening. The description of the headache together with the findings on neurological examination determine the appropriate management.

Scenario

Mrs Angela Coombes, aged 31 years.

Please undertake a focused history and examination of this lady who has presented to A&E with a headache.

History and examination

A good history is the key to diagnosis with examination usually being normal in patients with *primary headache* (migraine, tension-type headache, cluster headache, trigeminal neuralgia and hemicrania continua – continuous headache on one side of the head).

- Consider a diagnosis of *migraine* in patients with recurrent, severe, disabling headache associated with nausea, photophobia, spreading visual, sensory and/or motor symptoms and a normal neurological examination. Migraine is characteristically unilateral, pulsating, builds up over minutes to hours, and is aggravated by routine physical activity.
- Consider a diagnosis of *tension-type* headache in patients with recurrent, non-disabling bilateral headache and a normal neurological examination.
- Consider the diagnosis of *cluster headache* in patients with frequent, brief, severe, unilateral headaches in a trigeminal distribution with ipsilateral cranial autonomic features such as tearing.

Secondary headache

'Red flag' symptoms/signs need to be sought:

- New headache in patient aged >50 years.
- Headache that develops within minutes (thunderclap headache) may be the only sign of subarachnoid haemorrhage.
- Inability to move a limb or abnormalities on neurological examination.
- Mental confusion.
- Recent trauma (that may precipitate subdural haemorrhage).
- Being woken by headache.

- Headache that worsens with changing posture, exertion, coughing, sneezing, straining: raising concern of raised intracranial pressure.
- Symptoms of giant cell arteritis (GCA), including:
  - Unilateral headache, unresponsive to analgesics.
  - Scalp tenderness to palpation (usually localized over affected artery).
  - Visual loss/abnormalities.
  - Jaw or lingual claudication (pain in jaw or tongue on chewing that resolves afterwards).
- Neck stiffness and/or associated rash (meningitis).
- Fever.
- Pre-existing HIV (intracranial abscess), cancer (metastases), or risk factors for thrombosis.

❶ Top Tips

- Headache may also be caused by:
  - Pain arising from the neck muscles (cervicogenic headache)
  - Overuse of analgesic medications for chronic headache (medication overuse headache).

Investigations

- Blood tests (FBC, U&E, ESR, CRP, clotting):
  - ESR raised (often very high) in GCA
  - WCC/CRP raised in inflammatory states
  - Clotting studies pre-lumbar puncture
- Brain imaging: for all patients with 'red flag' features
- Lumbar puncture: for patients with suspected meningitis/encephalitis, subarachnoid haemorrhage with normal brain imaging and benign intracranial hypertension.

Treatment

- Migraine:
  - Aspirin 900mg or ibuprofen 400mg (or paracetamol in pregnancy) combined with an oral or rectal antiemetic to reduce symptoms of nausea and vomiting and to promote gastric emptying.
  - Oral triptans if previous attacks have not been controlled with simple analgesics.
  - Discuss the risks of medication overuse.
- Tension-type headache: aspirin or paracetamol.
- Cluster headache: subcutaneous/nasal triptans (as oral triptans will not be effective) and 100% oxygen if no contraindications.
- Hemicrania continua: oral indomethacin.
- Medication overuse headache: cessation of the overused medication with structured education about how medications may cause headache and warning about withdrawal symptoms.
  - Gradual withdrawal in patients on opioids.
- Secondary headache: treatment will be dictated by the cause.

Patient concerns

The patient is likely to be distressed by the symptoms of the headache and the worry of it being due to a sinister cause such as a brain tumour. The patient will also want to know what to do if the symptoms recur. The candidate needs to describe the differential diagnosis and management plan, based on the clinical findings, with appropriate reassurance in cases of benign primary headache and sympathetic explanation in cases where investigation of potentially sinister causes is warranted.

Viva questions

These will focus on the management of the specific diagnosis provided by the candidate but will also involve the candidate being asked questions such as *'Does this patient need a brain scan?'* or *'Can this patient be discharged safely?'*. The candidate should be aware that investigation is not indicated in patients with a clear history of migraine, no 'red flag' features and a normal neurological examination but, in contrast, 'red flag' features warrant urgent investigation.

📖 Further reading

Duncan CW, et al. Diagnosis and management of headache in adults: summary of SIGN guideline. *BMJ* 2008; **337**: a2329.

Edlow JA, et al. Clinical policy: critical issues in the evaluation and management of adult patients presenting to the emergency department with acute headache. *Ann Emerg Med* 2008; **52**:407–36.

Chest pain

Chest pain is a very frequent presenting acute medical complaint. The examiners would expect the candidate to perform well in this Station 5 scenario, as the symptoms may not only be suggestive of medical emergencies, but they should be well rehearsed in dealing with these common problems in their day-to-day practice.

> ### Scenario
>
> Mrs Edith Swain, age 58 years.
>
> This lady with a history of rheumatoid arthritis has been complaining of increasing chest pain. Please take a focused history and examine her appropriately.

History

Chest pain has a wide differential diagnosis and a focused history is important to making the correct diagnosis. The candidate needs to question the patient about the pain's:
- Site
- Radiation
- Character
- Severity
- Duration
- Frequency
- Precipitants
- Aggravating factors
- Relieving factors
- Associated symptoms e.g. palpitations, breathlessness, ankle swelling, cough, haemoptysis, dysphagia.

The rest of the history needs to be tailored to the probable cause of the pain. For example, if the pain appears to be cardiac in nature, the candidate needs to focus on relevant cardiac risk factors whilst if the pain is pleuritic in nature the history needs to be focused on respiratory features. If there is a history of musculoskeletal symptoms, then the candidate needs to pay attention to the social history and the ability of the patient to self-care.

Examination

The physical examination needs to be tailored to the most likely diagnosis and may be undertaken simultaneous to history taking. For example, in the patient with systemic sclerosis whose chest pain is due to dysphagia, the candidate should examine for features of the patient's connective tissue disease, whilst questioning about symptoms.

Investigations

These will again depend on the case but the candidate always needs to start with basic tests before moving on to more specialized investigations.

Treatment/patient concerns

Treatment will depend entirely on the specific case but the candidate will always be expected to address the patient's concerns such as:

• 'Have I got cancer, doctor?'
• 'Is it due to my heart?'
• 'Am I going to die, doctor?'
• 'Can I go home?'

The candidate needs to show sympathy and empathy and explain clearly the management plan with appropriate reasoning.

Viva questions

The survey undertaken by the authors demonstrated that in this case the viva will always focus on certain key questions:

What is the differential diagnosis?

What is the diagnosis?

What investigations would you undertake?

What would be your management plan?

How will you treat this patient?

Hypertension

Hypertension is classified as essential in 90–95% of cases with only 5–10% having a secondary cause affecting renal, endocrine or cardiovascular systems.

> ### Scenario
>
> Mr Timothy Tomlinson, age 59 years.
>
> This man has been referred by his GP for poorly controlled hypertension despite being on amlodipine 5mg OM. Please speak to the patient and carry out a focused physical examination.

History

Hypertension is usually asymptomatic unless 'accelerated' when it is associated with headache, drowsiness, confusion, nausea, vomiting and vision disorders, collectively referred to as hypertensive encephalopathy (caused by severe small blood vessel congestion and brain swelling and reversible if BP is lowered). The candidate needs to spend time asking about:

- Other vascular risk factors (diabetes, hyperlipidaemia, renal disease and cigarette/alcohol/recreational drug use).
- Medications that may cause hypertension e.g. steroids.
- Current and past anti-hypertensive use and side effect profile.
- History of hypertensive end-organ damage e.g. cerebrovascular disease.
- Family history of hypertension.

Examination

The physical examination needs to be tailored to the most likely diagnosis and the candidate needs to inspect the patient carefully to look for signs associated with secondary causes of hypertension e.g. insulin injection marks, Cushingoid facies, acromegaly. The candidate must palpate the radial pulse and auscultate the praecordium in addition to stating that they would measure the BP and perform fundoscopy (to assess for hypertensive retinopathy) and a urine dipstick examination (to assess for urinary protein, glycosuria and/or haematuria).

Investigations

Like the physical examination, these need to be tailored to the most likely diagnosis but in young hypertensives with no clear cause from clinical assessment, investigations for secondary causes need to be undertaken. In the first instance these include blood and urine screening tests and a renal ultrasound for renal/endocrine causes of hypertension.

British Hypertension Society guidelines also advise that patients should have an ECG and have their blood glucose and lipids checked.

Treatment

Patients should be treated in line with national guidelines as shown in Figs. 8.1 and 8.2 and viva questions will focus on these management pathways.

Causes of hypertension

Renal
- Chronic glomerulonephritis
- Chronic atrophic pyelonephritis
- Adult polycystic kidney disease
- Analgesic nephropathy
- Renal artery stenosis.

Endocrine
- Conn's syndrome
- Cushing's syndrome
- Phaeochromocytoma
- Acromegaly
- Thyrotoxicosis
- Hyperparathyroidism.

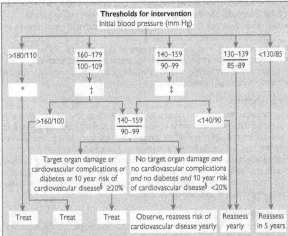

Fig. 8.1 Blood pressure thresholds for intervention.
Reproduced from British Hypertension Society guidelines for hypertension management 2004 (BHS-IV): summary, Bryan Williams, Neil R. Poulter, Morris J. Brown, Mark Davis, Gordon T. McInnes, John F. Potter, Peter S. Sever, Simon McG Thom. *BMJ*, **328**, pp.634–40, 2004, with permission from BMJ Publishing Group Ltd.

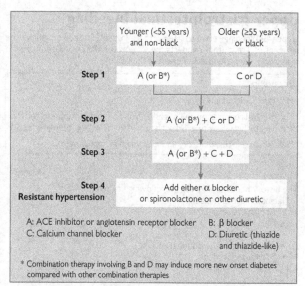

Fig. 8.2 Recommendations for combining blood pressure lowering drugs. Reproduced from British Hypertension Society guidelines for hypertension management 2004 (BHS-IV): summary, Bryan Williams, Neil R. Poulter, Morris J. Brown, Mark Davis, Gordon T. McInnes, John F. Potter, Peter S. Sever, Simon McG Thom. *BMJ*, **328**, pp.634–40, 2004, with permission from BMJ Publishing Group Ltd.

📖 Further reading

Williams B, *et al.*; The BHS Guidelines Working Party. British Hypertension Society Guidelines for Hypertension Management, 2004—BHS IV: Summary. *BMJ* 2004; **328**:634–40.

🔗 Useful website

NICE. *Hypertension: full guideline (CG127)*. London: NICE, 2011. Available at: http://guidance.nice. org.uk/CG127

Upper gastrointestinal bleeding

Upper GI bleeding refers to haemorrhage in the GI tract from above the ligament of Treitz (that connects the 4th portion of the duodenum to the diaphragm, near the splenic flexure of the colon).

> **Scenario**
>
> Mr Frank Colt, aged 41 years.
>
> The medical registrar on-call has asked you to see this man, referred this morning by his GP, with a 1-day history of vomiting and haematemesis.
>
> Please take a focused history and examine him appropriately.

History

The history needs to address the following key symptoms:

- Haematemesis ± melaena
  - Approximate volume
  - Frequency
  - Duration
  - Association with vomiting/retching
  - Previous episodes
- Nausea ± vomiting
- GI reflux
- Abdominal pain
- Contents/consistency of vomitus
  - Fresh blood
  - 'Coffee granules' indicating altered blood
- Contents/consistency of faeces: fresh blood suggests rapid upper GI bleed and/or lower GI bleeding
- Change in bowel habit (more likely to be present with lower GI bleeding)
- Assessment of patient's normal dietary intake
- Change in appetite
- Weight loss
- Liver disease
- Use of anti-platelets, anticoagulants, NSAIDs, anti-depressants, anti-hypertensives
- Alcohol and cigarette use.

Examination

The candidate is unlikely to be presented with a patient who is acutely unwell but the examination needs to focus on:

- Assessment of haemodynamic stability: pulse, BP (with postural change), JVP
- Inspection for peripheral stigmata of disease with gastrointestinal bleeding diathesis:
  - Chronic liver disease
  - Hereditary haemorrhagic telangiectasia (HHT)
- Focused GI examination:
  - BMI (weight/height²)/nutritional status
  - Lymphadenopathy/Virchow's node
  - Abdominal tenderness/mass

- Organomegaly
- Expression of need for rectal examination and inspection of any vomitus.

Investigations

- Blood tests: FBC, U&E, LFT, clotting, group & save/crossmatch.
- Endoscopy (OGD): investigation of choice that can also be therapeutic.
- Assessment of helicobacter pylori status by biopsy or urea breath test.

Treatment

Initial management

- Intravenous fluid/blood replacement to correct fluid/blood losses and restore BP.
- In severe bleeds (patients usually >60 years of age, with comorbidity, pulse >100/min, systolic BP (SBP) <100mmHg and/or Hb <10g/dL) patients require close monitoring with insertion of urethral catheter ± CVP line.
- Correct abnormalities of INR and platelets.
- Intravenous terlipressin in suspected variceal bleeding.

OGD (within 24 hours)

- Non-variceal bleeding: injection of adrenaline coupled with thermal or mechanical treatment to actively bleeding lesions, non-bleeding visible vessels and ulcers with an adherent clot.
- Variceal bleeding: band ligation for oesophageal varices and cyanoacrylate injection for gastric varices.[1]

Management after OGD

- Close monitoring to ensure adequate BP and urine output.
- Drug therapy:
  - PPI in bleeding from peptic ulcer disease.
  - Terlipressin, propranolol (if no contraindication) and antibiotics in suspected variceal bleeding.
- Referral for selective arterial embolization or surgery if continued bleeding after OGD.
- Balloon tamponade ± transjugular intrahepatic porto-systemic shunt (TIPS) if continued bleeding from varices after OGD.

Follow-up

- Peptic ulcers:
  - Avoid anti-platelets/NSAIDs.
  - *Helicobacter pylori* eradication for 1 week and a further 3 weeks of anti-secretory therapy in NSAID users.
- Oesophageal varices: repeat OGD and repeat endoscopic banding of varices.
- Gastric ulcers: follow-up OGD to confirm healing if suspicion of malignancy.

Patient concerns

Am I going to die? Am I going to vomit blood again? Will I need an endoscopy?

The candidate should provide objective predictive answers to these questions based on evidence-based scoring systems:

All patients presenting with acute upper GI bleeding should have a *Rockall score* calculated to identify risk of adverse outcome (Table 8.4).[2]

Table 8.4 Rockall score

Variable	0	1	2	3
Age	<60	60–79	>80	
Shock	None	Pulse >100	SBP <100	
Comorbidity	None		CCF, IHD major morbidity	Renal failure, liver failure, metastatic cancer
Diagnosis	Mallory–Weiss tear	All other diagnoses	GI malignancy	
Evidence of bleeding	None		Blood, adherent clot, spurting vessel	

Pre-endoscopy Rockall score	0	1	2	3	4	5	6	7
Mortality (%)	0.2	2.4	5.6	11.0	24.6	39.6	48.9	50.0

Post-endoscopy Rockall score	0	1	2	3	4	5	6	7	≥8
Rebled (%)	4.9	3.4	5.3	11.2	14.1	24.1	32.9	43.8	41.6
Mortality (%)	0	0	0.2	2.9	5.3	10.8	17.3	27.0	41.1

Whilst not as good as the Rockall score in predicting mortality, the *Blatchford score* has been demonstrated to be better at determining who will need a hospital based intervention. If all of the following parameters are present, the patient is at low risk of requiring endoscopic treatment: [3]

- Urea <6.5mmol/L
- Hb >13g/dL in men and >12 g/dL in women
- SBP >110mmHg
- Pulse <100/min.

Viva questions

What are the causes of haematemesis?

The most common cause of haematemesis demonstrated at endoscopy is peptic ulceration (Table 8.5). However, in up to 20% of patients presenting with upper gastrointestinal bleeding, endoscopy does not reveal a cause.[1]

Table 8.5 Cause and relative frequency of haematemesis found at endoscopy

Cause of bleeding found at endoscopy[1]	Relative frequency (%)
Peptic ulcer	44
Oesophagitis	28
Gastritis/erosions	26
Erosive duodenitis	15
Varices	13
Portal hypertensive gastropathy	7
Malignancy	5
Mallory–Weiss tear	5
Vascular malformation	3

Can this patient be discharged safely?

- Guidelines advocate that patients meeting all of the following criteria may be discharged safely with outpatient follow-up:
  - Age <60; SBP>100mmHg; pulse <100/min, no significant comorbidity (especially heart/liver disease); no witnessed blood loss.

References

1. Scottish Intercollegiate Guidelines Network. *Management of acute upper and lower gastrointestinal bleeding.* Edinburgh, SIGN, 2008.

2. Rockall TA, *et al.* Risk assessment after acute gastrointestinal hemorrhage. *Gut* 1996; **38**:316–21.

3. Blatchford O, *et al.* A risk score to predict need for treatment for upper gastrointestinal haemorrhage. *Lancet* 2000; **356**:1318–21.

Irregular pulse

Whilst any arrhythmia may feature in PACES, atrial fibrillation (AF) is the most common with a population prevalence of 0.5% at age 50–59 and almost 9% at age 80–89. AF is present in 3–6% of UK acute medical admissions.

> ## Scenario
>
> Mr David Clark, aged 59 years.
>
> This man has been complaining of palpitations and light-headedness. Please speak to the patient and carry out a focused physical examination.

History

- Palpitations (onset, frequency, precipitating factors e.g. exercise, caffeine)
- Chest pain*
- Breathlessness*
- Exercise tolerance*
- Ankle swelling
- Light-headedness/pre-syncope/syncope*
- Fatigue
- Vascular risk factors (hypertension, diabetes mellitus, hyperlipidaemia)
- Past history of cardiac/respiratory/thyroid/metabolic disease; stroke/TIA
- Drug/alcohol/cigarette use*
- Treatment (if any) to date
- Family history.

*Any correlation of these symptoms with the palpitations should be established.

Examination

- Inspection:
  - Mitral facies.
  - Permanent pacemaker.
  - Cardiac surgical scar(s).
- Inspection with appropriate subsequent focused examination:
  - Thyroid facies ± goitre.
  - Evidence of focal neurologic deficit as a result of cardioembolism.
- Focused cardiovascular examination concentrating on pulse rate, rhythm, volume and character, pulse deficit (difference between cardiac and radial pulse rates), BP, cardiac auscultatory findings and signs of cardiac failure.

Investigations

- Blood tests:
  - FBC for anaemia
  - U&E/Ca^{2+}/Mg^{2+} for electrolyte abnormalities
  - Glucose
  - Lipids
  - TFTs
- ECG
- 24-hour ECG (Holter monitoring)
- Echocardiogram
- Electrophysiological studies.

Treatment/patient concerns

The main goals of AF treatment are to prevent circulatory instability and stroke (see Fig. 8.3). Heart rate and rhythm control are principally used to achieve the former while antithrombotic treatment is used to decrease the risk of stroke. In emergencies, when circulatory collapse is imminent due to uncontrolled tachycardia, immediate cardioversion may be indicated.

AF may be defined as:

- First detected: only 1 diagnosed episode.
- Paroxysmal: recurrent episodes that self-terminate in <7 days.
- Persistent: recurrent episodes that last >7 days.
- Permanent: ongoing long-term episode.

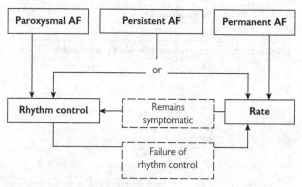

Fig. 8.3 AF treatment strategy decision tree.
Reproduced from: National Collaborating Centre for Chronic Conditions. *Atrial fibrillation: national clinical guideline for management in primary and secondary care.* London: Royal College of Physicians, 2006. Copyright © 2006 Royal College of Physicians. Reproduced with permission.[1]

- In patients with persistent AF:
  - A rate-control strategy is preferred in patients:
    - >65 years of age
    - With IHD
    - Contraindications to anti-arrhythmic drugs/cardioversion
    - Without cardiac failure
  - A rhythm control strategy is preferred in patients:
    - <65 years of age who are symptomatic
    - Presenting with lone AF (in the absence of other cardiovascular/respiratory disease)
    - With AF secondary to a treated/corrected precipitant (e.g. electrolyte disturbance)
    - With cardiac failure
- Beta-blockers should be used as a 1st-line anti-arrhythmic.
- Beta-blockers or rate-limiting calcium-channel antagonists should be preferred as rate-controlling monotherapy.
- Digoxin should be considered for rate control only in predominantly sedentary patients.

Anti-thrombotic treatment
Guidelines advocate the use of clinical prediction rules such as the CHADS$_2$ score (Table 8.6) to estimate the risk of stroke and whether or not treatment is required with anticoagulation or anti-platelet therapy.[2]

Table 8.6 CHADS$_2$ score

	Condition	Points
C	Congestive heart failure	1
H	Hypertension	1
A	Age >75 years	1
D	Diabetes mellitus	1
S	Prior stroke or TIA	2
CHADS$_2$ score	**Stroke rate per 100 patient years of aspirin**	
0	0.8	
1	2.2	
2	4.5	
3	8.6	
4	10.9	
5	12.3	
6	13.7	

In patients with CHADS$_2$ score of 0, aspirin is advised; in patients with CHADS$_2$ score of 1, aspirin or warfarin is advised (decided on an individual basis on the basis of risk:benefit in association with stroke risk factors); and in patients with CHADS$_2$ score ≥2, anticoagulation with warfarin is advised.

Viva questions

What are the causes of AF?
- Ischaemic heart disease
- Rheumatic heart disease
- Hypertensive heart disease
- Thyrotoxicosis
- Acute infection
- Electrolyte imbalance (e.g. hypokalaemia)
- Cardiomyopathy (toxic, metabolic, endocrine, collagen-disease related, infiltrative, infective, genetic, fibroblastic)
- Constrictive pericarditis.

How could you differentiate AF from other pulse irregularities?
An irregular pulse due to controlled AF is differentiated from that of multiple extrasystoles by the long pauses which occur in groups of 2 or more,

whilst with ectopic beats the compensatory pause follows a short pause, because the ectopic is premature. Exercise may abolish extrasystoles but worsen the irregularity of AF. AF may be difficult to distinguish from atrial flutter with a variable block, multiple atrial ectopics due to a shifting pace-maker and paroxysmal atrial tachycardia with block but, only in AF, is the rhythm truly chaotic.

References

1. NICE. *Atrial fibrillation: full guideline.* London: NICE, 2006.
2. Gage BF, et al. Selecting patients with atrial fibrillation for anticoagulation: stroke risk stratification in patients taking aspirin. *Circulation* 2004; **110**:2287–92.

Pyelonephritis

Scenario

Miss Tracy Bratcher, age 29 years.

This lady has presented to the Medical Admissions Unit with a 2-day history of worsening fever and abdominal pain. Please speak to the patient and carry out a focused physical examination.

History

Pyelonephritis is characterized by dysuria, pyrexia, rigors, flank pain, nausea and vomiting. The presentation may be non-specific with an extensive differential diagnosis and features of the pain need to be asked carefully. A history of dyspaerunia, genitourinary symptoms in sexual partners, urinary incontinence, confusion, a travel history, and a history of previous urinary tract infections or renal disease also need to be sought.

Examination

The patient is likely to be a young, previously fit and well individual, with the only positive findings being fever and loin/suprapubic tenderness. However, patients presenting with pyelonephritis may become septic and unwell and the candidate needs also to assess heart rate, BP and respiratory rate. The candidate should also state that they would perform a bed-side urine dipstick examination to look for urinary leucocytosis and nitrites (and/or blood and protein).

❶ Top Tips

- When stating that you wish to carry out urine dipstick examination, always specify what abnormality you expect to find, e.g. leucocytosis and nitrites in a patient with pyelonephritis or glycosuria in a patient with suspected diabetes.

Differential diagnosis

- Peritonitis, cholecystitis, appendicitis, renal colic, pelvic inflammatory disease, ectopic pregnancy, pneumonia.

Investigations

- Urine microscopy, culture and sensitivity
- Urine/blood pregnancy test
- Blood tests:
  - FBC for leucocytosis
  - CRP
  - U&E to assess for renal impairment
  - Glucose
  - Lactate
  - Blood cultures
- Renal tract ultrasound.

Treatment/patient concerns

There is no consensus on the definitions of grades of severity of pyelonephritis, but patients may be divided into those without signs of sepsis,* able to take oral antibiotics and suitable for outpatient management, and those requiring intravenous antibiotics and fluids in hospital. Antibiotic choice and duration is determined by local protocol. Most cases of community-acquired pyelonephritis are due to bowel organisms that enter the urinary tract such as *Escherichia coli* (70–80%) and *Enterococcus faecalis*. Hospital-acquired infections may be due to coliforms and enterococci, as well as other organisms uncommon in the community, such as *Klebsiella* and *Pseudomonas aeruginosa*.

Sepsis is defined by clinical evidence of infection plus systemic response indicated by 2 or more of the following systemic inflammatory response criteria:
- Temperature <36°C or >38°C
- Heart rate >90/min
- Respiratory rate >20/min or pCO_2 <4.16kPa
- WCC <4 ×10^9 or >12 × 10^9 or 'left-shifted' neutrophils.

Viva question

What factors predispose to urinary sepsis and pyelonephritis?

- Mechanical: structural abnormalities of the renal tract, vesicoureteral reflux, renal calculi, in-dwelling urethral catheter/renal tract stent, incomplete bladder emptying.
- Constitutional: diabetes mellitus, immunocompromised states, atrophic urethritis/vaginitis.
- Behavioural: change in sexual partner.
- Positive family history.

Peripheral vascular disease

Although peripheral vascular disease may be considered as a surgical rather than a medical problem, patients with cardiorespiratory disease often have symptoms of lower limb arterial insufficiency such that the RCP examiners deem peripheral vascular disease to be a suitable case for Station 5.

> **Scenario**
>
> Mr Hugo Cosky, age 89 years.
>
> This man has been complaining of worsening calf pain when walking. Please carry out a focused history and examination.

History

- Presenting symptoms:
  - Claudication:
    - Location: buttocks, hips, legs
    - Usually asymmetrical
    - Precipitating/aggravating/relieving factors
    - Exercise tolerance ('claudication distance')
    - Duration
    - Effect on lifestyle
  - Rest pain
  - Erectile dysfunction
  - Ongoing cardiorespiratory symptoms: chest pain, dyspnoea, palpitations, ankle swelling
  - Raynaud's phenomenon
  - Exclusion of neurological leg symptoms
- Vascular risk profile: ischaemic heart disease, cerebrovascular disease, hypertension, diabetes, hyperlipidaemia, cigarette smoking, alcohol use
- Previous vascular surgical intervention
- History of connective tissue disease
- Drug history: use of anti-thrombotic/anti-hypertensive/lipid-lowering agents
- Family history of vascular disease.

Examination

The physical examination needs to focus on assessment of the peripheral pulses but the candidate needs to demonstrate a comprehensive approach as outlined:

- Inspection for facial/hand signs of systemic sclerosis/SLE/rheumatoid disease.
- Inspection of the lower limbs for: skin colour, trophic changes (shiny skin, hair loss), pressure areas (lateral side of foot, head of 1st metatarsal, heel, malleoli), ulcers, peripheral cyanosis, gangrene, surgical scars, amputation.
- Assessment of temperature change along legs and capillary refill at toes.

- Assessment of pulses:
  - Femoral, popliteal, dorsalis pedis, posterior tibial.
  - Carotid, brachial, radial.
- Palpation for abdominal aortic aneurysm.
- Auscultation for bruits over aorta, iliac, femoral and popliteal arteries.
- Assessment for peripheral neuropathy.
- Buerger's test:*
  - Elevate leg and observe for peripheral pallor.
  - Then sit the patient upright and ask the patient to hang the leg over the side of the couch.
- State that you would also:
  - measure the BP and ankle-brachial pressure index.**
  - perform a urine dipstick examination for glycosuria.

Buerger's angle is the angle of elevation at which the leg becomes pale. In a limb with a normal circulation the toes stay pink, even when the limb is raised by 90°. In an ischaemic leg, elevation to 15–30° for 30–60 seconds may cause pallor. On returning the leg from the raised position, and hanging it over the side of the bed, the leg will revert to the pink colour more slowly than normal, and will pass through this pink colour to a red-orange colour (often known as *sunset foot*) due to the dilatation of the arterioles in their attempt to remove the metabolic waste that has built up. This will then revert to the normal colour.

**The *ankle–brachial pressure index* (ABPI, Table 8.7) is the ratio of the BP in the lower legs to the BP in the arms and is calculated by dividing the higher systolic BP in either of the dorsalis pedis or posterior tibial arteries [measured using Doppler ultrasound] by the higher of the 2 systolic BPs in the arms.)

Table 8.7 Ankle–brachial pressure index

>1.2	Arterial calcification (often in diabetes, renal failure)
1.0–1.2	Normal range
0.9–1.0	Acceptable
0.8–0.9	Some arterial disease
0.5–0.8	Moderate arterial disease
<0.5	Severe arterial disease

❶ Top Tips

- Be aware of Leriche's syndrome comprising of bilateral pain (buttock/lower limb), impotence, bilateral absent pulses and aorto-iliac bruit.

Differential diagnosis

- Sciatica
- Osteoarthritis of hip/knee
- Anterior tibial compartment syndrome
- Cauda equina syndrome.

Investigations

- Blood tests:
  - FBC for underlying thrombophilic tendencies such as polycythaemia and thrombocythaemia
  - U&E to assess for renal impairment
  - Glucose and HbA_1c for glycaemic control
  - Lipid profile
  - Autoantibody profile in young patients
- ECG
- Arterial Duplex ultrasound
- Angiography (CT-A, MRA or percutaneous contrast angiography).

Treatment

- Lifestyle advice and control of vascular risk factors as for TIA (Ⓞ p.464).
- Anti-thrombotic medication (anti-platelets unless patient has coexisting cardiac disease requiring anticoagulation).
- Treatment of claudication:
  - Supervised exercise programme
  - Pharmacological agents: cilostazol, pentoxifylline
  - Endovascular treatment, e.g. stenting, angioplasty
  - Bypass surgery.
- Treatment of critical limb ischaemia:
  - Parenteral prostaglandins
  - Thrombolysis
  - Endovascular treatment e.g. stenting, angioplasty
  - Surgery.

Patient concerns

The pain and discomfort associated with claudication vary from person to person. Patients affected worst will suffer from rest pain and may develop gangrene. Candidates should explain the pathophysiology and management of peripheral vascular disease to patients and be aware of the greatest patient concern of amputation.

Viva questions

What symptoms/signs would encourage you to involve surgeons acutely?
Any of the 6 P's with an acute history: *pain, paraesthesia, paralysis, pallor, pulselessness, perishingly cold.*

Why do patients with more severe disease often have pain at rest in bed?
In bed at night there is a physiological decrease in cardiac output and a reactive dilatation of skin vessels to warmth in bed.

What is phantom limb pain?
Phantom limb pain is pain appearing to come from where an amputated limb used to be. It is often excruciating and very hard to treat. The pain is described in various ways e.g. burning, aching, 'as if the limb is being crushed in a vice'. Suggested mechanisms for the pain include damage to nerve endings and subsequent erroneous re-growth leading to abnormal and painful discharge of neurons in the stump, and altered nervous activity within the brain as a result of the loss of sensory input from the amputated limb.

Deep vein thrombosis

Deep vein thrombosis (DVT) is a common condition presenting to emergency medical admissions units and unlike arterial thrombosis, venous thrombosis often occurs in normal vessels.

Scenario

Mrs Eva Robinson, age 40 years.

This lady complains of pain in her right calf and feels that it may be swollen.

Please take a focused history and examine her appropriately.

History

The history needs to focus on the calf swelling and pain in terms of the onset, rate of progression, and effect the symptoms are having on the patient's activities of daily living. The history should also include:
- Risk factors for DVT.
- Any contraindications to anticoagulation.
- Any symptoms of pulmonary embolism.

Risk factors for DVT

- Age
- Obesity
- Immobility/recent long-haul travel
- Previous venous thromboembolic disease
- Pregnancy/puerperium
- Oral contraceptive pill use
- Cigarette smoking
- Thrombophilia
- Recent surgery
- Underlying neoplasia/cardiac failure.

Examination
- The unilateral leg swelling should be compared with the other normal leg and any proximal extension into the thigh should be assessed. The calf in DVT feels bulky and indurated and moves 'en mass' causing discomfort when moved side to side. In the normal calf the muscle contours are clearly visible and a part of the muscle can be moved side to side without pain or affecting the rest of the calf.
- The candidate should also comment on the presence of superficial veins and any associated skin changes such as erythema, warmth or cyanotic hue.
- The presence of a knee effusion and pain or restriction of movement of the knee would suggest an alternative diagnosis.

Differential diagnosis

- The knee joint is normal in DVT, in contrast to other conditions such as a ruptured popliteal cyst or an arthopathy, which would cause knee swelling.
- Cellulitis, another differential diagnosis, would normally, but not always, be associated with a puncture mark as a portal of bacterial entry and more florid skin changes of erythema, often with vesicles, bullae and/or crusts on the skin surface. The overlying skin is also more shiny and warm compared with DVT.
- The candidate would be expected to be aware of clinical models and scoring systems to predict DVT as the diagnosis. The clinical model of Wells et al.[1] (Table 8.8) is well recognized, where a score >2 indicates a likely probability of DVT, but <2 indicates DVT to be unlikely:

Table 8.8 Wells' criteria for DVT[a]

Clinical characteristic	Score
Active cancer	1
Paralysis, paresis, or recent plaster immobilization of the lower extremity	1
Bedridden recently >3 days or major surgery within 12 weeks	1
Tenderness along the distribution of the deep venous system	1
Entire leg swollen	1
Calf swelling >3cm compared to the other leg	1
Pitting oedema confined to the symptomatic leg	1
Collateral (non-varicose) superficial veins present	1
Previous DVT	1
Alternative diagnosis at least as likely as DVT	−2

[a] Wells PS, Anderson DR, Rodger M, et al. Evaluation of D-dimer in the diagnosis of suspected deep-vein thrombosis. *NEJM* 2003; **349**:1227–35.

Investigations

- Venous Duplex ultrasound is the investigation of choice and should be emphasized.
- Blood tests should include:
  - FBC for underlying thrombophilic tendencies such as polycythaemia and thrombocythaemia.
  - D-dimer.
- Other investigations as guided by underlying predisposing aetiologies, e.g. neoplasia.

Treatment

Candidates need to emphasize the need to start anticoagulant treatment as soon as the clinical diagnosis of DVT is suspected, prior to obtaining the results of investigations. It is important to be aware of acute anticoagulation for DVT with subcutaneous low-molecular-weight heparin (LMWH), at a fixed dose determined by the patient's weight, and subsequent oral warfarinization that will require INR monitoring in an anticoagulation clinic. LMWHs have anti-factor Xa activity with an immediate anticoagulant effect and are administered once daily. In contrast, warfarin acts by inhibiting the vitamin K-dependent synthesis of clotting factors II, VII, IX and X and therefore takes 2–3 days before achieving its anticoagulant effect. In addition, when warfarin is commenced, it may promote clot formation temporarily because the levels of anti-thrombotic Protein C and Protein S are also dependent on vitamin K activity.

Current guidelines recommend a target INR of 2.5 for secondary prevention of DVT with warfarin for at least 6 weeks after calf vein thrombosis and at least 3 months after proximal DVT. For patients with temporary risk factors and a low risk of recurrence, 3 months of treatment is considered sufficient but for those with idiopathic DVT or permanent risk factors, at least 6 months' anticoagulaton is recommended.[2]

As warfarin is teratogenic it should be avoided in the 1st trimester of pregnancy. During this time LMWH should be used in these patients. LMWH has also been shown to be advantageous in patients with DVT complicating cancer.[3]

Patient concerns

The patient is likely to ask what is wrong with their leg and, suspecting a DVT, its life-threatening consequences. You should explain your differential diagnosis and management plan, including the investigation and treatment, with appropriate reasoning. The patient will want to know if they need to be admitted to hospital and you need to show the examiner that DVT may be managed on an outpatient basis through emergency medical admissions unit and anticoagulation clinic services.

Viva questions

Can you tell me about the predictive value of the D-dimer test?
The D-dimer blood test is part of a diagnostic strategy that includes clinical estimation of DVT and Duplex ultrasound imaging. A positive D-dimer indicates the presence of an abnormally high level of fibrin degradation products. In patients who are considered clinically unlikely to have DVT and who have a negative D-dimer test, the diagnosis of DVT can safely be excluded without the need for further diagnostic testing. However, in patients in whom DVT is clinically suspected, D-dimer testing may be falsely positive in the setting of pregnancy, recent surgery or trauma or other medical conditions such as infection or neoplasia, or falsely negative in patients already on anticoagaulant therapy. There are several different methods of testing for D-dimer with bedside qualitative testing kits available in addition to quantitative testing in hospital laboratories.

Which patients need more careful monitoring of warfarin treatment?
Factors that may affect the anticoagulant effect of warfarin necessitate close monitoring by more frequent INR assessment.

Factors increasing the effect of warfarin include:
- Broad-spectrum antibiotics such as tetracyclines which depress the normal intestinal bacterial flora that normally synthesize vitamin K, thus potentiating the effect of warfarin.

- Liver disease with impaired synthesis of clotting factors.
- Hyperthyroidism.
- Excessive use of alcohol.
- Drugs that displace warfarin from its binding site on plasma albumin, e.g. phenylbutazone.
- Drugs that inhibit liver microsomal enzymes that normally metabolize warfarin e.g. metronidazole.

Factors decreasing the effect of warfarin include:
- Hypothyroidism.
- Oral contraceptive use.
- Drugs that induce liver microsomal enzymes that normally metabolize warfarin e.g. barbiturates.

References

1. Wells PS, et al. Evaluation of D-dimer in the diagnosis of suspected deep-vein thrombosis. *NEJM* 2003; **349**:1227–35.
2. British Committee for Standards in Haematology guidelines on anticoagulation: http://www.bcshguidelines.com.
3. Lee AY, et al. Randomized comparison of low-molecular-weight heparin versus oral anticoagulant therapy for the prevention of recurrent venous thromboembolism in patients with cancer (CLOT) investigators. Low-molecular-weight heparin versus a coumarin for the prevention of recurrent venous thromboembolism in patients with cancer. *NEJM* 2003; **349**:146–53.

Useful website

NHS Prescribing Support Team. Drugs to watch with warfarin: http://www.nhssb.n-i.nhs.uk/prescribing/documents/Drugs

Rheumatology: Introduction

Rheumatology cases frequently occur in Station 5 of the PACES exam as they have relatively stable signs and provide a wide spectrum of clinical scenarios and a rich vein of questions due to the multi-system involvement of the connective tissue diseases (CTDs). Although such patients are relatively rare in day-to-day clinical practice, they are not in the context of the PACES exam, with both rheumatoid arthritis and scleroderma featuring within the top six cases within the authors' survey. Broadly the type of rheumatology case will fall into 1 of 3 categories:

- *Examination of hands* (rheumatoid arthritis, psoriatic arthritis, polyarticular gout, Raynaud's, scleroderma [particularly the limited variant]).
- *Assessment of a patient with a connective tissue disorder* with an emphasis on eliciting multi-organ involvement such as pulmonary fibrosis, pulmonary arterial hypertension, Raynaud's phenomenon, sicca symptoms, neuropathies, antiphospholipid syndrome.
- *Emergency rheumatology*, particularly as an increasing emphasis on the management of medical emergencies is a feature of the new format PACES exam. In the field of rheumatology such cases would include the acute hot joint and giant cell arteritis.

The following cases will be covered in this section

- Examination of hands:
  - Rheumatoid arthritis
  - Psoriatic arthritis
  - Jaccoud's arthropathy
  - Systemic sclerosis
  - Polyarticular gout
- Focused history and pertinent examination of a patient with CTD:
  - Systemic lupus erythematosus
  - Sjögren's syndrome
  - Systemic sclerosis
  - Dermatomyositis is covered within the context of inflammatory myopathy, neurology chapter (Ⓔ p.387)
- Emergency rheumatology:
  - The acute hot joint
  - Giant cell arteritis
- Ankylosing spondylitis
- Paget's disease.

Rheumatoid hands

Rheumatoid arthritis (RA) is a common disease, affecting 1% of the population with a predominance in women. This was the most frequent case encountered in our Station 5 survey. Furthermore, since patients with RA often attend A&E and may be on potentially immunosuppressive drugs, they are a fertile source of viva questions relevant to acute medicine.

Scenario

The wide variety of scenarios may direct the candidate to focus their history taking and examination to either specific joints or to specific complications of RA.

Example 1: Mrs Violet Edwards, aged 58 years.
This lady with longstanding arthralgia has experienced increased pain and tingling in her fingers. Please take a focused history and examine her appropriately.

Example 2: Mr Robindra Mitra, aged 29 years.
This man has had progressive pain on walking. Please take a focused history and examine him appropriately.

History

Key features addressed in the history should note the presence of any recent changes in the following:
- Joint pain and swelling:
  - Distribution – typically symmetrical (i.e. affecting the same groups of joints on each side).
  - Chronology of joint involvement.
  - Identification and more detailed history of currently symptomatic joints including how these are affecting activities of daily living (ADLs).
  - Complications – particularly any referred to in the introductory statement, e.g. carpal tunnel syndrome in Example 1.
- Early morning stiffness:
  - Typically in a symmetrical distribution.
  - Severity is determined by duration (particularly if lasting >60 minutes) and restriction of ADLs.
- Treatment (⊃ Treatment, p.494) that should include monitoring and reasons for discontinuation of any previous therapies.

2010 ACR/EULAR classification criteria for RA (definite RA scores ≥6)
- A. Joint involvement:
  - 2–10 large joints (1)
  - 1–3 small joints (2)
  - 4–10 small joints (3)
  - >10 joints (5)
- B. Serology:
  - Low +ve RF or anti-CCP antibody (2)
  - High +ve RF or anti-CCP antibody (3)
- C. Acute phase response, i.e. abnormal CRP or ESR (1)
- D. Duration ≥6 weeks (1)

The 2010 criteria focus on early diagnosis and treatment which has become increasingly important with the advent of more effective drug treatments over the past decade.

Hand examination for PACES

With the new Station 5, hand examination is usually one part of a longer case, so it is imperative that candidates practise to examine rapidly for arthritis in the hands.

- Key components of the look-feel-move system include:
  - *Look* carefully on both sides of the hands for signs of RA (listed in detail in ➲ Signs, p.493). Ask the patient to make a fist and turn their hands over to see if the fist is fully formed. Examine the elbows for rheumatoid nodules, plaque psoriasis, gouty tophi, surgical scars (see Fig. 8.4) and at the same time look for fixed flexion deformities at the elbows and subluxation of the wrists.
  - *Feel* systematically palpating all the joints for tenderness (metacarpophalangeal [MCP], proximal interphalangeal [PIP], distal interphalangeal [DIP], including thumbs and then wrists) as well as the boggy swelling of synovitis. These 2 features (tenderness and swelling) are key to determining whether an inflammatory arthritis is active.
  - *Move* to determine functionality, testing power grip in both hands ('Grip my fingers tightly') and fine dexterity ('Are you able to undo a button on your shirt?' or 'Can you pick up this coin?'). Examine range of movement particularly at the wrists in full extension and flexion.
- Ask yourself, what is the *distribution* of the arthritis?
  - Is it monoarthritis, oligo (4 joints or fewer), or polyarthritis?
  - Is it symmetrical or asymmetrical?
  - Does it affect large (wrists, elbows etc) or small joints (rest of the hand)?

For example, RA is a symmetrical polyarthritis affecting small and large joints, but sparing the DIP joints. Ankylosing spondylitis and other seronegative arthritides are typically an asymmetrical large joint oligoarthritis, while psoriatic arthritis can vary (➲ Psoriasis case p.497).

Patients who attend the PACES exam may have deformities from long-standing damage, yet their disease is frequently inactive – after all, if their disease was active, it could be painful for them to be repeatedly examined. Patients with longstanding RA may not have the typical deformities due to surgical correction, and therefore the candidate must examine closely for surgical scars (see Fig. 8.4). Note that a key manifestation of damage from arthritis is restricted range of movement. Sometimes, in cases of psoriatic arthritis, there is no obvious deformity, but the only evidence of past arthritis is restriction at a wrist or elbow or some DIP joints, which if not carefully examined, could lead to a candidate missing the diagnosis.

Signs

- Symmetrical deforming polyarthritis affecting all of the small joints of the hands, wrists and elbows, sparing the DIP joints.
- Ulnar deviation of the MCP joints.
- Boutonnière's and/or swan neck deformity.
- Z thumb.
- Piano key ulnar head.
- Rheumatoid nodules, most common at the elbows, but may occur over any pressure point.
- Commonest surgical scars (see Fig. 8.4):
  - Carpal tunnel decompression
  - Swanson's arthroplasty
  - Wrist arthrodesis
  - Ulnar styloidectomy
  - Wrist synovectomy
  - Tendon transfer (follows the line of a tendon).
- Extra-articular manifestations are less commonly seen with the more aggressive and early treatment of RA but include:
  - Haematological: anaemia (pallor of lower conjuctiva), splenomegaly (Felty's syndrome: RA + splenomegaly + neutropenia).
  - Skin: nodules, vasculitis, pyoderma gangrenosum.
  - Eye: scleritis, episcleritis, scleromalacia perforans.
  - Cardiovascular: valvular disease, pericarditis, conduction defects, myocardial infarction (accelerated atherosclerosis), myocarditis, heart failure.
  - Respiratory: pulmonary fibrosis (typically lower zones), pleural effusions, lung nodules, bronchiolitis obliterans.
  - Renal: amyloidosis.
  - Neurological: peripheral neuropathy, mononeuritis multiplex, compression neuropathies.
  - Compression neuropathies include:
    - Cervical myelopathy (atlanto-axial subluxation). Signs include spastic paraparesis, hyperreflexia, upgoing plantar response ± scar from previous surgery (may present in neurology section).
    - Ulnar neuropathy (elbow involvement).
    - Carpal tunnel syndrome (wrist involvement).

❶ Top Tips

- In rheumatological terminology, symmetry refers to the group of joints involved and does not specifically indicate the digits affected.
- For example, a patient with swelling of the 2nd & 3rd PIP and 2nd to 4th MCP of the right hand and 4th & 5th PIP and 3rd MCP of the left hand has symmetrical inflammation in their hands.
- If a scar overlies a joint, determine whether there is any movement of that joint – if not, the patient is likely to have undergone an arthrodesis.

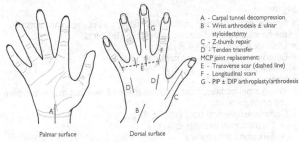

A - Carpal tunnel decompression
B - Wrist arthrodesis ± ulnar
    styloidectomy
C - Z-thumb repair
D - Tendon transfer
MCP joint replacement:
E - Transverse scar (dashed line)
F - Longitudinal scars
G - PIP ± DIP arthroplasty/arthrodesis

Palmar surface   Dorsal surface

Fig. 8.4 Surgical scars on hands of patient with rheumatoid/inflammatory arthritis
(With permission from Olivia Bessant).

Investigations

- Inflammatory markers: CRP, ESR – both elevated.
- FBC that may show:
  - Normochromic normocytic anaemia of chronic disease
  - Low WBC in Felty's syndrome.
- Rheumatoid factor is:
  - A series of antibodies which recognize the Fc portion of IgG.
  - Associated with more severe disease, increased mortality and extra-
    articular manifestations e.g. nodules.
  - Present in up to 5–10% of normals (increasing with age).
  - Over time, present in 80% of RA patients.
- Anti-CCP (cyclic citrullinated peptide) antibodies are:
  - a newer test with increased specificity for RA diagnosis (active TB
    can cause false +ve).
  - of increased positive predictive value for future development of RA.
- X-rays: key signs – periarticular osteopenia, erosions typically at the
  margins of the small joints, joint space narrowing, deformity.
- Power Doppler ultrasound or MRI to look for active synovitis.
- CXR: pulmonary fibrosis or pulmonary nodules.
- Lung function tests:
  - ↓ FVC due to kyphosis.
  - Restrictive defect: ↓ FVC, ↑ FEV$_1$/FVC ratio, ↓ TLCO due to
    pulmonary fibrosis.
- HRCT chest: non-specific interstitial pneumonitis (NSIP) (commonest)
  but usual interstitial pneumonitis (UIP), organizing pneumonia and
  bronchiolitis all occur.

Treatment

- Exercise, physiotherapy, occupational therapy, modification of home,
  mobility and dexterity aids.
- NSAIDs, COX-2 inhibitors.
- DMARDs:
  - Methotrexate
  - Sulphasalazine
  - Leflunomide
  - Hydroxychloroquine (antimalarial).
- Old drugs now rarely in use include gold and penicillamine.

Biologic therapies

- TNF blockade:
  - Infliximab, adalimumab and golimumab (anti-TNF monoclonal antibodies)
  - Etanercept (soluble TNF receptor antagonist)
  - Certiluzumab pegol (pegylated Fab construct)
- Newer biologic therapies:
  - Rituximab (anti-CD20 monoclonal antibody which depletes B cells)
  - Abatacept (CTLA4-Ig which blocks co-stimulation of T cells)
  - Tociluzimab (anti-IL-6 receptor monoclonal antibody).

Patient concerns

The patient may ask if they can be cured if they are prescribed injections.

The candidate should inform the patient that at present, RA cannot be cured. A significant proportion of patients may attain remission by use of drugs such as methotrexate, with or without a biological agent e.g. a TNF inhibitor. The word 'injection' should alert the candidate that the patient may well have read recent articles on the use of biological therapies in inflammatory arthritis (in newspapers or the Internet).

My aunt has RA and has undergone several joint replacements. Will I also need these operations?

The candidate should explain that current management is much more aggressive and that modern therapies are much more efficacious. This has resulted in far fewer patients having disease of the severity that necessitates joint replacement surgery.

I have been informed that the standard treatment for my condition will be methotrexate. My friend has also told me that methotrexate is a treatment for cancer.

Many of the therapies that are used to treat patients with RA were first used in other branches of medicine, such as haematology and oncology. However, we now use these drugs in much lower doses to suppress the activity of the immune system, rather than to treat a cancer. Therefore these drugs are employed for many differing conditions (e.g. inflammatory bowel disease).

Viva questions

How would you monitor a patient on DMARD therapy or anti-TNF?

Both DMARDs and biologic therapies require regular specialist review:
- Clinical: regular history and examination, looking for evidence of infection, especially TB, or complications including pulmonary fibrosis (methotrexate, anti-TNF).
- Blood tests for early detection of adverse effects, especially cytopenia and transaminitis: FBC, U&E, LFT at regular intervals, usually monthly for most DMARDs, but refer to specialist guidance.

What are the side effects of methotrexate?

- Hepatitis, alveolitis, stomatitis.
- Toxicity due to overdose: marrow suppression/pancytopenia leading to opportunistic infections (e.g. PCP).
- Methotrexate is given once weekly and the commonest cause of toxicity is being incorrectly prescribed or being taken as daily dose.

What is the treatment for methotrexate toxicity?
Folinic acid (works quicker than folic acid).

How do you manage a patient on anti-TNF treatment who presents to A&E with a minor infection such as cellulitis?
• Admit the patient
• Stop anti-TNF Rx
• Intravenous antibiotics
• Seek specialist advice.

NB The WBC is typically unaffected by anti-TNF.

List possible causes of anaemia in RA
Anaemia of chronic disease; GI damage due to NSAIDs and/or steroids; Felty's syndrome; renal amyloid; marrow suppression (methotrexate or other DMARDs); autoimmune haemolytic anaemia; associated pernicious anaemia.

How do you distinguish rheumatoid arthritis (RA) from osteoarthritis (OA) on x-ray?
• RA: juxta-articular osteopenia, erosions, symmetry, deformity.
• OA: sclerosis, osteophytes.
• Both: bone cysts, joint space narrowing.

How do you distinguish active from inactive arthritis?
Symptoms (increased pain, fatigue), swelling, joint tenderness, warmth of joints, raised ESR.
NB Disease activity may be masked in a patient taking NSAIDs.

Useful websites
Arthritis Care website: http://www.arthritisuk.com
National Rheumatoid Arthritis Society website: http://www.nras.org.uk
NICE: www.nice.org.uk/CG79
The Scottish Intercollegiate Guidelines Network: http://www.sign.ac.uk/guidelines

Psoriatic arthritis

Psoriatic arthritis (PsA) develops in 5–10% of patients with psoriasis, more commonly in those patients with nail involvement. Axial arthritis accounts for only 2% of cases of psoriatic arthritis. 70% of patients have skin psoriasis for >10 years before the development of PsA. In the remaining 30% of patients the arthritis precedes or coincides with the onset of skin psoriasis. The sex distribution is equal, except for the inflammatory spondyloarthropathy, where there is a 3-fold increased male predominance. The typical age of onset is between 35–50 years old. Having a first degree relative with PsA increases one's chance of developing the condition 50-fold, and a father with the disease confers twice the risk as a mother with the disease to a child.

> **Scenario**
>
> Mr Daniel Potter, 39 years old, is finding it more difficult to perform his job as a painter and decorator due to painful hands.
>
> Please perform a focused history and examination.

In the PACES examination, a patient with PsA is most likely to be encountered in the scenario of hand examination. The same approach to history, examination and functional assessment should be taken as outlined for a patient with RA (➔ p.491). Once a candidate has elicited a history of psoriasis in either the patient, or in their family history, further aspects of history and examination should include:

History
- Any episodes of:
  - inflammatory back pain
  - iritis
  - symptoms of inflammatory bowel disease e.g. bloody diarrhoea
  - enthesitis e.g. Achilles' tendonitis
  - plantar fasciitis (especially if bilateral)
- The joint distribution:
  - Smaller joints e.g. hands and feet.
  - Larger joints e.g. shoulders, elbows, knees. Enquire about the number involved. Oligoarthritis effects 1–4 joints and, in psoriatic arthritis, is often associated with massive effusions.
- Response to exercise and NSAIDs.

Examination
In addition the following examination should also be carried out:
- Nails for pitting/onycholysis/transverse ridging/hyperkeratosis and yellowing.
- Skin for psoriasis especially elbows, knees, nape of neck, hairline, umbilicus, natal cleft and any surgical scars (Koebner's phenomenon).
- Back for any restriction of movement or presence of sacroiliitis (➔ p.524).
- Auscultation of the precordium to exclude aortic regurgitation.

❶ Top Tips

- Sacroiliitis is often asymmetrical in psoriatic arthritis, whereas it is almost always bilateral in patients with ankylosing spondylitis.

Differential diagnosis

The differential diagnosis will vary according to the clinical subtype:
- DIP involvement: OA, particularly erosive OA.
- Rheumatoid distribution type: RA.
- Inflammatory spondyloarthropathy: ankylosing spondylitis, reactive arthritis, inflammatory bowel disease related arthropathy.
- Oligoarthropathy: reactive arthritis, sarcoidosis, gout.
- Dactylitis: gout, reactive arthritis, and sarcoidosis.
- Explosive onset of severe psoriasis with arthritis: consider HIV infection.

Investigations

- Radiographs of the symptomatic joints.
- Ultrasound or isotope bone scan if plain radiographs inconclusive.
- Blood tests should include:
  • FBC for anaemia.
  • Renal function (NSAID use).
  • Acute phase reactants although it is not uncommon for the ESR and CRP to be normal in PsA.
- HLA-B27 status.

Treatment

- NSAIDs in mild non-erosive disease.
- The DMARD sulphasalazine is helpful for the arthritis, but not skin disease.
- The mainstay of treatment is methotrexate, which is effective against both the skin disease and the arthritis.
- Leflunomide is also an effective treatment for the arthritis and to a lesser extent for the skin disease.
- Hydroxychloroquine is best avoided as it can exacerbate skin psoriasis.
- Steroids are used with caution as a significant flare of skin disease usually occurs on their withdrawal.
- Local cortisone injections are very effective for enthesitis.
- If the patient's disease is severe enough, then anti-TNF blockers can be prescribed, which are very effective in controlling the joint and skin involvement.

Patient concerns

- 'Can this be treated effectively?'
- 'Will I have to give up my job?'
- 'Will my children develop this disease?'
- 'Will I have to take medication for the rest of my life?'

Methotrexate and TNF-inhibitors are very effective treatments for PsA and one would expect the patient to remain in employment if treated appropriately and effectively. As PsA can be associated with HLA B27 there is an increased chance of offspring developing the disease i.e. a 50-fold increase if a first degree-degree relative has the disease. PsA very rarely goes into spontaneous remission and therefore the majority of patients will remain dependent on medication to control their arthritis.

Viva questions

In this patient with an inflammatory arthropathy of the hands, how can you differentiate between PsA and RA?

The following favour a diagnosis of PsA rather than RA:

- Asymmetry.
- Negative rheumatoid factor and anti-CCP antibodies.
- Presence of nail changes.
- Dactylitis (inflammation of entire finger or toe, leading to sausage digits).
- A family or personal history of psoriasis.

Do you know any HLA associations of psoriatic arthritis?

- HLA B38/B39 is associated with peripheral distal arthritis.
- HLA DR4 with a rheumatoid distribution subtype.
- HLA B27 with the sacroiliitis/spondyloarthropathy form.

What is the pattern of joint involvement in psoriatic arthritis?

The classification of Moll and Wright in 1973 described the following 5 subtypes of psoriatic arthritis, although considerable overlap between these clinical subtypes can occur:

- Rheumatoid-like pattern (symmetrical, persistently seronegative).
- Arthritis mutilans (destructive – shortened fingers, with resorption/telescoping of joints).
- DIP joint involvement.
- Oligoarthritis (asymmetrical, often with massive effusions).
- Spondyloarthropathy (sacroiliitis; resembling ankylosing spondylitis).

📖 Further reading

Goodman A. New psoriatic arthritis recommendations tailored to rheumatologists. [Medscape article from EULAR June 21 2010.] Available at: http://www.medscape.com/viewarticle/723884.

NICE. *Etanercept, infliximab and adulimumab for the treatment of psoriatic arthritis* (TA199). London: NICE, 2010.

SIGN. *Diagnosis and management of psoriasis and psoriatic arthritis in adults* (SIGN guidance 121). Edinburgh: SIGN, 2010.

Systemic lupus erythematosus and Sjögren's syndrome

Systemic lupus erythematosus (SLE) is a fairly common autoimmune disease with a strong female preponderance (female: male ratio 8:1). The patient is typically young (usually aged 20–40) and the disease is more common in certain ethnic groups including Africans (3× more common than in whites) and Asians. Its features can be wide-ranging such that it may crop up in any of the stations in the PACES exam, e.g. from hand or skin rash examination in Station 5 to a renal transplant as part of abdominal examination.

> ## Scenario
>
> As a multi-organ disease, a variety of scenarios exist involving patients with previously undiagnosed SLE or with a history of SLE who present with an acute complaint.
>
> E.g. Miss Olokunwe Mallon, aged 31.
>
> This lady has had SLE for a long time. She presents generally unwell to A&E, feverish and breathless. Please assess her and describe your management plan.

History and examination

Feeling unwell and feverish with associated breathlessness has a wide differential diagnosis in a patient with SLE and includes a chest infection (which may be opportunistic), a pulmonary embolism or active lupus itself. For history and examination related to dyspnoea ➔ Shortness of breath, p.459. Specific causes of dyspnoea in patients with SLE are highlighted in the Top Tips Box.

> ## ❶ Top Tips
>
> *Causes of breathlessness in SLE and connective tissue diseases*
> - PE
> - Pleural effusion
> - Pneumonia (may be opportunistic due to immunosuppression)
> - Pulmonary fibrosis
> - Reaction to biologic therapy (mimics ARDS)
> - Pericardial effusion
> - Acute MI
> - Cardiomyopathy
> - Renal failure causing pulmonary oedema
> - Neuromuscular – myositis causing ventilatory muscle weakness or Guillain–Barré syndrome (very rare).

History

- Arthritis: arthralgia with tenderness is almost universal. True inflammatory arthritis is typically non-deforming (Jaccoud's arthritis) – → Examination p.502.
- Mucocutaneous lesions: these can take many forms so it is important to ask about rashes especially on the face. These may come and go and so may not be present when you assess the patient. They may be photosensitive (provoked by sunlight). Alopecia is common and can either be diffuse hair loss associated with active disease, or patchy scarring alopecia which can lead to severe loss of hair (more common in Africans). Also, always ask about persistent mouth ulcers.
- Cardiorespiratory involvement: ask about breathlessness and chest pain, especially pleuritic. Sudden dyspnoea, syncope or haemoptysis may herald a PE.
- Renal disease: patients may develop swollen legs due to oedema, have had renal biopsies, renal replacement therapy or transplant. They may also be aware of proteinuria either during recent clinic visits or in the past.
- Myositis: overlap between connective tissue diseases is common and frequently missed even by specialists. Ask about muscle pain, tenderness or weakness.
- Neuropsychiatric: acute psychotic events are common as are multiple neurological lesions including mononeuritis multiplex, transverse myelitis and Guillain–Barré syndrome.
- Haematological: patients are predisposed to thrombotic events (both venous and arterial), particularly in patients with anti-phospholipid antibodies and candidates would be expected to enquire about any history of DVT, PE or miscarriage for example.
- Obstetric: recurrent miscarriage (fetal loss is usually before the 10th week of pregnancy) or pre-eclampsia can be features of antiphospholipid syndrome in the context of SLE.

ACR criteria for SLE (requires 4 or more)

- Malar rash
- Discoid rash
- Photosensitivity
- Oral ulcers
- Non-erosive arthritis
- Serositis, i.e. pleuritis/pleural effusion or pericarditis
- Renal disorder (persistent proteinuria or cellular casts indicating glomerulonephritis)
- Neurological disorder (seizures, psychosis, transverse myelitis, Guillain–Barré syndrome)
- Haematological disorder (haemolytic anaemia, leucopenia, lymphopenia, thrombocytopenia)
- Anti-nuclear antibodies (ANA)
- Other autoantibodies including anti-Sm, anti-dsDNA, antiphospholipid antibodies.

Candidates would also be expected to enquire what immunosuppressive therapy the patient is on.

Examination

Look for the following:
- General features of systemic disease e.g. lymphadenopathy or fever (temperature chart) which may be suggestive of infection or active lupus.
- Arthritis: inflammatory arthritis in SLE is typically non-deforming. In Jaccoud's arthropathy the fingers show deformities at rest, especially ulnar deviation and swan necks, which reverse when closed into a fist. However, overlap syndromes can cause a destructive arthritis, more typical of rheumatoid arthritis.
- Mucocutaneous features (➔ Cutaneous lupus case p.610) – have many forms, so look carefully for:
  - Malar rash: the classic symmetrical butterfly rash across the face.
  - Discoid lupus.
  - Vasculitis: a mottled vasculitic rash on the palms is frequently seen with active lupus.
  - Scarring alopecia: common in Africans and often hidden under a wig (or weave).
  - Mouth ulcers: often red and painful.
  - Overlap with other conditions such as scleroderma or dermatomyositis.
  - Livedo reticularis: a mottled reticular pattern caused by dilated medium-sized veins giving the skin a purplish lace-work appearance. Sometimes seen in association with antiphospholipid syndrome but also characteristic of polyarteritis nodosa.
- Cardiac involvement: valve incompetence due to Libman–Sacks endocarditis may cause AR or MR and require valve replacement; patients may show signs of heart failure.
- Lung involvement: pulmonary fibrosis or pleural effusions, or consolidation in the acute setting.
- Hypertension: often resulting from renal disease in patients with SLE.
- Urinalysis (for blood and protein) to exclude active renal disease; this critical bedside test is frequently forgotten!
- Renal disease: patients may be oedematous with nephrotic syndrome, show signs of being on renal replacement therapy i.e. AV fistula, haemodialysis lines/scars, peritoneal dialysis lines/scars, or have had a renal transplant
- Evidence of thrombotic events: wearing compression stockings to prevent further DVT, or swollen leg from current DVT
- Neurological: cranial nerve lesions, mononeuritis multiplex, transverse myelitis (looks like cord compression; ➔ neurology chapter p.351), rarely Guillain–Barré syndrome, optic atrophy
- Iatrogenic: Cushingoid from excessive steroid use

Sjögren's syndrome

Often misleadingly described as a milder version of SLE, Sjögren's not infrequently crops up as a station 5 case. Confusingly Sjögren's is most commonly secondary to another rheumatic disease e.g. RA or SLE.

Key features

- Dry eyes (xerophthalmia).
- Dry mouth (xerostoma) or tongue.
- Bilateral enlarged parotid glands (NB differential diagnosis: lymphoma, sarcoidosis, parotid tumour, mumps).
- Candidates would not be expected to perform *Schirmer's test*, but ought to be able to describe it: 5mm wide strips of sterile filter paper are hooked inside each lower eyelid and the patient asked to close their eyes. Normal secretion of tears causes moisture to migrate >15mm along the filter paper over 5min.

Key tests

The ENA antibodies Ro or La are typically positive, but rheumatoid factor and anti-dsDNA antibodies may also be seen. Diagnostic antibodies are present in ~60% of cases; if negative, a salivary gland biopsy (labial biopsy) is required to make the diagnosis.

Follow-up

Patients with primary Sjögren's syndrome (in the absence of other CTD) require long-term review, due to the 40-fold increased risk of lymphoma (usually B cell) over their lifetime.

Investigations

These are largely determined by the pattern of disease.
- Urine cytology for red cell casts.
- Inflammatory markers: ESR commonly elevated, CRP usually only elevated during serositis or infection.
- FBC: may show an array of haematological disorders including haemolytic anaemia, thrombocytopenia, lymphopenia; thus direct Coombs test and reticulocyte count also helpful.
- Immunological tests.
  - ANA: positive in >95% of cases, titre usually very high in SLE i.e. >1:320.
  - dsDNA: usually positive, may rise during flares.
  - ENA (extractable nuclear antigens): often positive, especially Ro, La, Sm(Smith), RNP.
  - Complement: low C4 and less commonly low C3 associated with renal involvement, both may fall during active flares.
  - Anti-phospholipid antibodies: high titres associated with secondary antiphospholipid syndrome.
  - NB Complete absence of autoantibodies is very unusual in SLE.
- CK: if raised suggests myositis.
- Pulse oximetry ± ABG if symptomatic with dyspnoea.
- CXR: fibrosis, effusions, cardiomegaly (can be a sign of pericardial effusion).

- VQ or CTPA if concerns of PE.
- Echo: valvular incompetence or vegetations, pericardial effusion.
- Skin biopsy: may show immune complex deposition (IgG/IgM and C3) at the dermal-epidermal junction.
- Renal biopsy: may show glomerulonephritis with evidence of immune complex (Ig and C3) deposition or microthrombotic disease. PACES candidates would not be expected to discuss the complex classification system for defining lupus nephritis histologically.

Treatment

Treatments which directly target the disease include:
- Steroids especially prednisolone, often long term.
- Antimalarials: hydroxychloroquine.
- Immunosuppressants:
  - Azathioprine
  - IV cyclophosphamide
  - Mycophenolate mofetil
  - Methotrexate.
- Biologics: rituximab (anti-CD20 monoclonal antibody which depletes B cells).
- IV Ig: frequently used for serious flares, e.g. neurological complications or where sepsis cannot be ruled out such as on ITU.
- Plasmapheresis: rarely used for severe cases.

For secondary antiphospholipid syndrome, warfarin or LMWH are commonly used. For renal disease, ACE inhibitors or angiotensin II receptor antagonists may reduce proteinuria. Statins are commonly used as patients with SLE are at substantially increased risk of atherosclerotic vascular events (all patients with SLE should undergo cardiovascular risk assessment as part of their routine management). Patients with SLE may also need to be treated for diabetes as a consequence of long-term steroid therapy.

Consider broad-spectrum IV antibiotics if patient septic and neutropenic or recently received potent immunosuppression e.g. cyclophosphamide.

Patient concerns

As with any other multisystem disease, the concerns raised will be dependent on which systems have been affected in a particular patient. Many patients will also be worried about their offspring being affected, particularly as SLE affects women of childbearing age. Although genetic factors are important in causing SLE, it is vital to reassure the patient that the risk of a child inheriting exactly the required genes to cause SLE is actually very small. Patients are frequently concerned about side effects of medications especially corticosteroids and the effects of immunosuppressants on fertility. In addition due to the risk of teratogenicity, patients should be counselled not to conceive while on nearly all immunosuppressants (except azathioprine and hydroxychloroquine).

Viva questions

What investigations are helpful to determine if this patient's lupus is active?

- Urinalysis for blood and protein ± urinary protein:creatinine ratio
- Urine cytology for red cell casts
- U&E
- ESR
- FBC to look for cytopenias
- Anti-dsDNA antibodies
- Complement C3 & C4.

What are the major risks of cyclophosphamide? What can be done to prevent them?

- *Infection* There are 2 major issues:
  - Reactivation of latent infections due to immunosuppression. It is therefore necessary to screen for Hep B, Hep C, HIV and TB prior to therapy.
  - Bone marrow suppression – usually seen at 8–10 days after each infusion (check FBC).
  - Additionally it is important that all other immunosuppressants are stopped during cyclophosphamide therapy (except steroids, which should be tapered as rapidly as feasible).
  - Regular oral septrin prophylaxis for opportunistic infections such as *Pneumocystis jiroveci (carinii)* should be prescribed.
- *Bladder toxicity* Haemorrhagic cystitis was a well recognized feature of cyclophosphamide therapy but is now much rarer, given the use of oral mesna taken immediately before and after each infusion of cyclophosphamide. It also reduces the risk of subsequent bladder cancer.
- *Malignancy* Risk is dependent on cumulative dose. Patients who have been treated with cyclophosphamide should be under long-term surveillance for malignancy of all forms.
- *Infertility* Variable risk dependent on cumulative dose and age. Ovarian failure risk is substantially reduced if a short course of only 6 doses of IV cyclophosphamide is used, with each infusion at a reduced dose. Expert advice is required. Men can opt to freeze sperm samples for future use. An ovarian protection regimen can be employed using gonadotrophin analogues, to minimize ovarian toxicity.
- *Other risks* Nausea, vomiting, reversible alopecia, teratogenicity.

Note that oral cyclophosphamide has a higher risk of all of these toxicities and thus for most conditions pulsed IV therapy is preferred.

📖 Further reading

Bambacle AS, Appel GB. Update on the treatment of lupus nephritis. *J Am Soc Nephrol* **21**:1–8.
Bertsias G et al. EULAR recommendations for the management of SLE. Report of a task force of the eular standing committee for international clinical studies including therapeutics. *Ann Rheum Dis* 2008; **67**:195–205.

🕸 Useful website

Christine M. Bartels et al. SLE. Emedicine.medscape.com/article/332244

Painful hands: systemic sclerosis

Systemic sclerosis (SSc), a connective tissue disorder characterized by thickening and fibrosis of the skin, displays considerable variation in its severity and heterogeneity in the degree of other organ involvement. The female:male ratio is 3:1 and most commonly involves the age group 35–65 with no ethnic bias.

The scleroderma spectrum of disorders encompasses:

- Raynaud's phenomenon: secondary to autoimmune disorders (systemic sclerosis, SLE, Sjögren's, MCTD); note that the primary form is not associated with CTD and is far more prevalent.
- Localized scleroderma:
  - Morphoea.
  - Linear scleroderma.
  - En coup de sabre (type of linear scleroderma that presents on the frontal or frontoparietal scalp).
- Systemic sclerosis:
  - Limited cutaneous systemic sclerosis (lcSSc; skin involvement distal to knees and elbows, facial involvement, but the trunk is spared)
  - CREST (Calcinosis, Raynaud's, (o)Esophageal hypomotility, Sclerodactyly, Telangiectasia), a subgroup of lcSSc
  - Diffuse cutaneous systemic sclerosis (dcSSc; skin involvement proximal to the elbows and knees).

✤ Common Pitfalls

- Scleroderma refers to the skin manifestation which occurs in SSc, the multi-organ CTD. Candidates frequently interchange these 2 terms.
- The diagnosis of CREST is too frequently applied by candidates who either do not display all of the 5 features, or in whom the scleroderma extends proximal to the MCP joints (i.e. more extensive than sclerodactyly).

Scenario

Mrs Susan White, age 43.

This lady has developed painful cold hands. Please take a focused history and perform an appropriate examination.

History

This scenario should prompt the candidate to consider Raynaud's phenomenon and, in a woman of this age, secondary rather than primary Raynaud's. Therefore the approach to the patient should be to elicit the classical history of Raynaud's phenomenon and determine the underlying connective tissue disease (Table 8.9).

Raynaud's phenomenon

The classic triphasic colour changes of Raynaud's phenomenon (white to blue to red, with pain during the erythematous phase) should be elicited as follows:

- Colour changes:
  - 'Do your hands change colour?'

- If so, 'What colour?'
- 'When does this happen?'
- Features suggesting severe, pathological Raynaud's:
  - Extent of hand involvement: whole hand rather than just finger tips.
  - Ulceration: past or present, or other chronic skin changes.
  - Involvement of other peripheries: nose and ears (however toes are commonly involved, even in milder cases).
  - Occurrence in a warm environment.
  - Slow recovery time.

Whilst eliciting this history, candidates should look for features of underlying CTD:
- Sclerodermatous facies (tight shiny skin, microstomia, telangiectasia, beaked nose)
- Malar rash
- Scarring alopecia
- Hands: swollen joints/sclerodactyly/calcinosis
- Bottle of water/artificial tears/chewing gum near bedside.

History of:

Co-existent inflammatory arthropathy:
- 'Are your joints painful?' If so, 'Which ones?'
- 'Do your joints swell?'
- 'Are these symptoms more marked during any time of the day or night (diurnal variation)?'

Table 8.9 Causes of secondary Raynaud's

CTD	Discriminatory features
Systemic sclerosis	Scleroderma
	SOB secondary to pulmonary fibrosis and/or PAH[a]
	Dysphagia/dyspepsia/diarrhoea (3Ds!)
SLE	Malar rash and/or photosensitivity/scarring alopecia
	Jaccoud's arthropathy
	Oral ulceration
Dermatomyositis	Heliotope rash/Gottron's papules/periungual erythema
	Proximal myopathy
MCTD[b]	Features of SLE
	Features of scleroderma
	Muscle pain/tenderness with associated proximal weakness (i.e. features of polymyositis)
Sjögren's syndrome	Xerophthalmia (dry eyes)/xerostomia (dry mouth)
	Fatigue
	Non-erosive small joint polyarthropathy

[a] Pulmonary arterial hypertension. [b] Mixed connective tissue disease – an overlap syndrome combining SLE, systemic sclerosis, myositis.

Screening questions for underlying connective tissue disease
- 'Do you have any rashes; if so, does it worsen on sun exposure?'
- 'Are you losing hair?'
- 'Do you suffer from mouth ulcers?'
- 'Do you have dry eyes and/or a dry mouth?'
- 'Are you short of breath?' (pulmonary fibrosis and/or PAH)
- 'Do you have difficulty swallowing?' (oesophageal dysmotility); 'Do you suffer with heartburn?'
- 'Do you have diarrhoea and/or have you lost weight?' (bacterial overgrowth and malabsorption secondary to hypomotility of the bowel)
- 'Are your muscles painful or weak?'
- 'Do you have difficulty rising from a chair, or getting in and out of a bath/car?' (proximal myopathy)

❶ Top Tips

- The most common patient for this scenario would be a patient with limited SSc (previously known as CREST).
- The absence of Raynaud's phenomenon makes a diagnosis of systemic sclerosis extremely unlikely.
- The Raynaud's may precede the onset of CREST (limited cutaneous systemic sclerosis) by several years. In contrast, in diffuse systemic sclerosis, Raynaud's and other organ involvement commonly coincide.
- Many patients who do not experience dysphagia do suffer with heartburn, but this history will only become evident on direct questioning.

Examination

Whilst talking to Mrs White candidates should look for features of scleroderma such as microstomia and facial telangiectasia but also look for features of the other connective tissue diseases included in the differential for a patient presenting with secondary Raynaud's phenomenon (see Table 8.9).
- Hands:
  - Sclerodactyly
  - Inflammatory arthritis
  - Jaccoud's arthropathy
  - Digital ulcers
  - Subcutaneous calcinosis
  - Cutaneous vasculitis
  - Periungal erythema (dermatomyositis)
  - Gottron's papules (dermatomyositis)
- Cardiorespiratory:
  - Bibasal, fixed, fine end-expiratory crepitations of pulmonary fibrosis
  - Left parasternal heave of RVH and loud P_2 of pulmonary hypertension.

❶ Common Pitfalls

- Remember to screen for coexistent pulmonary fibrosis and/or pulmonary hypertension as these determine the severity of the condition and the prognosis for the patient.
- Pulmonary fibrosis may respond to immunosuppression (cyclophosphamide) and pulmonary hypertension can now be treated.

❶ Top Tips

- The examination must be focused to demonstrate to the examiner that the candidate has a narrow differential and knows the important organ systems that can be affected by connective tissue disease associated with secondary Raynaud's phenomenon.

Features of systemic sclerosis

- Raynaud's phenomenon is one of the earliest features: its absence should make the diagnosis unlikely.
- Sclerodactyly.
- Microstomia.
- Abnormal nailfold capillary loops (ideally via capillaroscopy).
- Digital ulcers (in 50% of patients).
- GIT involvement:
  - Oesophageal dysmotility in 70–90% of patients.
  - Small bowel and large bowel involvement in 50% of patients: can lead to bacterial overgrowth, malabsorption and chronic diarrhoea.
- Pulmonary involvement:
  - Is the leading cause of morbidity and mortality in SSc due to the development of interstitial lung disease (ILD) and pulmonary hypertension.
  - NSIP is the most common pattern of ILD, although UIP may be present; both lead to exertional dyspnoea, hypoxaemia and a non-productive cough with bibasal crepitations.
  - Development of pulmonary hypertension is associated with fatigue, palpable loud P_2, parasternal heave (secondary to RVH), murmurs of pulmonary and tricuspid regurgitation, elevated JVP and peripheral oedema.
- Scleroderma renal crisis:
  - Sudden onset of severe arterial hypertension, headache, visual disturbance, seizures, congestive cardiac failure, microangiopathic haemolytic anaemia, thrombocytopaenia and accelerated oliguric renal failure.

Investigations

- Positive ANA in 90% of patients; anti-Scl-70 (anti-topoisomerase) in 40% of patients with dcSSc and anti-centromere antibodies in 80% of patients with lcSSc.
- Nailfold capillaroscopy: enlarged capillaries, microhaemorrhages, dropouts.

- Lung function tests: decreased transfer factor.
- HRCT: features of ILD.
- Echo for RVH and increased pulmonary pressures.
- Radiographs may demonstrate acro-osteolysis of terminal phalanges, subcutaneous calcinosis (in CREST variant); erosive arthritis is rare.

Treatment

- There is no proven effective treatment to prevent disease progression.
- Calcium antagonists and iloprost infusions for Raynaud's. Limited evidence that fluoxetine and losartan may also have a beneficial role for Raynaud's.
- Iloprost infusions, endothelin receptor antagonists and sildenafil are helpful in the healing of digital ulcers.
- Methotrexate and mycophenolate may be beneficial in treating the skin thickening.
- Cyclophosphamide can improve skin thickening, stabilize pulmonary function and has been associated with increased survival.
- Clinical trials are ongoing in the USA and Europe and suggest a positive outcome from autologous stem cell transplantation.

Patient concerns

Can this condition be cured?

Although systemic sclerosis cannot be cured, in the majority of patients, the disease is slowly progressive over years. The candidate will need to consider the particular system involved and explain the treatment option available. In most cases, treatment is directed toward control of symptoms. Disease progression is less responsive to immunosuppression than the other autoimmune athritides/vasculitides.

Will my children inherit this disease?

All autoimmune diseases demonstrate an increased incidence of other autoimmune conditions in close relatives. As SSc is not hereditary the patient can be reassured that their children are not at increased risk of developing this condition.

Viva questions

This young patient has Raynaud's phenomenon. How would you determine if it is primary or secondary?

- Determine any other symptoms of connective tissue disease i.e. rashes, joint pain with swelling, dysphagia, dyspnoea.
- Autoantibodies.
- Careful examination of nail folds (or capillaroscopy if available).
- Late onset or acute onset (primary Raynaud's usually manifests in teenage years).

What is the presentation and management of scleroderma renal crisis?

The prognosis of scleroderma renal crisis is poor, with a substantial risk of death. It is more common in diffuse SSc, especially if it presents with sudden onset severe Raynaud's/sclerodactyly, which in its early stages manifests as hard, swollen, puffy hands. It may also be precipitated by corticosteroids. Renal crisis clinically presents with acute hypertension, abruptly rising creatinine, sometimes with evidence of microangiopathic haemolytic anaemia. Treatment involves ACE inhibitors, supportive management in HDU/ITU and iloprost infusions.

How do you differentiate cutaneous vasculitis from telangiectasia?
Cutaneous vaculitis will not blanche when pressed.

📖 Further reading

Derrett-Smith EC, Denton CP. Systemic sclerosis: clinical features and management. *Medicine* 2010; **38**:109–15.

🖙 Useful websites

Denton C. Renal complications of systemic sclerosis. [Video] http://www.dailymotion.com/video/xcrs6r_c-denton-renal-complications-of-sys_tech
Schwatz RA. Systemic sclerosis: http://emedicine.medscape.com/article/1066280-overview

Polyarticular gout

Polyarticular gout could present in Station 5 as a differential diagnosis of painful joints. Candidates would be expected to recognize the presence of chronic tophaceous lesions. The emphasis should be on the history, particularly with reference to predisposing factors, and the discussion will centre on the further management. Acute monoarticular gout will be covered under acute hot joint (➔ p.516).

Gouty arthritis is the most common form of arthritis in men over the age of 40. The overall male:female ratio is 4:1. The prevalence of gout increases with age and increasing serum urate concentrations, although only 15% of patients with hyperuricaemia develop gout.

There are 4 stages of gouty arthritis:
- Asymptomatic hyperuricaemia
- Acute gouty arthritis
- Intercritical gout
- Chronic tophaceous gout.

As the candidate is most likely to encounter such a patient in the scenario of hand examination the same approach to history, examination, and functional assessment should be taken as outlined for a patient with RA (➔ p.491).

> ### Scenario
>
> Mr George Windsor, 63 years old, is finding that his hands are increasingly painful and he is having great difficulty in using his hands for any fine movements.
>
> Please perform a focused history and examination.

Once a candidate has elicited a history suggestive of gouty arthritis in the patient, further aspects of history and examination should include:

History
- The age of onset of symptoms (if at a young age, the candidate must enquire with regard to renal function and any relevant family history).

- The frequency and duration of attacks; classically an attack will last between 3–10 days, but can be terminated quickly if appropriate treatment is initiated at the onset of the first symptoms.
- The distribution of joint involvement:
  - The first attack of gout is usually monoarticular and, in 85% of cases, involves the hallux, arch of foot or ankle.
  - 50% of cases at presentation involve the hallux and this joint will eventually become involved in >90% of cases (i.e. podagra, gout which involves the big toe).
- Diurnal variation in attacks: the beginning of a flare of gout usually commences in the middle of the night or in the early morning.
- Response to treatment: usually only high dose colchicine, steroids or a strong NSAID e.g. naproxen (but not ibuprofen) will be sufficient to alleviate the pain.
- Precipitants/triggers:
  - Excess alcohol
  - Excess purine ingestion e.g. shellfish, oily fish, legumes
  - Haemorrhage
  - Infection
  - Trauma
  - Surgery
  - Radiotherapy
  - Dehydration.
- Predisposing medical conditions:
  - Renal impairment
  - Hypothyroidism
  - Myeloproliferative and/or lymphoproliferative disorders
  - Polycythaemia rubra vera
  - Hyperparathyroidism
  - Diabetes mellitus
  - Diabetes insipidus
  - Barter's syndrome
  - Sarcoidosis
  - Psoriasis
  - Hyperlipidaemia
  - Obesity.

Drug history

- Drugs that increase urate level:
  - Thiazide diuretics
  - Low-dose aspirin
  - Theophylline
  - Ciclosporin
  - Levodopa
  - Ethambutol
- Drugs that decrease urate level:
  - Losartan
  - Fenofibrate.

Examination

Classically, acutely inflamed joints in gout will be erythematous and tender, with overlying shiny, desquamating skin. With a history of recurrent attacks, some joints may display these acute signs, whilst others show more chronic tophaceous changes. Alternatively, the patient may have only chronic changes, or indeed, no overt signs of gout.

Typically, gouty arthritis of the hands has an asymmetrical distribution. The candidate should examine the hands as outlined on ➔ p.492.

The following additional examination should also be carried out:

- Examination for tophi on:
  - Digits of hands and feet
  - Extensor surface of forearm, particularly along tendon sheaths
  - Elbow
  - Achilles tendon
  - Pinna.
- Look for olecranon bursitis.
- Inspect ulceration carefully:
  - Tophi may ulcerate extruding white chalk-like monosodium urate crystals.
  - Previous ulceration and extrusion of crystals from tophi may leave scars and sinus formation.
- Look at a temperature chart, as gout may be accompanied by a low grade pyrexia.
- Measure the BP: gout can lead to renal impairment and renal impairment itself, the most common predisposing factor for gout, may result in hypertension.

Investigations

- Assessment of serum urate, lipids, and renal and thyroid function.
- Radiographs of the symptomatic joints:
  - Punched out lateral erosions with sclerotic margins and overhanging edges ('mouse-bite erosions').
  - The joint space is preserved until late in the disease.
  - No juxta-articular osteopenia (c.f. other inflammatory arthritides).

Treatment

- NSAIDs/COX inhibitors, colchicine or short course of steroid for control of the acute attack.
- Allopurinol is prescribed for prophylaxis in the following indications:
  - If there are significantly frequent attacks i.e. >3 per year.
  - Presence of erosions.
  - Presence of tophi.
  - Renal impairment secondary to sodium urate kidney stones.
- Allopurinol should not be commenced during an acute attack, as it will prolong the attack, but there is no need for allopurinol to be discontinued during an attack.
- Sulphinpyrazone and probenecid are rarely used due to their side effect profile.
- Febuxostat, a new powerful xanthine oxidase inhibitor, is usually used if there is insufficient response or intolerance to allopurinol.

- Benzbromarone, a uricosuric drug, may be used in the presence of significant renal impairment on a named-patient basis.
- In severe cases synthetic uricases are used by monthly IV infusion and IL-1 antagonists can be employed intermittently for severe flares unresponsive to other treatments.

Patient concerns

- 'Can this be treated effectively?'
- 'Can I avoid medication if I alter my diet/lifestyle?'
- 'Will I have to take medication for the rest of my life?'
- 'Will my children develop this disease?'

Dietary factors may account for up to 15% of the body's serum urate. Alcohol increases the synthesis of urate by accelerating the degradation of ATP and decreases the renal excretion of urate by increasing the production of lactic acid. Lifestyle modifications are important but the majority of patients will require urate-lowering medication for the rest of their lives. Tophi will only resolve if the serum urate is reduced to the lower limit of the normal range, or a synthetic uricase is administered (humans and Dalmatians lack the uricase enzyme). Gout can, however, be successfully managed due to effective medications. Inherited causes of gout are vanishingly rare and therefore patients' children can be reassured.

Viva questions

Which medical conditions are associated with undersecretion of urate?

90% of patients with gout are undersecretors of urate (and 10% are over-producers of urate). The following conditions are associated with under-secretion:

- Renal disease (including polycystic kidney disease, lead nephropathy (saturnine gout))
- Ketoacidosis/lactic acidosis
- Respiratory acidosis
- Hyperparathyroidism
- Hypothyroidism.

What is the mechanism of action of allopurinol and why is not helpful in an acute attack of gout?

Allopurinol inhibits the enzyme xanthine oxidase that catalyses the conversion of hypoxanthine to xanthine and xanthine in turn to uric acid. It is an analogue of hypoxanthine and inhibits the enzyme by substrate competition. Allopurinol is converted to alloxanthine by xanthine oxidase and this metabolite is an effective non-competitive inhibitor of the enzyme. The pharmacological action of allopurinol is largely due to alloxanthine.

The result of the action of allopurinol is that the concentration of insoluble urates in tissues, plasma and urine decreases while that of the more soluble xanthines and hypoxathines increases. Hypoxanthine and xanthine are in turn converted into adenosine and guanosine monophosphates that cause feedback inhibition of amidophosphoribosyl transferase, the first and rate-limiting enzyme of purine biosynthesis. Allopurinol, therefore, decreases both uric acid formation and purine synthesis.

Initiation of allopurinol therapy may lower serum urate levels rapidly with the potential for urate reabsorption from tissue deposits, provoking an acute attack of gout.

What important drug interactions do you know in the management of gout?

- Allopurinol and azathioprine: mercaptopurine, the active metabolite of azathioprine, is normally metabolized by the xanthine oxidase pathway. By inhibiting this enzyme pathway, allopurinol increases the effect of mercaptopurine that may result in toxic bone marrow suppression.
- Allopurinol and warfarin: the effect of warfarin is increased due to inhibition of its metabolism.
- Colchicine and statins: colchicine increases the risk of myopathy in patients taking lipid-regulating medication.
- Colchicine and ciclosporin: the combination may result in nephrotoxicity and/or myopathy.

Who was Podagra?

She was a daughter of Bacchus (the God of wine) and Aphrodite and was known as the foot torturer in classical mythology.

📖 Further reading

Jordan KM et al. British Society for Rheumatology and British Health Professionals in Rheumatology guideline for the management of gout. *Rheumatology* 2007; **46:**1372–4.
Zhang W. et al. EULAR evidence based recommendations for gout: Part II. Management. *Ann Rheum Dis* 2006; **65**(10):1312–24.

The acute hot joint

An acutely inflamed joint is a medical emergency. At best, this will be an acute attack of gout, which if left, will self terminate within 7–10 days or, at worst, a septic arthritis which, if left untreated, will result in destruction of the joint and potentially death of the patient from sepsis.

The candidate will be expected to take a thorough history to try and elucidate the cause, perform an appropriate focused examination and then answer vital questions as regards management.

> **Scenario**
>
> Mr Andrew Garrod 56 years old, has presented to A&E with an acutely painful swollen left knee. Please take a focused history and examine appropriately.

History

The history needs to focus on:
- The differential diagnosis for the acute hot joint including:
  - Septic arthritis
  - An acute attack of gout
  - An acute attack of pseudogout (most commonly knee or wrist)
  - A monoarticular presentation of a polyarticular condition (psoriatic arthritis, reactive arthritis, acute sarcoidosis, IBD-related arthropathy).
- Rarer conditions to consider include:
  - Palindromic rheumatism (a forerunner of RA in 50% of patients)
  - Avascular necrosis (steroids, sickle cell anaemia)
  - Coagulopathy (anticoagulation, haemophilia, Christmas disease)
  - Pigmented villonodular synovitis (PVNS)
  - Foreign body synovitis (history of penetrating injury e.g. rose thorn synovitis)
  - Whipple's disease
  - Synovioma.
- Age of the patient (at onset of arthritis):
  - In children consider juvenile inflammatory arthritis.
  - In young adults consider seronegative inflammatory arthritides, trauma, gonococcal septic arthritis, and reactive arthritis (secondary to *Chlamydia, Campylobacter, Salmonella, Shigella,* or *Streptococcus*).
  - Older adults are more likely to have a crystal arthropathy avascular necrosis.
- The speed of onset of symptoms;
  - Within minutes: consider fracture or traumatic derangement of the joint.
  - Several hours to 1–2 days: consider infection, crystal arthropathy, inflammatory arthritis and palindromic rheumatism.
  - Insidious onset over days to weeks: consider reactive arthritis, mycobacterial or fungal infection (ethnicity/immunosuppression), osteoarthritis, tumour.
- Specific questions related to underlying aetiology:
  - Is there any history of previous episodes? – gout, pseudogout, palindromic rheumatism.

- Is there any history of trauma?
- Is the patient anticoagulated or has a known coagulopathy? – haemarthrosis.
- Has the patient been treated with a prolonged course of corticosteroids? – avascular necrosis or infection.
- Is there any history of mouth ulcers, colitis or psoriasis? – seronegative arthritis.
- Is there any history of preceding infection? – septic or reactive arthritis.

Examination

- The joint should be examined for the 4 cardinal signs of inflammation i.e. erythema, swelling, heat and pain.
- The candidate should elicit the range of passive and active movement and the degree of pain that this causes.
- The candidate must then examine for the extra-articular features of the spondyloarthropathies.
  - Skin rashes including psoriasis, keratoderma blenorhagicum, erythema nodosum
  - Oral ulcers
  - Iritis.
- Look for tophi or any evidence of any previous joint involvement.
- Specific examination for the knee (performed with patient supine) including:
  - A McMurray test, which assesses meniscal tears: flex the knee maximally and then rotate the knee into the varus position. Whilst feeling the medial joint line, extend the knee maximally to detect a medial meniscal tear. Then, to test for a lateral meniscus tear, rotate the knee into the valgus position and feel the lateral joint line whilst extending the knee. This test initially traps a torn meniscus between the tibia and femur. Palpation of a pop (which may also be audible) during extension of the knee, particularly if associated with pain, indicates meniscal injury.
  - Assessment of the stability of the collateral ligaments: Flex the knee to ~30°. To test the medial collateral ligament, hold the ankle over the medial malleolus, whilst placing pressure over the lateral aspect of the knee with the other hand. Repeat this procedure by holding the ankle over the lateral malleolus and placing pressure over the medial aspect of the knee to test the lateral collateral ligament. Excess movement of the knee indicates collateral ligament instability.
  - Assessment of cruciate ligaments: flex the knee to ~90° and, having asked permission, sit on the patient's foot. Try and pull the patient's tibia anteriorly and then posteriorly, ensuring that the hamstrings are relaxed. Positive anterior or posterior drawer test i.e. excess movement of the tibia in relation to the femur indicates instability of the anterior or posterior cruciate ligaments.

Investigations

- Radiographs: often normal in acute conditions.
- The joint must be aspirated to:
  - Exclude infection.

- Confirm a crystal arthropathy.
- Assess for blood staining that may indicate PVNS, synovial chondromatosis or synovioma.
- Mycobacterial infection will only be detected in 70% of cases by joint aspirate but in 95% of cases of synovial biopsy.
- Synovial biopsy is also useful for PVNS, synovial chondromatosis, synoviomas, sarcoid arthritis, foreign body synovitis and fungal infections.
- Blood tests should include:
  - FBC, CRP and ESR to assess the degree of inflammation.
  - Serum rheumatoid factor, ANA, HLA-B27, serum ACE and serology for Lyme disease.
  - Serum urate level.
  - Blood culture and sensitivity.
- PA CXR for TB and sarcoidosis and dedicated views of the sacroiliac joints as these may demonstrate sacroilitis which may be asymptomatic in a patient with a spondyloarthropathy.
- MRI: for avascular necrosis, osteomyelitis, PVNS, trauma.
- Isotope bone scan: for avascular necrosis, stress fracture and osteomyelitis.
- Arthroscopy: enables direct visualization of any internal derangement or synovial abnormality, facilitates a synovial biopsy and washout.

Treatment
- This will be determined by the underlying condition.

❶ Top Tips
- A septic arthritis cannot be excluded by being able to move the affected joint passively.
- Septic arthritis can be polyarticular.
- An abnormal joint is more prone to infection and therefore RA or gout and septic arthritis can coexist.

Patient concerns
Can this be cured or is my joint permanently damaged?
Prompt and appropriate treatment will prevent damage to a joint from infection, crystal arthropathy or an inflammatory arthritis – hence the need to determine the cause very quickly.

Is this the start of a generalized arthritis?
A monoarticular presentation of a polyarticular condition is less common than a crystal arthropathy, septic arthritis or reactive arthritis. The commonest monoarticular presentation of a polyarticular inflammatory arthritis is that of psoriatic arthritis and if thorough history and examination is performed, then psoriasis can be found in 70% of such cases.

Viva questions
What are the absolute contraindications to aspiration of an acutely inflamed joint?
- A prosthetic joint should only be aspirated in theatre.
- Overlying cellulitis.
- Overlying psoriatic plaque (increases the chance of a septic arthritis).
- Excess anticoagulation (INR of up to 3 should not cause any problems).

- Coagulopathy: will require clotting factor replacement.

Having obtained a joint fluid aspirate, which investigations should be ordered?

- Urgent Gram stain and cell count.
- MC&S.
- Cytology for crystals (strongly negatively birefringent [monosodium urate] or weakly positively birefringent [calcium pyrophosphate] in gout and pseudogout respectively).
- Zeil–Neilson stain and culture for AAFB.

📖 **Further reading**

Baer AL. The approach to the painful joint treatment and management. http://emedicine. medscape.com/article/336054 22 November 2010.

Coakley G. et al. BSR & BHPR, BOA, RCGP and BSAC guidelines for management of the hot swollen joint in adults. *Rheumatology* 2006; **45**:1039–41.

Giant cell arteritis and polymyalgia rheumatica

Giant cell arteritis (GCA), also known as temporal arteritis, is a large-vessel vasculitis, which occurs almost exclusively in patients aged >50, with increasing incidence with age. It is more common in Northern Europeans. GCA and polymyalgia rheumatica (PMR) represent 2 ends of the spectrum of the same condition. During viva questions, the emphasis is more often placed on GCA for 2 key reasons: firstly because this is a common emergency scenario whose correct management is necessary to prevent the risk of acute blindness and stroke; secondly the ability of the clinician to take a careful and probing history is critical to making the correct diagnosis. In our survey of Station 5 cases, PMR was not infrequently encountered, including in conjunction with RA, or in the context of discussions related to differential diagnosis of RA and other cases.

Scenario 1

Mrs Anthea Holloway, 75 years old, presents to the emergency department with unilateral headache and blurred vision in her left eye. Take a brief history and examine her as necessary.

Scenario 2

Mr Timothy Singer, 79 years old, describes aching shoulders and being too stiff to lift his arms above his head. Please take a focused history and examine appropriately.

History

Giant cell arteritis

The typical patient presents with cranial symptoms: superficial headache, usually unilateral and localized to the region of the temporal artery (and not the forehead). The headache is unresponsive to simple analgesics. Two key symptoms help to distinguish this headache from other more benign forms: scalp tenderness and jaw claudication. It is important to ask specifically which areas of the scalp are tender, as these overlie the arteries affected (usually temporal artery, but the occipital artery can also be affected). Jaw and/or tongue claudication may be present and must be distinguished from pain on chewing that arises from the temporomandibular joint. Sinister symptoms include diplopia or visual disturbance, such as amaurosis fugax, transient field loss or severe blurring of central vision indicating impending arterial occlusion. Blindness when it occurs is abrupt and painless. Constitutional symptoms of fever or weight loss may also occur. Note that 40% of patients with GCA may actually present primarily with symptoms of polymyalgia rheumatica with little or no cranial symptoms.

Polymyalgia rheumatica

This is classically described as proximal myalgia and stiffness affecting the shoulders and pelvic girdle which is usually bilateral, symmetrical and of sudden onset (patients often describe awakening one morning with these intense symptoms). Notably, actual muscle strength is unimpaired. Inflammatory stiffness worse in the morning or after rest is often a prominent feature.

- Ask whether the patient has difficulty lifting their arms above their head and why.
- Ask whether he/she has difficulty rising from a chair/getting out of a bath or alighting from a car.
- Ask whether their joints are swollen to help exclude a diagnosis of RA (so called 'polymyalgic onset RA,' which may present with symptoms difficult to differentiate from PMR, particularly in the elderly).

> **❶ Top Tips**
>
> - PMR may mimic the following conditions:
>   - Inflammatory arthritis e.g. RA
>   - Muscle diseases e.g. polymyositis/dermatomyositis
>   - Paraneoplastic syndrome
>   - Hypo- or hyperthyroidism
>   - Infective endocarditis
>   - OA
>   - Bilateral frozen shoulder
>   - Depression.

Examination

Giant cell arteritis

Tortuous temporal arteries are a common finding with age and the clinician is actually looking for thickening of the arterial wall, suggestive of an underlying inflammatory process, with local tenderness. Visual loss occurs in 15% of patients, due to ischaemic optic neuritis. GCA is a generalized vasculitis which can also affect the aorta and its major branches and patients may have asymmetrical or absent peripheral pulses. Key points to look for:

- Thickened, inflamed and often tender temporal arteries.
- Check visual acuities and fields.
- Fundoscopy to look for the blurred, swollen disc of acute optic neuritis, central retinal artery occlusion or optic atrophy.
- Check the peripheral pulses in the head, neck and limbs for tenderness, enlargement, signs of thrombosis and rarely bruits (e.g. subclavian, renal arteries).

Polymyalgia rheumatica

Key signs to look for:
- Rule out myositis: muscle power is unimpaired; no signs of Gottron's papules, heliotrope rash, or evidence of lung fibrosis.
- Very important to examine both shoulders to exclude a more simple musculoskeletal explanation for shoulder pain (usually unilateral; if bilateral often (but not always) asymmetrical) e.g. glenohumeral OA (globally restricted shoulder movements and/or crepitus) or rotator cuff tear (painful arc on abduction).
- Examine the hands and wrists to look for synovitis – symptoms mimicking PMR may actually be an early manifestation of RA.

❶ Top Tips

- There may appear to be weakness on examination of proximal muscles due to the stiffness and pain experienced by patients with PMR on testing power.
- If patients are warned that it is important to assess power of shoulder abduction for a few seconds, the majority will be willing to undergo this short discomfort: 'It may be a little painful, but it is important to check the strength in your arms. On the count of three, please hold your arms up just for a couple of seconds. One, two three . . . now relax.'

Investigations

- The most critical investigations are both the ESR, which tends to be very high (often >100mm/h), and CRP, which is also usually elevated. It is extremely rare for GCA or PMR to occur with both of these tests within normal limits.
- Other blood tests include FBC (may show normochromic, normocytic anaemia), U&E, LFT, ferritin (may be elevated due to acute phase response), CK, autoantibodies including ANA, rheumatoid factor and anti-CCP (to exclude RA), blood cultures if infective endocarditis is suspected.
- A temporal artery biopsy is important for histological diagnosis, although this test *must not delay* the initiation of steroid therapy. A sufficient length (3–4cm) of artery should be removed surgically and examined for granulomatous changes at intervals along its length, since the disease is often patchy with skip lesions. Whilst a positive biopsy

is the gold standard for diagnosis, a negative biopsy does not exclude GCA.

- If diagnostic uncertainty remains, then PET scanning may be indicated. This will identify the extent of the arteritis and on occasions may even reveal clinically unsuspected cases.
  Further tests may be necessary as clinically indicated to exclude other causes of headaches e.g. CT brain to exclude a tumour or brain abscess in a subacute presentation.
- In cases with constitutional symptoms, it is important to screen carefully for underlying malignancy (mandatory in the younger patient) or infection (CXR, breast or rectal examination, PSA, blood cultures, echocardiogram, etc).

Management

A compelling history with significantly abnormal ESR or CRP is sufficient to start treatment with high dose steroids, most commonly oral prednisolone 60mg daily (although studies report a variety of starting doses ranging 40–80mg). If visual symptoms are present then pulsed methylprednisolone may be indicated.

Patient concerns

The patient may ask if they will need long-term or permanent steroid therapy. Explain that treatment over a couple of years is to be expected, initially at a high dose, but that the steroid dose will be reduced gradually and cautiously during this period. Warn patients not to reduce the dose of steroid by themselves. Patients should be advised that if during a dose reduction, they re-develop their symptoms, they should return to their prior dose.

A small proportion of patients (about 1/3) are resistant to weaning the final few milligrams of prednisolone and require long-term steroid treatment (usually ≤5mg). Some patients may require steroid sparing therapy with a disease modifying drug e.g. azathioprine or methotrexate.

Viva questions

What symptoms help to distinguish giant cell arteritis from other forms of headache?

- Characteristic cranial symptoms of GCA:
  - Headache precipitated by brushing hair.
  - Scalp tenderness overlying the temporal (or rarely occipital) artery.
  - Jaw claudication.
  - Abnormal tongue sensation or altered taste.
  - Visual disturbance.
- Presence of constitutional symptoms: fever, weight loss, malaise.
- Exclude other diagnoses: not a thunder clap headache.
- Unresponsive to simple analgesics; steroid therapy leads to immediate resolution of symptoms (otherwise reconsider diagnosis).

How do you treat GCA?

If the diagnosis is suspected from the history and either ESR or CRP are significantly elevated, high dose steroids must be started to prevent the risk of blindness, typically oral prednisolone 60mg daily.

A typical regimen for slowly tapering steroid therapy would be:

- Reduce by 5mg every week until reaching 30mg daily.
- Then reduce by 2.5mg every week until reaching 20mg daily.
- Then reduce by 2.5mg every 4 weeks until 10mg daily.
- Then reduce by 1mg every 4 weeks down to zero.

Regular monitoring of symptoms, ESR and CRP should guide the patient's regimen (too rapid tapering may result in recurrence of symptoms and subsequent consequences).

To whom would you offer bone protection, how would you investigate them and what would you prescribe to them?

With glucocorticoid-induced osteoporosis the greatest bone loss occurs at the start of steroid treatment. The average age of a patient with GCA/PMR also places them at risk of osteoporosis, particularly the female patients. It is therefore prudent to commence osteoporosis prophylaxis in the form of a bisphosphonate when the steroids are commenced and to perform a DEXA scan at the end of steroid treatment to determine if anti-osteoporosis treatment is still required. The first line of treatment should be alendronic acid as this is licensed for the prevention of steroid induced osteoporosis and is also licensed for treating male patients.

📖 **Further reading**

BSR & BHPR Guidelines for the Management of Polymyalgia Rheumatica (PMR). Available at: www.pmr-gca-northeast.org.uk/assets/pmr_resource_9.doc.

Ankylosing spondylitis

Ankylosing spondylitis is a chronic inflammatory disease affecting the sacroiliac joints and spine (axial disease) and not infrequently peripheral joints (appendicular disease). Typical of a rheumatological inflammatory disorder, it may involve multiple systems and the candidate may encounter ankylosing spondylitis patients in other stations e.g. cardiology – aortic regurgitation; neurology – cervical myelopathy, cauda equina syndrome; gastroenterology – inflammatory bowel disease.

> **Scenario**
>
> Mr Boris Atherton, 22 years old, has increasing difficulty mobilizing and performing his job as a car mechanic. Please take a focused history and examine appropriately.

History

The history needs to focus on the reason for difficulty in mobilizing:

- Is it weakness?
- Is this muscle or joint-related (e.g. suggested by pain ± stiffness)?
- Could his job be exacerbating the problem (e.g. long hours, cold garage, lots of bending, manual work)?

The history also needs to focus on:

- Age of onset of symptoms.
- Any relevant family history of inflammatory back pain, psoriasis, iritis, inflammatory bowel disease.
- Diurnal variation of symptoms, including duration of early morning stiffness.
- Presence or absence of any associated features, including psoriasis, bloody diarrhoea, acute eye inflammation.
- Any current or previous episodes of enthesitis e.g. Achilles tendonitis, plantar fasciitis (especially if bilateral), shoulder or elbow involvement.
- The joint distribution: cervical/dorsal/lumbosacral back pain and any peripheral joint involvement.
- Whether any pain is localized or radiates to the limbs.
- Treatment to date, including response to exercise and NSAIDs.

❶ Top Tips

Sacroiliac joint pain is classically felt in the buttock and radiates down the back of the thigh, but does not extend distal to the knee; sciatic pain can radiate all the way down the posterior aspect of the leg and the plantar aspect of the feet.

Examination

Always ask the patient to walk first. The precise order of further examination will be guided by the instruction, e.g. the cervical spine should be examined next in a patient presenting with neck symptoms before proceeding to examine the low back.

- A general visual survey should note the presence of walking aids and/or prism spectacles.
- Look at the eyes for iritis and the skin for psoriasis.
- The candidate should ask the patient to rise from the chair, walk several metres, turn and walk back:
  - Observe for hyperextension of the cervical spine and loss of the normal lumbar lordosis, resulting in a protuberant abdomen.
  - Note any stiffness and whether the patient turns with the torso and cervical spine fixed (as opposed to looking over his shoulder as he turns).
- Active cervical spine movements should be elicited; remember to examine 6 directions of movement – flexion, extension, lateral flexion left & right, lateral rotation left & right.
- Assess low back movements:
  - In the 6 directions (as for cervical spine): forward flexion, extension, lateral flexion, left & right, and lateral rotation, left & right. Strictly speaking, lateral rotation arises from movement of the thoracic spine.
  - Perform Schober's test: stand behind the patient and identify the 'dimples of Venus' which correspond to the posterior superior iliac spines. Place a finger half way between these points. Having asked the patient's permission, mark two lines, one 10cm above and the other 5cm below this point. Ask the patient to flex forward as far as possible and measure the increase in the distance between these lines. An increase of <5cm (i.e. <20cm between the 2 marks) indicates a positive Schober's test result (~50% increase would be expected in a normal healthy adult).
- The candidate should then perform specific tests for ankylosing spondylitis:
  - Chest expansion at the 4th intercostal space (normal >2.5cm).
  - Finger to floor distance on forward flexion (normal <10cm).
  - Occiput to wall distance (normal 0cm). Similarly measurement of the distance from wall to the tragus of the ear is routinely monitored in rheumatology clinic to look for disease progression.

Common Pitfalls

- Always use a tape measure to make accurate recordings rather than trying to 'guestimate' measurements.
- When examining the back:
  - Expose the patient's back by removing their top and loosening trouser belt if necessary.
  - Examine the patient from the back, but ensure that they can see you when giving instructions (i.e. you may need to go around to face your patient and return to their back to do this).
- Fix the patient's pelvis whilst examining the range of movement of the low back:
  - This will eliminate movements arising from the lower limb joints, in an attempt to compromise the restricted movement from the spine.
  - When examining lateral rotation, the spine can be fixed by asking the patient to sit on the edge of the bed.
- Always carry out the 6 simple low back movements before proceeding to Schober's test.

- With the patient in the supine position perform FABER's test:
  - Cross the leg of the symptomatic side so that the foot lies as proximal as possible on the opposite knee/thigh. This manoeuvre places hip in **F**lexion **AB**duction and **E**xternal **R**otation.
  - Apply gentle pressure with one hand on the medial (superior) aspect of the knee of the affected side whilst stabilizing the position of the pelvis by holding the opposite anterior superior iliac spine with the other hand.
  - FABER's test is positive if tenderness is elicited in the sacroiliac joint, hip or buttock, indicating active sacroiliitis or hip disease.
- Examine the cardiovascular system for:
  - Pulse rate (heart block 1st to 3rd degree; patient may have a pacemaker).
  - Valvular lesions especially AR.
  - Apex beat (cardiomyopathies).
- Listen at the apex of the lungs for pulmonary fibrosis.
- The BP should be elicited, as well as urine dipstick (renal impairment e.g. due to the long-term use of NSAIDs and risk of secondary amyloidosis or IgA nephropathy).

Differential diagnosis

- Psoriatic spondyloarthropathy.
- Inflammatory bowel disease-related spondyloarthropathy.
- Scheuermann's disease (a self-limiting skeletal disorder).
- Diffuse idiopathic skeletal hyperostosis (DISH).
- Differential diagnosis of radiographic sacroiliac (SI) joint abnormalities
  - Osteitis condensans ileii (characterized by a triangular area of sclerosis in the iliac portion of the sacroiliac joint)
  - Degenerative
  - Infection
  - Gout
  - Hyperparathyroidism
  - Paget's disease
  - Paraplegia (if longstanding, may have calcification of SI joint and intervertebral discs)
  - Neoplastic metastases.

Investigations

- Radiographs of the lumbosacral spine with dedicated (Ferguson) views of the sacroiliac joints and PA CXR for apical fibrosis (consider pulmonary function tests and HRCT of thorax).
- MRI if plain radiographs inconclusive (more sensitive than isotope bone scan).
- Blood tests should include:
  - FBC for anaemia.
  - Renal function (NSAID use and possibility of secondary amyloidosis/IgA nephropathy).
  - Acute phase reactants.
- HLA-B27 status.

Treatment

- The mainstay of treatment is physiotherapy and NSAIDs (which if taken regularly may have a disease-modifying effect).
- The DMARD sulphasalazine may be helpful in appendicular disease.
- DMARDs and steroids are usually ineffective in axial disease.
- Local cortisone injections are very effective for enthesitis (inflammation at the site where a tendon inserts into a bone).
- If disease activity, as determined by the BASDAI (Bath Ankylosing Spondylitis Disease Activity Index) is severe enough on 2 occasions 3 months apart, then the patient would qualify for treatment with anti-TNF therapy.

Patient concerns

- 'Can this be treated effectively?'
- 'Will I have to give up my job?'
- 'Will my children develop this disease?'
- 'Will I have to take medication for the rest of my life?'

Patients should be reassured that, with appropriate physiotherapy and NSAIDs, the majority of patients with ankylosing spondylitis maintain a near normal lifestyle. Patients should be encouraged to carry out regular, daily, life-long physiotherapy which will help to maintain spinal movements and mobility, and to continue with their activities of daily living, although high-impact sport should be avoided. They should also be encouraged to inform their employers regarding their diagnosis, so that any necessary work assessment and adjustments can be initiated.

The introduction of biologic therapies over the past decade has provided a significant clinical response to those patients who had previously had inadequate response to conventional therapies.

Viva questions

What is the value of the HLA-B27 test in a patient with back pain?

- 90% of Caucasian patients with ankylosing spondylitis will be HLA-B27 positive; this drops to 50–80% in other ethnic groups.
- The presence of HLA-B27 in the normal population is latitude dependent i.e. 15–20% in Scandinavians, 3% in North American blacks and <1% in Africans and Asians.

Can you reassure him that his children will not develop the condition?

2% of HLA-B27 positive individuals develop ankylosing spondylitis but this figure rises to 15–20% if a 1st-degree relative has the disease.

Do bisphosphonates have a role in the treatment of ankylosing spondylitis?

Intravenous pamidronate may have a role as a disease modifier but is unlicensed and has been superseded by the advent of anti-TNF agents. There is an increased risk of osteoporosis in patients with ankylosing spondylitis and it is often missed in the male patients. (DEXA readings at the spine will be artefactually elevated due to syndesmophyte formation; therefore interpret on hip and forearm).

Bisphosphonates are prescribed prophylactically for a period of 3 months to a patient undergoing arthroplasty surgery in order to minimize the chance of postoperative extra-articular soft issue calcification.

What advice should be given to a patient with ankylosing spondylitis who receives anti-TNF treatment?
- Always inform any doctor/dentist that they are on the treatment.
- Stop the treatment 2 doses before any surgery.
- Stop the treatment if there is intercurrent infection.
- Always seek urgent medical advice should they suspect an infection.
- Be up to date with vaccinations (influenza, swine flu, pneumovax).

📖 **Further reading**

BSR guidelines for prescribing TNFα blockers in adults with ankylosing spondylitis. London: BSR, 2004
Kiltz U et al. ASAS/EULAR recommendations for the management of ankylosing spondylitis: the patient version. Ann Rheum Dis 2009; **68**:1381–6.
NICE. Adulimumab, etanercept and infliximab in ankylosing spondylitis (TA143). London: NICE, 2008.

Paget's disease

This case more commonly cropped up in the previous short cases for MRCP but has still been reported in surveys of candidates who have been through the most recent Station 5 of PACES. Paget's disease is characterized by accelerated bone turnover with the result that deformity and enlargement of specific bones occurs. Its incidence increases with age, from 2–3% over the age of 40, becoming much more common over 70. Early diagnosis and the advent of treatment with oral bisphosphonates has meant that patients are now more rapidly treated in primary care; thus the severe cases common in the MRCP will become progressively unusual.

Scenario 1

Mrs Hilda Jones. This 68-year-old lady is having difficulty walking. Please take a focused history and examine appropriately.

Scenario 2

Mr Arthur Hopkirk. This 81-year-old man has been having problems with his hearing and vision. Please take a focused history and examine the cranial nerves.

History

Only a 1/3 of patients are symptomatic; the majority are diagnosed as an incidental finding on x-rays or chronically elevated alkaline phosphatase of bony origin. Bony pain (80%), joint pain (50%) and slowly developing bone deformities are the main symptoms. Patients can also present with a spontaneous fracture typically affecting the femur, tibia, humerus or forearm.

Examination

Although Paget's disease can affect any bone in the skeleton, it has a predilection for the pelvis and sacrum, lumbar and thoracic spine, femur, tibia, skull and humerus. The disease is usually polyostotic (affecting multiple bones simultaneously) but is monostotic in ~20%.
Key skeletal signs to look for:
- Enlargement of the skull (look for asymmetry).

- Bowing and enlargement of a tibia (sabre tibia) which may be warmer than the other side.
- Kyphosis.

Further examination is dictated by searching for potential complications of Paget's disease. This is a classic viva question and, as always in PACES, it is important to be systematic.

Complications of Paget's disease

- **Skeletal:** bone pain, deformity, fracture.
- **Neurological:** deafness (due to auditory nerve entrapment), other cranial nerve palsies, spinal stenosis, headaches, optic atrophy, cerebral ischaemia as part of a steal syndrome (compared to normal bone, blood flow in pagetic bone is increased 3-fold) or subsequent to cervical artery compression.
- **Cardiac:** may precipitate angina, hypertension, rarely high-output heart failure.
- **Malignancy:** osteogenic sarcoma (1%), fibrosarcoma, benign giant cell tumour.
- **Metabolic:** hypercalcaemia, nephrocalcinosis.

Treatment

Paget's disease was previously treated with a 3-day course of daily IV pamidronate given every few years but nowadays it is more common for GPs to prescribe a 2-month course of oral risedronate or single-dose IV zoledronate. More rarely Paget's can be treated with calcitonin. Surgery may be required to prevent progression of neurological complications or where the disease encroaches on a joint.

Patient concerns

The patient may be worried about their persistent pain, usually overlying the bony involvement. It is important to determine the cause of the underlying pain and target treatment appropriately. Patients with nerve entrapment or coexistent OA should respond to a step-up management starting with simple analgesics and anti-inflammatories. Bony pain due to Paget's disease responds poorly to these measures however, but generally responds to the bisphosphonate or calcitonin treatment.

Possible viva questions

Which tests are helpful in Paget's disease?

- Serum alkaline phosphatase is frequently highly elevated, though not always.
- Serum calcium and phosphate should be normal and hypercalcaemia is only seen with immobilization or fracture.
- PTH is normal.
- Plain x-rays have a characteristic appearance showing:
  - Osteolytic or osteoblastic lesions, or a mixture of the two.
  - Trabecular thickening of the inner aspect of the pelvis.
- Technetium bone scan shows regions of very high uptake which may be commonly mistaken for metastases or lymphomatous marrow infiltration in vertebral bodies.

- If available, urinary markers of bone turnover such as N-telopeptide may be useful, particularly if serum alkaline phosphatase does not reflect disease activity.

List important side effects of bisphosphonates
- Bone-related: bone pain, hypocalcaemia.
- GI tract: oesophagitis or oesophageal ulceration (important to warn patients to take their tablet(s) in the morning with a glass of water at least 30min prior to food, and not lie down for 30min after ingestion).
- There is some controversy over the association of bisphosphonates with gastro-oesophageal cancer: one meta-analysis showed an association but a larger meta-analysis demonstrated no association. Therefore, bisphosphonates should be avoided in patients with a prior history of gastroesophageal cancer or Barrett's oesophagus.
- Systemic: fever, flu-like symptoms, arthralgia, myalgia.
- Dental: rarely, osteonecrosis of the jaw (usually in those patients with pre-existing poor dentition).

📖 Further reading

Selby PL, et al. Guidelines on the management of Paget's disease of bone. Bone 2002; **31**:366–73.
Scarsbrook A et al. UK guidelines on the management of Paget's disease of bone. Rheumatology 2004, **43**:399–400.

🕸 Useful website

Shiel WC Jr et al. Paget's disease of bone. Available at: http://www.medicinenet.com/pagets_disease/article.htm

Ophthalmology: Introduction

Ophthalmology is now primarily encountered in Station 5 of the PACES examination, although it may also feature as an important aspect of cranial nerve examination in the neurology station. A recent survey suggests that 2 out of every 5 candidates encountered an ophthalmic case. With station 5 holding 1/3 of the marks, being comfortable assessing ophthalmic conditions is therefore very important.

This chapter is divided into 2 parts. The first describes history and examination techniques relevant to ophthalmological assessment for the PACES examination. The second highlights those ophthalmology scenarios most frequently encountered by candidates.

Ptosis, nystagmus, and cranial nerve palsies are covered in the neurology chapter and should be read in conjunction with this section.

Cases

- Sudden loss of vision: diabetic vitreous haemorrhage.
- Gradual visual loss: retinitis pigmentosa.
- Subacute visual loss: optic atrophy.
- Sore prominent eye with visual disturbance: thyroid eye disease.
- Visual field defect 1: bitemporal hemianopia.
- Visual field defect 2: homonymous hemianopia.
- Double vision: third nerve palsy.
- Anisocoria: Horner's syndrome.

Ophthalmic history and examination techniques

As with all assessments it is wise to start with the history of presenting complaint. Certain general initial questions can be useful:

General initial questions

- Duration of symptoms.
- Rate of progression (e.g. sudden onset strongly suggests a vascular aetiology whereas gradual onset might indicate a compressive lesion).
- Whether the complaint is monocular or binocular.
- Whether there is any associated pain and/or systemic symptoms.
- Whether symptoms are constant or intermittent; if intermittent, establish any diurnal variation, e.g. myasthenia gravis worse as day progresses.
- What effect the visual loss/diplopia is having on the patient's activities of daily living.

> **❶ Top Tips**
>
> - It is essential to determine whether loss of vision is monocular or binocular. For example, in relation to optic atrophy, monocular loss of vision might be compressive, ischaemic or demyelinating, whilst bilateral involvement could be toxic, nutritional or inherited.

Initial examination

Once you have elicited the history of presenting complaint start examining the patient.

- Inspect the patient, initially at a distance, then closer. Look for:
  - Props such as a white stick or Braille suggesting poor visual acuity (a striped white stick suggests the patient is both blind and deaf).
  - Ptosis: look at where the upper eye lid bisects the iris.
  - Pupils: observe pupillary size, asymmetry or pupil irregularity.
  - Eye position: check whether eyes are conjugate (point in the same direction) or disconjugate in the primary position of gaze.
  - Proptosis: observe from above for globe protrusion.
- Further examination will be determined by the presenting complaint and the signs observed on initial inspection. Candidates should continue the examination with the technique which will elicit the most signs.

Common presenting complaints

The following list should serve as a guide to commencing the examination:

- Reduced vision in one or both eyes: Ophthalmoscopy
- Reduced peripheral vision: Visual fields
- Double vision: Eye movements
- Eyes appear prominent: Eye movements and lids
- Both eyes uncomfortable: Eye movements and lids
- Pupils are unequal: Pupils.

Continue the focused history, related to the presenting complaint, whilst extending the examination to elicit further relevant signs. Examine the eyes but do not forget the rest of the patient. Be flexible in your approach and always remember to explain to the patient each step of your examination. Cover all relevant points in the history and examination, although you do not need to be comprehensive. The aim is to collect enough information to either confirm your diagnosis or focus your differential list, as well to determine an appropriate management plan. Therefore once you have determined the main problem (e.g. diabetic retinopathy) look for specific features that will change the way you manage the patient (e.g. presence of diabetic maculopathy, neovascularization or diabetic nephropathy).

If initial inspection is fruitless, proceed according to the presenting complaint or with the formal sequence of neurological examination:

• Visual acuity.
• Colour vision, if Ishihara plates available.
• Fields to confrontation.
• Eye movements: tracking and saccadic movements.
• Pupillary light reflexes: if abnormal, check for response to accommodation.
• Fundoscopy.

Patient concerns

Patient concerns are likely to centre on loss of vision and the impact that this will have on the patient's lifestyle e.g. their ability to drive, work, read, and carry out activities of daily living. The effect of the patient's visual loss (or diplopia) on these important activities should be determined during any Station 5 consultation.

Frequently the patient can be reassured that treatment for their condition is available to minimize further loss of vision and, in most cases, that they will not become 'blind' in the sense of losing sight completely. Some patients may become legally blind – now referred to as 'severely visually impaired' – implying that they are unable to do any work for which vision is required. Specific patient concerns are addressed in the individual scenarios where appropriate.

If the patient is likely to have significant long-term visual disability, they should be advised that there are a number of organizations which provide support for blind and partially sighted people, e.g. Royal National Institute of Blind People (http://www.rnib.org.uk).

Visual acuity

Asking the patient to read small print on a newspaper (with reading glasses if used) can be a convenient basic assessment of reading vision. Distance vision is usually performed with a Snellen chart. This is read at 6m. Sometimes reduced size Snellen charts are available and are read at 2m or 3m (as appropriate; see Fig. 8.5). This is equivalent to a full size chart read at 6m.

• Make sure the patient is wearing their distance glasses if required.
• Test one eye at a time, covering the other eye. Ask them to read down the chart. When they start having difficulty encourage them to take an educated guess at the letters. If they get more than half of the letters correct then they have achieved that line on the chart.

- Score them as follows, according to the lowest line read satisfactorily:
  - If they see the '6' line, reading at 6m, then score them as 6/6 (pronounced six over six).
  - If they only saw up to the 12 line, score them as 6/12.
  - If you use a half size chart at 3 meters you can still say 6/12.
- If vision is worse than 6/6, a pinhole can be used, keeping distance glasses on (although this may not necessarily be required in PACES).
  - If the vision improves significantly, then the initial reduction in vision is usually due to refractive error or cataract.
  - If the vision remains below 6/6, even with pinhole, then this is usually due to retinal, optic nerve or cortical pathology.
- If they cannot see the top line (6/60) establish the visual acuity in the following order:
  - Ability to count fingers at 1m.
  - Detection of hand movement.
  - Light being shone into the eye (cover the other eye well)

Vision can be scored as 'counting fingers' (CF), 'hand movements' (HM), 'perception of light' (PL) or 'no perception of light' (NPL) respectively.

❶ Top Tips

- It is important to perform visual acuity quickly in order to have enough time for the rest of the examination.
- To save time ask your patient to go directly to the lowest line they can read, rather than reading the whole of the chart.
- A clear view of the chart is best achieved if the patient (rather than the doctor) holds the pinhole. Ask them to move it to find the clearest view through the hole.

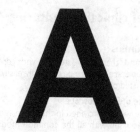

A

60

OX

36

HVT

24

VOTH

18

TMUAX

12

YUXAHV

9

AUTHYMXV

6

Fig. 8.5 Reduced Snellen chart (to be held 2 metres away from the patient).
Reproduced from PassPACES Courses Ltd.

Examining the fundus

Examiners understand that candidates are not ophthalmologists and fundal signs in Station 5 are likely to be relatively easily seen so long as the ophthalmoscope is used properly.

Basic features of the ophthalmoscope

An ophthalmoscope will be provided in the exam (where required). It is best to familiarize yourself with all the common models, or to take your own to the exam. All ophthalmoscopes have basic features in common:

- On/off/dimmer switch.
- Viewing hole.
- Focus dial. This changes the lens in the viewing hole. Red numbers correct for short sightedness; black or green numbers correct for long sightedness. As a general guide if you:
  - Do not wear distance glasses/contact lenses: set dial to zero.
  - Wear distance glasses/contacts: set the dial to zero.
  - Wear distance glasses, but will take them off while using the ophthalmoscope: set the dial to roughly your glasses prescription.
- Light setting switch. Use the largest round white light in your exam.

Holding the ophthalmoscope

- When examining the patient's right eye, hold the ophthalmoscope in your right hand and examine with your right eye. Vice versa for left.
- Hold the ophthalmoscope vertically. Rest the top against your brow (or glasses). Rest your hand (holding the battery case) against your cheek. This will steady the ophthalmoscope against you, preventing you from losing your view through the viewing hole.
- Always keep your index finger on the focus dial. This allows you to easily get your view into focus while looking into the eye.

Examining the patient

- The patient should be seated with you standing.
- The candidate should either:
  - a) Ask the patient to fix their gaze on a distant object, ideally high on the wall. This raises the eyes and lids, making the examination easier. Commence the examination approximately 15° temporal to their direction of gaze. This method is preferable if the eye has not been dilated as otherwise, the patient may try to accommodate to focus on the ophthalmoscope, making it difficult for the candidate to focus on the retina, or
  - b) Ask the patient to look directly at the light of the ophthalmoscope, in which case they will be looking directly at the fovea (the centre of the macula) when they visualize the fundus.
- Check the red reflex at arms length from the patient. If the red reflex is either absent or reduced, this indicates an opacity in the ocular media e.g. cataract or vitreous haemorrhage.
- Move towards the patient, keeping the red reflex in view. When the red reflex fills your entire view look for a blood vessel.
- Adjust the ophthalmoscope to correct the patient's refractive error. Rotate the focus dial in one direction. If the vessel becomes more blurred then rotate in the other direction until it becomes sharp.

- Follow the vessel towards the disc. Consciously note the '3 Cs' of the disc:
  - *Colour:* pale colour indicates optic atrophy
  - *Cup:* large cup indicates glaucoma.
  - *Contour:* blurred contour indicates disc swelling.
- Follow the superotemporal arcade vessels away from the disc and then back towards the disc (Fig. 8.6). Repeat for the inferotemporal, superonasal, and inferonasal vessels.
  - While following these vessels ask yourself if you see any features suggestive of disease (haemorrhage, exudate, pigment, atrophy, vessel changes).
  - Do not forget to look around the vessels for laser scars or bone spicule pigmentation.
- Look at the macula. Either ask the patient to look at the light, or move temporal to the disc while the patient looks straight ahead. Again consciously ask yourself if you see pathology.
- Ask the patient to look up, down, left and right, to examine the far periphery. This usually provides little further information.

❶ Top Tips

- Get your eye as close as possible to the viewing hole and the ophthalmoscope as close as possible to the patient. Like looking through a keyhole, the view is much better the closer you are.
- As vessels join each other they form a 'V' shape. The point of the 'V' shows the direction of the disc.
- Traditionally one is taught to examine the macula at the end of the examination, after examining the far periphery. However time is short in Station 5 and pathology is far more likely to be found in the macula region than the far periphery.
- When looking at the macula many candidates feel that they are out of focus. If the disc is in focus, the macula will also usually be in focus. A healthy macula is relatively featureless compared to the rest of the retina, being devoid of large vessels. Have a careful look – if you cannot see anything at all, there is probably no pathology to be seen.

⬥ Common Pitfalls

- Being unfamiliar with the ophthalmoscope, especially:
  - Switching it on (beware those that require a button to be pressed).
  - Not setting the focus dial correctly before starting.
  - Not checking the light setting switch (select the largest round white light).
  - Not getting close enough to the patient. This is one of the most common mistakes. Being close will considerably widen your field of view.
  - Not using your free hand to steady yourself. Place it on the back of the patient's chair, their shoulder, or on their forehead (ask permission first). Being steady on your feet will prevent you from losing your view as you move around the eye.

- Holding the patient's lid up throughout the examination, preventing blinking. This is likely to cause the patient discomfort, due to the front of the eye drying. Ask the patient to look up. This will help lift the lid. On looking down the lid can be lifted temporarily. In general most patients will be very familiar with the examination and will be able keep their eyes open for you.

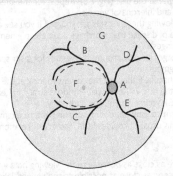

Fig. 8.6 Diagram of the right fundus. **A**, optic disc. **B**, superotemporal vessels. **C**, inferotemproal vessels. **D**, superonasal vessels. **E**, inferonasal vessels. **F**, macula. (Region surrounded by the superotemporal and inferotemporal vessels; shown by dotted line. At the centre of the macula is the fovea.) **G**, peripery. Everything outside the macula. Divided (naturally by blood vessels) into superior, inferior, nasal, and temporal regions.

Visual fields

When assessing visual fields by confrontation you are comparing the patient's visual field with your own. Therefore it is important that you perform the assessment exactly halfway between the patient and yourself. Imagine a sheet of glass halfway between you and the patient. Every part of the exam should be performed on this imaginary sheet of glass.

- Sit directly opposite the patient, 1m away.
- While talking observe for signs of systemic disease, including hemiparesis, acromegaly and cerebellar disease (multiple sclerosis).
- Assess for visual inattention. Ask the patient to look at the bridge of your nose, with both eyes open, while you place your index fingers just inside the outer limits of your temporal fields. Then move your fingers in turn and then both at the same time and ask the patient to point to the finger that moves. If there is visual inattention, the patient will only point to one finger when you move both at the same time.
- Next assess the monocular visual fields. Ask the patient to cover their left eye while you cover your right. Ask the patient to look at your uncovered eye whilst you look at theirs. Imagine a vertical and horizontal line running through their pupil. These vertical and horizontal midlines divide the visual field into four quadrants (Fig. 8.7). They are extremely useful in determining if a field defect is neurological or not, and which part of the brain is involved (Fig. 8.8).

- Using a white hatpin, or a pen with a white end, place it at central fixation (in front of the patient's pupil). Ask the patient if they can see the target. If they cannot, either a central scotoma is present, or they have generally poor vision (if required, use a larger target). Having asked the patient to say 'yes' when they first see the target, bring it slowly in at a 45° angle, in a straight line, from the far periphery to in front of the patient's pupil. When the target appears, always continue to the pupil, asking the patient if it disappears. This prevents you from missing a central scotoma. Repeat for the other eye. If necessary remind the patient to look at your eye at all times.
- Once the field defect has been detected, assess where the borders of the defect lie, particularly with regard to the vertical and horizontal midlines. Take the target and place it in the blind area. Move towards the 'seeing area', asking the patient to tell you when they first see it. In a central scotoma move radially out in different directions. In a hemianopia move horizontally from blind to seeing, testing the vertical midline both above and below central fixation. Moving vertically from blind to seeing tests the horizontal midline.
- An enlarged blind spot is usually asymptomatic. Associated disc swelling will usually be detected using an ophthalmoscope. Therefore testing for an enlarged blind spot is of little diagnostic use.
- A red hatpin or target is excellent at detecting red desaturation in the central 30° visual field. Red desaturation is suggestive of optic nerve disease as the cause of poor vision (as opposed to macular disease).

> ❶ **Top Tips**
>
> - Do not move the target too fast, especially in the peripheral field. This can lead to inaccuracies in the size of the field.
> - It is best to remove the patient's glasses. Lenses can alter the size of the visual field and thick frames can get in the way of the vision. However if the patient is very short sighted, and cannot see the target without glasses, keep them on. Beware that the field may be smaller with the spectacles on.
> - If they cannot see your eye ask them to look at your face or towards your voice.
> - Do not cross the vertical or horizontal midlines, as your intention is to test only one quadrant at a time.
> - Remember the imaginary piece of glass. You may need to reach forwards in the periphery, bending the elbow as you reach the centre.

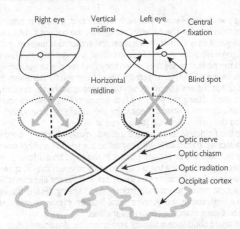

Fig. 8.7 Diagram representing the visual field and associated visual pathways. Note that the visual field of each eye can be divided into 4 quadrants by the vertical and horizontal midlines, both of which intersect at the point of fixation. The field to the right of the vertical midline travels to the left side of the brain (and vice versa). The fields above and below the horizontal midline travel to the temporal and parietal lobes respectively.

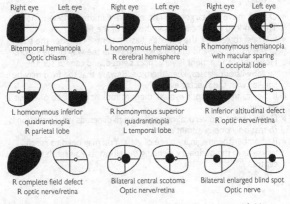

Fig. 8.8 Visual field defects with location of pathology. Patient's visual fields are displayed from the doctor's perspective (i.e. patient's right eye is on the left side).

Eye movements

Examination of the eye movements, incorporating the findings from 2 eyes, looking in 9 positions of gaze, and using 12 muscles may appear a daunting task. Looking for patterns will however, simplify the interpretation of these signs.

- While talking observe for any signs of thyroid disease (proptosis, lid retraction, goitre, thyroid acropachy), cerebellar disease indicating possible multiple sclerosis (nystagmus, intention tremor), or a myasthenic or myotonic facial appearance.
- Ask the patient to look at a pen torch held straight ahead at approximately 50cm. Be careful not to shine it directly into their eyes. Observe the corneal light reflexes. They should both lie slightly nasal of centre. Asymmetry suggests deviation. Ask yourself the following 3 questions:
  - *Are the eyes straight?* Look for a convergent squint (sixth nerve palsy) or 'down and out' eye (third nerve palsy). Vertical deviation, in the absence of other thyroid or myasthenic features, suggests a fourth nerve palsy, which may also result in a head tilt.
  - *Are the lids equal?* The upper lids normally rest 2mm below the superior limbus (junction between the sclera and the cornea) while the lower lids rest at the inferior limbus. The patient must be looking straight ahead. Look for a low (ptosis) or high position (retraction) of the eyelid. Particularly compare the position of one lid with the other. They should be symmetrical to within 1mm. A ptosis with a 'down and out' eye ± a dilated pupil (third nerve palsy) is abnormal. Unilateral ptosis could also indicate myasthenia. The bilateral symmetrical partial ptosis of myotonic dystrophy or the subtle unilateral ptosis of Horners syndrome may be easy to miss. Look for lid retraction ± ocular deviation/proptosis (thyroid eye disease).
  - *Are the pupils equal?* Look for a dilated pupil (compressive third nerve palsy) or a constricted pupil (Horner's).
- Ask the patient to keep their head still, follow the light with their eyes, and say if they see double.
  - Move light up and down, looking for lid retraction, lag and restricted up gaze (thyroid eye disease).
  - Then move in an 'H' shape to examine the 6 cardinal positions of gaze. Test to extremes of gaze, carefully watching for asymmetry in eye position and corneal light reflex in each position of gaze. Question regarding diplopia in each position.
  - Extraocular muscles work in pairs, one muscle in each eye, to move the eyes in a particular direction. They are yoked together like a pair of oxen pulling a plough (see Fig. 8.9).

❶ Top Tips

- If double vision is found, determine in which direction(s) of gaze it is at its worst. This should be the direction of action of an affected muscle(s).

- Is the diplopia side by side (horizontal diplopia suggesting weakness of a medial or lateral rectus muscle) or one on top of each other (vertical diplopia)?
- There may be obvious limitation of movement of a specific muscle to explain the diplopia, such as the lateral rectus in a sixth nerve palsy.
- If it is not clear which of a pair of muscles is affected it is possible to establish which eye has the limited movement by asking the patient to cover one eye, whilst looking in the direction in which their diplopia is at its worst. The patient will always perceive the outermost (peripheral) image to originate in the eye with the limitation of movement.

- Ask yourself whether the signs seen fit a pattern consistent with a cranial nerve weakness.
- If not consider complex ophthalmoplegia (e.g. thyroid eye disease or myasthenia gravis). Look for further evidence of ocular myasthenia by asking the patient to maintain upgaze – they may complain of diplopia or develop ptosis after a few seconds (➲ p.379).

❶ Top Tips

- Remember to keep things simple with the following 4 questions:
  - Which eye is most affected by limited movement?
  - Is it affected more on looking up or down?
  - Is it affected more on looking left or right?
  - Are there any associated lid or pupil changes that fit a pattern?

- If no extraocular palsy has yet been revealed at this point, move on to test saccades (fast eye movements). Ask the patient to look quickly from a hand held on the right to a fist held on the left. Asymmetry in speed of movement is suggestive of internuclear ophthalmoplegia (multiple sclerosis; ➲ p.359). Test saccades looking up and down.
- The final part of the examination involves testing convergence. Bring a target from 30cm slowly towards the nose.

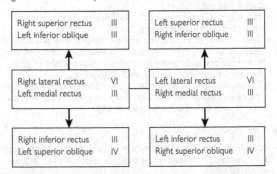

Fig. 8.9 Cardinal positions of gaze, muscles involved and nerves supplying them. Patient's eye movements are displayed from the doctor's perspective (i.e. patient's right eye is on the left side).

Pupils

In order to assess the pupils you need a bright pen torch and a dimly lit room. Dim lighting allows the pupils to dilate as much as possible while the bright torch allows them to constrict as much as possible. This makes pupillary reactions easier to see. However, if the room is too dark, it will be difficult to assess consensual pupil reactions, particularly in patients with dark irises.

- While talking observe for signs associated with Horner's syndrome:
  - Wasting of the small muscles of the hand (Pancoast's tumour, syringomyelia).
  - Scars suggesting neck surgery or trauma.
  - Palpate for cervical lymphadenopathy.
- Look for other associated signs including:
  - Nystagmus, intention tremor, ataxic dysarthria: multiple sclerosis.
  - Hemiparesis (with third nerve palsy): Weber's syndrome.
  - High stepping gait (with Argyll Robertson pupils): tabes dorsalis.
- With the room lights on, stand to the side of the patient and ask them to look into the distance. Observe the pupil size and shape. Ask yourself:
  - **Are the pupils equal?** Unequal pupils (anisocoria) indicates a motor rather than sensory abnormality. A dilated pupil suggests a compressive third nerve palsy or Adie's pupil, whilst a constricted pupil suggests a Horner's syndrome.
  - **Are the eyes straight?** Look for a 'down and out' eye (third nerve palsy).
  - **Are the lids equal?** Look for a ptosis with a 'down and out' eye (third nerve palsy) or lid retraction (thyroid eye disease).
- Dim the lights as much as possible while still being able to see the pupils. Ask yourself if the pupils are still equal?
  - Anisocoria may become more apparent in either a brightly lit or dimly lit room.
  - The abnormal pupil is the one that shows limited dilation from light to dark (Horner's syndrome) or limited constriction from dark to light (third nerve palsy, Adie's pupil).
  - Bilateral poor constriction/dilatation may result from Argyll Robertson pupils, opiates or pilocarpine eye drops.
  - Argyll Robertson pupils are usually small and irregular; they do not react to light but constrict slowly to accommodation.
  - Homes–Adie pupil is a clinical diagnosis of exclusion, which may be associated with absent ankle reflexes (Adie's syndrome); usually idiopathic, but may be associated with Sjögren's syndrome.
- If no abnormality is detected by this point, it is likely that there is an afferent (sensory) defect.
- Keeping the room dimly lit, test for a direct light reflex by observing the right eye while shining light in the right eye first. Failure/sluggish constriction indicates either an afferent (sensory) defect or an efferent (motor) defect on the right. Test for a consensual light reflex by observing the left eye while shining light in the right. Failure/sluggish constriction in the presence of an abnormal direct reflex on the right indicates an afferent (sensory) defect on the right. Failure/sluggish constriction in the presence of a normal direct reflex on the right indicates an efferent (motor) defect on the left (Fig. 8.10). Now repeat direct and consensual reflexes for the left eye.

- Now assess for a relative afferent pupillary defect (RAPD; Marcus–Gunn pupil) using the swinging light test. Swing the pen torch back and forth, shining the light for three seconds in each eye. This allows enough time to spot delayed dilatation that can occur in a mild relative afferent pupillary defect (➲ The RAPD and Fig. 8.10).
- A unilateral optic neuropathy, or a markedly asymmetrical bilateral optic neuropathy, produces an RAPD. If an RAPD is found, proceed to fundoscopy to examine for optic atrophy (➲ p.561). Remember that a patient may have both a sensory and a motor defect.
- Finally assess constriction to accommodation. Ask the patient to look into the distance, then close to a target held 30cm away at eye level. Watch for the constriction of accommodation.

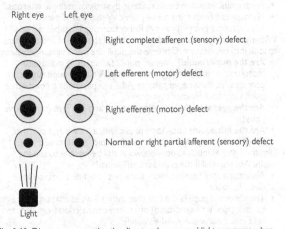

Right eye   Left eye

Right complete afferent (sensory) defect

Left efferent (motor) defect

Right efferent (motor) defect

Normal or right partial afferent (sensory) defect

Light

Fig. 8.10 Diagram representing the direct and consensual light responses when light is shone into the right eye. Patient's pupillary reactions are displayed from the doctor's perspective (i.e. patient's right eye is on the left side).

The RAPD

Having established that there is no efferent (motor) defect (the pupils are equal in both light and dark) the swinging light test is used to elicit the presence of a relative afferent pupillary defect (RAPD). Swinging the light from one eye to the other, enables the testing of one pupil's responses 'relative' to the other – i.e. looking for an afferent (sensory) defect. The key features are (see Fig. 8.11):

- Shining light on one eye leads to bilateral pupillary constriction. The candidate should concentrate only on the side on which the light is shone.

- On moving across to the other eye both pupils dilate, until the contralateral eye is reached, when dilatation halts and constriction re-occurs. If the contralateral eye is:
  - abnormal, with a mildly damaged optic nerve, constriction may be poor relative to the normal side. Mild defects may only become apparent after a few swings as the nerve 'fatigues'.
  - moderately affected, constriction may be absent.
  - severely affected, dilation continues.
- On returning to the healthy eye, constriction occurs as normal.
- The swinging light test is sensitive for 3 reasons:
  - Halting dilatation, and then inducing constriction (as in the swinging light test), is much harder than inducing constriction from standstill (as in the direct reflex). This makes the test more demanding.
  - The repetitive nature of the test makes mild defects clearer over time as the nerve 'fatigues'.

By comparing one eye with the other subtle differences can be seen. This is analogous to identical twins, whose differences are easier to see when stood next to each other.

> **❶ Top Tips**
>
> - Asymmetry of pupil size suggests a motor (efferent) defect of the pupils, rather than a sensory (afferent) defect due to optic neuropathy. The Edinger–Westphal nucleus projects to both eyes so even if one eye is blind light falling on the fellow eye will stimulate both pupils. Therefore, the pupils should remain equal in all lighting conditions.
> - Always stand to the side of the patient. This avoids inadvertently inducing accommodative pupillary constriction.
> - A wealth of information can be determined just by turning the room light on and off. Careful observation is vital.
> - Shine light straight and use a bright pen torch. If illumination varies during examination this can make the pupillary responses vary.
> - Partial afferent (sensory) defects can give rise to normal direct and consensual responses. Defect may only become apparent after 3–4 swings of the swinging light test (delayed dilatation).
> - When performing the swinging light test look for asymmetry in pupillary reactions. Pupillary 'bounce' or slight dilatation after constriction can be seen in normal young patients. However this is seen equally in both eyes. The dilatation of an RAPD is asymmetrically seen in one eye only.
> - Long standing Adie's pupils may become constricted (little old Adie).
> - Beware the glass eye – if there is no pupillary response and you cannot perform fundoscopy, this is the most likely cause.

⚫ Common Pitfalls

- An afferent pupil defect may be missed if the torch is moved either too quickly or too slowly during the swinging light test.
- Beware that some 10–20% of the population have physiological anisocoria. The difference in pupil size is typically ≤1mm, and this difference remains the same in both light and dark conditions; in pathological anisocoria the difference is >1mm and becomes greater in either light or the dark conditions.

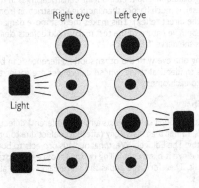

Fig. 8.11 Diagram representing the swinging light test in the presence of a left relative afferent pupillary defect. Patient's pupillary reactions are displayed from the doctor's perspective (i.e. patient's right eye is on the left side).

Sudden loss of vision: diabetic vitreous haemorrhage

Information for candidates

- You will be asked to see 2 patients at this station. The clinical information about one of these patients is given in the box. You should have a second sheet giving you information about the other patient.
- You have 10 minutes with each patient. The examiners will alert you when 6 minutes have elapsed and will stop you after 8 minutes.
- In the remaining 2 minutes, one examiner will ask you to report abnormal physical signs (if any), your diagnosis or differential diagnosis, and your plan for management (if not already clear from your discussion with the patient).

Your role: you are the medical doctor on call.

Patient name: Mr. Jayantilal Patel – age 57 years.

This gentleman presented to the A&E department with a sudden loss of vision.

Your task is to assess the patient's problems and address any questions or concerns raised by the patient.

- You should assess the problem by means of a relevant clinical history and a relevant physical examination. You do not need to complete the history before carrying out appropriate examination.
- You should respond to any questions the patient may have, advise the patient of your probable diagnosis (or differential diagnoses) and your plan for investigation and treatment where appropriate.
- You have 8 minutes to complete the task.

Information for patient

The doctors sitting the examination have been asked to assess your problem. They will have 8 minutes to ask you about the problem and any other relevant issues. They will also examine you. During the examination they may ask to look at the back of your eyes with an ophthalmoscope. They should explain to you what they think is wrong and what action should be taken and answer any questions you have, for example about the diagnosis, tests that may be needed, or treatment. One of the examiners will ask them to describe any abnormal examination findings and give their diagnosis. Your history is described as follows:

You are: Mr. Jayantilal Patel – age 57 years.

Your problem: loss of vision due to haemorrhage in the vitreous (the jelly filled compartment) at the back of your right eye.

You have been diabetic for 14 years. You were initially treated with tablets, but for the last 5 years you have been using insulin.

You manage your own business importing and distributing clothing manufactured in India and the Far East. As a result you work long, irregular hours and travel extensively.

You find it hard to control your blood sugar levels under these circumstances and have also failed to attend 2 recent appointments in the Eye Clinic because you had work commitments.

You have been told that you have diabetic changes in your eyes, but you have not, until now, had any problems with your vision.

Today you woke up with almost no sight in your right eye.

You should ask why your vision has deteriorated, what treatment may be necessary and how urgently an eye specialist will see you. You are very concerned that you are going to become blind.

Information for examiners

Patient: Mr. Jayantilal Patel – age 57 years.

Examiners should discuss and agree the criteria for pass and for fail in the competencies being assessed.

As a general guide, candidates would be expected to:

- Determine that Mr. Patel is diabetic and enquire about his blood glucose and BP control.
- Assess the visual acuity.
- Perform fundoscopy and comment on the reduced red reflex in the right eye and signs of severe non-proliferative (pre-proliferative) diabetic retinopathy in the left eye.
- Test for an afferent pupillary defect.
- Examine the visual fields.
- Explain to the patient that he has had a vitreous haemorrhage, a potentially serious diabetic eye complication and that he needs urgent referral to an ophthalmologist (within 2 weeks).
- Emphasize the need for tight glycaemic control and regular ophthalmology reviews.
- Offer to arrange a follow-up appointment with a diabetic physician.

The lead examiner should:

- Advise the candidate after 6 minutes have elapsed that 'You have 2 minutes remaining with your patient'.
- Ask the candidate to describe any abnormal physical findings that have been identified.
- Ask the candidate to give the preferred diagnosis and any differential diagnosis that is being considered.
- Any remaining areas of uncertainty e.g. regarding the plan for investigation or management of the problem may be addressed in any time that remains.

History

In the absence of trauma, sudden loss of vision is virtually always due to a vascular event of some kind. This event may affect the vitreous, the retina, the optic nerve, or another part of the visual pathway, such as the occipital cortex.

An appreciation of the anatomy of the visual pathways (Fig. 8.7) is essential to localize the site of the lesion underlying the patient's symptoms.

Causes of sudden visual loss
- Vitreous haemorrhage
- Retinal artery occlusion
- Retinal vein occlusion
- Haemorrhagic ('wet') age-related macular degeneration
- Ischaemic optic neuropathy
- Pituitary apoplexy
- Cerebrovascular disease (stroke)
- Trauma.

Retinal detachment and optic neuritis cause rapid, but not sudden, loss of vision, usually over several hours or days.

Flashing lights and the appearance of floaters typically precede retinal detachment. It presents as a dark curtain that starts peripherally and progressively covers more of the patient's vision. Fundoscopy reveals a pale grey, elevated area of retina.

Optic neuritis usually causes progressive visual loss, frequently associated with pain on eye movements (➲ Multiple sclerosis, p.337).

Establish whether Mr Patel's loss of vision affects one or both eye(s)
If sudden visual loss is due to cortical disease (stroke) it should affect both eyes, causing a homonymous visual field defect (hemianopia/quadrantinopia). Patients sometimes mistake a left/right homonymous hemianopia for loss of vision in the left/right eye.

If visual loss is unilateral
- There may be an 'altitudinal' field defect (loss of the whole of the upper or the whole of the lower visual field) suggesting a branch retinal artery occlusion or anterior ischaemic optic neuropathy.
- The patient may describe the appearance of dark floating spots (a 'cobweb', 'curtain' etc), which suggests a vitreous haemorrhage.
- An associated headache (classically non responsive to simple analgesics) may indicate that the vascular occlusion is secondary to *giant cell arteritis*. If so ask about jaw and lingual claudication, as well as generalized symptoms such as anorexia and weight loss, which may overlap with features associated with polymyalgia rheumatica. An urgent ESR should be requested (➲ Rheumatology p.519).

Enquire about risk factors for vascular occlusion, particularly diabetes and hypertension and about any previous history of cardiovascular disease (e.g. angina, myocardial infarction, stroke).

> **❶ Top Tips**
>
> - For virtually all ophthalmology cases it is worth asking whether the patient is diabetic, as this is relevant for both sudden and gradual loss of vision, as well as for diplopia caused by cranial nerve palsies (which are frequently vascular in origin) and even for visual field loss, which may be due to cerebrovascular disease.

Having ascertained that Mr. Patel is diabetic, candidates should enquire about his medication, his blood glucose and BP control, and whether he is under regular review by an ophthalmologist or undergoing annual photographic screening through the Diabetic Retinopathy Screening Service. Patients with diabetic retinopathy frequently have nephropathy and vice versa.

Examination

Whilst talking to Mr. Patel candidates should look for signs associated with management of his diabetes. The patient may have a drug chart, medications or a blood glucose testing kit at their bedside.

Visual acuity

- Acuity should always be assessed separately for each eye
  (● p.533).
- Loss of acuity is generally proportional to the amount of damage to the macula area of the retina or those fibres of the optic nerve that are associated with the macula. Acuity may also be severely reduced in conditions that obscure the fundus, such as cataract and vitreous haemorrhage, depending on the density of the opacity.

Visual fields

If the history suggests loss of peripheral vision the field of vision should be determined in each eye by confrontation.

- Confrontation visual field testing should be performed in each of 4 quadrants (upper and lower, nasal and temporal) to assess the peripheral visual fields.
- Central visual fields, including the size of the blind spot, should be tested horizontally and vertically.

Pupil reactions

If the pupils have not been dilated with mydriatics:

- Test for an afferent pupillary defect.
- Pupil reactions will be normal in most patients with bilateral visual loss.
- A relative afferent pupillary defect (RAPD) either indicates optic nerve disease or widespread retinal damage. Ischaemic optic neuropathy will, therefore, usually cause an afferent pupillary defect, whereas 'wet' macular degeneration or diabetic maculopathy will not.
- Vitreous haemorrhage and cataract usually scatter light, but do not prevent all light reaching the fundus and pupil reactions should be normal unless a second pathology is present.

Fundoscopy

Fundoscopy should be performed as discussed on ● p.536. In particular, candidates should assess:

- The red reflex – if absent or reduced, this suggests a vitreous haemorrhage.
- The retina.

Vitreous haemorrhage will lead to a reduced red reflex in the affected eye. (Cataracts also diminish the red reflex, but cause very gradual visual loss.) If the haemorrhage is dense it may completely obscure the retina. If there is a fundal view, retinal neovascularization may be found. The fellow eye should be carefully examined for signs of diabetic retinopathy.

❶ Top Tips

(See Figs. 8.12 and 8.13 [➲ Plates 1 and 2]).

- In patients with diabetic retinopathy:
  - The macular region should be assessed for the presence of exudates close to fixation (potentially clinically significant maculopathy).
  - New vessels are most frequently seen on the optic disc or 1 of the 4 major veins that run from the disc to each quadrant of the retina.
  - New vessels are usually finer and more tortuous than normal vessels. They may branch in an abnormal fashion (normal vessels always split into 2) and cross over existing vessels (normal veins may cross arteries, but they do not cross each other).

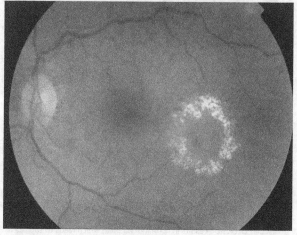

Fig. 8.12 Diabetic maculopathy. Diabetic maculopathy frequently manifests as rings of exudate around areas of oedema (circinate exudates).
With permission from Moorfields Eye Hospital. See also Plate 1.

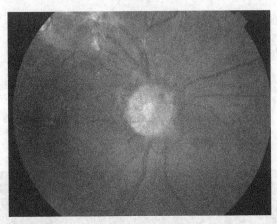

Fig. 8.13 Proliferative diabetic retinopathy. This fundus photograph shows florid new vessels on the optic disc (NVD). Frequently neovascularization is more subtle and may also be seen arising from vessels elsewhere (NVE), typically from one of the four major veins that run from the disc to each quadrant of the retina.
With permission from Moorfields Eye Hospital. See also Plate 2.

Patient concerns

The patient is likely to be worried about becoming blind. The candidate should seek to allay his fears by reassuring him that treatment is available that may restore his vision. It is however important to stress that regular attendance at the ophthalmology clinic, as well as optimal glycaemic control, is essential to reduce the risk of visual loss.

Diabetic retinopathy

Diabetic mellitus causes a microangiopathy that results both in a) vascular occlusion and b) leakage of plasma constituents out of damaged vessels.

Vascular occlusion results in retinal ischaemia, which leads to the release of angiogenic factors (principally VEGF – vascular endothelial growth factor) that drive the growth of new vessels.

Since diabetic retinopathy (DR) has been shown to be more frequent and more severe in patients with poor glycaemic control and high BP, all patients with DR should be counselled about measures to improve their diabetic control and their general health (❷ Diabetes mellitus and diabetic foot, p.579).

❶ Top Tips

- Diabetic retinopathy may progress very rapidly during pregnancy.
- All women with diabetes who become pregnant should be assessed for the presence of retinopathy at least once per trimester and be reviewed more frequently if significant retinopathy is detected.
- Patients with significant retinopathy frequently also have other microvascular complications of diabetes, so candidates must enquire about renal function and diabetic neuropathy.

Grading of diabetic retinopathy

Grading helps to predict risk of progression to sight-threatening, high-risk proliferative disease and determine the appropriate interval for review.

Most ophthalmologists now use a classification of DR employed by the Early Treatment of Diabetic Retinopathy (ETDRS) Study (➔ Useful websites, p.554). Mild to moderate non-proliferative background retinopathy (NPDR) roughly equates to 'background retinopathy' and severe to very severe NPDR roughly equates to 'pre-proliferative retinopathy'.

The risk of progression to sight-threatening high-risk proliferative DR is:
- 1% per year for mild NPDR: review in 12 months.
- 4% for moderate NPDR: review in 6–9 months.
- 8% for severe NPDR: review in 4–6 months.
- 17% for very severe NPDR: review in 3–4 months.
- *Background retinopathy:* early signs of localized retinal ischaemia include microaneurysms (dots) and blot haemorrhages.
- *Pre-proliferative retinopathy:* more widespread ischaemia leads to the development of fluffy 'cotton wool spots' (microinfarcts), venous calibre abnormalities, such as venous dilation, beading, loops and intraretinal microvascular abnormalities (IRMA).
- *Proliferative retinopathy:* extensive ischaemia leads to the growth of new vessels. These new vessels are fragile and prone to haemorrhage into the vitreous or the pre-retinal space (between the vitreous and the retina), where the blood tends to settle inferiorly, forming large crescent shaped haemorrhages.
- *High-risk proliferative disease* is defined as new vessels on or adjacent to the optic disc >1/4 of the area of the disc in size or any new vessels (on the disc or elsewhere) associated with vitreous or preretinal haemorrhage. It requires urgent (within 2 weeks) panretinal photocoagulation (laser) treatment.

Panretinal photocoagulation

The principle behind laser treatment in proliferative DR is to reduce the production of angiogenic factors, principally VEGF, and to remove this stimulus for the growth of new blood vessels. Laser burns are applied to all four quadrants of the peripheral retina beyond the major vascular arcades.

Initially around 2000 laser burns are applied, usually in 2 or 3 sessions, but treatment should be repeated until new vessels are observed to be regressing. Side effects may include reduced night vision and visual field loss. Damage to the patient's field of vision is minimized by spacing laser burns at least one burn width apart, but if repeated applications of laser are required patients may eventually suffer significant loss of peripheral vision and be rendered ineligible to drive (➔ p.557 regarding DVLA).

Diabetic maculopathy

- Diabetic maculopathy may occur irrespective of the severity of retinopathy.
- Diabetic maculopathy is caused by oedema from leaking capillaries and/or ischaemia due to capillary loss. Central visual loss may occur due to macular oedema, which is usually accompanied by exudate formation,

or macular ischaemia, which may be difficult to detect clinically. Unexplained visual loss may, therefore, be due to ischaemia.

• Treatment is indicated when maculopathy threatens the fovea (centre of the macula). Isolated microaneurysms around the fovea without clinical evidence of oedema do not merit treatment, but warrant regular review.

• Exudates in the macular area frequently form rings around areas of oedema (circinate exudates) or lines radiating out from the fovea (see Fig. 8.12 → Plate 1).

Clinically significant macular oedema, requiring laser treatment, is defined as:

• An area of retinal thickening, any part of which is at or within 500μm of the fovea. (Retinal thickening is difficult to detect by a direct ophthalmoscope and would not be expected of a PACES candidate.)

• Exudates at or within 500 μm of the fovea, if associated with adjacent retina thickening.

• Retinal thickening ≥1 disc area, any part of which is within 1 disc diameter of the fovea.

Focal laser treatment is usually applied to the centre of circinate exudates and around microaneurysms that are a source of leakage. If macular oedema is more diffuse a macular 'grid' treatment, in which laser burns are applied at regularly spaced intervals throughout the oedematous area, may be performed. Apart from improving general health there is no treatment available for ischaemic maculopathy.

Viva questions

How should this patient's retinopathy be managed?

• This depends on the severity of the retinopathy (see grading listed on → p. 553) and the presence or absence of significant maculopathy.

• Patients with background retinopathy can frequently be reviewed in the community by annual photographic screening (Diabetic Retinopathy Screening Service).

• If there are pre-proliferative changes or maculopathy, onward referral to the hospital eye service is required (within 13 weeks).

• Patients with proliferative retinopathy should be referred within 2 weeks for pan-retinal photocoagulation.

• Good control of both blood sugar levels and BP is very important because this significantly reduces the risk of visual loss due to diabetic retinopathy.

📖 Further reading

Mohamed Q, et al. Management of diabetic retinopathy: a systematic review. *JAMA* 2007; **298**(8):902–16.

🔗 Useful websites

Early Treatment of Diabetic Retinopathy (ETDRS) Study: http://clinicaltrials.gov/ct2/show/ NCT00000151

Royal College of Ophthalmologists DR Guidelines (text & figures): http://www.rcophth.ac.uk/page. asp?section=451&sectionTitle=Clinical+Guidelines

UK National Screening Programme for Diabetic Retinopathy: http://www.retinalscreening.nhs. uk/pages/

www.diabeticretinopathy.org.uk (Birmingham Eye Hospital site): http://medweb.bham.ac.uk/easdec/

Gradual visual loss: retinitis pigmentosa

The term retinitis pigmentosa (RP) refers to a group of inherited disorders of the retina that cause progressive and frequently severe loss of vision. RP affects approximately 1 in 3000–4000 people.

- Initial symptoms include difficulty with night vision (nyctalopia) and a gradual reduction in the field of vision, resulting in a tendency to trip over objects. The age at presentation is variable as there are many different genetic forms of RP (genetic heterogeneity), but is usually between the ages of 10–30 years.
- In more advanced cases, reading (central) vision and colour vision may be affected.
- The rate of visual deterioration is also variable, but is generally very slow with changes occurring over years rather than months.
- Many people retain a central 'tunnel' of useful vision and are able to continue reading until late in life.

Scenario

Patient name: Mr. Michael Scott – age 37 years.

This gentleman has suffered gradual loss of vision. Please take a focused history and examine him appropriately.

History

Since the diagnosis is not initially known candidates should, during the 5 minutes allocated for preparation, make a list of differential diagnoses for gradual visual loss and prepare appropriate questions:

Causes of gradual visual loss
- Cataract
- Age-related macular degeneration
- Diabetic maculopathy
- Glaucoma
- Retinitis pigmentosa
- Optic atrophy – compressive, toxic or nutritional.

Candidates should seek to establish whether Mr Scott's loss of vision:
- Affects one eye or both; clearly, since RP is an inherited disease it should affect both eyes.
- Is primarily central (difficulty with reading) or largely peripheral (difficulty getting around, bumping into things, tripping over).
- Is much worse in dim light ('night-blindness').
- Has required or benefited from any treatment (e.g. eye drops/laser).

It should become apparent that Mr. Scott's visual problems primarily or initially involved a reduction in his peripheral field of vision. If the candidate can establish a clear history of 'night-blindness' this is strongly suggestive of RP.

Loss of peripheral vision may be due to:
- Retinitis pigmentosa (constricted visual fields)

- Glaucoma (constricted)
- Laser photocoagulation (constricted)
- Branch retinal artery/vein occlusion affecting periphery (usually unilateral)
- Ischaemic optic neuropathy (usually unilateral)
- Cerebrovascular disease (homonymous)
- Chiasmal lesion (bitemporal)

Loss of central vision may be due to:

- Diabetic maculopathy
- Age-related macular degeneration
- Optic neuropathy: demyelinating/compressive/toxic/nutritional
- Cataract
- Branch retinal artery/vein occlusion affecting macula (usually unilateral).

Elicit a family history

If RP is suspected (or confirmed by the patient) the candidate should ask specifically whether any of Mr. Scott's family are affected by this condition. Over half of all patients have family members affected by RP.

❶ Top Tips

- Since RP can be inherited as an autosomal dominant, autosomal recessive, sex-linked recessive or a mitochondrial disorder it is crucial to determine the mode of inheritance in a particular family as genetic counselling is impossible without first establishing the mode of inheritance.

In the UK the figures for inheritance of non-syndromic RP are:

- ~50% sporadic (no family history – probably recessive).
- ~25% have only siblings affected (probably recessive).
- 15–20% have affected parents or children (dominant transmission).
- 5–10% have only male relatives affected, with no male-to-male transmission (X-linked recessive).

❖ Common Pitfalls

Recessive RP

- Remember that an individual affected by a recessively inherited disease can only transmit one disease-causing allele of a specific gene to his or her offspring.
- The risk of children being affected is not 25%.
- Whether children are affected will depend on whether their other parent carries a disease-causing allele of the same gene.
- Unless the affected individual and his/her partner are genetically related (a consanguineous relationship) the chance of the partner being a carrier of a disease-causing allele will depend on the 'carrier frequency' of these alleles in the community, which is frequently 1/100 or less. 1 in 4 children born to parents who are both carriers will be affected.

All the syndromic forms of RP (➜ Syndromes associated with RP, p.558) are inherited as autosomal recessive traits with the exception of Kearns–Sayre syndrome, which is transmitted as a mitochondrial disorder.

Patient concerns

Establish how the patient is affected by his poor vision

- Night blindness places few restrictions on patients residing in brightly lit modern cities, but may be a severe handicap in a rural setting.
- Peripheral visual field loss may render the patient ineligible to drive which can lead to a significant social handicap.
- RP is a progressive disease and many patients will eventually also experience difficulty with central vision, for example with reading.
- Some patients with RP suffer severe visual loss and need help with the normal activities of daily living.

❶ Top Tips

- In the UK the DVLA demands strict visual standards for driving.
- For a Group 1 (private car) license the patient must be able to read the letters on a number plate at a distance of 20m (corresponding to a binocular visual acuity of approximately 6/10 Snellen acuity).
- Patients must also have a visual field of at least 120° on the horizontal and no significant defect in the binocular field that encroaches within 20° of fixation either above or below the horizontal meridian.

Examination

Whilst talking to Mr. Scott candidates should look for signs associated with poor visual acuity. The patient may have a Braille book and/or a white stick at their bedside.

Visual acuity

Acuity should always be assessed separately for each eye. If the patient cannot read even the biggest print their ability to 'count fingers', to observe 'hand movements' or to perceive light should be assessed.

Visual fields

In RP bilateral, symmetrical constriction of the patient's visual fields would be expected.

❶ Top Tips

- A patient's visual field can be assessed so long as they have light perception in either eye; in this situation use a pen torch to assess the visual field.

Fundoscopy

The typical fundoscopic features of RP are (see Fig. 8.14 ➜ Plate 3):
- Peripheral retinal pigmentation, classically in a 'bone-spicule' pattern (like the branches of a tree) although it may also take the form of multiple small black spots.
  This pigment is bilateral and more prominent in the retinal periphery.

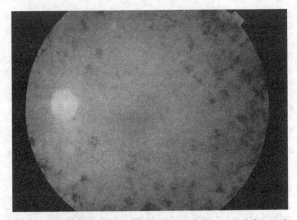

Fig. 8.14 Retinitis pigmentosa. This fundus photograph shows retinal pigmentation, attenuation of retinal vessels and pallor of the optic disc.
With permission from Moorfields Eye Hospital. See also Plate 3.

- Attenuation (narrowing) of retinal vessels.
- Pallor of the optic disc.

General examination
RP is associated with several systemic syndromes. It is essential to consider these and examine the patient appropriately.

> **① Top Tips**
>
> - Remember that RP is associated with systemic disorders.
> - *Commonest associated feature is hearing loss* (look for hearing aid).
> - Check hands and feet for polydactyly (Lawrence–Moon–Bardet–Biedl syndrome).
> - Consider tests of cerebellar function e.g. finger–nose coordination.
> - Offer to carry out a full neurological examination (to elicit signs of neuropathy caused by Refsum's syndrome).

Syndromes associated with RP
- Usher syndrome:
  - Congenital (usually) neurosensory deafness
- Refsum disease (a disorder of phytanic acid metabolism):
  - Deafness
  - Cerebellar ataxia
  - Peripheral neuropathy
  - Cardiomyopathy
  - Icthyosis
  - Palpable peripheral nerves
- Lawrence–Moon–Bardet–Biedl syndrome:
  - Deafness
  - Polydactyly

- Short stature
- Learning disability
- Hypogonadism
- Renal disease
- Diabetes
- Kearns–Sayre syndrome:
  - Chronic progressive external ophthalmoplegia (bilateral symmetrically reduced eye movements)
  - Cardiac conduction defects
  - Inherited as a mitochondrial trait.

Investigations

- Automated or Goldman perimetry (visual field assessment).
- Electrophysiology (electroretinogram/pattern electroretinogram – determines current severity of retinal damage and has prognostic implications).
- Audiology (if hearing loss suspected).
- Phytanic acid levels (Refsum disease).
- Molecular genetic analysis (may be appropriate for genetic counselling in some families – especially X-lined RP due to severity of disease in affected males and difficulty determining carrier status in females).

Treatment

- Treatments aimed at halting or reversing the progression of retinal disease are still in experimental stages. For most patients there is no treatment available.
- Patients may be eligible for partial sight/blind registration by an ophthalmologist. This enables access to benefits including social service support and reduced public transport costs (useful if can no longer drive).
- Magnifying glasses/devices can help with reading (refer to optometrist/ Low Vision Aid clinic).

New developments

- Gene therapy: experimental; human studies in progress, some success.
- Photosensitive retinal implants ('bionic eye') – experimental; human studies in progress, vision limited to perception of light/darkness/large objects only.

Viva questions

What syndromes are associated with RP?

(→ Syndromes associated with RP, p.558 for features of each syndrome.)
- Usher syndrome
- Refsum disease
- Lawrence–Moon–Bardet–Biedl syndrome
- Kearns-Sayre syndrome.

What is the risk that this patient's children will be affected by RP?

This will depend upon the pattern of inheritance:
- *Autosomal dominant:* 50%.
- *Autosomal recessive:* depends on patient's partner (→ p.556).

- *X-linked recessive:* a man's sons inherit his Y chromosome and will be unaffected. All his daughters will inherit his X chromosome and will be carriers of the disease (some may become mildly affected in later life).
- *Mitochondrial:* since all the mitochondria in an embryo are derived from the egg (those in the tail of the sperm do not enter the egg), mitochondrial disorders are inherited through the maternal route. Affected men cannot transmit the disease to their offspring. The sons and daughters of an affected woman are all at risk. The severity of the disorder in these individuals may be related to the proportion of their mitochondria that carry the disease-causing mutation.

Useful websites

British Retinitis Pigmentosa Society: http://www.brps.org.uk/
Online Mendelian Inheritance in Man: http://www.ncbi.nlm.nih.gov/sites/entrez?db=omim
Retnet (Retinal Information Network): http://www.sph.uth.tmc.edu/Retnet/

Subacute visual loss: optic atrophy

The optic nerve is comprised of axons that originate in the ganglion cell layer of the retina and project to the lateral geniculate body in the midbrain. These axons are heavily myelinated and, once damaged, do not regenerate.

Patients with optic neuropathy may be encountered in the neurology station or in Station 5.

> ### Scenario
>
> Miss Samantha Pritchard – age 24 years.
>
> This lady has suffered a deterioration in vision in her left eye.
>
> Please assess the patient's problems and address any questions or concerns raised by the patient.

Optic atrophy has many possible causes, the frequency of which depends on the age of the patient. In younger patients optic atrophy is most commonly due to demyelination whereas in those >50 years of age an ischaemic cause is more likely.

History

❶ Top Tips

- The differential diagnosis of optic atrophy should be structured according to:
  - The speed of onset of visual loss: sudden loss suggests an ischaemic cause, subacute loss demyelination and gradual deterioration a compressive lesion (e.g. pituitary tumour) or a toxic/nutritional cause.
  - Whether optic atrophy is unilateral or bilateral: unilateral optic atrophy may be ischaemic, compressive or demyelinating, whilst bilateral involvement suggests demyelinating, toxic, nutritional or inherited optic nerve disease.

Visual loss in optic neuropathy is usually painless
- Sudden visual loss associated with headache may be due to arteritic anterior ischaemic optic neuropathy and the patient should be questioned about other features of GCA (e.g. weight loss, jaw claudication, headaches – ⊃ p.519).
- Pain on eye movement typically occurs in optic neuritis.
- Constant periocular pain may indicate a localized inflammatory process such as sarcoidosis or Wegener's granulomatosis.

Examination

Initial assessment of subacute visual loss should include:
- Visual acuity: optic neuropathy frequently presents with loss of central vision, leading to reduced visual acuity.
- Pupillary reactions: test for an afferent pupillary defect.
- Fundoscopy: optic disc changes may include:
  - total pallor
  - temporal pallor (sometimes seen in demyelination, toxic neuropathy and nutritional deficiency)
  - bow-tie pallor (compression of the optic chiasm)
  - cupping (glaucomatous optic atrophy).

Further assessment if optic atrophy is detected may include:
- Colour vision: may be reduced.
- Visual fields: some lesions (e.g. a pituitary tumour) may give rise to peripheral visual field loss with relatively well preserved visual acuity.
- Eye movement:
  - Inflammatory and compressive lesions may also involve oculomotor nerves, particularly at the orbital apex (⊃ Superior orbital fissure syndrome, p.363), so eye movement examination may also be relevant
  - Patients with MS may exhibit an internuclear ophthalmoplegia (⊃ p.359)
- If an underlying systemic disease is suspected, such as MS, a brief non-ocular examination such as assessment of cerebellar function may also be appropriate.

❶ Top Tips

- A unilateral optic neuropathy frequently produces a RAPD.
- A RAPD may occur in the presence of massive retinal damage, such as a total retinal detachment, but *not* due to localized retinal diseases which lead to poor visual acuity, such as diabetic maculopathy or age-related macular degeneration.

Causes of optic atrophy

- Hereditary: optic atrophy may occur in isolation, both as:
  - A slowly progressive (over years), frequently dominant trait.
  - A relatively rapidly progressive (over days/weeks) condition e.g. Leber's optic neuropathy.

Optic atrophy may also occur as part of an inherited syndrome such as DIDMOAD (diabetes insipidus, diabetes mellitus, optic atrophy and deafness).

- Compressive lesions of the optic nerve (listed in anatomical order from anterior to posterior):
  - Tumours within the optic nerve (optic nerve glioma, optic nerve sheath meningioma).
  - Intra-orbital pathology such as dysthyroid eye disease.
  - Inflammatory masses at the orbital apex e.g. sarcoid or Wegener's granulomatosis. (NB these disorders may also cause ischaemic damage to the optic and oculomotor nerves.)
  - Lesions of the anterior cranial fossa (e.g. frontal meningioma, mucocele, metastasis).
  - Bilateral optic atrophy may occur when the chiasm is compressed by a pituitary macroadenoma or craniopharyngioma.
- Ischaemic:
  - Non-arteritic: the exact aetiology is unclear but systemic risk factors appear to be very similar to those associated with thrombo-embolism e.g. hypertension, diabetes, hyperlipidaemia, ischaemic heart disease.
  - Arteritic: GCA must be excluded.
- Demyelination: MS and neuromyelitis optica (Devic disease – ➲ p.340).
- Inflammatory:
  - Non-infective (orbital apex sarcoid or Wegener's granulomatosis).
  - Infective (TB, syphilis, Lyme disease, measles, mumps, varicella, fungal).
- Nutritional/toxic:
  - Deficiency of vitamin B12.
  - Tobacco, methanol and drugs (e.g. ethambutol).
- Other:
  - Traumatic optic nerve avulsion, transection, optic nerve sheath haematoma and optic nerve impingement by a bony fragment can all lead to optic atrophy.
  - Consecutive atrophy occurs in response to extensive ganglion cell damage in retinal disorders such as central retinal artery occlusion and retinitis pigmentosa.
  - Glaucoma results from a combination of high intraocular pressure and poor ocular perfusion. This causes a pale disc due to loss of nerve fibres, leading to an increase in the size of the optic cup.

Investigation

The choice of investigations depends on the presumed aetiology. If the onset was sudden a cardiovascular assessment may be indicated, whereas a gradual loss of vision will frequently necessitate neuroimaging.

- Formal perimetry (e.g. Humphrey 30-2 or 60-2)
- Electrophysiology: visually-evoked potentials (see following section)
- MRI of the brain and orbits with contrast
- CT scan of the orbits with contrast (if bony involvement suspected)
- Blood tests: glucose, ESR, vitamin B-12 levels, ANA, antiphospholipid antibodies, syphilis serology
- Cardiovascular examination (pulse (AF), BP)
- Carotid Doppler ultrasound study
- Temporal artery biopsy (if appropriate).

Visually evoked potentials (VEPs)

VEPs assess optic nerve function and can confirm that visual loss is due to optic neuropathy rather than retinal disease. In optic neuritis, the VEPs are delayed (have an increased latency) and a reduced amplitude. Compressive lesions tend to reduce the amplitude of the VEPs, while producing a minimal shift in the latency.

Treatment

Management depends entirely on the aetiology of optic neuropathy. In some cases optic nerve damage may be at least partially reversible, for example, visual recovery is often seen following removal of a pituitary macroadenoma. However, after an ischaemic optic neuropathy, visual recovery is usually very limited and management centres on preventing further cardiovascular events.

- Steroid treatment: may be used in optic neuritis, where it speeds up visual recovery, but does not affect the eventual visual outcome.
- Steroids are essential in the management of arteritic anterior ischaemic optic neuropathy to prevent further vascular occlusions.
- Vitamin B12 replacement should be used where deficiency is identified.

Patient concerns

The patient may enquire about the possible underlying diagnosis (e.g. MS) and this should be treated sensitively.

A diagnosis of MS requires evidence of lesions 'disseminated in time and space' so this cannot be confirmed based upon optic neuritis alone. If additional lesions are seen in the MRI scan the probability that the patient has MS is increased (⊃ p.337).

Viva questions

What are the causes of optic atrophy?

Causes of optic atrophy (order reflects likely frequency in PACES):
- Unilateral:
  - Demyelination
  - Ischaemic
  - Compressive
  - Inflammatory
  - Traumatic
  - Glaucomatous
- Bilateral:
  - Demyelination
  - Chiasmal compression
  - Glaucomatous
  - Inherited
  - Nutritional
  - Toxic.

How would you manage this patient?

- Suspected demyelination:
  - Investigations should include an MRI scan with gadolinium enhancement and VEPs.
  - Steroid treatment should be considered if visual loss is acute.

- Ischaemic optic neuropathy:
  - Investigations should include an urgent ESR and temporal artery biopsy (if appropriate).
  - BP, cardiovascular examination, carotid Doppler, blood glucose, ANA, and further investigations as appropriate.
  - High dose IV/oral steroid treatment is required for arteritic anterior ischaemic optic neuropathy (AION).
  - Management of non-arteritic AION is similar to the management of stroke.

Sore prominent eye with visual disturbance: thyroid eye disease

Sore gritty eyes and intermittent visual disturbance are classical symptoms of tear film disturbance. As candidates are typically examined on medical conditions which have ocular manifestations, the following causes of tear film disturbance should be considered:

- Thyroid eye disease (TED):
  - Lacrimal gland damage causing decreased tear production.
  - Conjunctival swelling, lid retraction and proptosis leading to increased tear evaporation.
- Sarcoidosis: lacrimal gland damage causing decreased tear production.
- Primary Sjögren's syndrome.
- Secondary Sjögren's syndrome:
  - RA
  - SSc
  - SLE
  - Graft-versus-host disease.

TED is due to autoimmune inflammation of the extra-ocular muscles and retro-orbital fat. It is usually associated with an overactive or underactive thyroid, although it may present both before, during or after this episode. Risk factors include female sex, middle age, smoking, autoimmune thyroid disease, HLA-DR3 and HLA-B8.

Scenario

Mrs Jean Talbot – age 45 years.

Mrs Talbot has a 1-month history of gritty sore eyes with bilateral inter-mittent visual disturbance.

Please assess the patient's problems and address any questions or concerns raised by the patient.

General observation

Specifically look for systemic features associated with dry eyes:

- Lid retraction, proptosis, thyroid acropachy ± goitre, tremor, pretibial myxoedema (TED).
- Lacrimal gland swelling ± erythema nodosum (sarcoid).

- Rheumatoid hands.
- Microstomia, beaked nose, sclerodactyly and tight skin changes of SSc.
- Malar rash, alopecia, cushingoid appearance (SLE).

General initial questions

On general observation the candidate should note features suggestive of TED. In the PACES examination, TED may also present with:
- Eyes appear prominent (lid retraction, proptosis).
- Double vision (extraocular muscle restriction).
- Unilateral progressive visual loss (optic nerve compression).

Initial examination

Examine eye movements and lids (→ p.541)
- Asymmetrical limitation of eye movements (esp. upgaze):
  - Inflammation and fibrosis of extraocular muscles.
- Lid retraction, lid lag and lid swelling.
  - The upper lids normally rest 2mm below the superior limbus (junction between the sclera and the cornea) while the lower lids rest at the inferior limbus. Any degree of 'scleral show' (visible sclera when looking straight ahead due to a raised lid) is abnormal.
  - Lid lag can be seen as a delay in lid depression following downgaze (also indicative of hyperthyroidism).

Check for proptosis
Stand behind the seated patient and tip their head back so that the lids/eyes become visible in front of the eyebrows. Compare the position of the lids/eyes with the brow. Compare right with left. The key feature is asymmetrical forward prominence of the lid/eye compared with the brow.

Focused history

Be sure to enquire about the following:
- Progressive asymmetrical visual loss (optic nerve compression).
- Double vision (affects ability to drive).
- Thyroid status (e.g. cold/heat intolerance, weight; → Examination of thyroid status, p.590).
- Past medical history of thyroid disease including treatment:
  - Surgery, radioiodine.
  - Drug history of thyroxine, antithyroid drugs.
- Smoking (associated with significantly worse TED outcome).

Focused examination

Exclude optic nerve compression (medical emergency)
- Visual acuity and pupils: RAPD (→ p.533 and → p.543).
- Fundoscopy if suspect optic nerve compression; look for early disc swelling or late disc pallor (optic atrophy).

Exclude corneal exposure (medical emergency)
Assess the ability to close the eyes fully on gentle blinking: inability to close (due to lid retraction and proptosis) can lead to corneal exposure, infection and permanent loss of vision.

Systemic examination

Elicit the systemic signs of Grave's disease including (covered in more detail on ➔ p.583):

- Goitre (Grave's disease is commonly associated with TED).
- Assessment of thyroid status (➔ p.590).
- Associated signs (thyroid acropachy, pretibial myxoedema).

Classification of TED

There are many classifications used. A popular one with physicians/endocrinologists is the 'NOSPECS' classification:

- 0   N   No signs or symptoms
- 1   O   Only signs, no symptoms
- 2   S   Soft tissue involvement
- 3   P   Proptosis
- 4   E   Extraocular muscle involvement
- 5   C   Corneal involvement
- 6   S   Sight loss (decreased visual acuity).

Investigation

This should be divided into ophthalmic and systemic:

- Ophthalmic:
  - Orbital imaging: thickened extraocular muscles without tendon involvement. CT gives better bony resolution for planning orbital decompression; MRI (T2 STIR) gives better soft tissue resolution.
  - Orthoptic review: formally document eye movements and field of binocular single vision (i.e. area where no diplopia is seen).
- Systemic:
  - Thyroid function tests: TSH and T_4 (T_3 active metabolite if strong clinical suspicion with otherwise normal biochemistry).
  - Thyroid autoantibodies: anti-TSH receptor, anti-thyroid peroxidase, anti-thyroglobulin.

Differential diagnosis of thyroid eye disease

- TED: asymmetrical ocular deviation, proptosis, lid retraction
- Orbital mass: unilateral, ptosis (not retraction), non-tender
- Orbital cellulitis: unilateral, ptosis (not retraction), tender
- Orbital fracture: history of trauma, enophthalmos (not proptosis)
- Myasthenia gravis: ocular deviation, ptosis, no proptosis.

Management

Acute disease (active orbital inflammation with evolving signs)

- Tear film lubrication.
- Systemic immunosuppression (steroids ± steroid sparing agents) if significant disease (troublesome diplopia, risk of optic nerve compression or corneal exposure).
- Cessation of smoking.
- Optimize control of thyroid function (usually requires block and replace therapy; ➔ p.584).

- Optic nerve compression (medical emergency):
  - Systemic immunosuppression (steroids ± steroid sparing agents).
  - Surgical decompression of orbital apex if systemic immunosuppression fails.
  - Orbital radiotherapy acutely in conjunction with steroids.
- Corneal exposure (medical emergency):
  - Tear film lubrication.
  - Systemic immunosuppression (steroids).
  - Surgical decompression of orbit or lid lengthening surgery if listed measures fail.

Burnt-out disease (quiescent orbital inflammation with stable signs)

Once stable, surgery is often performed to improve cosmetic appearance and minimize diplopia. 3 stages are performed in the following order (although patient may not require all 3 stages):
- Orbital decompression – indicated if significant proptosis.
- Squint surgery for diplopia.
- Lid lengthening surgery for lid retraction.

Patient concerns

- Patients may be concerned about the prominent appearance of their eyes. Reassure patients that TED usually burns out within 1–5 years, following which surgical procedures are often possible and can result in considerable cosmetic and functional success.
- Patients may also be worried about sight loss. Patients should be reassured that the long-term outlook for vision is good, so long as appropriate and timely management of sight threatening complications (optic nerve compression, corneal exposure) is provided during the acute phase.

Viva questions

What is the patient's thyroid status?

Patients with dysthyroid eye disease are frequently hyperthyroid, but they can be euthyroid or hypothyroid. TED can present both before, during or after episode of hyper/hypothyroidism. Candidates should assess thyroid status in addition to examining the eyes (➔ p.590).

How would you manage this patient?

Candidates should discuss treatment of any sight-threatening eye disease, but also describe management of the patient's underlying condition including drug therapy and surgery if appropriate.

Visual field defect 1: bitemporal hemianopia

The location of a visual field defect should identify the anatomical location of the underlying pathology (Ⓢ Fig. 8.7 and 8.8). This information can help select the correct imaging modality, focus the scan on the right area, and interpret the scan with accuracy.

❶ Top Tips

- Field defects due to neurological disease situated at or behind the optic chiasm will usually respect the vertical midline because the lesion affects one side of the brain.
- Field defects due to retinal or optic nerve disease may cross the vertical midline, but may respect the horizontal midline, e.g. branch retinal artery occlusion, due to the distribution of the retinal vessels (Ⓢ Fig. 8.6).

Neurological disease causes 'negative' defects (patient unaware of gap in vision, except when object disappears into it) as opposed to the 'positive' defects of retinal disease (patient aware of shadow covering part of vision). Therefore symptoms can be rather non-specific.

> **Scenario**
>
> Mr James Mitchell, aged 51 years, has a 1-month history of visual problems. He can see out of both eyes but notices things sometimes disappear.
>
> Please take a focused history and examination. Please also address any questions or concerns raised by the patient.

General observation

Specifically look for systemic features associated with visual disturbance:
- Acromegaly
- Nystagmus, intention tremor, ataxic dysarthria (MS)
- Hemiplegia (stroke)
- Potential vascular risk factors: tar staining of fingers, obesity, corneal arcus.

General initial questions

Do not forget to ask general initial questions (Ⓢ p.532) in order to clarify the presenting complaint. Specifically ask whether the visual symptoms affect the central (reading/TV) vision, or the peripheral (navigational) vision.

Initial examination

Examine visual acuity and visual fields (Ⓢ p.533 and 538)

Map out edges of field defect. Do they respect the vertical or horizontal midlines? (suggesting a neurological cause):
- A bitemporal hemianopia may extend up to the vertical midline but does not usually cross it.
- A bitemporal hemianopia can start superiorly (pituitary tumours compress the inferior chiasmal fibres first) or inferiorly (craniopharyngiomas compress the superior chiasmal fibres first). Inferior chiasmal fibres originate from the inferior retina, which receives images from the superior visual field and vice versa.

Focused history

Bitemporal hemianopias are usually due to compression of the optic chiasm (Table 8.10). Therefore a focused history including the following features should be undertaken:

- Local pressure effects:
  - Headache
  - Double vision (cranial nerve III, IV, VI involvement)
- Symptoms of hypopituitarism:
  - Symptoms of hypothyroidism (➔ p.588)
  - ↓ FSH, LH: ↓ libido, men: erectile dysfunction, women: ↓ menses.
  - ↓ ACTH: tiredness, depression, abdominal pain (➔ Addison's, p.596).
  - ↓ GH: dry wrinkly skin, reduced well-being.
- GH secreting tumour: enlarged hands, feet (shoe size), tongue (➔ p.592).
- Prolactinoma:
  - men: galactorrhoea, ↓ libido, erectile dysfunction,
  - women: galactorrhoea, ↓ libido, ↓ menses.
- ACTH secreting tumour: rarely causes pressure effects.

Focused examination

Assess local pressure effects

- Assess eye movements (cranial nerves III, IV, VI; ➔ p.541).
- Assess facial sensation (cranial nerve V_1).

Assess hormonal effects

- Signs of acromegaly.

Table 8.10 Differential diagnosis of bitemporal hemianopia

Chiasmal compression	From below	Pituitary adenoma
		Pituitary apoplexy
	From above	Craniopharyngioma
	Other	Meningioma
		ICA aneurysm
Non-chiasmal causes	Tilted optic discs	
	Nasal retinitis pigmentosa (rare)	

Investigation and management

- MRI pituitary fossa.
- Hormonal level measurement: prolactin, IGF-1, ACTH, cortisol, TFT, LH/FSH, testosterone (males), short Synacthen® test, glucose tolerance test (acromegaly), water deprivation test (diabetes insipidus).
- Start hormonal replacement as needed.
- Surgery: trans-sphenoidal, transfrontal (if suprasellar extension).
- Radiotherapy for residual or recurrent adenomas.
- Prolactinoma: dopamine agonist is 1st line (bromocriptine, cabergoline).

Visual field defect 2: homonymous hemianopia

Another commonly encountered visual field defect is a homonymous hemianopia. As the majority are due to stroke, a focused history and examination is aimed at cardiovascular risk factors, additional neurological findings and secondary prevention – see stroke and TIA management and secondary prevention ➔ p.323.

> **Scenario**
>
> Mr Jonathan Miles, aged 63 years, has a 2-day history of visual problems affecting the right side of his vision.
>
> Please take a focused history and examination. Please address any questions or concerns raised by the patient.

General observation and initial questions
As for bitemporal hemianopia (➔ p.568).

Initial examination
Examine visual acuity and visual fields (➔ p.533 and 538)
- Map out edge of field defect comparing it with the vertical midline.
- Note if the visual field defect shows macular sparing (➔ Figure 8.8):
  - The 'macular' visual cortex receives its blood supply from terminal branches of the posterior and middle cerebral arteries.
  - The posterior cerebral artery supplies the remaining visual cortex.
  - Hence in posterior cerebral artery obstruction the middle cerebral artery 'spares' the ipsilateral macular visual cortex.
  - The presence of macular sparing is highly suggestive of an occipital lobe lesion. However not all occipital lobe lesions exhibit macular sparing.

Focused history and examination
The candidate should establish features specifically related to a stroke or TIA (➔ Stroke, p.323, and ➔ Transient ischaemic attack, p.462) e.g. history of weakness or dysphasia, risk factors and any previous management. A brief motor and sensory assessment, functional status and determination of underlying aetiology (e.g. pulse for AF, auscultation for carotid bruits) should be conducted. The history obtained should direct the examination for any further suspected neurological deficit (Table 8.11).

Investigation and management
(➔ Stroke, p.323.)
   A CT or an MRI brain scan is the key diagnostic test. The presence of additional neurological findings may help to localize the lesion. Macular sparing, if present suggests an occipital lesion.

Table 8.11 Differential diagnosis of homonymous hemianopia

Infarction	Disease in artery	Atheroma, vasculitis, thrombus
	Embolic disease	Cardiac origin:
		Atrial fibrillation, mural thrombus
		Valve disease
		Vascular origin:
		Carotid stenosis (ant. circulation)
		Vertebral disease (post. circulation)
Haemorrhage	Disease in artery	
Mass lesion	Tumour	
Demyelination	MS	
Other	Migraine, trauma	

Patient concerns

Can I still drive?

You must advise the patient to contact the DVLA. The DVLA will assess the ability to drive, but until that is done the patient must *not* drive. In a homonymous visual field defect, the areas of visual loss in the 2 eyes overlap. Therefore, even with both eyes open, a debarring field defect may remain.

Will my vision get better?

In some cases vision does improve, for example after removal of a lesion compressing the optic chiasm or a meningioma in the occipital cortex. Improvement following stroke is usually limited.

Viva questions

How would you investigate the cause of this patient's visual field defect?

Neuroimaging (of the pituitary region or optic radiations/occipital cortex) and cardiovascular examination/investigations as appropriate.

Double vision: third nerve palsy

> ## Scenario
>
> Mrs Margaret Nwosu, aged 68 years, has a 2-week history of double vision and drooping of the left eyelid.
>
> Please assess the patient's problems and address any questions or concerns raised by the patient.

The history given is highly suggestive of a left third nerve palsy. Diagnosing a third nerve palsy is not difficult. It has a classic appearance of a 'down and out' eye and ptosis. The skill comes in determining the cause of the condition, some of which are potentially fatal.

General observation

On general observation specifically look for signs of:
- Ipsilateral dilated pupil (compressive third nerve lesion)
- Contralateral hemiparesis (Weber's syndrome)
- Nystagmus, intention tremor, ataxic dysarthria (MS).

General initial questions

Clarify the presenting complaint. Specifically ask whether the onset of symptoms was:
- Sudden (minutes; vascular or trauma)
- Rapid (days; demyelinating)
- Gradual (weeks; compressive).

Initial examination

Examine eye movements and lids (➋ Table 8.12, p.541 and 565)
- Third nerve palsies have a classic 'down and out' appearance. Sometimes in the presence of a fourth nerve lesion the eye may just be 'out' (abducted) as the only functioning nerve is the sixth.
- Medial and superior gaze are most markedly affected.

Exclude a compressive cause (see also ➋ Focused examination, p.573)
Examine the pupils looking for a dilated pupil (➋ p.543). Compressive lesions affect both the superficial pupillary fibres and the deep motor fibres of the nerve, whereas ischaemic lesions tend to only affect the motor fibres.

Focused history

A focused history specifically checking for the following details:
- Cardiovascular risk status: BP, diabetes, cholesterol, smoking.
- History of headache or pain. Pain is classically associated with compressive lesions but may also occur in vasculitic lesions.
- GCA symptoms if ≥50 years old.
- Any other neurological features: weakness, numbness, reduced vision.

Focused examination

Exclude complex lesion (brainstem or compressive pathology)

It is vital to look for associated neurology, especially:

- Fourth nerve involvement: ask the patient to look down and away from the side of the lesion. The affected eye fails to adduct, although it can be seen to intort (rotate inwards) if the fourth nerve is intact. This intorsion can be difficult to see.
- Second nerve involvement: test visual acuity, test for an afferent pupillary defect and look at ipsilateral optic disc (for atrophy) to exclude involvement of the optic nerve.
- Briefly assess power in the arms and legs: Weber's syndrome – ipsilateral third and contralateral hemiparesis (basal midbrain lesion). Benedict's syndrome – ipsilateral third and contralateral ataxia (paramedian midbrain lesion).

Table 8.12 Differential diagnosis of an ocular deviation with ptosis

IIIrd nerve palsy	Solitary, pupil sparing third	Microvascular infarction
	Compressive lesion	Posterior communicating artery aneurysm
		Internal carotid artery aneurysm
		Meningioma, parasellar tumour
	Brainstem infarction	Weber's, Benedict's syndrome
	Brainstem demyelination	MS
	Other	GCA, trauma, congenital
Other	Myasthenia / orbital mass / inflammation / cellulitis / fracture	

Investigation and management

The key decision is whether the third nerve palsy is a compressive and/ or complex lesion. Management of these lesions is much more aggressive than the management of solitary microvascular infarctions. Missing a compressive lesion can lead to the death of a patient (e.g. aneurysm rupture).

Compressive/complex lesion

- Urgent MRI/MRA/CT angiogram (aneurysm) or MRI (brainstem lesion).
- If aneurysm found – urgent neurosurgical referral.
- Management depends on lesion found (meningioma, brainstem infarct).

Solitary pupil sparing third (microvascular origin)

- If history of cardiovascular risk factors:
  - Cardiovascular work up: BP, glucose, lipids, (ESR, CRP if ≥50 years).
  - Optimize cardiovascular risk factors.
  - Review in 3 months, by which stage many patients will have recovered. If no improvement, investigate further with MRI.

- If no history of cardiovascular risk factors: manage as above but perform MRI at initial presentation to exclude compressive cause due to the absence of causative risk factors.

❶ Top Tips

- As a general rule in cranial nerve palsies always check the nerve above and below (in palsy of III check II and IV, in palsy of VI check V and VII).
- Pupillary involvement in a third nerve palsy strongly suggests a compressive lesion, whilst a normal pupil reaction is usually (but not exclusively) associated with microvascular disease.

Viva questions

How would you manage a patient with a third nerve lesion with pupillary involvement due to a posterior communicating artery aneurysm?

Urgent referral to neurosurgery with a view to intervention (endovascular coiling, surgical clipping).

What complications can arise from a posterior communicating artery aneurysm?

- Rupture of the aneurysm leading to a SAH, the mortality from which can be as high as 50%. Of those who survive, a significant proportion suffer major neurological morbidity.
- Local pressure effects on the third nerve.

Anisocoria: Horner's syndrome

Unless specifically sought, Horner's syndrome is a condition that is easy to miss. The anisocoria is subtle and more difficult to appreciate in a brightly lit room. The ptosis is only 1–2 mm. Careful observation is vital.

> **Scenario**
>
> Mrs Jenny Pearson – age 58 years.
>
> This lady has noticed that one pupil is smaller than the other. She notices this when doing her makeup.
>
> Please assess the patient's problems and address any questions or concerns raised by the patient.

General observation

On general observation specifically look for signs of:
- Ocular deviation, ptosis (third nerve palsy).
- Cranial nerve lesion, hemiparesis, wasting of the small muscles of the hands, cervical lymphadenopathy, neck scars (Horner's).
- High stepping gait (tabes dorsalis – Argyll Robertson pupils).
- Nystagmus, intention tremor, ataxic dysarthria (MS).

General initial questions

Clarify the presenting complaint. Specifically ask when the inequality in pupil size was first noticed. Old photos can help clarify the time of onset.

Initial examination

Examine the pupils (➔ p.543)
- Affected pupil is smaller (more noticeable in dim illumination) and reacts to light and accommodation. Mild ptosis (1–2mm).
- Ipsilateral iris hypochromia suggests congenital or longstanding lesion.

Examination of eye movements (➔ p.541)
- Contralateral lid retraction (thyroid eye disease) can be mistaken for ipsilateral ptosis.

Focused history

A focused history should specifically address:
- Any other neurological symptoms to suggest involvement of other cranial/peripheral nerves. This can help locate the site of pathology.
  - Ipsilateral facial anhydrosis localizes the lesion to proximal to the bifurcation of the carotid artery i.e. lesion of 1st- or 2nd-order neuron (see below).
- History of malignancy, especially:
  - Lung (smoking, cough, weight loss)
  - Thyroid
  - Lymphoma.
- Pain: headache, neck pain, arm pain.
- Neck trauma or surgery (e.g. central line insertion).

Focused examination

Determine the location of pathology

Sympathetic innervation to the eye consists of a 3-neuron arc. The 1st-order neuron originates in the ipsilateral hypothalamus and descends through the brainstem to the cervical cord at the level of T1/T2. The 2nd-order (pre-ganglionic) neuron projects from the spinal cord to the superior cervical ganglion. The 3rd-order (post-ganglionic) neuron travels via the internal carotid artery to the orbit and innervates the dilator muscle of the iris.

❶ Top Tips

- As the course of the sympathetic pathway from the hypothalamus to the eye is very long, any associated signs will enable more focused imaging studies to be chosen.

- 1st-order neuron examination: hemiparesis, cranial nerve palsies, wasting of the small muscles of the hands (syringomyelia).
- 2nd-order neuron examination: wasting of the small muscles of the hands (Pancoast's), cervical scars, nodes or masses, carotid bruit (common carotid dissection).
- 3rd-order neuron examination:
  - Carotid bruit (internal carotid dissection).
  - Eye movement examination (❷ p.541), visual acuity (❷ p.533), fundoscopy (optic atrophy and diabetic retinopathy).
  - (Cavernous sinus pathology [thrombosis, tumour] can cause lesions of cranial nerves III, IV, V_1 & V_2, and VI – ❷ p.364.)

Investigation and management

Pupil investigations

- Confirm diagnosis of Horner's syndrome:
  - Cocaine (4%): no/poor dilation in affected eye at 60min.
  - Apraclonidine (0.5%): miosis of normal pupil and relative mydriasis (dilatation) of affected pupil due to denervation hypersensitivity.
- Determine site of lesion:
  - Hydroxyamphetamine (1%) stimulates the release of stored noradrenaline from the post-ganglionic neuron. If this is intact the pupil will dilate, otherwise the affected pupil will remain miosed.
  - 1st/2nd-order lesion: normal dilation of affected eye.
  - 3rd-order lesion: no/poor dilation of affected eye.

Systemic investigations

- 1st-order neuron: MRI brain/spine.
- 2nd-order neuron: CXR, CT thorax, lymph node biopsy, MRI/MRA of head/neck, carotid Doppler.
- 3rd-order neuron: MRI/MRA of head/neck, carotid doppler, MRI cavernous sinus/orbits.

Management

- Treat underlying cause.
- Ptosis can be surgically corrected if patient cosmetically concerned.

Patient concerns

The patient may ask what is causing their unequal pupils. The candidate should explain that the nerve controlling the pupil size and eyelid position travels a long way from the brain to the eye. The next step is to determine what is causing this to happen. If a partial ptosis of the lid remains then a small operation can lift the eyelid. The pupil size difference does not require treatment.

Viva questions

What are the causes of Horner's syndrome? (Table 8.13)

Table 8.13 Differential diagnosis of Horner's syndrome

1st-order neuron	Brainstem	Stroke, tumour, demyelination
	Spinal cord	Syringomyelia, tumour, trauma
2nd-order neuron	Lung apex	Pancoast's tumour
	Neck	Tumour in cervical nodes
		Surgery, trauma
		Common carotid dissection
3rd-order neuron	Internal carotid artery	Dissection
	Cavernous sinus	Thrombus, tumour
	Orbit	Tumour
Congenital		

Endocrinology: **Diabetes mellitus and diabetic foot**

Diabetes results in a combination of vascular and neuropathic insults to the feet, thus resulting in increased susceptibility to ulceration and infection. The diabetic foot is a common and often chronic problem, which is therefore a relatively frequent Station 5 scenario.

> ### Scenario
>
> Mr. Matthew Simpson aged 44 years.
>
> This gentleman has cellulitis around a recurrent ulcer on the plantar aspect of his right foot. He was diagnosed with diabetes 23 years ago and is on Lantus® 20 units OD and NovaRapid® TDS. His last HBA1c was 10.7%. Please see and advise.

A candidate would be expected to quickly examine the feet and take a history focused on the diabetic foot, before undertaking a more general diabetic review.

Initial history and examination

During the initial history ask about:
- Systemic symptoms e.g. fever.
- Previous ulcers, trauma or infection.
- Sensation in the feet (walking on cotton wool) and in the ulcer, painless ulcers are classically neuropathic. NB The candidate should not assess the sensation in the ulcer during their PACES exam.
- Any painful 'electric shock' symptoms (painful neuropathy).
- Footwear.
- If the feet are checked regularly.
- Any issues caused by the foot ulcer on work and quality of life.

Simultaneously examine the feet:
- Ask to remove any dressings!
- Inspect for any callus, deformity and ulceration (including between the toes).
- Assess the nails observing for source of infection.
- Palpate the dorsalis pedis and posterior tibial pulses – if absent check popliteal and femoral pulses.
- Assess temperature by running the back of your hand across the feet.
- Observe for any hair loss in the legs and feet.

When examining the ulcer:
- Inspect the base and classify it as granular, fibrotic or necrotic.
- Bone at the base of the ulcer suggests osteomyelitis; areas of necrosis imply peripheral vascular disease (PVD).
- Note any oedema.
- Assess colour (erythema) and odour (infection).
- Sensory modalities should also be assessed (distally working proximally) ➔ Sensory exam p.312. Check all modalities, including light touch, vibration, pinprick and proprioception.
- Examine footwear and ensure appropriate.

History

A general diabetic review should now be undertaken and should include:

- Duration of diabetes and any specific concerns.
- Occupation, hobbies and the impact of diabetes on these.
- Infections: in particular oral or genital candidiasis.
- Medications and any side effects, including:
  - Metformin: indigestion, headache and diarrhoea.
  - Pioglitazone: oedema.
  - Gliclazide: hypoglycaemia.
- Patient's own understanding regarding their BP, cholesterol, HbA1c.
- Hypoglycaemic episodes, including their frequency, precipitating events and if any required assistance.
- The patient's blood sugar readings and how they might be improved – long-acting insulin influences fasting glucose and short-acting insulin determines the glucose level before the next meal.
- Symptoms of complications: angina, stroke, claudication, neuropathic symptoms, visual disturbance and erectile dysfunction.
- Retinal screening (annually), and previous microalbuminuria/proteinuria.
- Driving and if the DVLA and their insurers are aware of their diabetes. Ask if they always check their blood sugars before driving and have glucose available in the car at all times.
- Smoking – encourage to stop!

❶ Top Tips

- When examining the diabetic foot, be vigilant for Charcot arthropathy.
  In chronic Charcot arthropathy the plantar medial arch may often become depressed, producing a characteristic widening of the mid-foot, and the feet may be abducted at the ankles. These deformities cause new pressure points that lead to further ulcerations.
- In women with diabetes of childbearing age always ask about any plans for pregnancy and take the opportunity to stress the need for optimal control (HbA1c <7) for 3 months pre-conception, pre-pregnancy folic acid and the need to stop ACE inhibitors and statins. (ACE inhibitors cause cardiovascular defects and nervous system malformations; the evidence against statins is less clear, but there is a potential association with neurological and skeletal malformations.)

Examination

- Assess BP.
- Inspect insulin injection sites for lipohypertrophy.

Closing statement

- Ask to dip the urine for protein and glucose.
- Offer to perform fundoscopy.

Differential diagnosis

The main differential here is ischaemic vs. purely neuropathic ulcer:

- Plantar location makes a neuropathic ulcer more likely.
- Absent foot pulses is suggestive of an ischaemic ulcer.
- Both ischaemic and neuropathic factors may be contributory.

Investigations

- Swab ulcer including deep swabs.
- FBC, U&E, CRP, fasting lipids, TFT, HbA1c, urine ACR.
- Doppler to assess vascular supply.
- Plain foot x-ray may reveal osteomyelitis.
- MRI is often needed to exclude osteomyelitis.
- Consider bone biopsy if ongoing infection.

Treatment

- Pressure relief 'offloading' – this orthotic input is essential particularly for plantar ulcers. This may necessitate the use of a below knee plaster of Paris.
- Appropriate treatment for PVD e.g. revascularization.
- Broad-spectrum antibiotics covering staphs, streps and anaerobes if any suggestion of infection. Antibiotic therapy should be continued for 3 months if bone visible or x-ray changes suggestive of osteomyelitis. Adjust microbial therapy according to blood and deep culture sensitivities.
- Surgical review if evidence of deep tissue infection.
- Encourage optimal glycaemic control.

Patient concerns

Patients may be concerned about the possibility of amputation. It is important to highlight, that through a combination of good foot and ulcer care, tight glycaemic control and antibiotic treatment, amputation may be avoided. It is also important to be sensitive about any other issues that are highlighted during the consultation e.g. erectile dysfunction, driving concerns etc.

Viva questions

What are the symptoms of diabetes?
- Thirst, polyuria, polydipsia
- Weight loss
- Blurred vision
- Recurrent infections particularly urinary tract and skin, and oral and genital candidiasis.

What conditions can cause neuropathic ulcers?
- Diabetes
- Leprosy
- Tabes dorsalis
- Amyloidosis
- Alcoholic neuropathy
- Hereditary neuropathies (e.g. Charcot–Marie–Tooth)
- Drugs
- Deficiencies e.g. B12, thiamine.

How would you manage an obese patient with Type 2 DM?
- Multi-disciplinary team support: dietician input, exercise advice.
- Drugs:
  - Metformin
  - Orlistat (reduces the absorption of dietary fat).

- Exenatide (Byetta®) or Liragultidue (Victoza®) are incretin (GLP-1) mimetics which stimulate insulin secretion, slow emptying of the stomach and inhibit production of glucose by the liver. They also suppress appetite and aid weight loss.
- Surgery: gastric band, gastric bypass.

What are the causes of secondary diabetes?

- Steroid use
- Polycystic ovarian syndrome
- Hyperthyroidism
- Chronic pancreatitis
- Cystic fibrosis
- Haemochromatosis
- Acromegaly
- Phaeochromocytoma
- Cushing's syndrome
- Glucagonoma.

What are the symptoms of autonomic neuropathy?

- Dysregulated sweating including gustatory
- Constipation with bacterial overgrowth
- Gastroparesis with vomiting
- Diarrhoea
- Postural hypotension
- Bladder and erectile dysfunction
- Cardiac dysrhythmias.

What different types of neuropathy are seen in diabetes?

- Progressive sensory
- Mononeuritis e.g. cranial nerves
- Pressure palsies e.g. carpal tunnel syndrome
- Amyotrophic
- Autonomic.

📖 Further reading

Lavin N. *Manual of Endocrinology and Metabolism*, 4th edn, pp.589–615. Philadelphia, PA: Lippincott Williams & Wilkins, 2009.

McDermott M. *Endocrine Secrets*, 5th edn, pp.9–34. Amsterdam: Elsevier, 2009.

Sam AH, Meeran K. *Endocrinology and Diabetes (Lecture Notes)*, pp.215–34. Chichester: Wiley-Blackwell.

🔊 Useful websites

Diabetic Driving Advice: http://www.diabetes.org.uk/Guidetodiabetes/Living_with_diabetes/Driving/Informing_the_DVLA/

Diabetic foot examination techniques: http://http://www.ccjm.org/content/69/4/342.full.pdf

Diabetes and sexual function: http://www.diabetes.org.uk/Professionals/Education_and_skills/Sexual-dysfunction/

Thyroid: hyperthyroidism (Graves' disease)

Graves' disease is an autoimmune disorder caused by the development of thyroid-stimulating hormone receptor antibodies. It is responsible for 65–70% of cases of hyperthyroidism and is a very common Station 5 scenario.

> ### Scenario
>
> Mrs Francesca Dean.
>
> This 31-year-old lady has been increasingly anxious of late. She has also been complaining of heat intolerance and increasing weight loss. She has also noticed a change in the appearance of her eyes. Please see and advise.

A candidate would be expected to quickly identify, from the eye signs on initial inspection and the information in the scenario, that this case is thyrotoxicosis secondary to Graves' disease.

Initial history and examination

- From the end of the bed observe for obvious goitre or exophthalmos.
- Look for palmar erythema.
- Feel the patient's palms, with the backs of your own hands, for heat and sweating.
- Inspect the hands for thyroid acropachy (clubbing, digital swelling accompanied by periosteal reaction).
- Ask the patient to hold their arms outstretched and assess for tremor.
- Feel the pulse for 15 seconds and note the rate and rhythm (be vigilant for AF).

Whilst undertaking this part of the examination, ask the patient about:
- Duration of symptoms and effect on work and quality of life.
- Previous episodes and any treatment received.
- Easy irritability, nervousness and insomnia.
- Degree of the weight loss and whether there was increased appetite.
- Dislike for hot weather, heat intolerance, excessive sweating.
- Palpitations: frequency, rate and rhythm.
- Any neck pain or tenderness (if present suggests thyroiditis).
- Any symptoms in relation to the patient's eyes e.g. diplopia, pain, watery eyes, altered red colour perception (e.g. red roses appear bleached out/or traffic lights less distinct; rare, but if present may signify optic nerve compression).
- Ask about medication – specifically amiodarone and lithium.
- In women of childbearing age enquire whether they have had any recent pregnancies, or whether they have any pregnancy plans.

Specific history for Graves' disease

Important to ask about:
- Personal and family history of thyroid and other autoimmune diseases.
- Responsibilities for caring for young children or planning pregnancy (this will influence suitability for radioiodine treatment).

- Urinary incontinence. As radioiodine is excreted in urine, a temporary catheter may be indicated in those with urinary incontinence.
- Smoking (exacerbates thyroid eye disease).

Specific examination related to Graves' disease

Eyes

The ocular manifestations of Graves' disease and their management are described in more detail on p.564.

- Proptosis (forward displacement) look from above and the side. Exophthalmos is the specific term used for proptosis in the context of Graves' disease.
- Lid retraction (sclera visible above the upper limbus of the cornea).
- Soft tissue signs of active eye disease – red eyes (scleral injection), chemosis (conjunctival swelling), periorbital oedema.
- Lid lag (ask the patient to follow your finger and then move it along the arc of a circle from a point above their head to a point below the nose: the movement of the lid lags behind that of the globe).
- Extraocular movements: (➲ p.541) Observe for any ophthalmoplegia and ask the patient to report any diplopia.
- Ask to assess visual acuity.

❶ Top Tips

- The 4 manifestations of Graves' eye disease are swelling/soft tissue signs, proptosis, diplopia and optic nerve compression, which can all occur on their own, or in any combination.
- Thyroid eye disease is usually asymmetric and does not necessarily correlate with thyroid status.

Neck

- Carefully inspect the neck whilst the patient swallows a sip of water – only a goitre or a thyroglossal cyst will rise on swallowing.
- Inspect the neck for a thyroidectomy scar, which typically forms a ring around the base of the neck (often hidden in a neck crease or covered by a high necklace).
- Dilated veins over the upper part of the chest wall may suggest retrosternal expansion of the goitre and subsequent thoracic inlet obstruction.
- Palpate from behind with the patient's neck slightly flexed. Rest the fingers of both your hands over the gland and feel for the lobes and the isthmus and estimate its size. Note the normal thyroid should be impalpable. If palpable try to feel for the lower border of the thyroid – absence of this may signify retrosternal extension.
- Assess for any lymphadenopathy.
- Percuss the chest – to assess for retrosternal goitre.
- Auscultate the thyroid (a bruit is indicative of hyperthyroidism most likely Graves' disease).

To complete the examination check for:
- Proximal myopathy (ask the patient to stand with their arms folded).
- Pre-tibial myxoedema.

- Finally assess the ankle reflexes (slow relaxing in hypothyroidism; brisk in hyperthyroidism).

Differential diagnosis

The two most common diagnoses will be Graves disease (clues – eye signs and history of autoimmune disease) and toxic multinodular goitre (including toxic single nodule).

- Neck pain or recent childbirth may suggest thyroiditis.
- Drug induced – enquire about iodine/radiographic contrast medium, amiodarone, lithium, interferon therapy.
- Gestational thyrotoxicosis.
- Rare causes of thyrotoxicosis include factitious thyroxine usage, struma ovarii (ovarian tumour) and immune recovery during treatment of leukaemia or HIV. These treatments can cause transient antibodies in individuals predisposed to Graves' disease.

Investigations

- TSH, T_3, T_4
- Thyroid auto-antibodies (and anti-TSH receptor antibodies if available)
- It may be necessary to perform a thyroid uptake scan in individuals with thyrotoxicosis and a small goitre, but no eye signs and negative antibodies (→ p.587 and Table 8.14).

Treatment

Correcting hyperthyroidism

- Drugs:
  - Carbimazole and propylthiouracil most commonly prescribed in the UK.
  - Given by 'titration' or 'block and replace'. Typically in the titration regime, an initial dose of carbimazole 30–40mg is tapered down over 4–8 weeks to a maintenance dose of 5–10mg. In the block and replace regime typically 40mg of carbimazole is used initially and 100mg of levothyroxine added when the free T_4 is in the normal range (usually after 4 weeks) to prevent hypothyroidism.
  - Treatment course for both regimes is typically 18 months.
  - Warn about rash (1:10) and risk of agranulocytosis (1:200; should mouth ulcers develop, stop carbimazole immediately and check neutrophil count).
  - 50% relapse rate in Graves' disease after completion of drug course.
- Radioiodine:
  - Commonest treatment in the USA.
  - >1 dose may be required.
  - Likely to result in long-term hypothyroidism.
  - May exacerbate eye disease.
- Surgery:
  - Effective.
  - May result in hoarse voice (following damage to laryngeal nerves).
  - Results in long-term hypothyroidism.
  - May cause damage to parathyroid glands.

Treatment of symptoms

Non-selective beta-blockers e.g. proponalol (NB caution in asthma/COPD).

Treatment of Graves' ophthalmopathy
➲ Viva questions below.

Patient concerns
Few patients will be concerned about the weight loss! Firm reassurance is needed that many of the psychological side effects (anxiety, irritability) will improve on treatment. Women with Graves' eye disease will be particularly distressed by the cosmetic changes and this needs sensitive management.

Viva questions
What are the causes of hyperthyroidism?
- Graves disease.
- Toxic multinodular goitre (including toxic single nodule).
- Thyroiditis (subacute, post-partum or 'silent' autoimmune thyroiditis).
- Ectopic thyroid tissue.
- Over replacement with levothyroxine.

How is proptosis quantified?
Quantified using a Hertel's exophthalmometer, readings >20mm are suggestive of proptosis.

How would you manage a patient with Graves' ophthalmopathy?
- Even clinically mild Graves' ophthalmopathy can be cosmetically very distressing for patients and needs to be handled pro-actively and sensitively. All patients should be advised to stop smoking. Lubricating eye drops and raising the head of the bed may also help. It is essential that the patient is kept euthyroid; both raised TSH and raised thyroid hormone levels are associated with a worse clinical outcome in Graves' ophthalmopathy.
- Active eye disease is indicated by soft tissue signs (scleral injection, chemosis and periorbital oedema), pain behind the eyes and changing appearance, and indicate that the patient may respond to immunosuppression (e.g. steroids).
- Patients with diplopia or significant proptosis need ophthalmological assessment and are best managed in a joint clinic. Exposure keratitis may be relieved by lateral tarsorrhaphy (partial closure by suturing the lateral aspect of the upper and lower eyelids). Diplopia may be relieved by prisms or surgery to the extra-ocular muscles. Worsening ophthalmopathy may be an indication for IV steroids, orbital decompression and/or orbital irradiation.
- Any change in visual acuity or colour vision needs immediate ophthalmological input and should be treated with high dose intravenous corticosteroids, immunosuppression, orbital irradiation, and occasionally orbital decompression.

What do you know about the use of radioiodine in patients with Graves' eye disease?
Radioiodine may exacerbate thyroid eye disease and is therefore contraindicated in patients with active or severe ophthalmopathy. Radioiodine may however be used in patients with mild dysthyroid eye disease with steroid cover following treatment. As radioiodine treatment can occasionally precipitate ophthalmopathy in the absence of previous thyroid eye disease,

patients should be appropriately consented when considering radioiodine treatment.

📖 **Further reading**

Daniels GH, Dayan CM. *Fast Facts: Thyroid Disorders*, pp.26–68. London: Health Press Ltd, 2006.
Toft A. *Understanding Thyroid Disorders*, pp.8–14. Poole: Family Doctor Publications Ltd, 2008.

🖰 **Useful websites**

Overview on Graves: http://www.thyroid.org/patients/brochures/Graves_brochure.pdf
Information on thyroid eye disease: http://www.tedct.co.uk

Thyroid: hyperthyroidism (toxic multinodular goitre)

Toxic multinodular goitre is the second most common cause of hyperthyroidism after Graves' disease. It is particularly common in elderly patients. Patients may present with symptoms of thyrotoxicosis or because they have noticed the goitre.

> **Scenario**
>
> Mrs Lauren Hepworth aged 75.
>
> This lady has noticed a swelling in her neck, it is not painful, but is causing her some concern. She has also felt increasingly anxious of late and has had some palpitations.

From the information in the scenario and a quick general inspection it should be obvious to the candidate, that the diagnosis is most likely thyrotoxicosis secondary to toxic multinodular goitre.

Initial history and examination

The initial history to be taken will be the same as for Graves' disease (→ p.582).

Specific history for toxic multinodular goitre

Important to address obstructive symptoms:

- Dysphagia or stridor (may require surgical intervention or if severe, a surgical emergency).
- Hoarse voice – as a result of compression or malignant infiltration of the recurrent laryngeal nerve.
- Pain with rapid enlargement suggests bleeding into nodule.

Examination

Proceed as for Graves' disease (→ p.583). It should be noted however:

- There should be no eye signs other than lid lag.
- The thyroid gland may be causing proportionally more symptoms than its apparent size due to significant retrosternal extension of the goitre.
- Be particularly vigilant for any tracheal deviation, SVC obstruction, and for AF.

Differential diagnosis: hyperthyroidism

→ p.584.

Investigations

- TSH, T_3, T_4 – note in toxic multinodular goitre subclinical hyperthyroidism (suppressed TSH normal T_3 and T_4) is relatively common.
- Thyroid auto-antibodies (and, if available, anti-TSH receptor antibodies) should be negative.
- Thyroid ultrasound is helpful for detecting impalpable nodules.
- CT thorax and neck are useful for large goitres to assess for compression.
- Nuclear scintigraphy (thyroid uptake scans) to determine if nodules are functioning (Table 8.14). Non-functioning nodules are more likely to be malignant.
- Fine-needle aspiration (increasingly ultrasound-guided).
- Pulmonary function tests: flow volume loop assess for compression of large airways (→ p.30).

Table 8.14 Interpreting thyroid uptake scans

High uptake	Low uptake
Graves' disease (diffuse uptake)	Thyroiditis
Toxic multinodular goitre (focal uptake)	Iodine/amiodarone-induced hyperthyroidism
Toxic adenoma (focal uptake)	Factitious: people taking levothyroxine

Treatment

- Radioactive iodine: may cause transient enlargement before reduction in goitre.
- Surgery: particularly if compressive symptoms.
- Anti-thyroid drugs are not a viable long-term option for toxic multinodular goitre as thyrotoxicosis recurs when treatment stops.
- If the TSH is normal and patient is unsuitable for radioactive iodine or surgery, then small doses of levothyroxine can be given to suppress TSH levels and reduce the chance of the goitre enlarging. However this is not a very effective treatment.

Patient concerns

As for Graves' disease (bar the eye changes). If there is a significant goitre patients may be concerned about cosmetic appearances.

Viva questions

What are the indications for treatment in non-toxic multinodular goitre?

- Compression and obstruction – trachea, oesophagus, venous outflow
- Cosmetic
- Marked intra-thoracic extension.

Explain the difference between hot and cold nodules?

A cold nodule has diminished uptake when compared to surrounding thyroid tissue, whereas a hot nodule has increased uptake with suppressed uptake in thyroid tissue. Hot nodules are never malignant; a small proportion (5 – 10%) of cold nodules are.

What is the differential diagnosis of a solitary thyroid nodule?

- Thyroid cyst
- Thyroid adenoma
- Thyroid carcinoma
- Metastatic cancer
- Lymphoma
- Sarcoma
- Parathyroid cyst.

📖 Further reading

Lavin N. *Manual of Endocrinology and Metabolism*, 4th edn, pp.434–47, Philadelphia, PA: Lippincott Williams & Wilkins, 2009.

🔗 Useful website

Overview of toxic multinodular goitre: http://emedicine.medscape.com/article/120497-overview

Thyroid disorders: hypothyroidism

Hypothyroidism is common and affects between 5–10% of the UK population. It presents with a variety of non-specific symptoms and is diagnosed by thyroid function tests. It is an uncommon PACES scenario.

> **Scenario**
>
> Mrs Caroline Martin aged 78.
>
> This lady has been increasingly forgetful and tired of late. She has also been gaining weight. Please see and advise.

Whilst the symptoms stated are very non-specific, the weight gain should suggest an underactive thyroid problem.

Initial history and examination

Initial inspection may reveal coarse facial features, peri-orbital oedema and hair loss as further evidence to support hypothyroidism.

Specific history for hypothyroidism

Important to ask about:

- Dry skin and hair loss
- Cold intolerance
- Constipation
- Peripheral oedema
- Tingling and paraesthesia in the hands (carpal tunnel syndrome)
- Neck swelling (if present ask about compressive symptoms – ➔ p.586)

- If appropriate, menstrual disturbances (typically menorrhagia)
- Snoring and early morning headache (hypothyroidism is associated with obstructive sleep apnoea)
- Medication – in particular amiodarone
- Personal and family history of thyroid disease and other autoimmune diseases (e.g. diabetes mellitus, pernicious anaemia)
- Abdominal pain, skin pigment changes (see Top Tips box).

Examination

The signs of hypothyroidism are frequently subtle and are generally found only with careful inspection (Table 8.15).

Hands

Bradycardia.

Head and neck

- Coarse, brittle hair – with evidence of hair loss
- Coarse facial features
- Periorbital oedema
- Jaundice
- Macroglossia
- Goitre (➲ Examining the thyroid – specific examination related to Graves' disease p.583).

Table 8.15 Overview of symptoms and signs in hypo/hyperthyroidism

Sign/symptom	Hypothyroidism	Hyperthyroidism
Weight	Gained	Reduced
Temperature preference	Cold intolerance	Heat intolerance
Palpitations	Bradycardia	Tachycardia, AF
Mood and cognition	Depressed	Anxious
	Poor memory	Irritable
	Poor concentration	
Bowel movements	Constipation	Diarrhoea
Skin and hair	Dry, pale skin	Sweating
	Dry, coarse hair	Hair loss
	Hair loss	
	Loss of lateral eyebrows	
Muscles and movements	General aches	Tremor
	Muscle stiffness	Proximal muscle weakness
	Slow relaxation of muscles	
Menstruation	Heavy periods	Lighter periods

Chest and abdomen

Percuss for:
- Pleural effusion
- Abdominal distension, ascites (uncommon).

Lower limbs
- Non-pitting oedema (myxoedema)
- Pitting oedema of lower extremities
- Hyporeflexia with delayed relaxation (a sign of hypothyroidism or myotonia).

Examination of thyroid status

The new station 5 format makes it unlikely that a sole examination of thyroid status will be required. Thyroid status can be readily determined using part of the examination techniques described in this chapter. To quickly examine thyroid status:

- Assess the patient's demeanour – are they anxious (hyper) or withdrawn and apathetic (hypo).
- Feel the patient's palms, with the backs of your own hands, for heat and sweating (hyper).
- Ask the patient to hold their arms outstretched and assess for tremor.
- Feel the pulse for 15 seconds and note the rate and rhythm (be vigilant for AF). AF or tachycardia (hyper) or bradycardia (hypo).
- Assess for lid lag (hyper).
- Auscultate for the presence of thyroid bruit, which indicates increased vascularity, suggesting hyperthyroidism secondary to Graves' disease. Auscultation should be carried out over the goitre. (A goitre itself does not signify hyperthyroidism.)
- Assess for proximal myopathy – this occurs with both hypo- and hyperthyroidism, but resolves in each case with treatment.
- Finally assess the ankle jerks – slowly relaxing reflexes imply hypothyroidism.

❶ Top Tips

- A slick way of completing the thyroid status examination is to ask the patient to stand up with their arms folded (thereby assessing proximal myopathy) and then to kneel onto a chair to proceed to examine ankle jerks.
- This approach enables these 2 (often poorly performed!) examinations to be carried out in a succinct manner.

Differential diagnosis

The most common cause of hypothyroidism in the UK is auto-immune disease. Other causes include thyroiditis, drugs (e.g. amiodarone), iatrogenic (e.g. previous radioiodine), and thyroidectomy. As there is a wide list of non-specific symptoms there is a large differential diagnosis for hypothyroidism. Notable conditions include Addison's disease, depression and chronic fatigue syndrome.

❶ Top Tips

- Hypothyroidism and Addison's disease can coexist. Hypothyroidism has a relatively protective effect on Addison's disease. If thyroid hormone replacement is given alone, this can precipitate an adrenal crisis. It is therefore important to ask about some symptoms more consistent with Addison's disease such as abdominal pain and postural symptoms.
- Addison's disease can also cause an isolated raised TSH in the absence of thyroid disease (other thyroid hormones will be normal)

Investigations

- TSH and T_4.
- TPO antibodies.

Treatment

Levothyroxine replacement and adjust according to TSH. Caution in the elderly (➋ Viva questions, see below). Once maintained on a steady dose, annual blood tests are advisable (however no firm consensus exists).

Patient concerns: hypothyroidism

- Most patients will be concerned about weight gain and low mood. They should be given reassurance that these should resolve on treatment.
- Emphasize that lifelong treatment will be required.

Viva questions

What are the causes of hypothyroidism?

- Hashimoto's thyroiditis (autoimmune; most common).
- Following thyroid ablation, by surgery or radioiodine.
- Thyroiditis: post-transient hyperthyroid stage.
- Drugs: amiodarone, lithium, interferon, anti-thyroid drugs (!).

Tell me about hypothyroidism in pregnancy

Hypothyroidism, particularly in the first 12 weeks of pregnancy, has been shown to have detrimental effects on fetal neurodevelopment. It is also common for thyroid hormone requirements to rise substantially during pregnancy, with the range of dose increments being 25–50%. Women with pre-existing thyroid disease should have their TFT checked at least every trimester with a typical target range for TSH of 0.5–2.0mU/L. After delivery the patient can return to their pre-pregnancy dose, with immediate effect.

Tell me how you would initiate levothyroxine replacement therapy in an elderly patient with hypothyroidism

Elderly patients may have been hypothyroid for some time before diagnosis as many of the symptoms of hypothyroidism can be wrongly attributed to the aging process. Furthermore they may have coexisting IHD and it is therefore prudent to start with a low initial dose of levothyroxine e.g. 12.5–25 μg/OD and titrate up cautiously, by 25 μg every 2–4 weeks.

What is myxoedema coma?

A severe form of hypothyroidism resulting in altered mental status, hypothermia, bradycardia and hyponatraemia. Cardiomegaly, pericardial effusion, cardiogenic shock and ascites may also be present. It may be a consequence of long-term undiagnosed hypothyroidism or it may be precipitated by an insult, e.g. infection, silent MI, surgery or major tranquillizers.

📖 Further reading

Daniels GH, Dayan CM. *Fast Facts: Thyroid Disorders*, pp.26–68. London: Health Press Ltd, 2006.

Lavin N. *Manual of Endocrinology and Metabolism*, 4th edn, pp.589–695. Philadelphia, PA: Lippincott Williams & Wilkins, 2009.

McDermott M. *Endocrine Secrets*, 5th edn, pp.414–512. Amsterdam: Elsevier, 2009.

🖰 Useful websites

British Thyroid Foundation website: http://www.btf-thyroid.org

American Association of Clinical Endocrinologists guidelines: https://www.aace.com/pub/guidelines

Acromegaly

Acromegaly is an uncommon condition, resulting from excessive production and secretion of growth hormone, usually from a pituitary macroadenoma. It is frequently encountered in the PACES examination.

Scenario

Mr. Robin Dewar, age 48 years.

This gentleman with a past medical history of hypertension has recently become concerned about pain and tingling in his hands.

During their introduction to the patient, a candidate would be expected to quickly identify the underlying diagnosis of acromegaly, with subsequent carpal tunnel syndrome from the observational findings.

Initial history and examination

The history needs to focus on the nature and duration of symptoms, and the rate of progression. The initial history needs to cover:

- Duration of symptoms and effect on quality of life/work
- Which fingers are most affected
- If the symptoms are worse at night
- If there is any neck or shoulder pain.

Whilst obtaining these details, a good general inspection should identify enlargement of the facial features, the hands and the feet (➔ p.593).

History

- Ask if the patient and/or their relatives have noticed any changes in their appearance over time. In particular ask about old photographs, shoe/ring sizes.

- Sweating (see Top Tips box).
- Symptoms of hyperglycaemia – e.g. thirst (⟳ p.580).
- Hypertension.
- Daytime somnolence, early morning headaches (OSA).
- Change in bowel habit/rectal bleeding.
- Trouble with peripheral vision/bumping into objects.
- Weakness, particularly proximal.
- Joint pains – in particular hips and knees.

Examination

It is key to identify both disease phenotype and complications.

Hands

- Large and doughy (spade like) with thickened skin; sweaty hands imply active disease.
- Oedema, prominent superficial veins, absence of rings.
- Loss of thenar eminence and sensation in median nerve distribution (⟳ CTS, p.371).
- Tinel's test.
- BM testing marks.

Head and neck

- Goitre.
- Kyphosis (osteoporotic fractures due to hormonal imbalance).
- Proximal muscle weakness (check shoulder abduction).
- Oedematous eyelids.
- Prominent supra-orbital ridges.
- Bi-temporal hemianopia (from compression of optic chiasm).
- Marked enlargement nose and ears.
- Proganthism (protrusion of the lower jaw).
- Fullness of the lips.
- Macroglossia.
- Poor dentition, widened interdenticular spaces.
- Surgical scars:
  - Transphenoidal surgery (inside the nose, around the philtrum and underside of upper lips).
  - Transcranial (forehead or side of head).

Chest and abdomen

- Gynaecomastia
- Displaced apex beat (cardiomegaly)
- Acanthosis nigricans
- Multiple skin tags.

Lower limbs

Ask patient to stand up with arms folded (assessing legs for proximal myopathy).

Closing statement

- Ask to measure BP, look at the chart and dip the urine for glycosuria.
- Offer to palpate the abdomen (for colonic masses and hepatosplenomegaly). Offer PR examination if history indicative.

❶ Top Tips

- Ensure the patient's main problem (in this case paraesthesia) is dealt with properly before focusing on the other features of acromegaly.
- The candidate should be presenting not only a diagnosis of acromegaly but whether it is active/inactive – remember sweating, skin tags, hypertension and peripheral oedema imply active disease.
- Remember to demonstrate that you have considered there may be coexisting hypopituitarism.

Differential diagnosis

Classical acromegaly should not raise any alternative diagnosis.

Investigations

- Failure of growth hormone (GH) to suppress to <2nmol/L following an OGTT. (Random GH measurements are not diagnostic because of the episodic secretion of GH, its short half-life, and the overlap between GH concentration in individuals with and without acromegaly.)
- IGF 1: used to monitor disease progression.
- MRI pituitary (no need for lateral skull x-rays!).
- Formal Goldman or Humphrey visual fields.

Test anterior pituitary function

- Check T₄ (TSH unhelpful in pituitary disease).
- LH, FSH and testosterone/oestradiol (ensure FSH/LH appropriate).
- Short Synacthen test, ACTH and cortisol levels (ensure ACTH appropriate).

Treatment

- Surgery: candidates need to emphasize that surgery is the treatment of choice, and trans-sphenoidal surgery is usually the best option.
- Radiotherapy can be used as an adjunct to surgery and in those unfit for an operation, but may take many years to have full effect.
- Drug therapy is often used preoperatively and can also be a useful adjunct to surgery.
  - Somatostatin analogues (e.g. octreotide) reduce GH secretion but do not significantly reduce tumour size. Valuable role in reducing hypersecretion post surgery.
  - Dopamine agonists (e.g. bromocripine) only effective in <20% of cases.
  - Pegvisomont, a competitive GH antagonist, normalizes IGF1 levels and rapidly improves active symptoms. Although well tolerated, it is expensive and has to be given subcutaneously. It does not reduce tumour size.

Patient concerns

Most patients will be primarily concerned about their appearance. It is important to counsel them that most physical features do not regress after treatment. Features of active disease can, however, regress (sweating, skin tags and peripheral oedema of the hands and feet). It is equally important to be sensitive about any complications that may have been identified and the need for other tests e.g. colonoscopy.

Viva questions

What are the complications of acromegaly?

- Diabetes
- Hypertension
- Cardiomyopathy
- OSA
- Colonic polyps/bowel cancer
- OA
- Hypercalciuria.

What signs and symptoms may indicate active disease?

- Sweating
- Skin tags
- Hypertension
- Peripheral oedema.

What may be the significance of a raised calcium?

- A raised calcium may indicate MEN 1 (Werner's syndrome; 2 or more of pituitary tumour, islet cell tumour, parathyroid tumour, adrenal tumour).
- MEN2A medullary thyroid cancer (90%), phaeochromocytoma (50%), parathyroid adenoma (20–30%)
- MEN 2B medullary thyroid cancer (90%), phaeochromocytoma, marfanoid habitus

What role is there for growth hormone in medical treatments?

GH is used in childhood cases of short stature secondary to Turner's syndrome and GH deficiency, but has no role in constitutional short stature. GH therapy in hypopituitarism improves well-being, lipid profile and bone mineral density, as well as possibly reducing cardiovascular mortality.

What are the causes of macroglossia?

- Acromegaly
- Amyloidosis
- Hypothyroidism
- Down's syndrome.

What are the complications of pituitary surgery?

- Diabetes insipidus (may be transient)
- SIADH (transient)
- Hypopituitarism
- CSF leak
- Intracranial bleeding.

📖 Further reading

Khandwala HM. *Acromegaly*. [Medscape article, 2011.]. Available at: www.emedicine.com/MED/topic27.htm

Sam AH, Meeran K. *Endocrinology and Diabetes (Lecture Notes)*, pp.95–99. Chichester: Wiley-Blackwell.

🔊 Useful websites

Acromegaly.org website: www.acromegaly.org

National Endocrine and Metabolic Diseases Information Service website—acromegaly: http://www.endocrine.niddk.nih.gov/pubs/acro/acro.aspx

Addison's disease

Addison's disease (primary adrenal insufficiency) can either present with an insidious and progressive course, or with an acute Addisonian crisis. Diagnosis requires a high index of clinical suspicion, as many patients present with non-specific symptoms, particularly with the chronic presentations. Patients look well but feel ill – 'tired and tanned'.

Scenario

Mr. Adam Hagger aged 46.

This gentleman has become increasingly tired and fatigued of late. His wife has also commented he has become increasingly tanned.

A candidate would be expected to quickly establish the underlying diagnosis from details in the scenario and pigmentation seen on inspection.

Initial history and examination

Focus on the nature and duration of the tiredness and fatigue and the rate of their progression. Candidates should clarify:
- The duration of tiredness and fatigue, and effect on quality of life/work.
- If tiredness is present all day or just towards the end of the day.
- If there is sleep disturbance, depressive symptoms.

Simultaneously examine for any obvious pigment changes or vitiligo.

History

Specifically ask about:
- New skin pigmentation changes and if disproportionate to sun exposure (distribution will also include skin not exposed to sun).
- Change in the pigment of existing scars.
- Exhaustion.
- Weight loss.
- Symptoms of postural hypotension.
- Loss of appetite, abdominal pain, vomiting or diarrhoea.
- Widespread muscle and joint pain.
- Amenorrhoea may be a feature in females.
- Personal and family history of autoimmune disease e.g. thyroid disease, diabetes. In those with type 1 diabetes mellitus, ask about insulin requirements – these may decrease as patients develop Addison's disease.
- Travel abroad and TB contacts (➜ pages 51 and 203).
- Previous abdominal surgery – specifically adrenalectomy.

Examination

- The key is to rapidly identify and explore pigmentation changes.
- Hyperpigmentation is diffuse, but more marked in certain areas. Examine specifically for hyperpigmentation in:
  - Palmar creases (normal in darkly pigmented people).
  - Lips and buccal membranes – particularly bluish black discolorations.

- Exposed and pressure areas (feet, elbows, take off the patients watch and also inspect around the belt and brasserie lines).
  - Non-sunexposed areas.
  - Scars.
- Sparse body hair (due to loss of androgens in complete adrenal failure).
- Be vigilant for coexisting vitiligo, as well as other autoimmune diseases e.g. thyroid.
- Auscultate chest (➔ p.50).
- Examine for abdominal scars (especially of bilateral adrenalectomy; occasionally performed via an anterior (rooftop) approach).
- Visual field defect (➔ p.538; classically bitemporal hemianopia) may be present if anterior pituitary function is compromised by an enlarged pituitary tumour such as a prolactinoma.

Closing statement

Ask to measure lying and standing BP.

Differential diagnosis

From the history and examination it should be clear that the diagnosis is primary hypoadrenalism. If possible speculate whether it is autoimmune (most common) or TB (➔ Viva questions, p.598). If a patient has pigmented changes, secondary hypoadrenalism is unlikely.

Investigations

- Short Synacthen test will highlight failure of the adrenal glands to produce sufficient quantities of cortisol.
- Blood cortisol levels are sampled before, and at 30 and 60 minutes after 250 μg of tetracosactide (IM or IV).
- A normal response is a basal cortisol in the reference range, a cortisol rise of > 170nmol above the basal result and/or a peak cortisol >530nmol/L.
- Note that a random cortisol level, although a useful indicator of adrenal function, should not in itself be relied upon as an accurate estimate of adrenal function. In particular, severely malnourished or septic patients can have very low plasma cortisol levels as cortisol is usually very highly protein bound.
- ACTH: raised in primary hypoadrenalism.
- Other blood tests should include:
  - Adrenal auto-antibodies.
  - Electrolytes: hyponatraemia, hyperkalaemia.
  - Blood glucose: looking for hypoglycaemia.
- CXR: to assess for TB.
- CT/MRI adrenals: depending on the history.

Treatment

- Glucorticoid replacement: hydrocortisone in divided doses classically 20mg in the morning; 10mg at night (see also Top Tips box)
- Mineralocorticoid replacement: fludrocortisone for postural hypotension, may cause peripheral oedema.
- Androgen replacement: may improve overall well-being and restore any decline in libido.

❶ Top Tips

- It is important to stress to the examiner (and the patient if practical) the necessity of regular life-long hydrocortisone replacement therapy. It is also important to highlight the need for a steroid alert card and medic alert bracelet (these should also be noted whilst examining the patient). The patient should also be aware of the need to increase the dose when under physiological stress (e.g. surgery, infection).
- If bilateral adrenalectomy scars are present and the patient has diffuse tanning it is important to examine for visual field defect (looking for bitemporal heminaopia) – Nelson's syndrome (➲ Viva questions, p.599).

Patient concerns

Firm reassurance should be given that the patient's symptoms should greatly improve on treatment. Emphasize the need for lifelong treatment and increased doses of steroids when ill.

Viva questions

What are the causes of hypoadrenalism?

- Primary:
  - Autoimmune adrenalitis
  - Granulomatous: TB, histoplasmosis, sarcoidosis
  - Amyloidosis
  - Haemochromatosis
  - Metastatic infiltration
  - Thrombotic disease
  - Congenital adrenal hyperplasia
  - Adrenoleukodystrophy (rare, X-linked inherited disorder therefore, more common and severe in males, resulting in progressive brain damage, failure of the adrenal glands and eventually death)
  - Iatrogenic: following bilateral adrenalectomy
- Secondary:
  - Anterior pituitary failure.

How may a patient with an acute Addisonian crisis present?

- Addisonian crisis is often characterized by nausea and vomiting with accompanying hypotension.
- Hypoglycaemia and confusion may or may not be present.
- If cardiovascular compromise is significant, the patient may present in shock and may be centrally cyanosed.

What diseases are associated with Addison's disease? (listed in order of frequency)

- Vitiligo
- Autoimmune thyroid disease (Hashimoto's and Graves')
- Diabetes mellitus
- Pernicious anaemia
- Coeliac disease
- Premature ovarian failure
- Hypoparathyroidism.

What are the polyglandular autoimmune syndromes?
- Type I:
  - Mild immune deficiency (causing chronic mucocutaneous candidiasis), hypoparathyroidism and Addison's disease.
  - Patients may also have organ-specific autoimmune diseases.
  - Due to mutations in the autoimmune regulator (*AIRE*) gene.
- Type II (Schmidt's syndrome): Addison's disease, type 1 diabetes mellitus and thyroid disease (hypo or hyperthyroidism).
- NB Do not confuse the autoimmune polyglandular syndromes with the multiple endocrine neoplasia syndromes (➍ p.595).

What is the mechanism of hyperpigmentation in adrenal failure and can you name some other causes of hyperpigmentation?
The pituitary gland produces a pre-hormone called pro-opiomelanocortin which is cleaved to ACTH and MHS (melanocyte stimulating hormone). In adrenal failure, the negative feedback loop of adrenal hormones (especially cortisol) on the pituitary is lost, therefore the ACTH precursor is produced in excess, leading to higher than normal levels of MSH. MSH stimulates melanocytes resulting in pigmentation.

Other causes of hyperpigmentation include:
- Racial
- Sun exposure
- Uraemia
- Haemochromatosis
- Primary biliary cirrhosis
- Porphyria cutanea tarda.

What is Nelson's syndrome?
Nelson's syndrome is the rapid enlargement of a pituitary adenoma accompanied by very high ACTH levels and hyperpigmentation (due to excess pro-opiomelanocortin production). The tumour may compress the optic chiasm causing visual field defects. It can occur after bilateral adrenalectomy for Cushing's disease, with loss of the negative feedback loop.

Who was Thomas Addison and why is he so famous?
Thomas Addison was a physician of great renown in the 19th century, who described the following conditions, either alone or in collaboration with others:
- Addison disease* and Addisonian crisis
- Pernicious anaemia (eponymously known as Addisonian anaemia)
- Adrenoleukodystrophy (known as Addison–Schilder syndrome)
- Primary biliary cirrhosis (known as Addison–Gull syndrome)
- Allgrove syndrome (isolated glucocorticoid adrenal failure, achalasia and alacrima – described by Allgrove and colleagues[1] more than a century after Addison)
- Addison's keloid syndrome (now known as morphea)
- Appendicitis.

(*NB Addison's first description of adrenal failure was in the context of TB of the adrenal glands.[2])

He suffered from tremendous bouts of depression and committed suicide in 1860, shortly after his retirement.

References

1. Allgrove J et al. Familial glucocorticoid deficiency with achalasia of the cardia and deficient tear production. *Lancet* 1978; **1**:1284–6.
2. Addison T. On anaemia: disease of the supra-renal capsules. *London Medical Gazette* 1849; **8**:517–18.

📖 Further reading

Lavin N. *Manual of Endocrinology and Metabolism*, 4th edn, pp.257–65. Philadelphia, PA: Lippincott Williams & Wilkins, 2009.

🖰 Useful websites

Australian Addison's Disease Association Inc website: http://www.addisons.org.au/core.html
Addison's Disease Self-Help Group website: http://www.addisons.org.uk/info/i_index1.html

Cushing's syndrome

Cushing's syndrome results from an excess of endogenous or exogenous steroid hormone. Cushing's disease is Cushing's syndrome that specifically results from excess ACTH secretion from an adenoma of the pituitary gland with consequent overstimulation of the adrenal glands. Cushing's syndrome is therefore a wider term, and may also be ACTH-dependent (e.g. ectopic production from a small cell carcinoma of the lungs) or ACTH-independent (e.g. adrenal tumours). Cushing's syndrome may be encountered in the PACES exam, either in Station 5 or as an iatrogenic consequence of treatment for other common PACES conditions!

> ### Scenario
>
> Mr. Richard Tyler aged 58.
>
> This gentleman with hypertension, has been complaining of increasing weight gain and leg weakness and finds climbing stairs particularly difficult. He has also recently been diagnosed with diabetes (diet controlled). Please see and advise.

This scenario may seem difficult at first, but the combination of hypertension, weight gain, proximal muscle weakness and diabetes is highly suggestive of Cushing's. (NB Candidates may only be presented with 2 or 3 of these symptoms.)

Initial history and examination

A quick general inspection may reveal central obesity and a plethoric face.

History

Ask about:

• Duration of symptoms, rate of progression and effect on quality of life.
• The nature of the leg weakness and about urinary or faecal incontinence (unlikely in Cushing's syndrome).
• Clarify exercise tolerance.
• Duration of hypertension.

- Symptoms that led to a diagnosis of diabetes.
- Weight gain and distribution (does the patient feel it has particularly affected the face, neck and torso?).
- Easy bruising, skin thinning and new stretch marks.
- Other proximal muscle weakness patterns, such as getting out of a low chair and raising their arms.
- Any depressive symptoms (low mood, early morning waking).
- Establish whether the patient is taking steroids, and if so, the dose and the underlying condition being treated e.g. COPD.

Examination

- Assess for increased adipose tissue in the face, upper back (at the base of neck/inter-scapular fat pad; avoid the term 'buffalo hump'), and above the clavicles (supraclavicular fat pads). Also note any facial plethora, thin skin and bruising. Steroid acne (papular or pustular lesions) over the face, chest and back, may also be present.
- Signs related to an underlying steroid-responsive disease e.g. SLE.
- Inspect the abdomen, buttocks, lower back, upper thighs, upper arms and breasts for violaceous striae. Also note any evidence of bruising.
- Palpate the abdomen: however adrenal masses are very unlikely to be palpable.
- Examine the tone and power in the legs, particularly for proximal weakness (ask the patient to stand up with their arms folded).
- Carefully assess for a sensory level and check plantars (should both be normal).

☞ Common Pitfalls

- Although the diagnosis may seem obvious, it is important to demonstrate safety as a doctor and being vigilant for 'red flags'. History and examination to exclude cord compression is essential here.

Closing statement

- Ask to measure the BP.
- Say you would like to perform a PR examination to assess anal tone.

Investigations

Confirmation of hypercortisolism

- Overnight dexamethasone suppression test (1mg dexamethasone at midnight and check 9.00am serum cortisol. This test is considered abnormal if the cortisol level is >50nmol/L).
- 3 × 24-hour urine free cortisol measurements.
- Ideally both tests should be done and if negative Cushing's is very unlikely.

If positive proceed to:

Identification of the cause of Cushing's syndrome

- Plasma ACTH level: ACTH levels should be undetectable in adrenal Cushing's but will be inappropriately 'normal' or elevated in pituitary (Cushing's disease) or ectopic Cushing's syndrome.
- High dose dexamethasome suppression test (give 2mg dexamethasone 6-hourly for 48 hours and measure a baseline cortisol and a 48-hour

cortisol. Cortisol levels should fall by >50% of baseline in pituitary Cushing's, but not adrenal or ectopic.
- Corticotropin releasing hormone (CRH) test will cause a rise in cortisol in 90% of individuals with pituitary Cushing's but should not cause a rise in individuals with adrenal or ectopic Cushing's.

Radiological localization (only proceed after biochemical confirmation)
The fact that both pituitary and adrenal incidentalomas are common complicates assessment if biochemical confirmation is not secure.
- Adrenal CT: incidentalomas can cause problems in diagnosis.
- MRI pituitary: will identify 50-80% of ACTH secreting microadenomas.

If there is uncertainty whether it is due to pituitary or ectopic ACTH, use inferior petrosal sinus sampling (sometimes pituitary microadenomas may be too small to see on MRI).

Consider HRCT chest to look for ectopic source of ACTH.

Differential diagnosis
- Alcoholism
- Obesity
- Depression.

Treatment
Most patients will be started on metyrapone whilst awaiting definitive treatment.
- Treatment of pituitary Cushing's:
  - Transphenoidal resection
  - Pituitary radiotherapy
  - Bilateral adrenalectomy (rarely done)
- Treatment of adrenal Cushing's:
  - Adrenalectomy
- Other options include:
  - Ketoconazole
  - Mitotane (if Cushing's caused by adrenal carcinoma)

Patient concerns
Patients are most likely to be concerned about their appearance and weight gain. These are likely to partially improve with treatment but may not completely regress.

In the patients with Cushing's syndrome secondary to steroid therapy, it is important to explain that controlling the underlying disease (e.g. inflammatory bowel disease) is important, although at a later stage steroid sparing agents can be introduced. Patients may still require intermittent courses of steroids.

Viva questions
What are the causes of hypercortisolism?
- Exogenous steroids
- Pituitary adenoma (Cushing's disease)
- Adrenal adenoma/hyperplasia
- Adrenal carcinoma
- Ectopic ACTH (e.g. small cell carcinoma of the lungs).

What is pseudo-Cushing's?

Pseudo-Cushing's syndrome is usually due to alcoholism or depression. Patients can display the signs, symptoms and abnormal hormone levels seen in Cushing's syndrome, but there is no intrinsic problem with the hypothalamic–pituitary–adrenal axis. Blood results and symptoms will normalize rapidly on cessation of the underlying cause e.g. cessation of drinking or remission of depression.

How can pseudo-Cushing's be distinguished from Cushing's syndrome?

This can be very difficult. CRH test after a low dose dexamethasone suppression test is reported to be of some value. This test utilizes the premise that suppression of ACTH by dexamethasone is greater in normal subjects and depressed patients than in patients with Cushing's disease. Therefore following suppression with dexamethasone, serum cortisol is not increased after CRH stimulation in depressed patients, but is increased in individuals with Cushing's disease.

Apart from the description of the syndrome, what was the claim to fame of William Cushing?

- He won the Pulitzer prize for writing a biographical account of the life of Sir William Osler (who was not only an iconic physician at Johns Hopkins but also Regius Professor of Medicine at Oxford).
- Cushing practised as a neurosurgeon at Johns Hopkins and a professor at Harvard Medical School. His mortality rate for hypophysectomy in the pre-antibiotic era was reported to be remarkably low, of the order of 5%.

📖 Further reading

Lavin N. *Manual of Endocrinology and Metabolism*, 4th edn, pp.802–7. Philadelphia, PA: Lippincott Williams & Wilkins, 2009. [Good summary of tests for Cushing's.]

McDermott M. *Endocrine Secrets*, 5th edn, pp.197–204. Amsterdam: Elsevier, 2009.

🔗 Useful websites

National Endocrine and Metabolic Diseases Information Service: http://www.endocrine.niddk.nih. gov/pubs/cushings/cushings.aspx [Cushing's syndrome.]

Pituitary Society: www.pituitarysociety.org/public/specific/cushing/cushings.pdf

Klinefelter's syndrome

Klinefelter's syndrome is the commonest sex chromosome abnormality, and a leading cause of hypogonadism and infertility in men. It is an unusual PACES case.

> **Scenario**
>
> Mr. Peter Kirkland aged 33.
>
> This gentleman is concerned about increasing breast tenderness and swelling. He and his wife have also been trying to conceive for the last 2 years.

Having introduced themselves to the patient, a candidate would be expected to quickly establish the underlying diagnosis of Klinefelter's from the combination of gynaecomastia and infertility in the scenario and a patient with tall stature on inspection.

History

- Infertility (**Ð** Top Tips, p.607).
- Gynaecomastia: duration and effect on the patient's quality of life.
- Other symptoms of hypoandrogenism: fatigue, weakness, erectile dysfunction, low shaving frequency.
- Tactfully enquire about any academic difficulties and behavioural problems.
- Ask about symptoms related to important differentials:
  - Difficulties with smell: Kallman's syndrome (**Ð** Viva questions, p.605).
  - Joint pain, change in skin colouration and diabetes: haemochromatosis (also causes hypogonadism).

Examination

- If practical measure the patient's height, patients with Klinefelter's usually tall and slim, but unlike Marfan's would not have arm span greater than height.
- Examine for gynaecomastia and any breast tenderness.
- Assess for paucity of facial and axillary hair.
- Auscultate the praecordium for mitral valve prolapse (**Ð** p.239) which occurs in 55% of patients.

Closing statement

Offer to perform a genital examination. Patients have generally quite well preserved secondary sexual characteristics, but small soft testes.

Differential diagnosis

- Kallman's syndrome.
- Other causes of hypogonadism: testicular disease, pituitary disease, haemochromatosis.
- Fragile X syndrome (much more severe learning difficulties).

Investigations

- Confirm primary gonadal failure (high LH/FSH, low testosterone)
- Karyotyping
- Echo for MVP
- Bone density.

Treatment

- Testosterone replacement therapy.
- Fertility assessment and assistance.
- Surgery for gynaecomastia.

Patient concerns

There are many erroneous pre-conceptions about Klinefelter's syndrome. These need to be addressed sensitively. Patients should be reassured that sexual functioning and orientation are normal. The majority of patients with Klinefelter's syndrome will be infertile except for those with significant mosaicism, who may be fertile. Testosterone treatment is, however, important to reduce the risk of complications, such as cardiovascular disease, hypercholesterolaemia and osteoporosis.

Viva questions

What is the commonest karyotype in Klinefelter's syndrome?
47 XXY in >80% of cases. XXXY and XYY variants also exist.

What is Kallman's syndrome?
Kallman's syndrome comprises of hypogonadotrophic hypogonadism, accompanied with anosmia or hyposmia. It is caused by reduced migration of gonadotropin-releasing hormone secreting neurons from the forebrain to the hypothalamus.

How can testosterone be given?
- IM injection (every 2–3 weeks or long-acting 3-monthly (newer preparations).
- Gel (applied to upper forearms).
- Patches.
- NB Oral preparations are insufficient to restore male testosterone levels.

What questions are important to ask in individuals presenting with a erectile dysfunction?
This needs to be handled tactfully and sensitively. It is important to assess libido early in the consultation as low libido suggests hypogonadism rather than penile neurovascular disease. A good early question to ask: 'Is the mind willing, but the body isn't or are neither particularly willing?'. This will allow a rapid (but relatively tactful!) assessment of libido.

It is essential to determine whether it is hormonal or psychosocial – a gradual onset suggests an organic cause whereas a sudden onset often suggests a psychological cause (e.g. depression, bereavement, stress, performance anxiety and relationship problems). Anorgasmia, intermittent episodes of low libido or variance between an individual's partners also suggest a psychosocial cause.

Ask about erection timing and quality. The presence of morning or nocturnal erections suggests a psychogenic cause.

📖 Further reading

Lavin N. *Manual of Endocrinology and Metabolism*, 4th edn, pp.315–16. Philadelphia, PA: Lippincott Williams & Wilkins, 2009

🔗 Useful website

Klinefelter Organisation: http://www.klinefelter.org.uk/

Infertility in female patients

Infertility itself or conditions causing it may unusually occur in the PACES. It is important to identify the likely underlying diagnosis and approach the issues around infertility sensitively.

Polycystic ovarian syndrome (PCOS)

- Commonest cause of infertility in women.
- Diagnosis (Rotterdam criteria) requires 2 out of 3 oligomenorrhoea/ ameonorrhoea, hyperandrogenism, polycystic ovaries on ultrasound.
- Clinical features include acne, hirsutism, male pattern baldness (from hyperandrogenism). Other features include obesity, acanthosis nigricans.
- Metformin improves both insulin resistance and period regularity.
- In women with hyperandrogenism the differential is PCOS, congenital adrenal hyperplasia (elevated 17-hydroxyprogesterone) or androgen secreting tumour (very elevated testosterone/DHEA-S).

Turner's syndrome

- Lack of secondary sexual characteristics e.g. pubic hair.
- Short stature.
- Widely spaced nipples.
- Webbed neck with low posterior hairline.
- Endocrine: increased incidence of diabetes and hypothyroidism.
- Cardiovascular: congenital lymphoedema, aortic dissection, bicuspid aortic valve, coarctation of the aorta, hypertension.
- Gastrointestinal: coeliac disease, angiodysplasia.
- Renal: horseshoe kidneys, aberrant vascular supply.
- Musculoskeletal: short 4th and 5th metacarpals, nail hypoplasia, high-arched palate.
- Skin: multiple pigmented naevi.

NB Noonan's syndrome has a similar phenotype to Turner's syndrome. Principal features include congenital heart defects, short stature, learning problems, pectus excavatum and a webbed neck. Unlike Turner's it is not a cause of infertility and can occur in men. It is an autosomal dominant inherited condition.

❶ Top Tips

- Important questions regarding infertility which must be addressed in a sensitive manner (for both men and women) include:
  - Pubertal development
  - Duration of infertility
  - Previous fertility (i.e. including those proceeding to ToP or spontaneous abortion) in the patient and their current or any previous partner.
- For men enquire specifically about:
  - Conditions which could lead to erectile dysfunction, including diabetes and neurological disorders (e.g. spinal pathology).
  - Childhood illnesses: testicular torsion, mumps, developmental delay or precocious puberty.
  - Galactorrhoea or visual-field disturbances (pituitary tumour).
- For women enquire about:
  - Amenorrhea and whether primary or secondary
  - Irregular menstruation
  - Symptoms of hypothyroidism
  - Previous sexual transmitted diseases
  - Galactorrhoea.

Dermatology: **Introduction to dermatological assessment**

Introduction

Skin conditions may present in Station 5 as either the main focus of a case or as an important cutaneous manifestation of a systemic disease, providing important clues as to the underlying diagnosis. It is important that the candidate demonstrates their understanding of how skin conditions can have a significant psychological effect on patients.

Examination

Although a candidate may be directed towards a particular cutaneous sign, it is very important that they should step back and perform a general skin examination, as this often gives vital clues which may reveal the correct underlying diagnosis. For example, if faced with a classic psoriatic plaque, a candidate's complete examination should include the nails, scalp, ears, neck and umbilicus, as well as asking to examine the groin. This more thorough approach will demonstrate that the candidate not only knows the diagnosis, but also has an understanding of the condition.

The candidate must appreciate that the appearance of inflammation varies with skin type. Pigmentary changes are prominent in darker skin types where inflammation can result in lasting patches of hypo- or hyperpigmentation.

Candidates should always look for relevant examination equipment that may be placed around the bedside. They should be familiar with Wood's light. This is a UV light source under which depigmented skin (e.g. vitiligo) appears bright white, some fungi (e.g. dermatophytes) fluoresce green and corynebacterium (e.g. underlying erythrasma) fluoresces coral pink.

Description

It is advisable for the candidate to describe their findings in a clear, concise and structured manner prior to reaching a diagnosis. The secret to this is morphology, configuration and distribution.

Morphology

The appearance of the individual lesions. Consider the colour, shape, size, margins, surface, texture and temperature.
Descriptive terms:
- Macule: impalpable colour change of the skin (e.g. freckle or vitiligo).
- Papule: raised, dome-shaped lesion, <0.5cm in diameter (e.g. lichen planus).
- Nodule: larger dome-shaped lesion, >0.5cm in diameter (e.g. acne).
- Plaque: plateau-like elevation above the skin surface (e.g. psoriasis).
- Vesicle: circumscribed, elevated, superficial cavity containing fluid, <0.5cm in diameter (e.g. herpes simplex or vesicular eczema).
- Bulla: circumscribed, elevated, superficial cavity containing yellowish fluid, >0.5cm in diameter (e.g. bullous pemphigoid).
- Pustule: circumscribed superficial cavity containing purulent exudates (e.g. acne vulgaris or folliculitis).

- Erosion: a superficial defect due to loss of part of the epidermis (e.g. pemphigus vulgaris).
- Ulcer: a deeper skin defect extending into the dermis or below (e.g. venous ulcer).

Configuration

How the individual lesions are related to one another. The candidate needs to consider whether the lesions are single, multiple, confluent, in groups, annular (in a ring), linear or evenly scattered.

Distribution

The areas of the body affected (e.g. extensor versus flexural surfaces, mucous membranes). The candidate must consider symmetry and think about aetiology, for instance, if the signs are in sun-exposed areas or over pressure points.

For example, you could describe lichen planus as flat-topped, violaceous papules found in groups on the flexor surfaces of the wrists.

Differential diagnosis

The dermatology section of this chapter will cover the conditions most commonly seen in the PACES exam. It is advisable for candidates to attend some dermatology clinics prior to their PACES examination, however a good colour atlas[1] can be used as an adjunct for revision, particularly if access to a number of dermatology clinics is not possible. As with all other PACES stations, simply reciting a long list of differentials is not adequate. The examiners will expect the list in order of likelihood and to justify why a certain condition might be more likely in a particular individual. Demonstrate your knowledge by giving reasons that support or negate each diagnosis.

Investigations and management

Basic investigations to consider in this station are skin swabs (bacterial and viral), blood cultures, scrapings for mycology, blood tests and skin biopsy for histology or immunofluorescence studies. These must be tailored to the individual condition. Management will be discussed at the end of each scenario.

Reference

1. Du Vivier A. *Atlas of Clinical Dermatology*, 3rd edn. London: Churchill Livingstone, 2002.

Cutaneous lupus erythematosus

Lupus erythematosus is an autoimmune condition that can present in a purely cutaneous form or in a systemic form (SLE) with or without cutaneous features.

> **Scenario**
>
> Ms Jane Smithey, aged 28 years.
>
> This lady has been referred to you with a rash on her face. Please perform a focused history and examination.

History

There is a great deal to cover in this scenario and the candidate needs to ask very specific, targeted questions. The history needs to focus on the rash and whether or not there are symptoms of systemic involvement. It should include:

Skin
- Duration of rash and individual lesions.
- Site of rash (malar, photosensitive distribution, discoid lupus often affects the ears).
- What do individual patches look like?
- Burning/itching.
- Do they leave scarring?
- Is it related to sunlight (photosensitive)?
- Associated hair loss.

Systemic
- Mouth ulcers
- Headaches
- Arthralgia
- Joint deformities
- Raynaud's phenomenon
- Hypertension
- Renal history
- Pleuritic chest pain
- Breathing problems (fibrosis)
- Anaemia
- Thromboses
- Miscarriages.

Other questions
- What medications are they on (some medications can induce lupus-like symptoms)?
- What treatments have they had and were they effective?
- Anyone else in the family with lupus or other autoimmune conditions?
- How is the condition affecting the patient and their activities of daily living?

Examination

This scenario is focusing on the skin in particular; other systems to examine are detailed in the SLE case (➲ p.500), with focused examination being guided by the history obtained. The candidate should examine the skin rash in question, but also the scalp (looking for inflammation and scarring alopecia), ears (especially affected in discoid lupus), the fingers and toes (for signs of Raynaud's phenomenon/infarction) and all other areas of the skin.

- Acute cutaneous lupus erythematosus:
  - Generalized photosensitive or malar rash (malar rash spares the nasolabial folds, is usually erythematous and raised dependent on disease activity).
  - Almost inevitably associated with systemic disease.
- Subacute cutaneous lupus erythematosus (more chronic):
  - Can take many different forms such as erythematous annular (ring-like) patches, papules or plaques.
  - Usually in a photosensitive distribution and only associated with systemic disease in ~50% of cases.
- Chronic cutaneous lupus erythematosus (e.g. discoid lupus erythematosus [DLE]):
  - Presents with fixed erythematous papules with raised edges and atrophic centres and plaques which often result in post-inflammatory hypo- or hyperpigmentation, severe scarring and alopecia; depigmentation may be particularly marked in black patients.
  - Commonly affects the head (look in ears) and neck.
  - Less commonly associated with systemic disease compared with acute and subacute cutaneous lupus erythematosus.

Differential diagnosis

The differential diagnosis is wide in cutaneous lupus – see Table 8.16.

> **❶ Top Tips**
>
> - If the candidate suspects discoid lupus they should always examine:
>   - The ears (looking for follicular plugging which resembles blackheads).
>   - The scalp for hair loss, asking sensitively whether the patient is wearing a wig ('May I ask if this is your natural hair?').

Investigations

- Urinalysis (looking for protein and blood, indicating renal involvement).
- FBC, U&E, LFT, CRP, ESR, complement.
- Serology (ANA, ENA, anti-dsDNA).
- Skin biopsy for histology and immunofluorescence.
- Further investigations depend upon clinical history.

Treatment

- Avoid the sun.
- Sun protection with high factor topical sun screens.
- Stop smoking (smoking can worsen lupus erythematosus and reduce the effect of hydroxychloroquine).
- Topical steroids (discoid lupus requires potent topical steroids e.g. clobetasol propionate).
- Topical tacrolimus.

Table 8.16 Differential diagnosis in cutaneous lupus

Differential	Distinguishing features
Malar rash	
Seborrhoeic dermatitis	Scaly, erythematous eczematous rash commonly over scalp, face (e.g. eyebrows, facial folds), sternum; may be sun-related, but no scarring
Rosacea	Erythema/telangiectasia over nose and cheeks with overlying papules and pustules. Exacerbated by heat, alcohol and spicy foods
Photosensitive rash	
Drug-induced	The candidate must take a detailed drug history. Examples include antibiotics (tetracyclines, quinolones), NSAIDs, diuretics (frusemide, bumetanide) and retinoids
Polymorphous light eruption	Very itchy, polymorphic erythematous rash developing 24–48 hours after sun exposure and fading over 1 week. No resultant scarring; often improves through the summer but recurs the following year
Actinic dermatitis/ photo-exacerbated eczema	Erythematous, scaly, itchy eczematous rash, worse in sun-exposed areas. No associated scarring
Discoid patches	
Discoid eczema	Circular patches of eczema, not photosensitive, no scarring
Psoriasis	➔ p.613
Fungal infections (e.g. tinea corporis)	Increased erythema and scaling at the margins of patches, often with central clearing. Not photosensitive, no scarring

- Anti-malarials (hydroxychloroquine, mepacrine).
- Prednisolone.
- Azathioprine.
- Mycophenolate mofetil.
- Cyclophosphamide/pulsed methylprednisolone.
- Camouflage make-up can be extremely helpful to patients.

Patient concerns

The patient will want to know their diagnosis and your intended investigation and management plan. They may be very distressed by the appearance of their skin, by their hair loss or concerned about the development of further lesions and the possibility of developing systemic disease.

Viva questions

What is the differential diagnosis for a scarring alopecia?

Discoid lupus, lichen planus (lichen plano-pilaris, LPP) and tinea capitis (more in children) are the 3 commonest causes of a scarring alopecia. The appearance of DLE and LPP on the scalp can be very similar, presenting with patches of inflammation and resulting scarring alopecia. Involvement elsewhere can help to differentiate the two. Lichen planus presents with very itchy flat topped, violaceous papules and plaques, most commonly on the wrists. Unlike DLE, it is not photosensitive and does not result in scarring outside of the scalp. Tinea capitis is most frequently diagnosed in children and is associated with significant scaling and erythema (as with tinea infections at other sites).

If a patient with DLE has negative autoantibodies at presentation, what is their chance of developing systemic lupus erythematosus in the future?
5%, whereas 25% of patients with systemic disease develop discoid patches at some stage during the course of their disease.

What are the potential side effects of chronic topical steroid application?
The commonest side effects are telangiectasia, skin atrophy, skin break-down and ulceration.

Psoriasis

Psoriasis is defined as a chronic, non-infectious inflammatory skin condition. It affects ~2% of the UK population.

Scenario

Mr David Turner, aged 45 years.

This gentleman has been referred to you with a skin rash. Please assess.

History

The history should focus on:
- The duration, distribution and progression of the skin lesions.
- Associated pruritus.
- Associated nail changes.
- Current and previous medication/management.
- Previous UV light treatment.
- Associated joint pain and stiffness.
- Any associated HLA B27 related symptoms e.g. symptoms of inflammatory bowel disease.
- Family history of HLA B27 disorders.
- Cosmetic concerns/psychological burden.

---

❶ Top Tips

- Always enquire about the family history which will be positive in 30% of patients. Despite the strong familial tendency, it does not follow a Mendelian pattern of inheritance.
- Psoriasis is a polygenic disorder and the aetiology is multifactorial i.e. environmental as well as genetic factors interact to produce the clinical features of psoriasis.

Examination

Skin

- Well demarcated, raised erythematous plaques with silvery scale (see Fig. 8.15 ➲ Plate 4).
- Single or multiple scattered lesions.
- Usually found symmetrically on extensor surfaces, scalp, umbilicus, groin and natal cleft (examine these areas carefully).

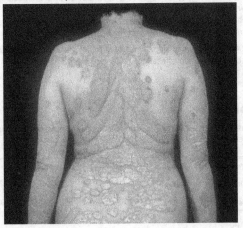

Fig. 8.15 Psoriatic plaques.
With permission from St John's Institute of Dermatology. See also Plate 4.

Nails

- Pitting (psoriatic pits are large, deep and irregularly scattered within the nail plate).
- Onycholysis (apparent splitting of the nail with distal nail plate detachment).
- Subungual hyperkeratosis (thickening of the nail plate).

Joints

- Mobility aids around the bed.
- Tender swollen joints, if active psoriatic arthritis; deformity with reduced function, if quiescent psoriatic arthritis (➲ Psoriatic arthritis, p.497).
- Severity of skin changes does not necessarily correlate with joint activity.

Patient concerns

This patient may be quite distressed at the development of the rash. He may need reassurance that this is not infectious and there are a wide variety of treatment options available. Furthermore, it is vital to address any underlying concerns regarding the psychological issues surrounding this diagnosis.

Management

Be supportive. Explain there is no cure but good control of symptoms is usually achievable.

Treatment

Topical

- Soap substitutes e.g. aqueous cream or Dermol®.
- Frequent emollient at least twice daily.
- Vitamin D analogues:
  - Inhibit proliferation and promote differentiation of keratinocytes.
  - Used as monotherapy as well as in combination with other treatments for psoriasis (e.g. topical steroids and acitretin).
- Salicylic acid: a keratolytic agent used alone or in combination with a topical steroid.
- Topical steroids: short-term use during inflammatory flares.
- Coal tar:
  - Antimicrobial, anti-inflammatory and anti-pruritic effects.
  - Also thought to suppress DNA synthesis, imparting an antiproliferative effect.
- Dithranol: cytotoxic and inhibits a variety of cellular functions leading to a reduction in keratinocyte proliferation.

Photo(chemo)therapy

- Indications for use include moderate to severe psoriasis not controlled by topical treatments.
- Used as monotherapy or in combination.
- Narrow band UVB (optimal irradiation currently available) is usually given for around 6 weeks at a time.
- Psoralen plus UVA phototherapy (PUVA) with psoralens applied topically or taken orally (penetrates deeper than UVB) and is usually given for around 6 weeks at a time.
- Acute effects include erythema, blistering and burning sensation.
- Risk of carcinogenesis represents the major long-term side effect.

Systemic

Indications for stepping up to a systemic agent include severe psoriasis and psoriasis resistant to topical treatments and photo(chemo)therapy:
- Retinoids (e.g. acitretin)
- Methotrexate
- Ciclosporin.

Biological

- Etanercept
- Ustekinumab
- Adalimumab
- Infliximab.

Indications for use include patients with severe psoriasis who have previously failed on conventional systemic agents.

❶ Top Tips

- Comment on complications of systemic therapy including:
  - Dry lips on acitretin.
  - Gum hypertrophy, hypertrichosis or sebaceous gland hyperplasia with ciclosporin.
  - Injection sites from etanercept or adalimumab.

Patient concerns

The patient will want to know their diagnosis and your management plan. They may be distressed by the appearance of their skin and female patients may want advice on which toiletries and make-up products to avoid. Patient should be advised to avoid abrasive facial 'scrubs' and cosmetics with irritants and instead use cosmetics with a moisturizing component, creams as opposed to gels, which have high alcohol content, or lotions, which have fewer emollients.

Viva questions

What are the 6 clinical presentations of psoriasis?

- Chronic plaque psoriasis.
- Guttate psoriasis (small, symmetrical and superficial papular lesions scattered over the body, especially the trunk).
- Hyperkeratotic palmo-plantar psoriasis.
- Flexural psoriasis (mainly affecting intertriginous areas).
- Erythrodermic psoriasis (generalized erythema and scaling, with risk of sepsis and cardiovascular compromise in severe cases).
- Pustular psoriasis (either limited to the palms and soles or generalized).

From a clinical perspective, psoriasis can be regarded as a spectrum of different cutaneous manifestations. At any one point in time, different variants can coexist in a particular individual.

What are the precipitating factors in psoriasis?

- Physical trauma (Koebner phenomenon).
- Infections (classically beta-haemolytic *Streptococcus*).
- Drugs (e.g. beta-blockers, antimalarials, lithium, NSAIDS and steroids).
- Psychological stress (although hard evidence for this is lacking).
- Alcohol.
- Tobacco.
- Climate (psoriasis tends to flare in cold climates, although some facial psoriasis is worsened by exposure to sunlight).

What are the two characteristic histological features seen in psoriasis?

- Epidermal hyperplasia (increased activity of the epidermis) with 'squared off' rete ridges.
- Inflammatory cell infiltrate (lymphocytes, macrophages and neutrophils) in both the dermis and epidermis.

What is the Koebner phenomenon?

Psoriasis appearing at the sites of trauma to the skin (e.g. surgical scar, site of phlebotomy, microtrauma to knees etc.).

How can you establish the severity and functional status of these patients?

This can be done using the PASI and DLQI:

- PASI: the Psoriasis Area and Severity Index is an objective assessment of the severity of psoriasis. It takes into consideration redness, scaling, thickness and area of involvement. Maximum score is 72. Whilst the PASI score is routinely measured in dermatology clinics and for clinical research purposes, this evaluation during PACES would not be expected.

- DLQI – the Dermatology Life Quality Index, assessed by patient questionnaire, is a subjective measure of the impact that any dermatological condition can have on a patient's life. Social and psychological problems are commonly associated with psoriasis.

🖉 **Useful websites**

British Association of Dermatology: http://www.bad.org.uk
The Psoriasis Association: http://www.psoriasis-association.org.uk

Neurofibromatosis

Neurofibromatosis (NF) is an autosomal dominant, inherited multi-system disease. There are two very distinct forms, type 1 and type 2.

Type 1

NF type 1, also known as von Recklinghausen's disease, is characterized by abnormalities of the skin, neurological system and the bones.

> **Scenario**
>
> Mr John Smithers, age 45 years.
>
> This gentleman is concerned as he is developing an increasing number of skin lesions. Please perform a focused history and examination.

History

Skin
- Duration, distribution and progression of the skin lesions.
- Previous excisions (neurofibromas can undergo sarcomatous change).

Neurological
- Radicular pain (nerve compression due to neuromas).
- Visual problems (secondary to optic gliomas).
- Hearing problems (secondary to acoustic neuromas).
- Epilepsy (usually secondary to CNS tumours).
- History of brain tumours (➲ Viva questions, p.620).
- Previous surgery (skin, nerves, spine, brain).
- Learning difficulties (can ask whether there were any problems at school, what age they left, what exams they passed; up to 50% may have mild intellectual impairment).

Bones
- Lordosis, kyphosis, dislocations, fractures.
- Independence/dependence for activities of daily living.

Other
- Hypertension (➲ Viva questions, p.620).
- Drug history (anti-epileptics, analgesics).
- Family history.

Examination

As with most examinations it is advisable for the candidate to start at the hands and work up the arms on to the head and neck, down the trunk and finish with the legs. Clinical signs to elicit include:

Skin

- Neurofibromas (soft tumours that can usually be pushed down into the panniculus 'button-holing'; Fig. 8.16 ⊃ Plate 5).
- Café-au-lait spots (light brown, evenly pigmented macules; Fig. 8.17 ⊃ Plate 6).
- Axillary (or generalized) freckling.
- Plexiform neuromas (large nodules containing multiple neurofibromas, 'bag of worms').
- Lipomas.
- Scars from previous surgery.

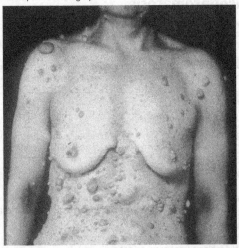

Fig. 8.16 Neurofibromatosis – neurofibromas.
With permission from St John's Institute of Dermatology. See also Plate 5.

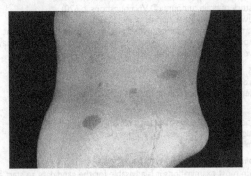

Fig. 8.17 Neurofibromatosis – café-au-lait spots.
With permission from St John's Institute of Dermatology. See also Plate 6.

Arm
- Ask for the BP.
- Look in the axillae.

Ears
Look behind the ears for hearing aids.

Eyes
With a pen torch the candidate should look for hamartomas (Lisch nodules) on the iris, which appear as small brown dots. If not visible with the naked eye, then the candidate should state that they would like to perform a slit lamp examination.

> **❶ Top Tips**
>
> - Remember to look behind the ears for hearing aids.
> - If evidence of a hearing deficit is found, examine the cranial nerves V, VI and VII (LMN) and look for cerebellar signs – these may be present if the patient has a cerebellopontine angle lesion (e.g. acoustic neuromas).

Diagnostic criteria
The National Institute of Health criteria confirms a diagnosis of neurofibromatosis type 1 in the presence of ≥2 of:
- ≥6 café au lait macules (>5mm in greatest diameter in prebubertal children and >15mm diameter in postpubertal individuals).
- ≥2 neurofibromas of any type or one plexiform neuroma.
- Freckling in axillary or inguinal regions.
- ≥2 Lisch nodules.
- Optic glioma.
- Distinctive osseous lesion, such as sphenoid dysplasia or thinning of long bone cortex, with or without pseudoarthrosis:
- 1st-degree relative with NF-1.

Type 2

This most commonly presents with hearing loss, tinnitus or balance problems as a result of unilateral or bilateral acoustic neuromas. Visual changes can occur secondary to optic nerve sheath meningiomas or juvenile cataracts. Cranial nerve symptoms can arise due to cranial nerve schwannomas. Cutaneous features are far less prominent than in type 1 NF. Patients with Type 2 NF, have fewer café-au-lait macules (usually <6), no axillary freckling and no Lisch nodules. They can develop multiple subcutaneous nodules (as seen in type 1); however histologically these are schwannomas and neurilemomas, rather than neurofibromas (as in type 1).

Diagnostic criteria for type 2 neurofibromatosis includes either of the following:
- Bilateral 8th cranial nerve masses (on CT or MRI).
- 1st-degree relative with NF-2 and either a unilateral 8th nerve mass or 2 of: neurofibroma, meningioma, glioma, schwannoma or juvenile posterior subcapsular lenticular opacity.

Differential diagnosis
- Single neurofibromas can occur individually without neurofibromatosis.
- Some café-au-lait macules may also be seen in other conditions including tuberous sclerosis and McCune–Albright syndrome.

Investigations
These are guided by clinical indication and include:
- Audiogram.
- Brainstem auditory evoked responses.
- CT/MR imaging.
- Skin/deeper tissue biopsy (if concerns regarding malignant transformation e.g. neurofibroma sarcoma).

Treatment
Treatment is based upon managing the complications of the condition and may include:
- Anti-hypertensives.
- Anti-epileptics.
- Educational help.
- Surgery – to remove benign or malignant tumours.
- Hearing aids.

Patient concerns
The patient will ask what is wrong with them. You should explain the diagnosis and your investigation and management plan. They may ask you about the inheritance of this disease, about other family members and the likelihood of their children suffering with the condition. As with all autosomal dominant conditions, if the partner does not carry the mutation then the likelihood of the patient's children inheriting the condition is 50%.

Viva questions

Name three causes of hypertension associated with neurofibromatosis?
- Renal artery stenosis
- Phaeochromocytoma
- Coarctation of the aorta.

On which chromosomes are the genes responsible for neurofibromatosis type 1 and type 2 located?
The gene for:
- NF-1 is located on chromosome 17 (17q11.2).
- NF-2 is located on chromosome 22 (22q12).

What is the most common central nervous system tumour occurring in NF-1?
Optic gliomas have been shown to occur in 15% of patients. Other neoplasms are rarer, such as schwannomas, astrocytomas and hamartomas.

What is Crowe's sign?
This refers to the axillary freckling seen in some patients with NF type 1.

Vitiligo

Vitiligo is an acquired, idiopathic disorder characterized by circumscribed de-pigmented macules and patches. The condition may progress, sometimes extending rapidly over a period of several months and then remain quiescent for many years. Functional melanocytes disappear from involved skin by a mechanism not, as yet, defined.

> ### Scenario
>
> Miss Santra Singh. Aged 22 years.
>
> This lady is concerned regarding the appearance of skin on her hands. Please assess.

History

Focused questions should include:

- Duration, distribution and rate of progression of skin lesions.
- Family history (36% of cases are familial).
- Associated autoimmune disorders including: type 1 diabetes mellitus, pernicious anaemia, hypothyroidism, hyperthyroidism and Addison's disease.
- Effect of sun exposure on lesions (the depigmented areas are more likely to burn).
- Current and previous management.
- Psychological burden.

Examination

Skin

- Well demarcated de-pigmented macules and patches surrounded by normal skin with a hyperpigmented border.
- Distribution is frequently localized to areas that are normally hyperpigmented such as: the face, dorsal hands, nipples, axillae, umbilicus, sacrum and anogenital regions.

> ### ❶ Top Tips
>
> - The lesions in vitiligo, particularly in people with paler skin types, may more easily be distinguishable:
>   - Using Wood's lamp to distinguish hyopigmentation from depigmentation; in vitiligo the skin will appear bluish.
>   - During the summer months or after a period of sun exposure, when the surrounding skin is more tanned.

Scalp

Alopecia areata of the scalp may be seen in association with vitiligo

> ### ❶ Top Tips
>
> - Look for signs of associated autoimmune disease, including thyroidectomy scars, needle marks (diabetes mellitus) and evidence of peripheral neuropathy (pernicious anaemia).

Treatment

The aims of vitiligo treatments are re-pigmentation and stabilization of the de-pigmentation process. Treatment response may be unsatisfactory.

- *Psychological:* the impact of this disorder on quality of life is very severe in many patients. Psychological support is important.
- *Skin camouflage:* cosmetics are extremely useful for concealing disfiguring patches, if socially and culturally acceptable.
- *Sunscreens* are important in all vitiligo patients.
- *Reversal:*
  - Narrowband UVB 2–3 times per week for many weeks: slow re-pigmentation initially from hair follicles is expected.
  - PUVA with psoralens applied topically or taken orally.
  - Super-potent topical corticosteroids for small localized areas.
  - Topical application of 0.1% tacrolimus ointment: may improve re-pigmentation, especially when used for a prolonged period of time.
- *Depigmentation:* in extensive vitiligo where only small areas of normally pigmented skin remain, skin-bleaching creams, such as hydroquinone derivatives, may help to even-up skin colour.

Viva questions

What disorders are associated with vitiligo?

Autoimmune disorders do occur in some patients. The strongest association is with thyroid dysfunction, either hypo- or hyperthyroidism (i.e. Graves' disease, Hashimoto's thyroiditis). Pernicious anaemia, Addison's disease, diabetes mellitus, and alopecia areata are also more frequent.

Is vitiligo familial?

~36% of patients have a positive family history and a genetic factor is undoubtedly involved. Inheritance may be polygenic or determined by an autosomal dominant gene of variable penetrance. The *NALP1* gene (located on chromosome 17p) has been implicated in vitiligo and other autoimmune conditions.

What is the histology of vitiligo?

There is marked absence of melanocytes and melanin in the epidermis.

Can you suggest any theories for the aetiology of vitiligo?

- Autoimmune destruction due to antibodies against the melanocytes, in addition to altered T-cell immunity.
- An intrinsic defect in the structure and function of melanocytes.
- Reduced melanocyte survival and dysregulation of melanocyte apoptosis.
- Destruction of melanocytes by neurochemical substances.

℘ Useful websites

The Vitiligo Society website: http://www.vitiligosociety.org.uk
Changing Faces website: http://www.changingfaces.org.uk

Pyoderma gangrenosum

Pyoderma gangrenosum is an uncommon, chronic, recurrent condition causing skin ulceration, frequently associated with underlying systemic disease. Diagnosis is based on typical clinical features and exclusion of other ulcerating diseases.

> **Scenario**
>
> Mrs Susan Lynch, aged 34 years.
>
> This lady has been referred to you with a non-healing ulcer on the left thigh. Please assess.

History

- Duration, distribution and progression of the lesions:
  - Lesions may increase in size rapidly.
- Associated pain.
- Associated symptoms e.g. fever, malaise, myalgia and arthralgia.
- Associated underlying systemic diseases including:
  - Inflammatory bowel disease
  - Myeloproliferative disorders
  - RA.

> **① Top Tips**
>
> - Remember to ask about underlying systemic diseases which are present in 50% of patients.
> - Enquire about injury or operations as pyoderma gangrenosum may localize in areas of skin damage.

Examination

- Initial lesion is often a tender papulo-pustule with surrounding erythematous or violaceous induration.
- Characteristic lesion is a necrotic ulcer with an undermined gun-metal grey border and purulent base (Fig. 8.18 ➲ Plate 7).
- Lesions may be solitary or multiple.
- Signs related to an underlying disorder e.g. rheumatoid hands.

Investigations

Pyoderma gangrenosum is often a diagnosis of exclusion as laboratory and histopathological findings are variable and non-specific. Consider the following:

- Skin biopsy for histology and culture (bacteria, viruses and fungi), as well as skin swabs (these are typically negative).
- Gastrointestinal studies including stool for occult blood, colonoscopy, biopsy and radiography.
- Haematological studies including FBC and bone marrow examination.
- Serological studies, including serum protein electrophoresis, ANA, ANCAs and anti-phospholipid antibodies.

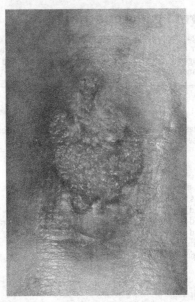

Fig. 8.18 Pyoderma gangrenosum.
With permission from St John's Institute of Dermatology. See also Plate 7.

Treatment
- Bed rest and elevation; consider compression bandaging.
- Topical therapy such as topical corticosteroids.
- High-dose systemic corticosteroids.
- Systemic therapy with ciclosporin or dapsone.
- Infliximab if the disease is refractory to other treatments.

The nature and intensity of the therapeutic approach depends on the number, site and depth of the lesions, the rate of expansion and appearance of new lesions, any associated disorder, the medical status of the patient and the risk and patient tolerance of prolonged therapy. Standard therapy is local or combined local and systemic corticosteroid therapy, with or without adjunctive systemic therapy.

Viva questions

What systemic diseases are associated with pyoderma gangrenosum?
~50% of patients have an associated condition. The most common associations are:
- Inflammatory bowel disease (especially UC)
- Crohn's disease
- Arthritis:
  - Seronegative arthritis
  - RA

- Haematological diseases including:
  - Acute and chronic myeloid leukaemia
  - Hairy cell leukaemia
  - Myelodysplasia
  - Monoclonal gammopathy.

Apart from cutaneous sites, what other sites are affected by this condition?

- Mucous membranes and peristomal sites:
  - Pyostomatitis vegetans is seen in patients with IBD and is characterized by a chronic, vegetative, sterile pyoderma of the labial and buccal musosa.
  - Peristomal pyoderma gangrenosum occurs at the sites of an ileostomy or colostomy in UC or Crohn's disease.
- Less common sites include the vulva, penis, and scrotum.

What are the 4 major clinical forms of pyoderma gangrenosum?

- Ulcerative
- Bullous
- Pustular
- Superficial granulomatous.

Is the histology diagnostic?

No. The histology is relatively non-specific. Features include neutrophilic infiltration, haemorrhage and necrosis of the epidermis. Clinicopathological correlation is important in diagnosis.

Necrobiosis lipoidica

Necrobiosis lipoidica is a rare and chronic skin condition that may be associated with diabetes mellitus. The underlying cause remains unclear. The granulomatous inflammation and fibrosis appears as yellow, atrophic lesions, almost exclusively on the shins.

> **Scenario**
>
> Mrs Catherine Brown, aged 28 years.
>
> This lady has been referred to you with skin changes on her shins. Please perform a focused history and examination.

History

The history should focus on:

- Skin changes.
- Site of changes.
- Do the affected areas break down?
- Duration of changes.
- Symptoms of diabetes/history of diabetes (and how this coincided with the onset of skin symptoms).
- Previous treatments (and their efficacy).
- Family history of similar skin changes or diabetes.

Examination

The characteristic patches usually start as erythematous papules and then expand and become yellow/brown, often atrophic, plaques with overlying dilated blood vessels. Palpation of the waxy plaques can be a helpful diagnostic aid (feels like candle-wax), but beware, as this may be painful. The patches can break down. They are most commonly found on the shins, and although they rarely occur elsewhere, a general skin examination is worthwhile.

> **❶ Top Tips**
>
> - Examine the patient for BM testing pricks and insulin injection sites, indicating associated diabetes mellitus.

Differential

This condition has a very characteristic appearance (as discussed in 'Examination').

Investigations

- Fasting glucose (i.e. if not already diagnosed with diabetes, screen for this condition).
- Skin biopsy (avoid if possible as these patches are prone to breaking down and ulcerating).

Treatment

If diabetic, optimize control (although this may not improve the skin). Treatment options are limited but the treatments listed are of some benefit:

- Topical treatments that may be used under occlusion to make them more effective:
  - Potent topical steroids (in inflammatory rather than atrophic stage).
  - Topical tacrolimus.
- Intralesional steroids.
- Oral steroids.
- Ciclosporin.

Patient concerns

The patient is often very concerned about the appearance and the possibility of the patches ulcerating.

Viva questions

If this lesion was biopsied, what histology would you expect to see?
Palisaded necrobiotic granulomatous inflammation within the dermis. Thickening of small and large vessel walls may be present.

What proportion of patients with necrobiosis lipoidica have diabetes mellitus?
It has been reported that up to 60% of patients have diabetes mellitis. The condition occurs in patients with both type 1 and type 2 diabetes. All patients should therefore be screened for diabetes.

What proportion of diabetics develop necrobiosis lipoidica?
Very few, in the region of 0.5%.

What other skin changes are associated with diabetes mellitus?
- Infections: bacterial (e.g. impetigo, abscesses), fungal (e.g. *Candida*).
- Ulcers: arterial (macrovascular disease) and neuropathic (microvascular disease); ➔ Diabetes mellitus and diabetic foot, p.578.
- Diabetic dermopathy: brown, scaly, indented patches appear most commonly on the shins. These patches do not require treatment and often resolve with improved diabetic control.
- Diabetic bullae: spontaneous blisters on the feet, legs and hands that usually heal spontaneously.
- Diabetic stiff skin: thick, waxy, discoloured (usually yellow) skin can develop over the hands and may result in restricted joint movements (diabetic cheiroarthropathy).
- Granuloma annulare: annular (ring-shaped) erythematous patches. These can be localized or more generalized.

Hereditary haemorrhagic telangiectasia

Hereditary haemorrhagic telangiectasia (HHT), formerly known as Osler–Weber–Rendu syndrome, is an autosomal dominant disorder characterized by epistaxis, cutaneous telangiectasia and visceral arteriovenous malformations.

> **Scenario**
>
> Mrs Judith Ransom, aged 38 years.
>
> This lady has been suffering from recurrent nosebleeds and is breathless on exertion. Please perform a focused history and examination.

History

- Epistaxis: ask about severity and frequency.
- Associated gastrointestinal bleeding.
- Family history.
- Repeated blood transfusions or oral iron therapy.
- Symptoms of cyanosis, fatigue or dyspnoea (pulmonary arteriovenous malformations).
- Recurrent headache or SAH (cerebral arteriovenous malformations – AVMs).

Examination

Skin

- Multiple telangiectasia present on the face, especially around the mouth (Fig. 8.19 ➔ Plate 8).
- Pallor (due to iron deficiency anaemia).

Nails

- Telangiectasia of the nail beds.

Mucosa

- Telangiectasia of the tongue and palate.
- Pale conjunctiva.

Visceral AVMs

- Auscultate for pulmonary bruits (pulmonary AVMs have a predilection for lower lobes) and hepatic bruits.
- Signs of high output cardiac failure caused by left-to-right shunting (occuring between hepatic arteries and hepatic veins in the setting of large hepatic AVM).
- Neurological sequelae of AVMs:
  - Mostly secondary to paradoxical emboli from pulmonary AVMs but may also result from vascular lesions within the brain e.g. leading to SAH.

❶ Top Tips

- Remember to assess for evidence of AVMs in the lungs, liver and brain.

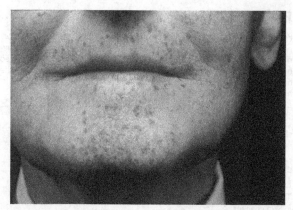

Fig. 8.19 Hereditary haemorrhagic telangiectasia.
With permission from St John's Institute of Dermatology. See also Plate 8.

Treatment

In mild cases, no treatment is needed. Individual lesions may be destroyed with cautery or laser. If epistaxis is problematic (recurrent/extensive) surgery may be needed. Usually treatment is limited to control of secondary anaemia. Pulmonary and other systemic arteriovenous malformations may be amenable to resection, ligation or embolization.

Viva questions

What are the clinical criteria for diagnosis?

Clinical diagnosis is made on the basis of Curacao criteria:
• Epistaxis: spontaneous, recurrent nose bleeds.
• Telangiectases: multiple, at characteristic sites i.e. lips, noses, fingers.
• Visceral lesions: gastrointestinal telangiectasia, pulmonary, hepatic, cerebral and spinal arteriovenous malformations.
• Family history: 1st-degree relative with HHT.

3 criteria indicate a definite diagnosis, 2 a possible or suspected case.

What are the complications of hereditary haemorrhagic telangiectasia?

• Gastrointestinal haemorrhage: AVMs, angiodysplasias and telangiectasias are found throughout the gastrointestinal system.
• Epistaxis.
• Pulmonary AVM resulting in haemoptysis, clubbing and embolic stroke.
• Iron deficiency anaemia.
• Headache and SAH.

What is the pattern of inheritance of hereditary haemorrhagic telangiectasia?

It is autosomal dominant due to mutations in endoglin (*ENG*) on chromosome 9 and activin receptor-like kinase 1 (*ACVRL1*) on chromosome 12.

℘ Useful website

HHT Foundation International: http://www.hht.org

Porphyria cutanea tarda

Porphyria cutanea tarda is caused by a deficiency of the enzyme uroporphyrinogen decarboxylase (UROD) leading to an accumulation of porphyrins in the skin and a resultant photo-induced dermatitis. It is characterized by bullae, milia and scarring over sun-exposed sites, most commonly the hands, forearms, face and ears. The most common form is sporadic; however an autosomal dominant inherited form exists.

> ### Scenario
>
> Mr Clive Brown, aged 45 years
>
> This man has been referred to you with blisters over his hands. Please perform a focused history and examination.

History
The history should focus on:
- Skin changes.
- Site of changes (sun-exposed areas).
- Duration of changes.
- Skin fragility.
- Scarring.
- Pigmentary changes (hyper- or hypopigmentation).
- Hypertrichosis (can occur over cheeks in this condition).
- Pre-disposing factors:
  - Alcohol intake: a high alcohol intake reduces the activity of UROD and hence worsens the condition.
  - History of hepatitis: often associated with the condition, possibly due to increased iron in the liver reducing UROD activity.
  - History of any liver problems e.g. haemochromatosis (for reason stated above).
  - Oestrogens that reduce UROD activity e.g. oral contraceptive pill.
- Previous treatment history (→ Treatment, p.631).
- Any family history of similar skin changes:
  - The condition is commonly sporadic but in order to identify autosomal dominantly inherited cases ask in detail about first degree relatives.

Examination
Look for bullae, erosions, milia, scarring and pigmentary changes in sun-exposed areas. The condition commonly affects the dorsa of the hands, forearms, face and ears but is also common over the lower legs and the dorsa of the feet in women.

Differential diagnosis
- Epidermolysis bullosa: inherited condition which usually presents at a young age and is associated with mechanically (traumatically) induced bullae
- Epidermolysis bullosa acquisita: autoimmune blistering disease affecting the skin (sites of trauma) and mucous membranes (unlike porphyria cutanea tarda)

- Erythropoietic porphyria: as well as cutaneous manifestations, porphyrins are deposited in enamel (teeth fluoresce red under Wood's light), eyes and bones (resulting in contractures and deformities)
- Pseudoporphyria: no actual porphyrin abnormality present in this condition but it mimics the cutaneous features seen in porphyria cutanea tarda:
  - Commonly caused by drugs (NSAIDs, doxycycline, diuretics and the oral contraceptive pill).
  - Occasionally associated with chronic renal failure.

Investigations

- Urine examination: urine fluoresces pink/coral red under Wood's light.
- 24-hour urine (looking for uroporphyrins).
- Skin biopsy (avoid if possible as these patches are prone to breaking down and ulcerating).

❶ Top Tips

- If a diagnosis of porphyria cutanea tarda is made then further investigations to consider would include:
  - Hepatitis screen.
  - Iron/ferritin levels (to exclude haemochromatosis).
  - Alphafetoprotein (to exclude hepatocellular carcinoma).

Treatment

- Removal of all contributory agents (e.g. alcohol and oestrogen-containing medications).
- Sun avoidance.
- Phlebotomy (iron stores in the liver inhibit the UROD enzyme and reducing hepatic iron via phlebotomy increases the activity of this enzyme).
- Anti-malarials (chloroquine) have been successfully used.

Patient concerns

The patient is often very concerned about the appearance and resultant scarring and needs to have the aforementioned management plan explained to them.

Viva questions

What age group is most commonly affected by this condition?

The average age of presentation for the sporadic (most common type) is 45. Familial forms present much earlier, usually by the age of 20.

Do you know some other causes of bullous lesions? (Table 8.17)

Table 8.17 Causes of bullous lesions

Diagnosis	Distinguishing features
Infection (cellulitis/ bullous impetigo)	Bullae localized to area of infection (tender, hot, erythematous, weepy, ± associated fever)
Arthropod bites	Detailed history required; distribution indicative (usually lower limbs)
Drug-induced	Detailed drug history required; may or may not be in sun-exposed areas
Bullous pemphigoid	Autoimmune condition; older age group; tense, fluid filled, intact blisters all over the body, especially acral sites
Pemphigus vulgaris	Autoimmune condition; more superficial, flaccid bullae; not usually intact but seen as superficial erosions
Epidermolysis bullosa	As stated under differential diagnosis
Epidermolysis bullosa acquisita	As stated under differential diagnosis
Stephen–Johnson syndrome/toxic epidermal necrolysis	Flaccid blisters associated with widespread erythema and desquamation; prominent mucosal involvement (eye/mouth/genitals); drug history crucial

MRCPI

Danny Cheriyan
Stephen Patchett

Introduction

The MRCPI part 2 clinical examination is the final hurdle in the membership trilogy, and can be viewed as a practical interview before entering higher specialist training. It is equivalent to the UK PACES; however, there are some important variations in its format, and this chapter will guide a candidate through the appropriate preparation required to succeed in the examination. Unlike the written examination, it affords examiners a relatively short period of time to judge a candidate's history taking and examination skills. They must also evaluate a candidate's ability to formulate differential diagnosis, investigations and management plans. The examiners will also 'get a feel' for the candidate's confidence, and their empathy in dealing with patients.

The examination is generally fair in that the examiners try to find out what the candidate knows, rather than try to catch them out. It is important to realize, however, that each examiner will vary in their personality, patience and style of examining. While some may forgive or overlook an outlandish candidate response during questioning, others may choose to further expose a potential weakness.

Aim

The aim of this chapter is to provide a comprehensive approach to the MRCPI 'long case'. The format and approach to MRCPI short cases will also be addressed in brief. Whilst the basic principles of history taking do not differ between the 2 examinations, it is important to note that candidates are given a fixed 15 minutes for the history-taking station on the PACES examination, whereas MRCPI candidates have 45 minutes for history and examination. In light of this, we have adapted the timing of the history-taking pro forma, permitting a more in-depth exploration of certain aspects of the history.

As a coherent presentation of the history and examination is crucial to the success of the candidate, particular importance has been given to not just *what to say*, but also *how to say it*. The first case, therefore, is a fully detailed dialogue between candidate and patient, and provides a foundation for the general manner of successful history taking. It also emphasizes the importance of using straightforward English to communicate with the patient whilst subsequently using medical terminology in presentation and discussion with the examiners.

MRCPI clinical examination format

5 marks for long case, 5 marks for short cases.

Marking system
- **5: Clear pass.** Competent in all aspects of history, examination, presentation and knowledge. This mark compensates for a 3 (redeemable fail) in the other section of the exam.
- **4: Pass.** Adequate presentation of the case, clinical examination, and clinical acumen; represents achievement of an adequate standard.
- **3: Redeemable.** Overall performance below required standard.
  - For example, this may be due to a poorly presented history (with accurate information), or sub-par knowledge of subject.
  - This mark may be compensated by achieving a 5 in the other section of the exam.
- **2: Fail.** Below standard in all respects.
  - Cannot pass MRCPI clinical with this mark.
- **1: Bad fail.** Candidate lacks skills and knowledge to pass the examination. This candidate will require specific training and supervision prior to retaking the examination.

Must achieve a combined total mark of at least 8 to pass.
- Candidates randomly assigned to long or short cases first.
- Real inpatients for long case.
- Outpatients may be recruited for short cases.

MRCPI short cases

As pathology and clinical signs do not differ between the PACES and MRCPI examinations, the information detailed in previous chapters of this book serve as an excellent adjunct in preparation for the MRCPI short cases. However, there are a few differences in the format of the examination which are detailed as follows:

Candidates will be subject to 5 short cases, each lasting approximately 6 minutes, and marked by 2 examiners. Typically 3 minutes is given to examine the salient features, and 3 minutes are then used for questioning by the examiners. It is important to note that the candidate is given an overall mark (1–5), which has been agreed by both examiners, based on the aforementioned marking scheme.

Typically candidates can expect to be examined on the following disciplines: neurology, respiratory, abdominal, cardiovascular, endocrinology and rheumatology. A patient with a dermatological condition will often have an associated systemic disease e.g. lupus pernio in sarcoidosis. Ophthalmology cases are also likely to be encountered in the context of a systemic illness, such as exophthalmos in thyroid eye disease.

Generally, the spectrum of cases range from spot diagnosis to eliciting physical signs. Cases will also vary from being straightforward to deliberately esoteric and challenging. Each candidate, however, is judged individually on the basis of the cases examined.

Examiners will usually direct candidates at the beginning of each case: 'Can you listen to this gentleman's heart?'. Always make it a point to start with the hands, with the anticipation that you will be moved on 'to the heart' quickly by the examiner. It is better to be directed later than asked if examining the hands is important. It is also crucial to 'read' your examiners, for unlike the PACES exam, the same 2 examiners will be present for each case. If they show frustration with the above method, i.e.: 'I thought I told you to listen to his heart . . .' then learn from this and amend your strategy for the subsequent stations.

❶ Top Tips

- Use observation skills during a focused examination, for example: while listening to the heart, be sure to feel the carotid pulse, assess the JVP, and look around for scars.
- Examiners may ask you to 'First observe, and then proceed with the examination you feel is appropriate'. This may sound difficult, but it is important not to panic. Observe carefully and deliberately. It is entirely reasonable to spend a whole minute (which can feel like an eternity) just looking. If the initial inspection does not reveal any abnormalities, then ask the patient to walk as this may give you a lead. An examiner may not always guide a candidate who chooses to examine the cranial nerves, having failed to notice a prominent goitre.
- Take the examination case by case; if one case seems to go poorly, leave it behind and focus on the next one.

MRCPI long case

Many candidates under-appreciate the importance of practising for the long case, possibly due to the assumption that 'on the job' patient interaction is sufficient. Unfortunately, while under pressure and with the added time constraints of the long case, candidates often find themselves poorly prepared on the day of the examination. Remember, an examiner is quickly able to identify those candidates who have practised time and time again from those who have not.

The remainder of this chapter will help you to prepare for the long case by exploring 15 cases from different disciplines, provide answers to commonly asked questions, and offer valuable insight into varying examiner styles. The cases will all be based on popular inpatient scenarios, and will vary from relatively straightforward to more complex, multisystem processes. In general, patients selected for this part of the examination will be able to give a reasonable history, and will have positive clinical signs.

The following page depicts a generic pro forma with suggested time allocations to various portions of the history. Each of the cases in this chapter also includes helpful questions that can be used to focus a difficult historian or case. The 15 cases included in this chapter will illustrate its application, along with strategies to approach the subsequent physical examination and presentation. This visual reference guide can be applied to almost any history-taking scenario and should be memorized by candidates for reproducibility in the examination, thus providing a structural framework with which the candidate can easily elicit all relevant information.

This timing pro forma is designed as a guide and may require slight deviation from the proposed time allocations. For example, a complex social history may be integral to the patient's overall presentation, and is therefore crucial to explore in more depth. It is imperative to use your judgement and experience to allow for this.

Time management

Each candidate will have 45 minutes of uninterrupted time with the patient prior to the arrival of the examiners. This must be used carefully in order to determine the most important parts of the history, elicit any clinical findings, and finally develop a strategy to present and manage the above. As there is no 'GP letter' or equivalent information sheet to direct the candidate before the long case, it is imperative to adopt a systematic and well-rehearsed approach to ensure the optimal use of time.

The allocated time is best used if divided into sections for:
- History (25 minutes)
- Examination (10–12 minutes)
- Preparation (8–10 minutes).

Long case history pro forma: (total 25 minutes)
(Recommended time in **bold and italics**.)
- Introduction, name, + age:
  - Introduce yourself to patient as always, establish rapport – *be nice!*
  - Let the patient know that you are a doctor trying for a higher qualification in an exam situation (they will have been asked to participate, but may not have understood the significance of the exam).
  - Listen carefully and interrupt appropriately.

❶ Top Tips

- Take *charge* of the history from the start – remember this is *your* exam.

- Presenting complaint (PC) (**1 minute**):
  - 'What brings you in *this* time?'
- History of presenting complaint (HPC) (**7 minutes**):
  - *Logically determine* the history of presenting complaint – have this written in a way you can present appropriately and *efficiently*.
  - Remember that you have a short amount of time to obtain a potentially long list of varied problems.
  - 'When were you last well?'
  - 'Have you attended any consultants or specialists for this/these problems?'
  - 'What was their impression?'
  - 'Did you receive a diagnosis?'
  - 'What treatment have you received? Did they work? (For any previous treatments ascertain why they were discontinued e.g. side effects, failure of treatment – primary or secondary.)
  - 'What investigations/scans have you had on this admission? Previously?'
  - 'How has this problem(s) affected your life – *what does it stop you from doing?*'
  - Complications of disease; complications (e.g. retinopathy in diabetes); monitoring of treatment and related conditions (e.g. other autoimmune diseases in a patient with hypothyroidism).
- Past medical history (PMHx) (**6 minutes**):
  - 'Do you have any other illnesses?' Make sure to cover all the common medical conditions (hypertension, diabetes mellitus, ischaemic heart disease, thyroid disease, rheumatic fever, epilepsy, TB).
  - If the patient has other coexistent conditions, ask questions to establish the duration, severity, complications, monitoring and treatment followed by relevant questions to a particular disease (for example: a diabetic patient should be asked specifically about blood glucose levels, HbA1c and hypoglycaemic episodes).
  - 'Have you ever been admitted to hospital in the past?' This question can yield surprising amounts of information.
  - 'Do you regularly go to any outpatient clinics?'

- Medications (**2 minutes**):
  - Be sure to comment on duration of treatment – e.g. iv antibiotics.
  - Medications prior to admission – have these changed now; if so, why?
  - Compliance.
  - Herbal remedies or over-the-counter medications.
  - Side effects of current medications, or other common medication classes (beta-blockers, statins).
  - Allergies.

❶ Top Tips

- If present, look at the medication record at the end of the bed.

- Social history (SHx) (**2 minutes**):
  - Smoking/alcohol/recreational drug use.
  - Employment, hobbies.
  - Do you live in a house or a bungalow?
  - 'Who is at home with you?' especially important for elderly patients.
  - 'Who visits you?'
  - 'Do you have enough support?'
  - Independence in activities of daily life.
  - Ask about sexual history if appropriate.
- Family history (FHx) (**1 minute**):
  - FHx should be limited to siblings, parents and 1st-degree relatives.
  - Age of onset of a chronic disease and age at time of death.
  - 'Is there anyone else in your family with this problem?'
  - Cancer.
  - Young/sudden deaths – particularly in cardiac cases.
- Systems review (ROS) (**2 minutes**):
  - *Quickly* cover each system.
  - Important not to get stuck here, as the majority of the problems should have already been elicited.
- Recap and final details (**4 minutes**):
  - Clarify details of HPC if there is time: 'Let me see if I have this right . . .'
  - 'Do you think I've missed anything?'
  - Is there anything else you need to tell me?
  - Here is a good time to ask about the plan for the patients hospital stay:
    – 'Has the team told you how long you will be in for?'
    – 'What tests are you waiting to have, or what results are awaited?'
    – If the patient is to be discharged shortly, what follow-up has been arranged?

❶ Top Tips

- Enquire about *multidisciplinary involvement*: 'Have you been seen by a physiotherapist, occupational therapist, dietician or social worker?'

Physical examination

A focused examination can and should be carried out in 10–12 minutes, and specific attention should be given to the organ system(s) pertaining to the history. Having a systematic method of examination will greatly reduce chances of missing an important clinical finding that may not have been detailed in the history. The following is a general approach to physical examination that can be applied to every case:

General examination

- Start from the end of the bed; look for clues around the bed (oxygen, walking stick, wheelchair, non-invasive positive pressure ventilation (NIPPV) machine, IV fluids).
- Note vital signs (BP, pulse, oxygen saturation, temperature).
- Quickly determine the patient's cognitive state (this should already have been noted during history taking). A formal mini-mental test score is useful to document if cognitive decline is suspected.
- Obvious scars, swellings.

> **❶ Top Tips**
>
> - It is important to be case specific. For example, if a patient had been on methotrexate as part of her treatment, it would be important to rule out clinically demonstrable side effects such as lung fibrosis and peripheral neuropathy.
> - The cardiovascular and respiratory systems are relatively succinct, and signs such as a murmur, an irregular pulse or Velcro-like crackles on auscultation should be elicited.
> - In diabetic patients fundoscopy should be attempted.
> - Peak flow should be performed in respiratory cases (or at least requested, along with a sputum sample).
> - Performing a detailed neurological examination in all cases will not be practical due to given time constraints.

Each of the illustrated cases that follow will highlight the key examination findings relevant to the particular case, as well as secondary or dual pathologies such as pulmonary fibrosis associated with rheumatoid arthritis.

General examination points

- *Physical status:*
  - Nutritional state
  - BMI (kg/m^2)
  - Pigmentation, jaundice, rashes
- *Hands:*
  - Clubbing
  - Deformity (symmetrical or asymmetrical)
  - Dupuytren's contracture
  - Leuconychia, koilonychia
  - Stigmata of infective endocarditis
  - Tar staining
  - Asterixis
  - Check pulse (rate, rhythm, character, radial-radial delay)
- *Head/neck/face:*
  - Cushingoid appearance
  - Icterus
  - Butterfly rash
  - Proptosis
  - Inspect mouth, dentition
  - Goitre
  - JVP
  - carotid pulse
  - Lymphadenopathy
- *Cardiovascular (CVS):*
  - Inspect closely for sternotomy or pacemaker scar
  - Apex beat
  - Heart sounds, murmurs, added sounds
- *Respiratory:*
  - Closely inspect for scars
  - Chest expansion
  - Percuss and auscultate lung fields
- *Abdominal:*
  - Scars
  - Organomegaly
  - Masses
  - Ascites
  - Caput medusae
  - Hernias
- *Central and peripheral nervous system (CNS and PNS):*
  - Cranial nerves II–XII
  - Peripheral sensation, motor function, coordination and reflexes
  - Gait where appropriate.

Preparation

At this stage approximately 35 minutes should have passed, leaving the candidate with 8–10 minutes to prepare prior to the arrival of the examiners. This time, though short, will make a significant difference to the overall examination. It is during this time that the presentation of the history and examination needs to be planned. Differential diagnosis, investigation and management should be considered. This is also a perfect opportunity to anticipate the often predictable questions that may arise pertaining to the case.

Finally, the examiners will have approximately 30 minutes with the candidate, during which time they will evaluate the history, assess clinical examination skills and test clinical acumen. Examiners are requested to give the candidates 8–10 minutes of uninterrupted time to present the case. The presentation of the history and clinical findings is perhaps the most important part of the examination. As each examiner has a different approach to questioning, it is important to practise presenting to a variety of senior colleagues to experience this spectrum.

℘ Useful website

MRCPI Part II General Medicine Clinical website: http://www.rcpi.ie/Examinations/Pages/ MRCPIPartIIGeneralMedicineClinical.aspx.

Case 1: Primary biliary cirrhosis (fully dialogued)

Candidate: *Good morning, my name is Dr. David Brown, thank you for agreeing to participate in this exam.*

Patient: No problem.

I might just quickly tell you that this exam is a very important part of our training, and I only have a short time to gather as much information about your medical history as possible. I may interrupt you from time to time, but it's only in the interest of getting the whole story. Please tell me if there is anything I miss or anything you feel is particularly important. After the history, I'll examine you as well. Is that ok with you?

Sure, that's fine doctor, go ahead.

Great, I'll start by taking your full name, age, and where you're from please.

Ms Sandra Murphy, I'm 45 and I'm from Dublin.

Ok Ms Murphy, may I ask you when and why you came into hospital on this occasion?

Well I've been unwell for a long time really. I was admitted 3 days ago. I've had liver problems for some time.

I see . . . But what was it in particular that made you come into hospital this time?

I've just been feeling more and more tired. I can't do anything at all.

I'm sorry to hear that. I'll get back to that in one moment if you don't mind – you said that your liver was the problem. Have you been attending a consultant's clinic for this problem?

Yes I have – Dr. Cole . . . I usually see him about once a month. In fact my GP called him up because he thought I looked dreadful, and I was told to come into the hospital.

I see . . . were you ever told what was wrong with your liver?

He said it was primary biliary cirrhosis (PBC) about 4 years ago. He told me it was to do with my immune system.

I understand. So you've been feeling very tired of late. Do you remember when you last felt well?

I was actually doing pretty well until the last month . . . then I just started getting progressively weaker.

---

❶ Top Tips

- Try to ask one question at a time, otherwise the patient may not give all the required information*!

(*Multiple questions may be asked in this sample case in the interest of space.)

Is your appetite gone? Have you lost weight?

Yes, I just don't have the taste for food, and I've lost about 1 stone in the last few weeks.

Have you been feeling sickly or even vomited? And has your bowel habit changed at all?

I feel a bit nauseated at the moment, but I haven't vomited. My stools are just the same.

Do you have any other complaints? Like pain, cough, fevers or itch?

Well I'm always itchy, but it is manageable. No pain, cough or fevers.

Do you have problems with a dry mouth or dry eyes?

Actually my eyes have been very dry recently too – I don't know why that is.

Any joint stiffness or pains?

Not particularly.

PMHx

Do you have any other medical conditions, Ms Murphy?

I have diabetes and high blood pressure.

When were you diagnosed with diabetes?

I was told that I only have mild diabetes about a year ago, it was picked up by chance. I'm just watching my diet.

I see, so do you check your blood sugars or take medications for it? Have you been seen by a diabetic specialist?

No, my GP takes care of it mostly.

Have you had your eyes checked within the last year?

No.

How about your blood pressure? Is it well controlled?

I'm not sure, I think so.

Have you had your thyroid function checked before?

I must have, but I'm not sure.

Ok . . . just a few more questions; have you had any other problems such as with your heart, asthma or high cholesterol?

I used to have high cholesterol, but now I take a tablet for it.

Have you been admitted for any operations or other procedures?

Well I had a camera test to look into my stomach 2 years ago, but I wasn't kept in for it. And I had a hysterectomy after the birth of my third child.

Did the doctors remove your ovaries?

I don't think so.

May I ask you what medications you take?

In the morning I take aspirin 75mg, one tablet of ramipril, ursodeoxycholic acid 250mg, colestyramine 2g, and Calogen®. I take another ursodeoxychoic acid 250mg at lunch and again at dinner. I take one more sachet of the colestyramine and atorvastatin 20mg at night.

Do you know what dose of ramipril you take?

No, it's just one tablet, sorry.

> **❶ Top Tips**
>
> * It is likely that patients will use commercial names such as Questran® and Ursofalk® instead of generic ones. *It is important to present generic names.*
> * Always check for a medication record at the end of the bed, and enquire if this list includes any new medications which have been commenced since admission.
> * Patients may not recall all dosages, and it is acceptable to state this.
> * If there is no record available, and the patient is not sure, prompt them with questions such as: 'do you take any blood pressure tablets, water tablets, tablets for cholesterol . . . etc.'

Thank you. Do you take any over-the-counter medications or herbal remedies?

No.

Are you allergic to any medications?

Not that I'm aware of.

Ok, just a few more questions, we're nearly there. Are you a smoker?

No, I never smoked.

How about alcohol, how many drinks would you have in a week?

I'd say on average about 4 glasses of red wine.

Are you working at the moment?

Yes I'm a librarian, but I've missed so much work because I've been unwell . . . and I get paid by the hour which doesn't help.

Are you finding it difficult to cope with finances because you are missing work?

Actually I recently received an inheritance from an aunt, so I'm fine for the moment.

I see. Are you married? Any children?

I got divorced 5 years ago, and I have 3 children living with me.

Ok. But do you feel like you need additional support at home at present?

No, my sister and her husband have been great, they help out loads with the kids. In fact, my kids are staying with them now.

That's very helpful. Do you have any family history of PBC?

Yes – two of my aunts on my mother's side had it, one of them passed away last year. She was 62.

I see. Are your parents alive? Are they well?

My mother is healthy at 82. My father died at 40, I think it was a heart attack.

I see. Is there any other medical illness in your family? Is there any history of thyroid disease, diabetes or lupus?

My sister has diabetes, she was diagnosed about 4 years ago and takes tablets.

Summary/recap

So Ms Murphy I'll just quickly go over what you've told me to make sure I have it right . . . you have a diagnosis of primary biliary cirrhosis for which you see Dr. Cole. You had been relatively well until last month, after which you began to feel excessively tired, lose your appetite, and lose weight. You also feel nauseated, but haven't been vomiting.

Have I missed anything or do you want to add anything more?

No I think you've covered it all really.

May I ask you then what has happened since your admission here . . . have you had blood tests or scans performed?

I've been getting bloods done every day, but I don't know what the results are yet. I had a scan of my tummy today, and I'm waiting for the result.

I see. Have you been seen by a dietician, physiotherapist, occupational therapist or social worker?

Yes, a dietician saw me and I've been given some extra drinks to take now.

Ok. You've been very helpful – I think I have asked all the questions I need for now. Would you mind if I go on to examine you?

No problem, go ahead.

Examination

At this stage approximately 25 minutes should have passed, leaving you with a further 20 for examination and preparation.

Examination should proceed in the format previously mentioned (starting with general inspection and moving to the hands etc.). This particular patient has liver pathology and therefore the following items must also be specifically addressed:

Specific examination points
- *General:*
  - Jaundice
  - Icterus
  - Spider naevi
  - Pigmentation
  - Scratch marks
- *Hands:*
  - Clubbing
  - Leuconychia

> - Dupuytren's contracture
> - Palmar erythema
> - Hepatic flap
> - Abdomen:
>   - Ascites
>   - Caput medusae
>   - Hepatomegaly
>   - Splenomegaly
>   - Testicular atrophy – male.

In view of her diabetes, it is warranted to check for peripheral neuropathy and perform fundoscopy. **Please note that it is not appropriate to perform genital or internal examination for the purpose of the MRCPI clinical examination.**

Thank you very much for your time Ms Murphy, I really appreciate it. If you don't mind, I'm going to take a few minutes just to compile my notes before the examiners arrive. If you feel like adding anything please do let me know.

At this stage, approximately 35 minutes should have passed, leaving the candidate with 8–10 minutes to prepare.

❶ Top Tips

- Though examiners may vary in style, they must mark candidates on 4 primary areas. These are:
  - Presentation of history (systematic presentation, accuracy)
  - Communication skills (with examiners, and patient)
  - Physical examination
  - Management and acumen
- The candidate will be given an overall mark of 1–6, agreed by both examiners, and based on these 4 categories.

Examiners arrive

Examiners: Ok Dr. Brown, talk me through your history and examination. Keep it brief please.

This is Ms Sandra Murphy, a 45-year-old lady from Dublin with known primary biliary cirrhosis, diagnosed 4 years ago. During a recent visit to her GP, she was advised to come into hospital for admission. She has been complaining of increasing fatigue and general malaise for the last month. She has a decreased appetite and has lost approximately 1 stone in this time period. She also complains of nausea and pruritus, but denies any vomiting, altered bowel habit, or any other specific symptoms such as pain, cough or fevers.

Her past medical history is significant for non-insulin dependent diabetes, hypertension and hypercholesterolemia. She has previously undergone a hysterectomy. Her diabetes was diagnosed approximately 1 year ago on routine testing; she does not check her blood sugars and is not taking oral hypoglycaemia agents. She has not had an ophthalmology review in the last year. The BP chart at end of bed shows her to be hypertensive since her admission. Both her diabetes and her hypertension appear to be under the supervision of the GP.

- *Medications:*

  - Aspirin 75mg OD
  - Ramipril 5mg OD
  - Atorvastatin 20mg OD
  - Ursodeoxycholic acid 250mg TDS
  - Colestyramine 2g BD
  - Calogen 30mL TDS
  - No allergies
- *FHx:*

  - 2 aunts have PBC
  - Sister has DM
  - Father had MI at 40
- *SHx:*

  - Mother of 3 (A+W), divorced
  - Librarian
  - Non-smoker
  - 8 units alcohol per week
  - No recreational drug use, no IVDU
  - 2-storey house, lives in Dublin, with kids
  - Not sexually active
  - Independent in activities of daily life (ADL)
  - Does not need support at present
- *ROS:*

  - Nil else of note

Medications listed above to be detailed by candidate at this point.

Ms Murphy has 2 aunts with PBC, one who died last year aged 62. Her mother is 82 and well, but her father died at age 40 of a presumed myocardial infarction. She also has a sister with non-insulin dependent diabetes.

In her social history, Ms Murphy is a divorced mother of 3, and she works as a librarian. Of late she has been missing work due to ill health. She is a non-smoker and consumes about 8 units of alcohol per week. Her sister helps to look after her children on a regular basis. She claims to have no financial difficulties and is not looking for extra support at present.

Her systems review was non-contributory.

***On examination** Ms Murphy was comfortable, but was notably cachectic. She was hypertensive with a BP of 165/90, and her pulse was regular at 72bpm. Her oxygen saturations and temperature were normal. There is generalized hyperpigmentation. She was alert, oriented and appropriate. Of note she has a cannula in her right antecubital fossa, through which she is receiving normal saline.*

She has clubbing and palmar erythema, but no evidence of asterixis. There are visible scratch marks and bruises on her arms. She has scleral icterus and multiple spider naevi on her upper chest. Her abdomen was soft with no evidence of ascites. She does, however have hepatomegaly, which appears to be nodular towards the midline. There was no evidence of caput medusae, and there was no other organomegaly.

Her cardiovascular examination yielded a grade 3/6 pan systolic murmur in the mitral area. She is in sinus rhythm and there is no evidence of cardiac failure. Her respiratory examination was unremarkable.

Neurological examination revealed moderate proximal myopathy in her shoulders and hips, but was otherwise normal.

Examination of her neck did not reveal a goitre, and she is clinically euthyroid. Fundoscopy was also normal.

In summary, Ms Murphy is a 45-year-old lady with PBC who has been feeling increasingly fatigued and is losing weight. She is also exhibiting symptoms of sicca syndrome. She is visibly cachectic and icteric and has evidence of nodular hepatomegaly. There is no evidence of hepatic encephalopathy. Of note she is also diabetic, hypertensive and has proximal myopathy.

---

❶ Top Tips

- Although the examiner has asked the candidate to present the history and findings, there is no reason to stop here. In fact, one should proceed with differential diagnosis, investigation and management unless stopped.

My differential diagnosis would include:
- *Hepatic malignancy, which could be either primary or secondary*
- *Progression of PBC*
- *Addison's disease*
- *Sicca syndrome/Sjogren's syndrome*
- *Subacute infective endocarditis*
- *Thyroid dysfunction.*

I would proceed to fully investigate this patient for these, along with a thorough evaluation of her hypertension, diabetic status and cardiac murmur.

Investigations (laboratory)
- FBC, LFT, U&E, albumin, Ca/PO_4/Mg^{2+}, Coagulation screen
- ESR, CRP
- Alpha fetoprotein
- Fasting lipids and blood sugar
- TFT
- HbA1C
- Hepatitis serology
- Autoimmune screen including anti-Ro and La antibodies (if these are not already known)
- Short Synacthen® test
- ACTH and cortisol levels
- Blood cultures
- 24-hour urinary protein
- Albumin-creatinine ratio

Investigations (other)
- CXR
- CT abdomen (triphasic CT for liver) ± MRI liver
- Liver biopsy (ultrasound- or CT-guided) if imaging yields a mass
- Oesophago-gastro-duodenoscopy (OGD)

- ECG and echocardiogram
- 24-hour ambulatory BP monitoring.

At this stage, it is likely that the examiners will ask questions either pertaining to the primary issue or secondary diagnosis. It is also possible for the examiner to ask the candidate to demonstrate a physical examination.

Viva questions

How do you diagnose PBC? What are the various stages of PBC?

- Antimitochondrial antibody (AMA) +ve; M2 subtype is highly specific.
- Raised alkaline phosphatase and GGT, mildly elevated AST and ALT.
- Raised immunoglobulins – particularly IgM.
- Liver biopsy, although not always required, shows granulomas around bile ducts.
- Stage 1: asymptomatic with abnormal liver function tests.
- Stage 2: symptomatic – lethargy, pruritis is prominent.
- Stage 3: decompensated PBC – ascites, jaundice, portal hypertension.

How is PBC usually treated?

- Ursodeoxycholic acid is the mainstay of treatment.
- The only known cure is liver transplantation.
- 5-year survival following transplantation is in excess of 80%.
- Other treatments are occasionally tried such as steroids, methotrexate or ciclosporin, but vast majority of patients remain on bile salt therapy alone.

What are some common associations with PBC?

- Sicca syndrome/Sjögren's (80%)
- Thyroid dysfunction, Raynaud's, arthralgias (20%)
- Addisons, SLE, myasthenia gravis (rare).

What factors would influence this patient's requirements for liver transplantation?

Signs and symptoms of end-stage liver disease:
- Increasing bilirubin with serum bilirubin >170 µmol/L
- Intractable ascites, recurrent spontaneous bacterial peritonitis (SBP)
- Encephalopathy
- Hepatopulmonary syndrome
- Incidental hepatocellular carcinoma
- Intractable pruritis and lethargy.

Please show us how you would demonstrate shifting dullness and asterixis in this patient

- ➔ Page 103 (shifting dullness) and 107 (asterixis).

We have just discovered that this lady has meticillin-resistant Staphylococcus aureus (MRSA) on a nasal swab. Would you tell her?

- She is entitled to know that she has MRSA.
- It is *important to reassure* her that MRSA, although notorious in the media, is usually harmless to most patients. The reason for concern is that it can cause potentially serious infection in patients who are immunocompromised.

- In accordance with hospital policy, we will treat her with nasal mupirocin (Bactroban®) and encourage the staff to use barrier protection (gloves and aprons) until she is clear on repeat swab.

Please obtain consent from this patient for a gastroscopy
- Explain indication (e.g. weight loss, decreased appetite, epigastric pain).
- Possibility of receiving intravenous sedatives/anxiolytics (midazolam).
- Biopsy.
- Complications are infrequent and usually minor (bleeding, infection, perforation, side effects of medication).
- Any questions?

Case 2: Stroke

> **History (key points: 25 minutes)**
>
> Mrs Samantha Parks.
>
> 68 years old.
>
> From Limerick.
>
> Brought into hospital by ambulance 2 weeks ago with left-sided weakness.

HPC
- Woke up 2 weeks ago with headache at 6am.
- Headache mild (3/10 severity) and global.
- Unable to get out of bed due to weakness in left arm and left leg.
- Decreased sensation left arm and face.
- Decreased vision, unable to quantify further.
- Husband noticed left facial droop.
- Slurred speech.
- Complained of nausea, but no vomiting.
- No loss of continence or seizure activity.
- Had been well the previous night – went to bed at 10pm.

> **❶ Top Tips**
>
> - Obtaining the precise time of symptom onset is crucial to the diagnosis and management of stroke.
> - The fact that this patient went to sleep at 10pm on the previous night and woke at 6am with symptoms rules out the option of thrombolysis.

PMHx
- 2 brief episodes of slurred speech in the last 6 months.
- AF past 8 years.
- Unsuccessful elective direct current cardioversion × 2.
- Hypertension.
- Previous history of alcohol abuse – stopped drinking 4 years ago.
- No history of diabetes, angina, intermittent claudication or abdominal aortic aneurysm (AAA).

❶ Top Tips

- In patients with AF, it is important to determine the duration, previous investigations (Holter, echocardiogram), procedures (MAZE, direct current cardioversion) and complications (direct or secondary to medications).
- In this case, it is important to know the presentation and subsequent management of the previous TIAs.

Medications

- Aspirin 300mg OD (stopped on admission)
- Digoxin 125µg OD
- Lansoprazole 30mg OD
- Ramipril 2.5mg OD
- Amiodarone 200mg OD (stopped 5 days ago)
- Dipyridamole/aspirin 200/25mg OD
- Atorvastatin 40mg OD (new)
- Folic acid 5mg OD (new)
- Nil known drug allergies.

❶ Top Tips

- If a patient is not taking a medication which you think is indicated, then ask them why. Why was this patient not on warfarin?

SHx

- Married, no children.
- Lives in 2-storey house with husband.
- Never smoked.
- History of alcohol abuse (>80 units per week for 10 years).
- Stopped drinking 4 years ago, still attends Alcoholics Anonymous.
- Retired 10 years ago (legal secretary).
- Independent in ADLs until admission.

FHx

- Father died when she was very young – unknown cause.
- Mother died following CVA aged 74.
- 1 younger sister (59) with SLE.

Systems review

- Non contributory.

Hospital management as per patient

- Blood tests
- CXR
- CT brain, refused MRI (severe claustrophobia)
- Carotid duplex/Doppler ultrasound
- Echocardiogram
- Physiotherapy
- Speech and language therapist
- Occupational therapist.

Examination: 10–12 minutes

Perform general examination as detailed on ➲ p.640.

Specific examination points

- *General:*
  - Note dominant hand
  - Nutritional status
  - Facial asymmetry
  - Obvious flexion/spastic posture
  - Note wheelchair/walking aid
- *CNS:*
  - Examine all cranial nerves
  - Carefully assess for hemianopias or diplopia
  - Assess speech
  - Assess cerebellar function
- *Fundoscopy:*
  - Hypertensive retinopathy
- *PNS:*
  - Tone, power, sensation, coordination and reflexes in 4 limbs
  - Assess gait if feasible
- *Cardiovascular:*
  - Pulse for AF
  - Carotid bruits
  - Cardiac murmurs
  - Peripheral pulses
- *Abdomen:*
  - Signs of chronic liver disease
  - AAA.

---

❶ Top Tips

- Look around the bed for clues such as wheelchairs, walking aids, signs for 'thickened fluids', all of which provide crucial information regarding the status of the patient.
- Sensory deficits (particularly joint position sense) are important in rehabilitation.

Summary

Mrs Parks is a 68-year-old lady who was brought into hospital with mild headache, left-sided weakness with paraesthesia, decreased vision and slurred speech. She was asymptomatic the previous night, and woke at 6am with these symptoms. Mrs Parks has presented to this hospital twice in the last 6 months with left facial droop and slurred speech, which were diagnosed as TIAs.

Her past medical history is significant for AF (8 years) which has been persistent despite 2 elective cardioversions. She also has hypertension, and a previous history of alcohol abuse.

On presentation Mrs Parks was on digoxin 125µg OD, aspirin 300mg OD, ramipril 2.5mg OD and amiodarone 200mg OD. Since admission her amiodarone and aspirin have been stopped, with the addition of dipyridamole/aspirin 200/25mg, atorvastatin 40mg OD and folic acid 5mg OD. She informs me that she previously took warfarin, but this was discontinued 6 years ago as the levels were 'difficult to control'. I suspect this was largely due to her heavy alcohol intake. Mrs Parks is a non-smoker, but had a 10-year history of alcohol abuse, which began following the death of her mother. She stopped drinking 4 years ago and still attends Alcoholics Anonymous. She is married and lives in a 2-storey house with her husband, who is fit and well. She has a positive family history for stroke (mother) and SLE (sister).

On examination, Mrs Parks has a left hemiplegic posture with notable facial asymmetry with smoothening of the nasolabial fold on the left. She has a walking aid next to her bed. She has an irregular pulse with a rate of approximately 80bpm and a right carotid bruit. Positive central neurological findings include a left homonymous hemianopia, left-sided neglect, left upper motor neuron facial nerve palsy with forehead sparing, and mild dysarthria. She has no evidence of receptive or expressive dysphasia, and though not examined, her swallow is intact. Peripherally she has increased tone and hyper-reflexia in the left arm and leg. Her left plantar is upgoing. The power has returned to normal in her leg; however her left arm remains 4/5 particularly on shoulder abduction and elbow extension. I do note that she is right handed. Her coordination and sensation are normal, and her handwriting is intact.

Despite her history of alcohol abuse, she has no history of cerebellar dysfunction or stigmata of chronic liver disease. Her cardiac and peripheral vascular examinations were unremarkable.

Differential diagnosis
- Non-dominant (right) anterior circulation embolic stroke
- Non-dominant (right) cerebral haemorrhage
- Tumour
- Subdural haematoma
- Encephalitis
- Connective tissue disease/vasculitis
- Temporal arteritis.

Investigations
- *Blood:* FBC, U&E, LFT, ESR, coagulation profile, fasting lipids + glucose, syphilis serology, autoimmune screen, TFT (on amiodarone).
- *Radiology:* CT brain (non contrast) ± MRI/MRA, carotid duplex, CXR.
- *Cardiac:* ECG, TOE.

Management
The onset of symptoms and time of presentation will greatly affect the management of acute stroke. Please refer to ➍ Stroke, p.323.

Viva questions
Have you heard of any recent developments in improving stroke treatment and outcome in Ireland?
The Irish Heart Foundation (IHF) recently published a 16-point manifesto which aims to improve treatment and outcomes in patients with stroke.

This manifesto covers improving patient education, improved medical diagnosis, dedicated stroke units, and improved patient after care services. This recent manifesto, published in November 2009 was prompted by the IHF National Audit of stroke care in 2008.

How would you best manage this lady's atrial fibrillation in this context?

This lady has twice failed cardioversion, and is not suitable to warfarin due to a long history of compliance issues. She also had a stroke while taking aspirin 300mg OD. AF increases the risk of stroke by 3–5% per year compared to the general population. While aspirin reduces this risk, it does not confer the same risk reduction as warfarin. Another consideration for this patient may be a MAZE procedure, ablation, or PLATO device as she has had unsuccessful cardioversions.[1,2]

This lady has a right-sided carotid bruit. Would you recommend an endarterectomy?

Carotid stenosis is an important risk factor for the development of stroke. The presence of AF is a complicating factor here, as the embolus may have been cardiac in origin. A TOE is required to rule out any cardiac thrombus. If this patient, on MR angiography or carotid duplex displayed >70% narrowing of the appropriate artery, then surgery would be recommended. If the stenosis is <70%, medical management, such as aspirin ± antiplatelet agents are recommended.[3]

Please examine this patient's lower limb proprioception.

Refer to ➔ p.312.

References

1. Wolf PA et al. Duration of atrial fibrillation and imminence of stroke: the Framingham study. *Stroke* 1983; **14**(5):664–7.
2. Hart RG et al. Meta-analysis: antithrombotic therapy to prevent stroke in patients who have nonvalvular atrial fibrillation. *Ann Intern Med* 2007; **146**(12):857–67.
3. Chaturvedi S et al. Carotid endarterectomy – an evidence-based review: report of the Therapeutics and Technology Assessment Subcommittee of the American Academy of Neurology. *Neurology* 2005; **65**(6):794–801.

✍ Useful website

Irish Heart Foundation website: http://www.irishheart.ie/.

Case 3: Optic neuritis

> **History (key points to elicit in 25 minutes)**
>
> Ms Susan O'Callaghan.
> 33 years old.
> From Dublin.
> Presented into A&E 3 days ago with blurred vision in her right eye.

HPC

- Noticed blurred vision with mild discomfort in right eye while driving to work in the morning (8am).
- Eyesight was normal the previous night, and on waking that morning.
- Eye not injected, inflamed or itchy.
- No diplopia.
- Vision became progressively worse over the next few hours, and at lunch time, she was advised to go to hospital by her colleagues.
- No headache, nausea, dizziness or tinnitus.
- No muscle weakness or sensory loss.
- Speech unaffected.
- No bladder or bowel incontinence.
- No recent history of flu like illness or travel.
- Only other complaint is worsening fatigue over last few weeks, which she attributed to her stressful job.
- 'Has never been to hospital before this.'

❶ Top Tips

- Perhaps the most important question in a case of suspected optic neuritis is a history of other neurological problems, such as sensory deficits, muscle weakness or incoordination in the past (which may or may not have been investigated).

PMHx

- Nil.

Medications

- Methylprednisolone 250mg IV QDS (day 3)
- Nil known drug allergies.

SHx

- Married, no children
- Uses barrier contraception
- Lives with husband in apartment
- Non-smoker
- Alcohol – 18 units/week
- Solicitor
- Sails competitively
- Plays league tennis weekly
- 'I love sports.'

> **① Top Tips**
> - Including details such as hobbies in the social history demonstrates important insight into the impact that a chronic disease can have both socially as well as professionally.
> - A patient who has an affected relative may have significantly greater anxiety regarding the disease course and outcome.

FHx
- Parents alive and well
- Sister (38) has psoriasis
- Maternal aunt (54) has MS – wheelchair bound.

ROS
- Non-contributory.

> **① Top Tips**
> - While this history may be highly suggestive of a demyelinating process, be sure to not to miss other potential causes for symptoms.
> - Her fatigue in this instance warrants thorough questioning to rule out thyroid dysfunction.

Hospital course
- Ophthalmology review, detailed eye examination (including formal visual field tests)
- Visual evoked potentials (awaited)
- MRI brain
- Blood tests
- Lumbar puncture
- Urine sample.

Examination (10–12 minutes)
Perform general examination as detailed on ➔ p.640. The following points are a guide to general neurology/ophthalmology examination and can be applied to this case.

> **Specific examination points**
> - *General:*
>   - Nutritional status
>   - Hand dominance
>   - Facial asymmetry
>   - Obvious flexion/spastic posture
>   - Note wheelchair/walking aid
> - *CNS:*
>   - Examine all cranial nerves, with particular emphasis on II, III, IV and V
>   - Assess speech
>   - Assess cerebellar function (PINARDS: *P*ast pointing, *I*ntention tremor, *N*ystagmus, *A*taxia, *R*omberg's test, *D*ysdiadochokinesia, *S*taccato speech)

- *Eyes:*
  - Visual acuity – pocket Snellen chart
  - Visual fields and eye movements
  - Colour vision – Ishihara cards (colour vision is often reduced in optic neuritis)
  - Fatiguability
  - Pupils (equal, round, reactive, accommodation)
  - Pupillary light reaction is often decreased in the affected eye, resulting in a relative afferent papillary defect (RAPD – Marcus Gunn pupil)
  - Fundoscopy (optic atrophy).
- *PNS:*
  - Tone, power, sensation, coordination and reflexes in 4 limbs
  - Assess gait
- *Cardiovascular:*
  - Pulse for AF
  - Carotid bruits
  - Cardiac murmurs.

Thyroid status: ➔, p.590.

❶ Top Tips

- Even though the pupils may not be adequately dilated, it is critical examine the fundus, and state that you have done so if appropriate to the case.

Summary

Mrs O'Callaghan is a 33-year-old solicitor from Dublin who presented into A&E 3 days ago with decreased vision in her right eye. It became progressively worse over the next few hours, and was associated with mild discomfort behind her eye. Her vision was normal that morning on waking, and she had never had this problem before. She denied diplopia, headache or dizziness. She denies muscular weakness, sensory deficits or problems with speech. She has no previous neurological complaints such as weakness or paraesthesia. Her other primary complaint is fatigue, which has been worsening over the last few weeks; however she attributes this to a stressful job. She has not been exhibiting any other classical features of thyroid dysfunction.

Mrs O'Callaghan has no significant medical history, no drug allergies and was on no medications on presentation to hospital. She is currently on day 3 of IV methylprednisolone 250mg QDS.

She is married and lives with her husband. They have no children. She is a non-smoker and drinks alcohol in moderation. She is a very active person – sailing and playing tennis competitively. She has a positive family history of MS in her maternal aunt, who is now wheelchair bound. Her systems review was non-contributory.

On examination Mrs O'Callaghan has a relative afferent pupillary defect affecting her right eye. Her visual acuity in her right eye is reduced at 6/12, but appears to have improved significantly since her admission. The acuity in her left eye was normal (6/6). Her cranial, cerebellar and peripheral neurological examinations were otherwise unremarkable. Her pulse is regular at 78bpm; she has no cardiac murmurs and no carotid bruits.

> **❶ Top Tips**
>
> • Aim to present positive findings confidently and precisely. As the rest of this patients' neurological examination was normal, it is perfectly acceptable to state it as described above. An examiner may get frustrated listening to detailed accounts of each 'normal' examination.
> • If you are asked specifically about a part of the examination, such as the cerebellar examination, it is then expected to discuss the components of the examination in detail (even if normal).

Differential diagnosis

• Optic neuritis affecting the right eye, which may be a presentation of MS.
• Compressive (pituitary lesion) or ischaemic optic neuropathy.
• Vascular occlusion, which generally results in sudden loss of vision (venous more common than arterial in younger age group). If venous occlusion, look for underlying causes (such as SLE and Behçet's disease).
• Sphenoidal wing meningioma.
• Acute disseminated encephalomyelitis (ADEM).
• Space-occupying lesion.

Investigations

• *Blood:* FBC, U&E, LFT, coagulation profile, ESR, CRP, $Ca^{2+}/PO_4/Mg^{2+}$, TFT, autoimmune screen, B12, folate.
• *CSF:* oligoclonal bands, elevated total protein (may be normal) with raised IgG index, raised myelin basic protein.
• *Radiology:* MRI brain with and without gadolinium (gadolinium is thought to enhance active lesions). High-resolution slices through optic nerves and chiasm should be requested.[1]
• *Others:* evoked potential testing (visual – most sensitive, auditory, somatosensory) can be helpful in diagnosing clinically silent lesions.

Management

Optic neuritis

The Optic Neuritis Treatment Trial (ONTT) was a multicentre randomized controlled trial performed in the USA between 1988–1991. It showed that most patients experience rapid visual recovery within 2 weeks after onset of symptoms (despite being on placebo, oral steroid, or IV steroids). IV methylprednisolone followed by a short course of oral prednisolone did result in significantly accelerated visual recovery, however did not improve the 6-month or 1-year outcome compared to placebo. The risk, of developing a second demyelinating event, consistent with MS, was found to be temporarily (but significantly) reduced.[2]

Multiple sclerosis

At this time point, a formal diagnosis of MS is not present, however up to 75% of female patients presenting with optic neuritis ultimately develop MS. It is crucial that investigations are carried out thoroughly to diagnose

MS, and that appropriate counselling and multidisciplinary care is instituted for the patient.

Refer to → p.339 for management details.

Viva questions

What do you know about acute demyelinating myeloencephalitis?

ADEM is a non-vasculitic inflammatory demyelinating condition that bears a striking clinical and pathological resemblance to MS. In most cases however, it is a monophasic illness of pre-pubescent children, and occurs following a febrile prodromal illness. A patient with neurological symptoms and the presence of multiple (>10) gadolinium enhanced lesions on MRI should be suspected of having ADEM. It is usually treated with high-dose steroids and IV Ig.[3]

What criteria do you know of to diagnose multiple sclerosis?

MacDonald Criteria (2001, revised in 2005) has replaced Poser criteria.[4]

Please examine this patient for a relative afferent pupillary defect

→ Ophthalmology, p.543

❶ Top Tips

- Remember to maintain a nasal light barrier with one hand as you shine the torch with the other. This will isolate the pupil you are testing.

Please assess this patient's speech

At this stage it is important to assess for staccato speech in keeping with cerebellar disease. At later stages, bulbar involvement may occur. The examination needs to be performed in the order of likely findings (staccato speech will usually occur before bulbar involvement is present).

References

1. http://emedicine.medscape.com/article/1146199-overview.
2. Beck RW, Gal RL. Treatment of acute optic neuritis: a summary of findings from the optic neuritis treatment trial. *Arch Ophthalmol* 2008; **126**(7):994–5.
3. http://emedicine.medscape.com/article/1147044-overview.
4. http://www.mult-sclerosis.org/DiagnosticCriteria.html.

Case 4: Pleural effusion

History (key points to elicit in 25 minutes)
Mr James Clark.
61 years old.
From Waterford.
History of increasing dyspnoea and chest discomfort.

HPC

- 3-month history of progressive dyspnoea on exertion.
- Initially very mild, but in week prior to admission developed into severe dyspnoea on minimal exertion, and mild dyspnoea at rest.
- 3-pillow orthopnoea, denies paroxysmal nocturnal dyspnoea (PND).
- Denies palpitations, syncope, ankle swelling.
- Also has left-sided chest discomfort – constant, pleuritic, 3/10 severity, for last 1 week.
- Cough for 1 month, non-productive, worse in the morning.
- Denies haemoptysis.
- No recent fevers/rigors.
- Unsure regarding weight loss.
- Generally feeling weak.
- Denies rashes or joint pain/swelling.
- No recent long haul flights.

❶ Top Tips

- Relevant negatives in your history are highly important, and will influence the formation of a differential diagnosis.
- If a patient is unsure regarding weight loss, questions such as 'Do your clothes still fit you properly?' or 'Are you using an extra notch on your belt recently?' may provide helpful information.

PMHx

- Hypercholesterolaemia.
- Hypertension.
- Negative for angina/ischaemic heart disease, diabetes, asthma, epilepsy, TB.
- No surgical procedures.

❶ Top Tips

- If you suspect a history of cardiac problems, it is important to ask patients if they have had an exercise stress test, echocardiogram or angiogram in the past.

Medications

- Bendroflumethiazide 5mg OD
- Atorvastatin 40mg OD

- Paracetamol 1g QDS/PRN
- Nil known drug allergies.

SHx

- Married, 4 children, 2 grandchildren (all well).
- Lives in bungalow with wife.
- No pets.
- Non-smoker (never smoked).
- Alcohol: 40 units per week (beer) since retirement, previously minimal.
- Retired 2 years ago (postman).
- Worked in a shipyard from age of 17–28, unsure regarding asbestos exposure.
- Independent in ADLs, though cannot mow lawn any more due to breathing difficulties.
- No foreign travel within last 2 years.

> **❶ Top Tips**
>
> - It is important to enquire specifically about previous occupations that may be related to the patient's presenting complaint.
> - As in this case, a patient may not volunteer the fact that he worked in a shipyard 40 years ago.

FMHx

- Father died from MI aged 63.
- Mother died from CVA aged 80.
- No siblings.

Systems review

- Symptoms of prostatic hypertrophy (frequency, nocturia × 3, poor stream, hesitancy).

Hospital course

- Blood tests (results unknown)
- X-ray and CT thorax
- Pleural tap (volume unknown).

Examination (10–12 minutes)

Perform general examination as detailed on **❸** p.640.

> **Specific examination points**
>
> - *General:*
>   - Nutritional status
>   - Fluid balance
>   - Signs of right-heart failure (cor pulmonale): raised JVP, peripheral oedema, ascites)
> - *Hands:*
>   - Clubbing
>   - Nicotine staining
>   - Asterixis

- Muscle wasting
- Associated pathology such as RA
- *Face:*
  - Evidence of Horner's syndrome
  - Chemosis
  - Central cyanosis
  - Butterfly rash
- *Neck:*
  - JVP
  - Cervical/axillary lymphadenopathy
- *Chest*
  - Scars, radiotherapy marks
  - Aspiration/pleural drainage sites (need to look carefully)
  - Chest expansion
  - Tactile vocal fremitus
  - Percussion:
    - *Dull*: pleural thickening/effusion
    - *Hyper-resonant*: emphysema
  - Auscultation:
    - Vocal resonance
    - Aegophony
    - Listen carefully for loud P2

❶ Top Tips

- This patient has a significant history of alcohol abuse, which warrants an abdominal and neurological examination (the latter including signs of cerebellar dysfunction – detailed in ➲ p.346).
- Paraneoplastic conditions can also result in neurological findings such as proximal myopathy and cerebellar disease (➲ p.78).

Summary

Mr Clark is a 61-year-old non-smoker who presented recently with progressively worsening dyspnoea. His symptoms began 3 months ago with mild dyspnoea on exertion. Within the last week, he has developed dyspnoea at rest. He is also complaining of mild, left-sided pleuritic chest pain, which has also been present for the past week. He has also recently developed 3-pillow orthopnoea, but denies PND. He denies palpitations, pre-syncope, syncope or ankle swelling. Mr Clark has also had a non-productive cough for the last month, which appears to be worse in the morning. He denies fevers or haemoptysis, and is unsure regarding weight loss.

His past medical history is significant for hypertension and hypercholesterolaemia, for which he takes bendroflumethiazide 5mg OD and atorvastatin 40mg OD.

Mr Clark is a lifelong non-smoker, but worked in a shipyard for 11 years when he was young. Of note he has been consuming approximately 40 units/week of alcohol since his retirement from the postal service 2 years ago. He has a positive family history of MI and stroke.

On examination, Mr Clark is a thin gentleman. He is clubbed. He has positive findings which include: decreased chest expansion (left), stony dull percussion note from left base to mid zone, decreased air entry and vocal resonance, bronchial breathing in left base, and aegophony at the upper level of the effusion. He has an aspiration mark on the left posterior chest wall.

Though he did not voice specific neurological complaints, Mr Clark has a marked intention tremor, impaired finger–nose coordination and dysdiadochokinesis. These are suggestive of cerebellar dysfunction.

❶ Top Tips

- If significant clinical signs (which may or may not be linked to the main presenting condition) are found during the examination, make sure you ask the patient further appropriate questions e.g. incoordination in a patient with cerebellar signs.

Differential diagnosis

- Pleural effusion secondary to:
  - malignancy (possibility of mesothelioma due to potential asbestos exposure)
  - TB
  - heart failure
  - connective tissue disease
- Pulmonary infarction/pulmonary embolism.
- Cerebellar disease (alcohol related or paraneoplastic).

Investigations

- *Blood:* FBC, U&E, LFT, coagulation profile, ESR, CRP, albumin, Ca^{2+}/PO_4/Mg^{2+}, arterial blood gas, TFT, PSA, autoimmune screen, B12, folate.
- *Radiology:* CXR, CT thorax (with biopsy if indicated), CT ± MRI brain.
- *Cardiac:* ECG, echocardiogram.
- *Others:*
  - Sputum culture
  - Pleural aspiration: protein, glucose, LDH, pH, amylase, microscopy and culture, TB culture
  - Bronchoscopy ± biopsy and lavage (for acid-fast bacillus)
  - Mantoux test.

Management

Treatment will be based on underlying cause and providing symptomatic relief.

❶ Top Tips

- It is important to note that the patient is entitled to seek compensation if the diagnosis is related to previous asbestos exposure.

Viva questions

What are Light's criteria?

These criteria are for determining if pleural fluid is transudate or exudates (protein content >3g/L) (sensitivity 100%, specificity of 72%):

- Ratio of pleural fluid protein to serum protein >0.5.
- Ratio of pleural fluid LDH to serum LDH >0.6.
- Pleural fluid LDH is >2/3 upper limit of normal for serum LDH.

What are the causes of transudates and exudates?

- Transudates:
  - Cardiac failure
  - Nephrotic syndrome
  - Liver failure
  - Hypothyroidism
- *Exudates*:
  - Bronchogenic carcinoma
  - Metastatic pleural disease
  - Pneumonia
  - TB
  - Connective tissue diseases
  - Pulmonary infarction
  - Mesothelioma.

Why might a pleural fluid amylase level be helpful?

Pleural fluid amylase levels are higher than serum concentrations in bacterial pneumonia and carcinoma. Pleural fluid amylase levels are also higher in adenocarcinoma compared to mesothelioma, and can be helpful when cytology cannot differentiate the two.

Based on his history, what else would you have included in this patient's treatment regimen?

This patient admits to significant alcohol consumption over the last 2 years. He may require psychiatric referral for further evaluation. On admission he should have been commenced on intravenous Pabrinex® to prevent acute Wernicke–Korsakoff syndrome, and would be likely to require a tapering dose of chlordiazepoxide to prevent delirium tremens.

You feel that this patient's cerebellar disease may be secondary to alcohol or to a paraneoplastic process. What other cause of cerebellar dysfunction do you know of?

- Demyelinating process (MS)
- Brainstem vascular lesion
- Space-occupying lesion (posterior fossa–cerebellar pontine angle tumour)
- Friedreich's ataxia
- Hypothyroidism
- Phenytoin toxicity
- Congenital malformations at the level of the foramen magnum.

Please demonstrate chest expansion

➲ Chapter 2, p.24.

Please consent this patient for a bronchoscopy
- Explain indication (e.g. cough, shortness of breath, chest discomfort).
- Possibility of receiving IV sedatives/anxiolytics (midazolam).
- Biopsy.
- Complications are infrequent and usually minor (bleeding, infection, pneumothorax, desaturation, side effects of medication).
- Any questions?

Case 5: Idiopathic pulmonary arterial hypertension (IPAH)

> **History (key points to elicit in 25 minutes)**
>
> Mrs Brenda Wilson.
> 32 years old.
> From Sligo.
> Referred by GP with progressive dyspnoea and recent collapse.

HPC
- Increasing dyspnoea on exertion over last 6 months; now short of breath on climbing stairs.
- Fainted 3 days ago after climbing 1 flight of stairs (husband present) and woke up after a few seconds.
- Second fainting episode in 2 weeks.
- Recently developed ankle oedema.
- No dyspnoea at rest, cough, haemoptysis, orthopnoea, chest pain, palpitations.
- No limb jerking, incontinence associated with fainting episode.
- Easily tired over the last few weeks.
- Sleeps well at night, no snoring.
- No recent flu like illness.
- No change in weight or appetite.
- No skin changes, photosensitivity, joint or muscular pains, mouth ulcers, dry eyes, dry mouth.
- No foreign travel/long-haul flights in last one year.

❶ Top Tips
- Ruling out multisystem conditions with general questions about rashes, muscular pain and fatigue is always important, as they can often be either directly responsible or associated with the patient's presentation.

PMHx
- Appendectomy 20 years ago
- No history of migraine or epilepsy
- No history of TIAs, CVA, PE, DVT or miscarriages.

Medications
- Oxygen via nasal prongs as required
- Oral contraceptive pill
- No drug allergies.

SHx
- Non-smoker, 10 units of alcohol per week
- Married, lives with husband in 2-storey house
- No children or pets
- Pharmacist.

FHx
- No history of clotting disorders
- Sister (age 39) has SLE.

ROS
- Nil of note.

Hospital course as per patient
- Blood tests
- CXR
- Chest CT
- ECG
- Echocardiogram
- Awaiting cardiac catheterization.

Examination (10–12 minutes)
Perform general examination as detailed on ➋ p.640.

Specific examination points

- *General:*
  - Nutritional status
  - Fluid balance
  - Respiratory rate
  - Evidence of cyanosis
  - Signs of right-heart failure (JVP, oedema, ascites)
  - Proximal muscle wasting
  - Scars
  - Legs (tender calf swelling – DVT)
- *Hands:*
  - Clubbing
  - Muscle wasting
  - Asterixis
- *Face:*
  - Chemosis
  - Central cyanosis
- *Cardiovascular:*
  - JVP (prominent A wave – RV hypertrophy, prominent V wave – TR)
  - Parasternal heave
  - Loud/palpable P2
  - Fixed or paradoxic splitting in severe RV dysfunction
  - TR

- *Chest:*
  - Chest expansion
  - Percuss and auscultate lung fields
- *Abdomen:*
  - Pulsatile hepatomegaly
- *Signs of connective tissue disease:*
  - Scleroderma.

Summary

Mrs Wilson is a 32-year-old pharmacist from Sligo who presented with fainting episodes, fatigue and a 6-month history of increasing dyspnoea on exertion. She fainted for the second time in 2 weeks after climbing the stairs. The episode only lasted a few seconds and was preceded by breathlessness. There was no associated chest pain, palpitations, vertigo, seizure or other neurological deficit. Her husband was present at the time.

Over the last 6 months, she has been increasingly breathless on exertion, and now has difficulty climbing 1 flight of stairs. She has no symptoms at rest, cough, haemoptysis or orthopnoea. She also has no arthralgia or myalgia, rashes, photosensitivity, appetite change or weight loss. She has not traveled abroad in the last year. In her past medical history she had an appendectomy 20 years ago. She has no history of miscarriage or thrombotic events.

Mrs Wilson was on the oral contraceptive pill on admission. She has no known allergies. She is a non-smoker, and lives at home with her husband in a 2-storey house. She has no children or pets, and has continued to work full time despite her symptoms. Her sister suffers from SLE, but her family history is otherwise unremarkable. Since her admission three days ago, Mrs Wilson has been receiving oxygen intermittently via nasal prongs.

On examination Mrs Wilson is a thin lady. She is in no distress and is well perfused. Her BP is 130/72, pulse 78 regular, and her oxygen saturation is 93% on room air. The positive findings on examination are an elevated JVP with prominent 'V' waves, a RV heave and paradoxical splitting of the second heart sound with a loud P2. Her respiratory examination was unremarkable.

● Top Tips

- Young patients with pulmonary hypertension often only present when signs of right-heart failure develop.

Differential diagnosis

- Idiopathic pulmonary arterial hypertension (IPAH) – formerly known as primary pulmonary hypertension.
- Pulmonary hypertension secondary to underlying connective tissue disease such as scleroderma.
- Pulmonary embolus.
- Chronic thromboembolic disease.

Investigations

- *Blood:* FBC, U&E, LFT, coagulation profile, ESR, CRP, D-dimer
  (⊕ Deep vein thrombosis, p.448), autoantibody screen, thrombophilia
  screen.
- *Radiology:*
  - CXR: may show dilated pulmonary vasculature (often normal).
  - HRCT thorax.
  - CT pulmonary angiogram (if suspicion of pulmonary emboli).
- *Others:* ECG (P pulmonale, RV hypertrophy or right axis strain),
  24-hour Holter monitor, echocardiogram, pulmonary function test,
  overnight oximetry (patients may have a history of daytime fatigue and
  somnolence), V/Q scan, 6-minute walk test, right heart catheterization
  (diagnostic criteria for IPHT: mean pulmonary artery pressure
  >25mmHg at rest, or >30mmHg with exercise).

Viva questions

What are the causes of pulmonary hypertension?

- Primary causes:
  - Idiopathic pulmonary arterial hypertension/primary pulmonary
    hypertension
- Secondary causes:
  - Collagen vascular disease
  - Left-to-right cardiac shunts (Eisenmenger's syndrome)
  - Stimulants like cocaine or methamphetamine
  - COPD
  - Obstructive sleep apnoea
  - Acute pulmonary embolism
  - Chronic thromboembolic disease
  - Left-heart disease
  - Pulmonary venous obstruction

Why would you perform overnight oximetry in a patient with pulmonary hypertension?

Nocturnal oxyhaemoglobin desaturations can occur in patients with pulmonary hypertension, even in the absence of obstructive sleep apnoea.[1]

What do you know about appetite suppressants and pulmonary hypertension?

Appetite suppressants, or anorexigens, such as fenfluramine and diethyl-
propion have been shown to increase the risk of developing pulmonary
arterial hypertension. The risk is higher when the drugs were used in the
previous year or for >3 months.[2]

What do you know about HIV and pulmonary hypertension?

Case series have shown that PAH occurs in approximately 1 in 200 patients
with HIV infection and that the prevalence has not increased in the last
20 years. Optimal retroviral therapy appears to improve haemodynamics.[3]

How would you manage IPAH? [4,5]

Early treatment is recommended because advanced disease is often less
responsive to medication.

- Treat underlying aetiology if possible
- Diuretics

- Oxygen therapy
- Anticoagulation with warfarin (target INR= 2; patients are at increased risk of pulmonary events)[4]
- Exercise (no improvement in haemodynamic measures, but increase in mean 6-minute walk distance and improved WHO functional class)[5]
- Prostanoids (epoprostenol, iloprost)
- Endothelin receptor antagonists (bosentan)
- Phosphodiesterase-5 inhibitors (sildenafil)
- Heart-lung transplantation – a viable option for patients with end-stage disease who fail maximal medical therapy.[6]

References

1. Minai OA et al. Predictors of nocturnal oxygen desaturation in pulmonary arterial hypertension. Chest 2007; **131**(1):109–17.
2. Abenhaim L et al. Appetite-suppressant drugs and the risk of primary pulmonary hypertension. International Primary Pulmnary Hypetension Study Group. NEJM 1996; **335**(9):609–16.
3. Sitbon O et al. Prevalence of HIV-related pulmonary arterial hypertension in the current antiretroviral therapy era. Am J Respir Crit Care Med 2008; **177**(1):108–13.
4. McLaughlin W et al. ACCF/AHA 2009 expert consensus document on pulmonary hypertension: a report of the American College of Cardiology Foundation Task Force on Expert Consensus Documents and the American Heart Association: developed in collaboration with the American College of Chest Physicians, American Thoracic Society, Inc., and the Pulmonary Hypertension Association. Circulation 2009; **119**:2250.
5. Mereles D et al. Exercise and respiratory training improve exercise capacity and quality of life in patients with severe chronic pulmonary hypertension. Circulation 2006; **114**(14):1482–9.
6. Gaine SP, Orens JB. Lung transplantation for pulmonary hypertension. Semin Respir Crit Care Med 2001; **22**(5):533–40.

Case 6: Methotrexate-induced pulmonary toxicity

History (key points to elicit in 25 minutes)

Mr Richard Davis.
44 years old.
From Dublin.
Presented to A&E 6 days ago with fever, cough and dyspnoea.

HPC

- Gradually progressive exertional dyspnoea over 1 month.
- Now has great difficulty climbing 1 flight of stairs.
- Non-productive cough for 1 month.
- Developed fever and severe breathlessness 24 hours prior to presentation.
- Anorexia for 2–3 days prior to presentation.
- No weight loss.
- Denied chest pain, palpitations or orthopnoea.
- No foreign travel.

PMHx

- Diagnosed with psoriatic arthritis 9 months ago; had plaque-like rash for several months prior to development of joint involvement.
- Commenced on steroids initially, but due to poor response placed on methotrexate, ~6 months ago.
- Insulin dependent diabetes diagnosed 30 years ago.
- Depression for past 10 years.

❶ Top Tips

- A recent diagnosis of a multisystemic illness should be fully explored, including presentation, treatment and complications.
- If you suspect the presentation is related to a recent diagnosis or new medication, ask the patient. They may share valuable information.
- Always ask diabetic patients about sugar control, HbA1c, ophthalmology review, and infections.

Medications

- Initially on IV hydrocortisone 100mg QDS for 3 days, now on tapering dose of oral prednisolone
- Co-amoxiclav 1.2g TDS IV
- Methotrexate 8 tablets per week (stopped on admission)
- Folic acid 5mg OD
- Citalopram 20mg OD
- Calcium with vitamin D
- Insulin glargine 12 units nocte, Novorapid® TDS
- Enoxaparin 20mg SC OD
- Nil known drug allergies.

SHx

- Lives with male partner of 10 years
- 20 pack-year smoking history
- No alcohol
- Interior designer
- Independent in ADLs
- Does not own birds or other pets.

FHx

- Father (smoker) died of lung cancer aged 68
- Mother alive and well
- Younger brother died aged 12 due to meningitis.

ROS

- Non-contributory.

❶ Top Tips

- In patients with underlying chronic illnesses, always ask regarding the disease status (active vs. quiescent).
- The history taking should be a multisystemic approach when relevant. In this case, appropriate questioning for extra-articular manifestations of the disease must be included.

Hospital management as per patient

- Blood tests
- CXR
- CT thorax
- Pulmonary function tests
- Vital signs and peak flow monitoring (may be available at the end of the bed).

Examination: 10–12 minutes

Perform general examination as detailed on ❷ p.640.

Specific examination points

- *General:*
  - Nutritional status
  - Fluid balance
  - Signs of right heart failure (cor pulmonale)
- *Hands:*
  - Clubbing
  - Nail pitting
  - Nicotine staining
  - Asterixis
  - Muscle wasting
  - Active joint disease
- *Neck:*
  - JVP
  - Tracheal deviation
  - Cervical/axillary lymphadenopathy

- *Face:*
  - Horner's syndrome
  - Chemosis (CO_2 retention)
  - Central cyanosis
- *Eyes:*
  - Diabetic or hypertensive retinopathy
- *Chest:*
  - Scars
  - Chest expansion
  - Tactile vocal fremitus
  - Percussion
  - Auscultation – carefully note quality of breath sounds, and character/timing of other sounds such as crackles
  - Vocal resonance, aegophony
  - Listen carefully for loud P2
- *Joints and skin:*
  - Quickly assess skin for evidence of psoriatic plaques and joints for active disease (tenderness and swelling)

❶ Top Tips

- Ask the patient to perform a peak flow (if available).
- An examination for peripheral sensory neuropathy is warranted in diabetic patients.

Summary

Mr Davis is a 44-year-old smoker who presented to hospital with respiratory distress and fever 1 week ago. Of note he has a recent diagnosis of psoriatic arthritis, and was commenced on methotrexate 6 months prior to admission.

Mr Davis has had progressive dyspnoea on exertion and a dry cough for the last month. In the 24 hours prior to admission, his symptoms worsened to severe breathlessness, dry cough and fever. He denies any rigors, diarrhoea or urinary symptoms. He has not travelled recently.

His past medical history includes the recently diagnosed psoriatic arthropathy, insulin dependent diabetes since childhood and depression. His diabetes is well controlled; he has regular follow-up with an endocrinologist and he has annual ophthalmology reviews.

His current medication includes a tapering dose of prednisolone, IV co-amoxiclav, folic acid 5mg OD, calcium and vitamin D supplementation, a combination of short- and long-acting insulin, citalopram 20mg OD and enoxaparin 20mg OD SC. On admission his methotrexate (20mg once weekly) was stopped and he was placed on a 4-day course of IV hydrocortisone 100mg QDS.

Mr Davis has a 20 pack-year smoking history, does not consume alcohol, and is an interior designer. He lives with his male partner of 10 years, and does not own birds or other pets. His father died of lung cancer at 68 years of age, and his mother has hypertension.

On examination Mr Davis was comfortable, afebrile and in no respiratory distress. He had nasal prongs *in situ* with 3L of oxygen and was maintaining saturations of 95%. His recent BP was 128/72. His pulse was 80 per minute and regular. Positive findings included bilaterally diminished chest expansion and fine, bibasal end-inspiratory crepitations that decreased when leaning forward.

Differential diagnosis

- Methotrexate-induced pulmonary toxicity
- Hypersensitivity pneumonitis (or extrinsic allergic alveolitis)
- Opportunistic pulmonary infection (PCP) secondary to HIV infection
- Pulmonary embolism.

Investigations

- Blood: FBC, U&E, LFT, ESR/CRP, coagulation profile, arterial blood gases, HIV serology, auto-immune screen, complement levels, blood cultures
- Radiology:
  - CXR
  - HRCT thorax (ground-glass appearance)
- Other: Bronchoscopy and BAL, urine culture.

Viva questions

What is the management for drug-induced pneumonitis?

The treatment of most drug-induced pulmonary disease is the immediate withdrawal of the offending agent, in this case methotrexate. Supportive measures such as steroids, oxygen and bronchodilators can be helpful. Of course smoking cessation and prompt treatment of coexisting respiratory infection is important. It is important to rule out other treatable causes of acute respiratory distress before this diagnosis is made.

What are some risk factors for developing MTX-induced pneumonitis?[1]

- >60 years of age
- Rheumatoid pulmonary disease
- Hypoalbuminaemia
- Smoking
- Diabetes.

What criteria have you heard of for the diagnosis of this condition?

Searles and McKendry criteria[2]:

- Major:
  - Hypersensitivity pneumonitis on histology, without infection
  - Radiological evidence of pulmonary interstitial disease
  - Negative blood and sputum cultures
- Minor:
  - Breathlessness <8 weeks
  - Non-productive cough
  - Oxygen saturation <90% on room air
  - DLCO <70% predicted for age
  - Leucocyte count <15,000 cells/uL.

Diagnosis made with 1 or 2 major criteria, plus 3 minor criteria.

References

1. Methotrexate-Lung Study Group. Risk factors for methotrexate-induced lung injury in patients with rheumatoid arthritis. A multicenter, case-control study. *Ann Intern Med* 1997; **127**(5):356–64.
2. Searles G, McKendry RJ. Methotrexate pneumonitis in rheumatoid arthritis: potential risk factors. Four case reports and a review of the literature. *J Rheumatol* 1987; **14**(6):1164–71.

Case 7: Cushing's syndrome secondary to ectopic ACTH (small-cell lung cancer)

History (key points to elicit in 25 minutes)
Mr David Rushmore. 68 years old. From County Mayo. Referred by GP with haemoptysis, fatigue and muscle weakness.

HPC

- Several episodes of haemoptysis in the last 2 weeks.
- Small amount of blood (tablespoon) each time.
- No chest pain, shortness of breath, fever or sweats.
- Chronic cough ('for years'), no purulent sputum.
- No obvious weight loss.
- Worsening fatigue over last 2 months.
- Difficulty getting out of chairs because of 'weak muscles' in his legs.
- No change in facial appearance, easy bruising or recent infections.
- No change in body habitus ('buffalo hump' or central obesity).
- More irritable over last few months (noted by his wife).
- No recent foreign travel.

❶ Top Tips

- Patients may not mention symptoms such as mood change unless directly asked.
- It is important to consider all aspects of the presenting complaint. If there is more than one, then each needs to be addressed thoroughly. Together they may provide a coherent clinical picture.

PMHx

- Splenectomy (1978) after road traffic accident.
  - Has received two vaccinations in the last 4 years, but doesn't remember which ones.
- Type 2 diabetes mellitus diagnosed 8 months ago (diet controlled).
- Hypertension.
- Hypercholesterolaemia.

Medications

- Ramipril 7.5mg OD
- Atorvastatin 20mg OD
- Aspirin 75mg OD

- Penicillin 1 tablet OD
- Allergic to erythromycin (rash).

SHx

- Married, no children, wife is healthy
- Heavy smoker (60 pack-year history)
- Minimal alcohol ('glass of wine at Christmas')
- Lives in bungalow
- Independent in ADLs.

FHx

- Both parents died of MI (mother aged 72, father aged 62)
- No siblings.

ROS

- No change in vision, or peripheral sensation
- Bowel habit remains normal
- No urinary dysfunction.

Hospital course as per patient

- Blood tests
- Urine collections
- CXR
- Bronchoscopy
- CT thorax
- Physiotherapy.

> **❶ Top Tips**
>
> - It may be helpful to ask the patient regarding specific tests, which may give you clues as to the working diagnosis, such as a 24-hour urinary cortisol collection, or overnight dexamethasone suppression test.

Examination (10–12 minutes)

Perform general examination as detailed on ➲ p.640.

> **Specific examination points**
>
> - *General:*
>   - Pigmentation
>   - Nutritional status
>   - Fluid balance
>   - Respiratory rate
>   - Proximal muscle wasting
> - *Hands:*
>   - Clubbing
>   - Nicotine staining
>   - Small muscle wasting
>   - Asterixis (unlikely to be found in this man without shortness of breath)

- *Face/neck:*
  - Horner's syndrome
  - Chemosis
  - Central cyanosis
  - Lymphadenopathy
- *Neurological:*
  - If suspecting Cushing syndrome examine for bitemporal hemianopia (uncommon as pituitary adenomas are often small tumours)
  - Tone, power, coordination, reflexes, sensation in 4 limbs
  - Fatigability
  - Gait ('waddling' in proximal myopathy)
- *Chest:*
  - Tracheal deviation
  - Expansion, tactile fremitus
  - Percussion
  - Auscultation
  - Listen for loud P2
- *Signs of cortisol excess:*
  - Proximal myopathy
  - Cushingoid facies
  - Dorsocervical fat pad
  - Skin fragility, bruising
  - Purple striae.

Summary

Mr Rushmore is a 68-year-old gentleman from County Mayo who was referred by his GP for a history of haemoptysis, fatigue and proximal myopathy. Mr Rushmore is a heavy smoker and has had several small episodes of frank haemoptysis in the last 2 weeks. He has a chronic cough, which he attributes to his smoking, but it has never been productive until recently. He denies shortness of breath, chest pain, fevers or weight loss. For the last 2 months, he has also become increasingly fatigued, and recently noticed difficulty in getting out of chairs due to the weakness in his legs. He denies features of cortisol excess such as infections, bruising or change in body habitus.

His past medical history is significant for an emergency splenectomy in 1978 following a road traffic accident, diet-controlled type 2 diabetes, hypertension and hypercholesterolaemia. His medications include ramipril 7.5mg OD, atorvastatin 20mg OD, aspirin 75mg OD and penicillin 1 tablet OD. He develops a rash after taking erythromycin. Mr Rushmore has had 2 vaccinations (in relation to his splenctomy) in the last 4 years, but is not sure what they were. He is married, and lives with his wife in a bungalow. To date he has been independent in his daily activities. He has a significant family history of cardiac illness, as both his parents died of MI. On systems review, Mr Rushmore has no complaints of visual deficits or neuropathy secondary to his diabetes.

On examination, Mr Rushmore is overweight and was comfortable at rest. His BP was 155/90 and his pulse was 82bpm and regular. Positive findings on clinical examination include finger clubbing, nicotine staining and proximal myopathy in his lower limbs. The rest of his neurological examination, including visual fields was normal. He did have evidence of purple abdominal striae, but has no other obvious features of cortisol excess.

Differential diagnosis

- Paraneoplastic syndrome – likely ectopic adrenocorticotropic hormone (ACTH) production from small-cell lung carinoma
- Lung cancer (primary or secondary).

❶ Top Tips

- Sepsis or chronic infection must always be considered in asplenic patients, however the presentation in this case makes this diagnosis less likely.

Viva questions

What are some common causes of Cushing's syndrome?

- Steroid use
- Pituitary adenoma (Cushing's disease)
- Ectopic ACTH production
- Adrenal adenoma.

Once hypercortisolism has been diagnosed, how would you determine its aetiology?

The January 2010 UpToDate guidelines recommend that once hypercortisolism has been established (usually by *low-dose dexamethasone testing*), the patient needs to be evaluated for:

- Primary adrenal disease vs. ACTH dependent tumour:
  - Check morning plasma ACTH level (normal range 20–80pg/mL).
  - Low plasma ACTH (<5pg/mL) in a patient with Cushing's syndrome is suggestive of ACTH – independent disease (thin-section CT adrenals is the next step in evaluation).
  - If plasma ACTH is >20pg/mL, it is likely that the disease is ACTH-dependent (due to pituitary disease or ectopic ACTH/CRH secretion).
- ACTH-dependent Cushing's syndrome:
  - High-dose dexamethasone testing should be performed initially (suppression of cortisol suggests pituitary adenoma – Cushing's disease).
  - If high-dose dexamethasone testing suggests Cushing's disease, then an MRI of the pituitary gland should be performed to confirm the diagnosis.
  - If MRI results are unclear (lesions <6mm) or other non-invasive tests are inconclusive, then petrosal sinus sampling and CRH stimulation should be performed.

- CRH stimulation test: most patients with Cushing's disease will show increased ACTH and cortisol within 45 minutes of IV CRH administration.
- Inferior petrosal sinus venous sampling is the most direct way to determine pituitary ACTH hypersecretion (a central to peripheral plasma ACTH gradient of ≥2 before CRH administration is diagnostic of a pituitary ACTH source).[1]

Do you think this patient should be on antibiotic prophylaxis given his history of splenectomy?

While it has generally been traditional practice to give asplenic patients life-long penicillin prophylaxis, current guidelines do not routinely recommend prolonged post-splenectomy prophylaxis in adults. This is due to lower incidence of adult sepsis and increasing problems with drug resistance. Administration of meningiococcal, pneumococcal and *H. influenzae* type b vaccines are advised.[2]

Please perform a visual field examination on this patient

Refer to ➔ p.538.

References

1. Oldfield EH et al. Petrosal sinus sampling with and without corticotropin-releasing hormone for the differential diagnosis of Cushing's syndrome. *NEJM* 1991; **325**(13):897–905.
2. Pasternack MS. Prevention of sepsis in the asplenic patient. UpTodate, January 2010. Available at: http://http://www.uptodate.com.

Case 8: Steroid-induced myopathy

> **History (key points to elicit in 25 minutes)**
>
> Mrs Jane Phillips.
> 64 years old.
> From Athlone.
> Referred by GP 2 days ago with shortness of breath, cough and fever.

HPC

- Chronic cough, productive of green sputum for last week.
- Fevers and chills.
- Shortness of breath on minimal exertion, wheeze.
- 'It's my COPD again.'
- No chest pain, palpitations, paroxysmal nocturnal dyspnoea or ankle swelling.
- Second admission during the last 6 months with similar symptoms.
- Has visited GP twice in between for shortness of breath; received short course of oral steroids both times.
- Admits to not taking her inhalers regularly – prescribed budesonide and formoterol after last admission but has not been compliant: 'I was told that they can weaken my bones'.
- Feels very weak at home, difficulty getting out of bed and chairs.
- Difficulty climbing stairs.
- Difficulty in reaching for things on shelf.
- Slight weight gain (2kg).
- No muscle pain or skin rashes.
- No sensory, visual or speech disturbance.
- No headaches.

❶ Top Tips

- If you suspect that a patient may have a chronic illness like COPD, then ask and clarify it early in the history.
- When a patient admits to non-compliance of medication, always find out specific reasons e.g. side effects.

PMHx

- COPD 'for many years'
- OA of knees
- Hysterectomy (emergency procedure following birth of 2nd child; ovaries preserved).

Medications

- Levofloxacin 500mg BD IV since admission
- Hydrocortisone 100mg QDS IV since admission
- Combivent® (salbutamol + ipatropium) 2.5mL nebulizer QDS
- Symbicort® 400/12 (formoterol + budesonide) – stopped on admission
- Salbutamol inhalers PRN at home (>10 puffs per day)
- Calcium + vitamin D BD since admission
- No drug allergies.

SHx

- Continues to smoke heavily – 40 pack-years
- Balanced diet with dairy products and fish
- No alcohol
- Widowed, husband died in car accident 8 years ago
- Lives alone, 2-storey house
- Independent in activities of daily life
- 2 sons, alive and well.

FHx

- Sister (age 59) has osteoporosis.

ROS

- No thinning of skin or easy bruising.
- No symptoms of inflammatory bowel disease/gluten intolerance.

Hospital course as per patient

- CXR
- Blood tests, including arterial blood gas
- ECG
- Respiratory nurse specialist review
- DEXA scan.

Examination (10–12 minutes)

Perform general examination as detailed on ➜ p.640.

Specific examination points

• *General:*
   • BP
   • Nutritional status
   • Fluid balance
   • Respiratory rate
   • Cyanosis
   • Signs of right-heart failure (JVP, oedema, ascites)
   • Proximal muscle wasting
   • Scars, radiotherapy marks
 • *Hands:*
   • Clubbing
   • Nicotine staining
   • Muscle wasting
   • Asterixis
 • *Face:*
   • Horner's syndrome
   • Chemosis
   • Central cyanosis
   • Rule out myasthenia with prolonged upward gaze
 • *Neurological:*
   • Bitemporal hemianopia – may indicate Cushing's disease (pituitary adenoma secreting ACTH)
   • Neck flexion and extension
   • Tone, power, coordination, reflexes, sensation in 4 limbs

- Fatigability
- Gait (waddling in proximal myopathy)
- *Chest:*
  - Expansion, tactile fremitus
  - Percussion
  - Auscultation
  - Listen for loud P2
- *Signs of glucocorticoid excess:*
  - Proximal myopathy
  - Cushingoid facies
  - Dorsocervical/interscapular fat pad
  - Skin fragility, bruising
  - Striae.

❶ Top Tips

- Neck flexors and extensors are strong muscles and can be severely affected in proximal myopathy.
- In patients with glucocorticoid-induced proximal myopathy, other features of Cushing's syndrome such as diabetes, moon facies, skin fragility and osteoporosis are often, *but not always*, found.[1]

Summary

Mrs Phillips is a 64-year-old lady from Athlone who was admitted to hospital 2 days ago with shortness of breath, cough and fevers. She is a heavy smoker and has an established history of COPD, with 2 admissions in the last 6 months. She has also visited her GP twice in between, and on each occasion, the dose of her oral steroids was increased. She admits to poor medication compliance, particularly to the formoterol/budesonide inhaler, which she was prescribed on her last admission to hospital. Her sister informed her that steroids cause osteoporosis, and hence she has not been keen to take the inhaler. Her lack of compliance with her steroid inhaler has resulted in regular courses of intravenous and oral steroids.

Mrs Phillips has also been complaining of significant difficulty in getting out of chairs and climbing stairs. More recently this proximal myopathy has been affecting her upper limbs as she finds reaching for items on high shelves difficult. She denies any muscular pains, sensory deficits, visual changes or symptoms associated with inflammatory bowel or coeliac disease. Her past medical history is significant for OA in her knees and an emergency hysterectomy (without oophorectomy) following the birth of her second child.

Her family history is significant for osteoporosis in her younger sister. She has a 40 pack-year smoking history, does not drink alcohol and has been living alone since the death of her husband 8 years ago. She has a balanced diet which includes both dairy products and fish. She has 2 sons who are both married and living in the UK. Mrs Phillips is able to manage her activities of daily life, however with her recent muscular weakness and difficulty climbing stairs, she has had to move her bedroom downstairs. She feels that she may benefit from a stair lift.

Her current medications are levofloxacin 500mg BD IV, hydrocortisone 100mg QDS IV, Combivent® nebulizers QDS and calcium with vitamin D. She has no drug allergies. Prior to admission she had been intermittently taking her formoterol/budesonide inhaler.

On examination, Mrs Phillips is hypertensive with a BP of 160/85, has cushingoid facies and coarse crepitations with bronchial breathing in her right lung base, which is consistent with a lower respiratory tract infection. Neurologically, she has a demonstrable myopathic gait and has grade 4/5 weakness in neck flexion and extension as well as proximal myopathy in her upper and lower limbs. Distal power in her limbs are well preserved.

Differential diagnosis

- Infective exacerbation of COPD and glucocorticoid induced proximal myopathy
- Paraneoplastic syndrome leading to proximal weakness
- Cushing's syndrome due to other causes (➔ p.602)
- Thyroid dysfunction
- Inflammatory myopathy (dermatomyositis, polymyositis)
- Myasthenia gravis
- Neuromuscular junction disease: Eaton–Lambert syndrome.

Investigations

- *Blood:* FBC, U&E, LFT, coagulation profile, ESR, CRP, $Ca^{2+}/PO_4/Mg^{2+}$, B12, folate, creatine kinase, thyroid function tests, 25-OH vitamin D
- *Microbiology:* sputum culture
- *Radiology:* CXR
- *Others:* ECG, peak flow, pulmonary function test, EMG and muscle biopsy, DEXA scan.

Management

This patient is obviously having compliance issues due to a misunderstanding of her medications. The risk of bone disease with inhaled steroids is comparatively low compared to the oral and IV steroid courses she now frequently requires. Patient education will be the first and foremost treatment modality.[2]

If they are able to tolerate a discontinuation in glucocorticoid therapy, virtually all patients will regain muscle strength within 3–4 weeks.[1]

Viva questions

What are the side effects of inhaled steroids?

- Dysphonia (hoarse voice) may occur in 50% of patients using metered dose inhalers. It is thought to be due to myopathy of the laryngeal muscles.[3]
- Oral thrush.
- Very rarely tongue hypertrophy and perioral dermatitis.

How would you definitively diagnose COPD?

COPD as a diagnosis needs to be considered in any patient who reports chronic cough, chronic sputum production or dyspnoea, with a history of smoking, or exposure to dust or inhaled chemicals. COPD is diagnosed when a patient with these typical symptoms is also confirmed to have airway obstruction (FEV_1/FVC <0.70) on pulmonary function tests.[4]

What staging system do you know about for COPD?

Gold staging system: reproduced from the Global Initiative for COPD:[4]

- I (mild): $FEV_1/FVC < 70\%$, $FEV_1 \geq 80\%$ predicted
- II (moderate): $FEV_1/FVC < 70\%$, $50\% \leq FEV_1 < 80\%$ predicted
- III (severe): $FEV_1/FVC < 70\%$, $30\% \leq FEV_1 < 50\%$ predicted
- IV (very severe): $FEV_1/FVC < 70\%$, $FEV_1 < 30\%$ predicted, or $< 50\%$ predicted with chronic respiratory failure.

References

1. Bowyer SL et al. Steroid myopathy: incidence and detection in a population with asthma. *J Allergy Clin Immunol* 1985; **76**(2 Pt 1):234–42.
2. Herzog, AG. Proximal myopathy associated with inhaled steroids. *JAMA* 1999; **281**:37.
3. Williamson IJ et al. Frequency of voice problems and cough in patients using pressurized aerosol inhaled steroid preparations. *Eur Respir J* 1995; **8**(4):590–2.
4. Global strategy for the diagnosis, management, and prevention of chronic obstructive pulmonary disease: Executive summary 2006. Global Initiative for Chronic Obstructive Lung Disease (GOLD). http://www.goldcopd.org.

Case 9: Amiodarone-induced hypothyroidism

History (key points: 25 minutes)

Mrs Julie Woods.
45 years old.
From Belfast.
Presented to A&E 3 days ago with dizziness and fatigue.

HPC

- Attended GP clinic 3 days ago due to weakness and fatigue.
- GP noticed very slow pulse rate and referred to A&E.
- General malaise for 2 months.
- Feels dizzy and tired all the time.
- No syncope, palpitations or chest pain.
- Has gained 1 stone in last 3 months.
- Intermittently constipated for last few weeks.
- Skin dry.
- Voice has become hoarse.
- No neck swelling, pain or recent flu-like illness.
- Thinks she is menopausal, no menses for 5 months.

❶ Top Tips

- While it is important to enquire about all the classical symptoms of hypo/hyperthyroidism, it is rare to find a patient with 'the full house of symptoms'.

PMHx

- Paroxysmal atrial fibrillation (PAF) diagnosed 1 year ago:
  - Presented to hospital with palpitations and chest discomfort, initially ECG was normal, but PAF subsequently diagnosed on Holter monitor.
  - Echocardiogram showed mitral stenosis; coronary angiogram normal.
  - Scheduled for yearly cardiology review.
- Rheumatic fever as a child.
- No previous history of thyroid disease.

Medications

- Warfarin 2mg OD, INR 'at the right level'; checked monthly
- Amiodarone 200mg OD (stopped on admission)
- Bisoprolol 1.25mg OD (on hold since admission)
- Levothyroxine 50µg OD (started yesterday)
- Nil known drug allergies.

SHx

- Married, lives with husband, no children
- 2-storey house
- Non-smoker, 14 units of alcohol per week
- Museum curator.

FHx

- Mother died age 80, had irregular heart beat, was on warfarin.
- Father – type 2 diabetes, otherwise well.
- 1 sister – alive and well.

ROS

- Non-contributory.

Hospital course as per patient

- Blood tests
- Urine pregnancy test – negative
- ECG: 'very slow heart beat'
- CXR
- Cardiac monitor
- Echocardiogram: does not know result.

Examination: 10–12 minutes

Perform general examination as detailed on ➋ p.640.

Specific examination points

- *General:*
  - Nutritional status
  - Character of voice (hoarse)
  - Coarse dry skin and hair
  - Loss of outer 1/3 of eyebrows
  - Puffy eyes
  - Amiodarone-induced skin pigmentation
  - Hands sweaty or dry?

- *Neck*
  - Scars – look carefully in neck creases
  - Goitre (ask patient to swallow water)
  - Inspect
  - Palpate
  - Auscultate for bruit
  - Precuss and elicit Pemberton's sign for retrosternal extension
- *Cardiovascular:*
  - Pulse rate and rhythm
  - Cardiac murmur (mitral stenosis)
  - Loud 1st heart sound
  - Mid diastolic murmur
  - Check for loud P2
- *Neurological:*
  - Proximal myopathy
  - Slowly relaxing reflexes, best seen with ankle jerk
  - Cerebellar disease
  - Carpal tunnel syndrome
  - Peripheral neuropathy
- *Thyroid status:*
  - Pulse rate/rhythm
  - Sweaty/dry skin
  - Tremor
  - Proximal weakness (occurs in both hypo- and hyperthyroidism)
  - Voice change, lid lag
  - Thyroid bruit
  - Reflexes.

❶ Top Tips

- In such cases, it is important to determine the patients current thyroid status and present your findings appropriately.

Summary

Mrs Woods is a 45-year-old lady who was referred to A&E by her GP with significant bradycardia, dizziness and fatigue. She has been feeling unduly tired for the last few months, and has noticed a 1 stone weight gain, dry skin, hoarse voice and intermittent constipation. She has not had her menses in 4–5 months and feels she is in the menopause. She does not voice any specific dislike to hot or cold weather.

Her past medical history includes a diagnosis of paroxysmal atrial fibrillation one year ago, for which she is on warfarin, amiodarone 200mg OD and bisoprolol 1.25mg OD. She had a normal coronary angiogram at that time, and an echocardiogram demonstrated mitral stenosis, which is likely due to her history of rheumatic fever as a child.

Her amiodarone was stopped on admission, and her bisoprolol is on hold. She was commenced on levothyroxine 50µg OD shortly after admission.

Mrs Woods is a non-smoker, drinks 14 units of alcohol per week and works as a museum curator. She is married, lives with her husband and has no children. Her family history is positive for cardiac arrhythmias (mother) and type 2 diabetes (father).

On examination Mrs Woods was comfortable, but had a rather flat affect. She had notably dry skin, coarse hair and puffy eyes. Her BP was 115/78 and her pulse was regular at 54 beats per minute. She had no palpable goitre on examination. Cardiac examination revealed a loud 1st heart sound and a low-pitched, rumbling mid diastolic murmur in the apex, which is consistent with mitral stenosis. Neurological examination revealed proximal myopathy in her upper limbs and slowly relaxing ankle reflexes. Overall, she is clinically hypothyroid.

Differential diagnosis

- Amiodarone-induced hypothyroidism resulting in symptomatic bradycardia.
- Spontaneous primary atrophic hypothyroidism.
- Subacute thyroiditis (typically has an initial hyperthyroid phase, and may have been related to her previous history of PAF).
- Beta-blocker-induced fatigue and bradycardia.
- Ortner's syndrome – hoarseness of voice caused by left vocal cord paralysis (associated with left atrial enlargement secondary to mitral stenosis).
- Addison's disease (though typically have weight loss) or other autoimmune disease.
- Depression.

Investigations

- Blood: FBC, U&E, LFT, TSH/T4, serum thyroglobulin (often increased), coagulation screen, short ACTH Synacthen test
- Cardiac: ECG, echocardiogram with Doppler
- Other: CXR, thyroid ultrasound (if goitre present).

Viva questions

How would you manage a patient with amiodarone induced hypothyroidism?

This is largely related to the severity of symptoms, although there is little published evidence as to best practice. Options are:

- Stop amiodarone and consider alternative management of underlying cardiac condition.
- Thyroxine replacement therapy.

Note that *UpToDate* guidelines (May 2009) suggest continuing amiodarone (unless it is ineffective in treating the arrhythmia), and establishing a euthyroid state by replacing thyroid hormone (grade 2C evidence – weak recommendation).

How soon should symptoms take to resolve?

Amiodarone has long half-life (40–100 days) so symptoms may persist for several weeks to months after withdrawal (if left untreated). With thyroxine replacement therapy the symptoms should resolve within a few days. Monitoring of thyroid function tests will be required to tailor the withdrawal of thyroxine as the amiodarone's effects diminish.

If this patient had long-standing undiagnosed hypothyroidism and underwent major surgery, such as mitral valve repair, what might you be concerned about?
- Myxoedema coma, which can be precipitated in patients with long-standing untreated hypothyroidism by a sudden stressful event e.g. surgery, concurrent illness.
- Uncommon but life threatening (untreated >50% mortality).
- Requires intensive care management.
- Intravenous thyroxine replacement ± glucocorticoid replacement.

What is Hashimoto's thyroiditis?
- A spectrum of autoimmune thyroid disease.
- Antibodies to thyroid-peroxidase (anti-TPO), antithyroglobulin.
- Results in hypothyroidism.
- Associated with diabetes, Addison's disease, pernicious anaemia, hypoparathyroidism, Graves' disease.

Please examine this patient's ankle reflexes
Slow relaxing reflexes are frequently present in a patient with clinical hypothyroidism. They are best demonstrated in the ankle or supinator reflexes. Brisk reflexes are often found in hyperthyroidism.

Please examine this patient's thyroid gland
Please refer to ➲ p.583.

Case 10: Infective endocarditis

> **History (key points to elicit in 25 minutes)**
>
> Mr David Burke.
> 28 years old.
> Homeless, from Dublin.
> Presented 5 days ago into A&E with fevers and rigors.

HPC

- Poor historian – 1-word answers, no eye contact.
- Complained of high fevers, sweats, fatigue and anorexia for 2 days prior to presentation.
- Non-productive cough for months.
- Intermittent intravenous drug use (cocaine), shares needles with his girlfriend.
- No history of chest pain, shortness of breath or weight loss.

> **❶ Top Tips**
>
> - A difficult historian is the 'nightmare' scenario that every candidate dreads, however, with a direct, confident and focused approach, most important issues can be addressed.
> - Think of yourself as taking the history in the emergency department for the first time – you need to be delicate, but firm in cases such as this. Asking about IV drug abuse early is important, as it will dictate the focus of your history.

PMHx

- Regular attendee of A&E with intoxication.
- Denies history of rheumatic fever.

Medications

- Vancomycin 1g BD day 5
- Thiamine 100mg TDS
- Chlordiazepoxide 20mg TDS (reducing dose)
- Allergic to penicillin (? reaction).

SHx

- Homeless
- Alcohol: 'A lot.' (unable to quantify)
- Heavy smoker
- Unemployed
- Multiple sexual partners
- Has a girlfriend, also an IV drug abuser, no contact since admission.

FHx

- Unknown.

ROS

- No diarrhoea
- No genitourinary symptoms.

Hospital course
- TOE
- Blood tests
- HIV test.

❶ Top Tips

- If a patient does not volunteer or seem to know what tests they have had, suggest likely procedures to them. E.g. 'did they put a camera down into your stomach?'.
- Ask about HIV, as consent would have been required.

Examination (10–12 minutes)

Perform general examination as detailed on ➲ p.640. The following points are a guide to general cardiovascular examination and can be applied to this case.

Specific examination points

- *General:*
  - Malnourished
  - Unkempt
  - Multiple tattoos
  - Try to position at 45° for examination
  - Note any scars or audible clicks
  - Fever/clammy skin
- *Hands:*
  - Splinter haemorrhages – remember to look at both fingers and toes
  - Osler's nodes
  - Janeway lesions (irregular painless erythematous vasculitic macules on palms and soles, most commonly occur in *S. aureus* infection)
  - Clubbing (historically found in subacute cases; now very rare due to treatment)
- *Eyes:*
  - Fundoscopy may reveal Roth spots (retinal haemorrhages with pale centres)
- *Cardiovascular:*
  - Pulse
  - JVP
  - Feel for cardiac thrills/heaves
  - Pansystolic murmur along left sternal border (tricuspid regurgitation); See Top Tips Box
  - Look for peripheral signs of embolic phenomena (petechiae, gangrenous toes)
- *Other:*
  - Examine abdomen for pulsatile hepatomegaly and splenomegaly
  - Examine joints for septic arthritis.

> **❶ Top Tips**
>
> • The vast majority of patients presenting with endocarditis will have a cardiac murmur, however the exception is tricuspid valve endocarditis, in which patients often do not have an audible murmur.[1]

Summary

Mr Burke is 28-year-old homeless man from Dublin who presented into hospital 5 days ago with fevers, sweats and general malaise. He is a poor historian and did not volunteer information readily. He complained of feeling unwell with fevers and sweats for 2 days leading up to his admission. He admits to intermittent IV cocaine use, and he shares needles with his girlfriend, whom he has not seen since admission. His other main complaint was a chronic non-productive cough, which has been present for several months. He denies chest pain, shortness of breath or weight loss.

Since admission Mr Burke has been on vancomycin 1g BD, thiamine 100mg TDS and a reducing dose of chlordiazepoxide. He is allergic to penicillin.

Mr Burke is also a heavy drinker and smoker, and has had multiple presentations to hospital with alcohol intoxication. Unfortunately, he does not want to stop drinking or using drugs. He is not in touch with family.

On examination Mr Burke is malnourished, but was otherwise comfortable at rest. His BP was 112/68, his pulse was 92 regular and his saturation was 99% on room air. He is currently afebrile. I note multiple tattoos over his body. His positive findings include Janeway lesions on his palms, a 6cm raised JVP with large v waves and a grade 3/6 pansystolic murmur on his left sternal border which is louder on inspiration. This is consistent with tricuspid regurgitation. He has no evidence of hepatosplenomegaly and does not appear to have signs of embolic phenomena.

> **❶ Top Tips**
>
> • Aim to present *positive* findings confidently and precisely.
> • Remember that this is a *real patient* with significant social and personal issues. If these are not addressed, there is a high chance that he will re-present in the future with similar problems. Asking him about why he abuses drugs and if he wants to stop will allow your examiner to see that you appreciate this.

Differential diagnosis

• Infective endocarditis; more specifically right-sided endocarditis, with *S. aureus*, related to IV drug abuse (❯ p.260)
• TB
• HIV seroconversion illness
• AIDS.

Investigations

• *Blood:* FBC, U&E, LFT, coagulation profile, ESR, CRP, Ca²⁺/PO4/Mg²⁺, B12, folate, HIV, hepatitis A, B, C.
• *Microbiology:* blood cultures (minimum 2 sets >12 hours apart; ❯ Table 5.10 for the Duke criteria for the diagnosis of definite IE, p.260), sputum and urine cultures.

- *Radiology:* CXR, consider liver ultrasound if LFT abnormal.
- *Others:* ECG, TTE, TOE, Mantoux test.

Management

For detailed management please refer to ➔ p.262.

Viva questions

Is transthoracic echocardiogram an acceptable diagnostic evaluation for infective endocarditis?

An echocardiogram should be performed in all patients who have moderate to high clinical suspicion of infective endocarditis (typical organism on culture, new murmur, fever).

For patients with a normal TTE (morphology and function), the likelihood of endocarditis is very low, and a follow-up TOE should be reserved for the following cases:[2]

- High clinical suspicion of endocarditis (persistently positive blood cultures and/or multiple minor criteria).
- Technically limited TTE study.
- If pulmonary valve endocarditis is suspected.

Some experts, however, believe that in suspected endocarditis, particularly those with staphylococcal bacteraemia, direct TOE should be performed.[3]

Actual practice will be dependent on the institution and quality/experience of TTE evaluation.

If this gentleman had MRSA grown in blood cultures, how long would you continue treatment?

Monotherapy for 6 weeks with vancomycin is the AHA (American Heart Association) and ESC (European Society of Cardiology) recommended therapy for native valve endocarditis, either for MRSA or coagulase negative staphylococci.[4,5]

What are some indications for surgery as a treatment of native valve infective endocarditis?

The 2006 American College of Cardiology/American Heart Association (ACC/AHA) guidelines on the management of valvular heart disease included recommendations for surgery in patients with native valve endocarditis. There is a general consensus that surgery is warranted for patients with active native valve IE who have one or more of the following complications:[6]

- Heart failure (HF), particularly if moderate to severe, that is directly related to valve dysfunction.
- Severe aortic or mitral regurgitation with evidence of abnormal haemodynamics.
- Endocarditis due to fungal or other highly resistant organisms.
- Perivalvular infection with abscess or fistula formation.

References

1. Sande, MA et al. Endocarditis in intravenous drug users. In: Kaye, D (ed) *Infective Endocarditis*, p.345. Raven Press, New York 1992.

2. Irani W et al. A negative transthoracic echocardiogram obviates the need for transesophageal echocardiography in patients with suspected native valve active infective endocarditis. *Am J Cardiol* 1996; **78**(1):101–3.

3. Heidenreich PA et al. Echocardiography in patients with suspected endocarditis: a cost-effectiveness analysis. *Am J Med* 1999; **107**(3):198–208.

4. Baddour LM et al. Infective endocarditis: diagnosis, antimicrobial therapy, and management of complications: a statement for healthcare professionals from the Committee on Rheumatic Fever, Endocarditis, and Kawasaki Disease, Council on Cardiovascular Disease in the Young, and the Councils on Clinical Cardiology, Stroke, and Cardiovascular Surgery and Anesthesia, American Heart Association – executive summary: endorsed by the Infectious Diseases Society of America. Circulation 2005; **111**(23):3167–84.

5. Horstkotte D et al. Guidelines on prevention, diagnosis and treatment of infective endocarditis executive summary; the task force on infective endocarditis of the European society of cardiology. Eur Heart J 2004; **25**(3):267–76.

6. Bonow RO et al. ACC/AHA 2006 guidelines for the management of patients with valvular heart disease. A report of the American College of Cardiology/American Heart Association Task Force on Practice Guidelines. J Am Coll Cardiol 2006; **48**:e1.

Case 11: Aortic stenosis

History (key points: 25 minutes)

Mrs Jane Brophy.
64 years old.
From Wexford.
Brought into A+E by ambulance 2 days ago with collapse.

HPC

- While walking to the local shops with her son, she became very breathless, developed chest pain and collapsed.
- No loss of consciousness or seizure activity.
- Gradually worsening breathlessness on exertion for the last 6 months.
- Now breathless walking around house.
- 3 pillow orthopnoea for past one week, no paroxysmal nocturnal dyspnoea.
- Central chest pain on exertion (similar to previous angina) for the last 3 months, seems to be getting worse, but no pain at rest.
- Has fainted twice at home in the last month, without other symptoms.
- Stopped attending cardiology clinics 2 years ago ('because I felt fine').

PMHx

- Myocardial infarction (MI) 8 years ago.
- Coronary stenting (post MI) – 2 stents.
- 'Mild heart murmur' according to GP.
- Non-insulin dependent diabetes × 15 years.
- Hypertension.
- Hypercholesterolaemia.
- No history of rheumatic fever, TIA, claudication or AAA.

❶ Top Tips

- In patients with significant cardiac histories, be sure to find out all the details surrounding any previous events.
- Do not assume that collapse is automatically related to aortic stenosis – other differential diagnosis such as epilepsy need to be ruled out.
- Including details such as time off clopidogrel or date of last exercise stress test will show the examiner that you are experienced and practical.

Medications

- Aspirin 75mg OD
- Clopidogrel 75mg OD (since admission)
- Bisoprolol 2.5mg OD
- Ramipril 2.5mg OD
- Metformin 500mg BD (on hold)
- Furosemide 40mg BD IV (since admission)
- Pravastatin 20mg OD
- Enoxaparin 20mg OD SC (since admission)
- Allergic to penicillin (anaphylaxis).

SHx

- Married, 2 adult sons (both married)
- Lives alone in bungalow
- Husband died 2 years ago, age 68 (gastric cancer)
- 20 pack-year smoking history (stopped smoking 5 years ago, but started again after husband died)
- 10 units of alcohol per week (wine)
- Retired teacher
- Until recently, independent in ADLs
- Excellent family support.

FHx

- Adopted, biological parents and siblings not known
- Children healthy.

ROS

- No weight loss, cough/haemoptysis.

Hospital course as per patient

- Admitted under cardiology team
- Blood tests
- CXR
- On cardiac monitor since admission
- TTE
- Coronary angiogram scheduled tomorrow.

❶ Top Tips

- Exercise stress testing is contraindicated in patients with symptomatic aortic stenosis due to safety issues.

Examination: 10–12 minutes

Perform general examination as detailed on ➔ p.640.

Specific examination points

- *General:*
  - BP (lying + standing)
  - Try to position at 45° for examination
  - Level of comfort at rest – respiratory rate
  - Nutritional status/fluid balance
  - Malar flush (mitral stenosis)
  - Thoracotomy scars; venous harvesting scars
  - Audible clicks (metallic valves)
- *Hands:*
  - Clubbing
  - Nicotine staining
  - Splinter haemorrhages
- *Pulse (use carotid);* in aortic stenosis:
  - Low volume
  - Slow rising
  - Anacrotic (notched upstroke) if severe
- *Cardiovascular:*
  - JVP
  - Apex beat; in aortic stenosis:
    – Heaving
    – Non-displaced (unless longstanding severe disease with LV dilatation or associated with aortic regurgitation)
  - Systolic thrill in aortic area (usually AV gradient >50mmHg)
  - S1 normal or soft
  - S2 soft or absent
  - Ejection systolic murmur radiating to carotids best heard in aortic area, but also at base (Gallavardin phenomenon)
  - Classically crescendo-decrescendo murmur
  - Auscultate lungs, and examine for sacrum and peripheral oedema
  - Check peripheral pulses and for AAA
- *Diabetic exam:*
  - Fundoscopy
  - Peripheral neuropathy
  - Autonomic neuropathy (lying and standing BP).

❶ Top Tips

- Remember dynamic manoeuvres while auscultating the praecordium.
- The severity of aortic stenosis is not necessarily determined by the intensity of the murmur, but rather the length/duration of the murmur and the timing of the peak.
- The later the 'peak' of the murmur and the longer the duration indicate more severe stenosis.

Summary

Mrs Brophy is a 64-year-old lady who was brought into A&E 2 days ago with a collapse that was preceded by shortness of breath and chest pain. She was walking to the shops with her son at the time. Mrs Brophy has been complaining of increasing dyspnoea on exertion for the last 6 months that has been associated with chest discomfort. Though she denies symptoms at rest, she now gets breathless while walking within her house, has new 3-pillow orthopnoea, and has fainted twice within the last month. She denies any palpitations or neurological symptoms.

Mrs Brophy has a significant cardiac history. She had an MI 5 years ago that was treated with primary percutaneous intervention and the insertion of 2 stents. She remained on clopidogrel for 18 months post MI, discontinuing this medication following advice from her cardiologist, and had a normal exercise stress test about 4 years ago. Mrs Brophy has a history of non-insulin dependent diabetes (15 years), hypertension, and hypercholesterolaemia. She continues to smoke heavily. Her diabetes is managed by her endocrinologist, whom she sees twice a year. She claims to have good sugar control and regularly gets her eyes checked. Unfortunately, she stopped attending cardiology outpatient clinics, as she was asymptomatic.

Her current medications include aspirin 75mg OD, clopidogrel 75mg OD, bisoprolol 2.5mg OD, ramipril 2.5mg OD, pravastatin 20mg OD and prophylactic enoxaparin. Her metformin was temporarily discontinued on admission. She has a severe penicillin allergy.

Mrs Brophy was widowed 2 years ago, and has 2 healthy sons, from who she gets excellent support. She currently lives alone in a bungalow. Her family history is unknown as she was adopted.

On examination Mrs Brophy was sitting comfortably at 45°, and was in no distress. Her BP was 118/82 with no postural change. Positive findings included a slow rising, low volume pulse (pulsus parvus et tardus), which was regular at 64bpm, and a non-displaced apex beat which was heaving in nature. On auscultation the 1st heart sound was normal, and the 2nd was very soft. There was a harsh ejection systolic murmur that was heard in the aortic area, radiated to the carotids and increased with expiration. There was no diastolic murmur. These findings are consistent with aortic stenosis. Of note she has no evidence of peripheral vascular disease, femoral bruits or AAA. Fundoscopy was normal and neurological examination did not reveal peripheral neuropathy.

Differential diagnosis

- Moderate to severe aortic stenosis resulting in angina, dyspnoea and syncope
- Ischaemic heart disease
- Cardiac arrhythmia
- Pulmonary embolism (less likely due to 6-month history of worsening dyspnoea).

Investigations

- *Blood:* FBC, U&E, LFT, coagulation profile, troponin & cardiac enzymes, HbA1C, fasting lipid profile, TFTs.
- *Cardiac:* ECG, TTE with Doppler, TOE (performed to determine suitability for valve repair), coronary angiogram, Holter monitor, 24-hour BP monitoring, lying/standing BP.
- *Other:* CXR.

Management

Aortic stenosis management is dependent on symptoms and severity of lesion (**Ɔ** p.229).

It is important to realize that when medically treating symptoms secondary to AS, such as pulmonary oedema, one must be careful not to critically lower cardiac preload.

This case highlights the importance of educating and involving patients with their care. It is very likely that this patient had documented aortic stenosis at her first presentation 5 years ago. If the importance to follow-up of this lesion had been explained to her, she may not have stopped attending clinics.

Viva questions

What typical ECG findings might you expect with this patient?

- LVH with strain pattern
- Left axis deviation
- Left bundle branch block
- Left atrial hypertrophy with p mitrale (late stage)
- May be normal.

What are some clinical signs of severity of aortic stenosis?

- Systolic thrill
- Heaving apex beat
- Soft or absent 2nd heart sound
- Narrow/reversed split 2nd heart sound
- Narrow pulse pressure
- Cardiac failure.

What are some complications of aortic stenosis?

- Sudden death
- Arrhythmias and conduction abnormalities
- Left ventricular failure
- Infective endocarditis
- Systemic embolization.

What precautions would you take if this patient needed endoscopy?

British Society of Gastroenterology guidelines (2009)[1] do not recommend routine antibiotic prophylaxis for the prevention of infective endocarditis in patients with valvular heart disease, or valve replacement. Severely immunocompromised or neutropenic patients should receive prophylaxis.

Reference

1. http://www.bsg.org.uk/clinical-guidelines/endoscopy/antibiotic-prophylaxis-in-gastrointestinal-endoscopy.html.

Case 12: Fistulating Crohn's disease

> **History (key points: 25 minutes)**
>
> Mr Michael Flemming.
> 29 years old.
> From Co. Wicklow.
> Presented 2 days ago with perianal pain and diarrhoea.

HPC

- 2/52 history of gradually worsening perianal pain, burning in nature.
- Initially bearable, now severe.
- Intermittent, generalized crampy abdominal pain.
- Pain worse with defecation.
- Loose stools, with urgency, not bloody.
- 12 bowel motions during day, 5 at night.
- 2 episodes of faecal incontinence in last week.
- Mild nausea, no vomiting.
- Approximately 1 stone weight loss in last month.
- Decreased appetite.
- Mild fever and general malaise, no rigors.
- No recent foreign travel.
- No new medications or recent antibiotics.

> **❶ Top Tips**
>
> - Always ask about nocturnal symptoms and incontinence – these can be indicative of severe disease.
> - It is important to know if these symptoms have ever occurred before, in which case a patient such as this is quite likely to be having a flare of their underlying condition.
> - First presentation vs. recurrence of symptoms also has a significant bearing on the differential diagnosis (e.g. infection vs. inflammatory bowel disease).

PMHx

- Depression, diagnosed 8 years ago following death of younger sister.
- Malaria – 3 years ago while visiting India.
- Appendectomy – age 9.

Medications

- Loperamide on a PRN basis prior to admission
- Fluoxetine 20mg OD
- IV hydrocortisone 100mg QDS since admission
- IV metronidazole 500mg TDS since admission
- Tinzaparin 3500IU SC OD
- Calcium carbonate 1 tablet OD.

> **❶ Top Tips**
>
> - Always ask about new medications commenced since hospital admission.

SHx
- Single
- Lives alone in apartment
- Taxi driver
- Smokes 20 cigarettes/day × 10 years (10 pack-years)
- Alcohol 24 units/week
- Independent in activities of daily life
- Good social support.

FHx
- Mother died 2 years ago of lung cancer (smoker)
- Father had TB 2 years ago, fully treated, now fine
- Sister died 8 years ago in road traffic accident
- No other siblings
- No history of IBD or HLA B27 diseases.

ROS
Denies any extra intestinal manifestations of IBD.

> **❶ Top Tips**
> - A history of *exposure* to TB (e.g. via a family member or endemic area) is important as this may influence management options (biological therapy).
> - In a case of suspected IBD, always ask for extra-gastrointestinal manifestations of disease such as joint pain, eye problems and rashes.

Hospital management as per patient
- Blood tests
- Stool samples
- Abdominal x-ray
- CT abdomen, pelvic MRI
- IV steroids and antibiotics.

Examination: 10–12 minutes
Perform general examination as detailed on ➔ p.640.

> **Specific examination points**
> - *General:*
>   - Nutritional status
>   - Signs of anaemia
>   - Oedema (sign of hypoalbuminaemia)
>   - Evidence of Mantoux test/BCG scar
> - *Hands:*
>   - Clubbing
> - *Face/mouth:*
>   - Aphthous ulcers
> - *Eyes:*
>   - Uveitis

- *Abdomen:*
  - Scars
  - Masses
  - Tenderness
  - Cutaneous fistulas
  - Always check perianal region
- *Skin:*
  - Erythema nodosum or pyoderma gangrenosum.

Summary

Mr Fleming is a 29-year-old gentleman who presented recently with a 1-week history of severe perianal pain, non-bloody diarrhoea and significant weight loss. He has never had any similar symptoms previously. He has also been complaining of lower back pain for the last 10 days. He is a heavy smoker, and has a family history of lung cancer and TB exposure. There is no family history of IBD or other HLA B27 related diseases. On examination, he is a thin, pale gentleman. He has several apthous ulcers in his mouth and tender sacroiliitis. His abdominal examination revealed a diffusely tender, but soft abdomen. His bowel sounds were present and normal. Examination of his perianal area revealed skin tags and several fistulous tracts. Since his admission he has been commenced on IV steroids, antibiotics and prophylactic LMWH. He has had several blood tests and scans, and is awaiting results.

Differential diagnosis

- Inflammatory bowel disease – specifically fistulating Crohn's disease
- Ileocaecal TB
- Diverticulitis
- Infectious diarrhoea
- Malignancy – consider colorectal adenocarcinoma or carcinoid tumour.

ⓘ Top Tips

- Always be specific when presenting the most likely differential diagnosis e.g. in this case: *fistulating* Crohn's disease.
- List differentials in order of probability, and mention if you think a differential is unlikely but important to consider, such as malignancy.

Investigations

Please refer to ⊃ p.166 for investigation and management of IBD.

Management

- IV fluids
- IV hydrocortisone
- Metronidazole 500mg TDS for treatment of perianal disease
- Infliximab (anti-TNF) therapy.

❶ Top Tips

- Unless the patient is likely to require an acute surgical intervention, keeping them nil by mouth is unnecessary. Oral diet *promotes* mucosal healing.
- Surgical review is highly important, particularly in the case of fistulating disease, where examination under anaesthetic and seton placement may be required.

Viva questions

Why is the history of TB exposure important?

This young gentleman may have latent TB, which could become active following Anti-TNF treatment. It is therefore imperative that such patients have a CXR prior to commencing therapy.

What is the role of infliximab in Crohn's disease?

Infliximab is a chimeric mouse-human monoclonal antibody against TNF and is effective in refractory and particularly fistulating disease.

A general administration guideline for fistulating disease is 5mg/kg at weeks 0, 2, and 6. The fistulating disease responds (closes) in approximately 2/3 of patients, usually within 2 weeks. The ACCENT II study showed that patients on 8-weekly infusions of infliximab had significantly higher rates of maintained remission (fistula closure) compared to placebo.[1] This study terminated at 54 weeks, hence there is currently no evidence base for continuing maintenance treatment beyond this stage. Infliximab is also immunogenic, and patients may develop antibodies after repeated administration, which can lead to quite serious infusion reactions.[2,3]

Do you know of any other anti-TNF agents useful in Crohn's disease?

Adalimumab (Humira®) may be less immunogenic than infliximab (CLASSIC I and II placebo controlled trials), and shown to be effective in induction and maintenance of remission in patients naïve to anti-TNF therapy (or those who have had allergic reactions to infliximab).[4]

Please demonstrate how you would examine this gentleman's abdomen

Refer to ❸ Abdominal examination, p.94.

Please explain the risks of infliximab therapy to this patient

Points to cover:

- Affects normal immune response → increased risk of infection.
- Allergic reactions.
- Rarely lymphoma, TB, lupus-like syndrome, demyelinating disorders.

References

1. Sands BE et al. Infliximab maintenance therapy for fistulizing Crohn's disease. *NEJM* 2004; **350**(9):934–6.
2. Present DH et al. Infliximab for the treatment of fistulas in patients with Crohn's disease. *NEJM* 1999; **340**(18):1398–405.
3. Carter MJ et al. Guidelines for the management of inflammatory bowel disease in adult. *Gut* 2004; **53**(Suppl V):v1–v16. http://www.bsg.org.uk/images/stories/docs/clinical/guidelines/ibd/ibd.pdf.
4. Hanauer SB et al Human anti-tumor necrosis factor monoclonal antibody (Adalimumab) in Crohn's Disease: the CLASSIC-I Trial. *Gastroenterology* 2006; **130**(2):323–33.

Case 13: Spontaneous bacterial peritonitis

History (key points: 25 minutes)

Mr Sam Peters.
49 years old.
From Dublin.
Admitted from outpatient clinic 2 days ago with fever and abdominal pain.

HPC

- Seen in hepatology outpatient clinic 2 days ago.
- Complaining of abdominal swelling and pain, malaise and fever.
- No rigors.
- Feeling generally unwell for the last 5 days.
- Anorexia, no weight loss.
- Mild nausea, no vomiting.
- Diarrhoea past 4 days, 6 motions per day, no nocturnal symptoms, no blood.

PMHx

- Alcoholic liver disease.
- Liver cirrhosis and ascites diagnosed 6 months ago.
- On waiting list for liver transplant.
- 3 previous therapeutic abdominal paracentesis – last one 4 weeks ago.
- Oesophageal varices, no previous upper GI bleed, last endoscopy 2 months ago.

Medications

- Propranolol 40mg BD
- Spironolactone 200mg OD
- Furosemide 40mg BD
- Lactulose 15mL TDS
- Salt restricted diet
- IV cefotaxime 2g TDS (since admission)
- Nil known drug allergies.

SHx

- 20 pack-year smoking history
- Significant history (20 years) of alcohol abuse, but stopped drinking completely 1 year ago
- Lives alone, separated from partner 4 years ago
- No children
- Unemployed, on social welfare.

FHx

- Mother died in road traffic accident shortly after his birth
- Father IHD – MI at age 58
- Only child.

ROS

- Extremely fatigued over last few weeks
- Feels confused at times.

Hospital course as per patient

- Blood tests
- Ascitic tap/diagnostic paracentesis
- Commenced on antibiotics
- Abdominal ultrasound.

Examination: 10–12 minutes

Perform general examination as detailed on ➔ p.640.

Specific examination points

- *General:*
  - Nutritional status
  - Mental status
  - Jaundice
  - Spider naevi
  - Abdominal distension and flank fullness
  - Gynaecomastia
- *Hands:*
  - Leuconychia
  - Clubbing
  - Palmar erythema
  - Asterixis
- *Abdominal:*
  - Paracentesis marks
  - Distension, full flanks
  - Caput medusae
  - Hepatosplenomegaly
  - Fluid thrill
  - Shifting dullness
- *Neurological:*
  - Proximal myopathy
  - Cerebellar disease.

Summary

Mr Peters is a 49-year-old man who was admitted from clinic 2 days ago with abdominal pain and fever. He was feeling generally unwell with abdominal swelling and pain for the previous 5 days. He is also complaining of associated fatigue, confusion, anorexia and nausea. During the last week, he has had about 6 loose bowel motions per day, with no nocturnal symptoms or PR bleeding.

Mr Peters has had a long-standing history of alcohol abuse, and was diagnosed with liver cirrhosis and liver failure about 6 months ago. Since that time he has required 3 therapeutic paracentesis for severe ascites, the last of which was 1 month ago. He has oesophageal varices, diagnosed 2 months ago on upper GI endoscopy. He has no history of GI bleeds. Mr Peters has abstained from alcohol since his diagnosis 6 months ago.

His medications include propranolol 40mg BD, spironolactone 200mg OD, furosemide 40mg BD and lactulose 15mL TDS. Since admission he has been commenced on cefotaxime 2g TDS IV. He is on sodium restriction.

Mr Peters is separated, lives alone, is unemployed and is receiving social welfare. He has no children and his family history is positive for ischaemic heart disease.

On examination, Mr Peters is notably icteric, with a distended abdomen. His vitals signs are stable and he is currently afebrile. He is alert and oriented with no signs of encephalopathy. He has evidence of leuconychia, palmar erythema and a hepatic flap. There are multiple spider naevi on his chest. Examination of his abdomen revealed a fluid thrill and shifting dullness, suggestive of ascites, and 3cm hepatomegaly. His abdomen was mildly tender, with no rebound or guarding, and bowel sounds were normal. Neurologically, Mr Peters has evidence of mild proximal myopathy in upper and lower limbs, but no signs of cerebellar disease.

Differential diagnosis

- Spontaneous bacterial peritonitis (SBP) with decompensated end stage liver disease
- Acute appendicitis
- Infectious diarrhoea
- Malignancy.

Investigations

- *Blood:* FBC, U&E, LFT (ALT, AST, alk phos, GGT), albumin, coagulation profile, CRP, blood cultures.
- *Radiology:* CXR, plain film of the abdomen, abdominal ultrasound – specifically Doppler study to determine patency of portal vein.
- *Other:* ascitic tap (neutrophil count, cytology, total protein/albumin, LDH, culture and microscopy), urine culture and microscopy.

Management of spontaneous bacterial peritonitis

An ascitic fluid neutrophil count of >250 cells/uL has a sensitivity of 93% and specificity of 94%. The following warrants treatment for SBP:

- Polymorphonuclear neutrophil (PMN) count >250 cells/uL with a positive bacterial culture result.
- Culture negative ascites (probable SBP) with PMN count >250 cells/uL.
- Monomicrobial non-neutrocytic ascites (PMN <250cell/uL) with a positive bacterial culture.

Empiric treatment with a 3rd-generation cephalosporin such as cefotaxime should be initiated immediately while awaiting ascitic tap results.

Viva questions

What organisms typically cause SBP?

- *Escherichia coli* (43%)
- *Klebsiella pneumoniae* (11%)
- *Streptococcus pneumoniae* (9%)
- Other streptococcal species (19%)
- Miscellaneous (10%).

❶ Top Tips[1]

- Anaerobic organisms are rare due to high oxygen tension of the ascitic fluid.
- Single organism contamination (92%); polymicrobial infection (8%).

What factors make a patient more susceptible to SBP?
- Cirrhotic patients in decompensated state.
- Low complement levels.
- Compromised synthetic function (low albumin, high INR).

Other than therapeutic paracentesis, what options are available to treat this patient's intractable ascites?
- Begin by optimizing medical therapy (diuretics and salt restriction).
- Peritovenous shunts (now very rarely used):
  - Leveen shunt & Denver shunt (peritoneal cavity to superior vena cava).[2]
- Transjugular intrahepatic portosystemic shunts (TIPS).
- Liver transplant – cirrhotic patients with diuretic resistant ascites have a 50% 6-month survival rate.

What is the significance of this patient's intermittent confusion?
Confusion in a cirrhotic patient is a worrying sign of hepatic encephalopathy. This can be precipitated by an underlying infection (such as in this patient). Other important causes are:
- GI bleeding
- Renal failure
- Constipation
- Medications (opiates, benzodiazepines, anti-psychotics).

Please demonstrate shifting dullness in this patient
Please refer to ➲ p.103.

References
1. Data from McHutchison, JG, Runyon, BA. Spontaneous bacterial peritonitis. In: Surawicz, CM, Owen, RL (eds) *Gastrointestinal and Hepatic Infections*, p.455. Philadelphia, PA: WB Saunders, 1995.
2. Bories P *et al.* The treatment of refractory ascites by the LeVeen shunt. A multi-centre controlled trial (57 patients). *J Hepatol* 1986; **3**(2):212–18.

Case 14: Post-transplant lymphoproliferative disorder (PTLD)

> **History (key points to elicit in 25 minutes)**
>
> Mr Michael Simmons.
> 37 years old.
> From Tipperary.
> Referred by GP with 2-day history of fever, axillary lymphadenopathy and swelling over renal transplant.

HPC

- General malaise and increasing fatigue in few weeks prior to presentation.
- 2 days of high fevers and sore throat.
- Noticed swelling in right axilla and presented to GP.
- Mild sweating at night.
- No cough or shortness of breath.
- No weight loss.
- No gastrointestinal symptoms.
- Normal urine output, no haematuria.
- No ankle swelling.
- Last felt 'well' about 2 weeks ago.
- Last visit to renal clinic was 6 weeks ago.
- No foreign travel in last 6 months.

> **❶ Top Tips**
>
> - Asking when a patient last felt well is a useful question, particularly when the onset of symptoms is gradual.
> - If the patient has a transplant, always find out when they received it, and when were they last seen in clinic.

PMHx

- Cadaveric renal transplant 9 months ago:
  - One episode of 'rejection' 6 weeks post transplant (diagnosed on renal biopsy) – treated with IV steroids and recovered well
- Chronic renal failure due to autosomal dominant polycystic kidney disease (ADPKD):
  - Haemodialysis via functioning left brachiocephalic arteriovenous fistula for 6 months prior to transplant
- Hypertension.

Medications

- Tacrolimus 1mg BD
- Mycophenolate mofetil 500mg BD
- Prednisolone 5mg OD
- Ganciclovir 1000mg TDS

- Ramipril 2.5mg OD
- Calcium carbonate 1 tablet OD
- No drug allergies.

Social history
- Married, 2 healthy children
- Computer programmer
- Non-smoker
- Alcohol – 14 units per week
- Lived in Africa for 6 months as a humanitarian worker 10 years ago.

Family history
- Mother has ADPKD (renal transplant at age 58), otherwise well
- No siblings.

Systems review
No symptoms of chronic steroid use or allograft dysfunction.

> **❶ Top Tips**
>
> - Transplant patients will often (*but not always*) know helpful information regarding their underlying disease, immunosuppressive medication and investigations. For example, if you are not sure about a particular medication they are on, *ask!*

Hospital course as per patient
- Blood tests including blood cultures and tacrolimus levels
- CXR
- Urine analysis
- Awaiting renal ultrasound and biopsy.

Examination (10–12 minutes)
Perform general examination as detailed on ❸ p.640.

Specific examination points

- *General:*
  - Nutritional status
  - Fluid balance, JVP, peripheral, sacral oedema
  - Temperature
  - Pulse, BP
  - AV fistula (bruit, thrill, puncture marks indicating recent use, aneurismal dilatation)
  - Tremor (associated with tacrolimus and ciclosporin use)
- *Lymphadenopathy:*
  - Submandibular
  - Submental
  - Pre/post-auricular
  - Occipital
  - Cervical
  - Supraclavicular
  - Axillary
  - Inguinal

- *Chest:*
  - Expansion
  - Percussion
  - Auscultation
  - Carefully examine apices
- *Abdomen:*
  - Examine renal allograft (note any masses, tenderness or bruits)
  - Hepato/splenomegaly
  - Examine native polycystic kidneys, noting if they are tender
- *Side effects of chronic glucocorticoid use:*
  - Oral/oesophageal *Candida*
  - Proximal myopathy
  - Cushingoid facies
  - Dorsocervical fat pad
  - Skin fragility, bruising
  - Striae.

Summary

Mr Simmons is a 37-year-old gentleman from Tipperary who presented with a recent history of fevers, axillary lymphadenopathy and swelling over his renal transplant. He last felt well 2 week ago, but has since become increasingly fatigued, and in the last few days has suffered from high temperatures, mild sweating at night, a sore throat and non-tender lymphadenopathy. He noticed the non-tender swelling over his transplant in the last few days as well. His urine output is normal and he denies haematuria. He has no cough, shortness of breath or gastrointestinal symptoms.

Mr Simmons had a cadaveric renal transplant 9 months ago for chronic renal failure secondary to ADPKD. He was on dialysis for a total of 6 months via a still functioning left brachial arteriovenous fistula. 6 weeks post transplant he suffered an episode of rejection, which was confirmed on biopsy, and subsequently responded well to IV steroids. He was last seen in clinic 6 weeks ago, and was told that his overall progress was satisfactory. His other past medical history includes hypertension, which was diagnosed 5 years ago.

He is married with two healthy children, is a computer programmer by trade, does not smoke and drinks about 14 units of alcohol per week. His mother who has ADPKD, received a renal transplant at age 58, and is otherwise well.

His current medications include tacrolimus 1mg BD, mycophenolate mofetil 500mg BD, ganciclovir 1000mg TDS, prednisolone 5mg OD, calcium carbonate 1 tablet OD, and ramipril 2.5mg OD. He has no known drug allergies.

Positive findings on examination included: a 3cm, non-tender, smooth lymph node in the right axilla, bilateral submandibular lymphadenopathy, a smooth, non-tender 3 × 4cm mass on the renal allograft.

Differential diagnosis

- Post-transplant lymphoproliferative disease (PTLD)
- Post-transplant infectious mononucleosis
- Miliary TB.

Investigations

- *Blood:* FBC, U&E, LFT, coagulation profile, ESR, CRP, $Ca^{2+}/PO_4/Mg^{2+}$, fasting lipid profile
- *Microbiology:* EBV serology, blood cultures, MSU, Mantoux test
- *Radiology:* CXR, renal ultrasound with Doppler, CT chest and abdomen
- *Others:* lymph node biopsy.

❶ Top Tips

- Suspected PTLD lesions should be biopsied to establish cell clonality, malignancy and the presence or absence of EBV.[1]

Viva questions

What risk factors for PTLD are you aware of?

Main risk factors include the degree of immunosuppression, time post transplant (highest risk during the first year), and recipient EBV serostatus. EBV negative recipients are at greater risk of developing PTLD from grafts of EBV positive donors. [2,3]

What types of EBV related lymphoproliferative disease are you aware of?

The first is a benign polyclonal lymphoproliferative disease, which presents similarly to infectious mononucleosis soon after starting immunosuppression. The second is also a polyclonal B cell proliferation that presents similarly to the first, but histologically has evidence of early malignant transformation. The third is a monoclonal B cell proliferation with malignant cytogenetic abnormalities that often presents with extranodal involvement.[4]

If this gentleman presented with a sudden onset headache, what would you be concerned about?

Subarachnoid haemorrhage from a berry aneurysm – a known association with ADPKD.

Other than PTLD, what other post transplant condition is this gentleman at risk of?

Post transplant diabetes mellitus is now a well recognized complication, which contributes to increased risk of infection and cardiovascular disease.[5]

References

1. Green M et al. Guidelines for the prevention and management of infectious complications of solid organ transplantation. *Am J Transplant* 2004; 4(Suppl)**10**:51.

2. Caillard S et al. Post-transplant lymphoproliferative disorders occurring after renal transplantation in adults: report of 230 cases from the French registry. *Am J Transplant* 2006; **6**(11):2735–42.

3. Smith JM et al. Risk of lymphoma after renal transplantation varies with time: an analysis of the United States Renal Data System. *Transplantation* 2006; **81**(2):175–80.

4. Nalesnik MA et al. The pathology of posttransplant lymphoproliferative disorders occurring in the setting of cyclosporine A-prednisone immunosuppression. *Am J Pathol* 1988; **133**(1):173–92.

5. Heisel O et al. New onset diabetes mellitus in patients receiving calcineurin inhibitors: a systematic review and meta-analysis. *Am J Transplant* 2004; **4**(4):583–95.

Case 15: 'Difficult' case

> **History (key points to elicit in 25 minutes)**
>
> Mr Frank Schneider.
> 78 years old.
> From Dublin.

On approaching and introducing yourself to Mr Schneider, it is immediately evident that he is unable speak clearly, but is alert, engaging and smiling.

A situation like this on the examination requires that you remain calm, assess the degree of impairment of communication and understanding in the patient, and assess patient comfort and safety.

'Mr Schneider I can see that you are having difficulty talking. Are you uncomfortable or in pain at the moment? Please nod or shake your head if you understand. Ok. As you may be aware, I need to ask you a few questions as part of my membership exam. I'll keep them simple and just nod or shake your head in response. Is that OK?'

Establish the patient's understanding

'Just before we start, I would like to ask you to follow a couple of simple instructions: Could you pick up the glass on your bedside?

Would you mind pointing to my tie with your right hand? Great.'

❶ Top Tips

- In the highly unlikely event that a patient is unable to give an adequate history, has significant dysphasia, or is confused, it is once again important to have a logical approach.
- Rarely, a case such as this is given to a candidate to assess their approach in a seemingly unfair, but also realistic scenario.
- It is fair to obtain a collateral history if available.
- If you genuinely feel that the case is inappropriate or that a patient is too unwell to continue, contact an invigilator.
- Establish the patient's understanding before starting to take the history.
- Reassure the patient intermittently during your history taking and examination that they are being helpful.

HPC

(Helpful questions to ask in this situation; each can be answered non-verbally).

- Did you come into hospital recently?
- Were you able to speak normally before you came into hospital?

- Did you suddenly lose the ability to speak?
- Did you wake up in the morning like this?
- Did it suddenly happen during the day?
- Was someone with you when this happened?
- Did you develop a headache?
- Any loss of vision?
- Any loss of muscle strength or sensation?
- Did you lose consciousness?
- Has this ever happened before?
- Were you doing fairly well before this event (establish baseline)?
- I would like to ask a few more questions regarding how you were before you came into hospital:
    - Were you able to walk normally?
    - Did you have any problems with your arms? If not, then ask more specific questions e.g. regarding specific actions such as writing, doing up a button or picking up a coin; these functions can also be examined.

PMHx
Ask about:
- Hypertension
- Hypercholesterolaemia
- Stroke/TIA
- Diabetes
- Myocardial infarction
- Atrial fibrillation.

Medications
- If available, look at the drug chart, but otherwise do not waste valuable time trying to get a detailed medication history.
- No drug allergies.

SHx
- Married, wife 'not well'
- Patient used to care for his wife
- Retired
- Smoker
- No alcohol
- Activities of daily living as above.

FHx
- Has this happened to anyone else in your family?

ROS
Ask directed questions, but do not waste too much time here if you have a reasonable idea as to the diagnosis. As this gentleman may have other cardiovascular pathology, be sure to ask about angina and claudication.

> **❶ Top Tips**
>
> - Remember that your examiner will be aware of the situation, therefore may not expect a very detailed history.
> - Does he have a carer (wife)?
> - Is the carer capable of looking after him? (Is she healthy?)

Hospital course as per patient

- Blood tests
- CT brain
- Carotid duplex
- Echocardiogram.

Examination (10–12 minutes)

For detailed examination → p.640 and Neurology, p. 287.

> **Specific examination points**
>
> - *General:*
>   - BP
>   - Note dominant hand
>   - Nutritional status
>   - Facial asymmetry; if present look for sparing of frontalis muscles indicating upper motor neuron pathology
>   - Obvious flexion/spastic posture
>   - Note wheelchair/walking aid
> - *CNS:*
>   - Examine all cranial nerves
>   - Carefully assess for hemianopias or diplopia
>   - Assess speech (Please → p.316 formal assessment of speech disorders)
>   - Assess cerebellar function
> - *PNS:*
>   - Tone, power, sensation, coordination and reflexes in 4 limbs
>   - Assess gait if feasible
> - *Fundoscopy:*
>   - Hypertensive retinopathy
>   - Diabetic retinopathy
>   - Ischaemic retina
>   - Optic atrophy (unilateral may indicate ischaemic aetiology)
> - *Cardiovascular:*
>   - Scars – median sternotomy and venous harvesting
>   - Pulse for atrial fibrillation
>   - Carotid bruits
>   - Cardiac murmurs
>   - Peripheral pulses
> - *Abdomen:*
>   - AAA
>   - Renal bruits.

❶ Top Tips

- The examination in this particular case will depend on clear instructions and good communication.
- Be logical – if a patient has receptive dysphasia (which should be apparent by this stage of the examination), then asking them to follow instructions such as eye movements or finger–nose testing may be a futile exercise.
- In such cases, passive examination such as observation of asymmetry, tone and reflexes will be much more helpful.

Summary

Mr Schneider is a 78-year-old gentleman from Dublin who presented recently with expressive dysphasia. Please note that this made the history challenging and I was unable to obtain a collateral account.

Mr Schneider was relatively well until the day he presented to hospital. He woke and found himself unable to speak properly and markedly weak on the right side of his body. His wife was with him at the time and she contacted the ambulance. He never lost consciousness, however he did have a headache and his vision was worse on the right side. He has never had symptoms like this before.

He has a history of hypertension and hypercholesterolaemia. He has no history of atrial fibrillation or stroke. I was unable to obtain a medication history from him today. Mr Schneider lives with his wife, who is in poor health, in a 2-storey house. Up until this admission he has been the primary carer for his wife. They only have a shower upstairs and do not have a stairlift, which means that social services and occupational health input will be very important. Prior to this incident, he was independent in ADLs.

On examination, Mr Schneider is right-handed, alert, oriented and was fully cooperative with the examination. Positive central neurological findings included an obvious expressive dysphasia with intact sensory component, right homonymous hemianopia and right-sided neglect. Positive peripheral neurological findings included hypertonia and hyper-reflexia on the right arm and leg, and right-sided hemiplegia with preserved sensory function. He has an upgoing right plantar. His coordination was impaired by his motor weakness on the right; however there was no apparent cerebellar dysfunction.

Differential diagnosis

- Left-sided (dominant) middle cerebral artery embolic stroke specifically involving the posterior inferior frontal gyrus (Broca's area)
- Left-sided (dominant) cerebral haemorrhage
- Cerebral neoplasm.

Investigations

- *Blood:* FBC, U&E, LFT, coagulation profile, ESR, CRP, fasting lipids, random blood glucose, treponemal serology
- *Radiology:* CT brain ± MRI brain, carotid duplex, CXR
- *Others:* ECG, echocardiogram.

Management

The onset of symptoms and time of presentation will greatly affect the management of acute stroke. Please refer to → p.334.

Viva questions

What do you know about global aphasia?

Global aphasia is a deficit in all aspects of language, and usually results in a person being mute and unable to follow commands. This results from large injury to the perisylvian area, affecting both Broca's and Wernicke's area, and often has an associated right-sided motor deficit and right-sided visual field defect with sparing of the macula.[1]

How would you assess a patients' cognitive status?

The Mini-Mental State Examination (MMSE) is a widely used and accepted test of cognition. It takes approximately 7 minutes to perform and tests areas including orientation, recall, language and constructional praxis. A score of <24/30 indicates dementia (or delerium), which in a large population based study gave a sensitivity of 87% and a specificity of 82%.[2]

What is the role of thrombolysis in the treatment of acute stroke?

Alteplase (tPA) is currently the only therapy for acute ischaemic stroke which is approved by the US food and drug administration and the European Union. As per results from the NINDS trial, treatment needs to be initiated within 3 hours of symptom onset, or within 3 hours of when the patient was last seen to be normal in cases which the onset time is unknown. Patients receiving tPA must fulfill inclusion and exclusion criteria, and may benefit from a significant 3-month functional outcome. Overall mortality did not vary between placebo and treatment groups in the trial, despite a 10-fold increase in symptomatic intracranial haemorrhage in the thrombolysis group.[3]

What do you know about thrombolysis between 3–4.5 hours after acute ischaemic stroke?

The benefit of using IV alteplase after the typical '3-hour window' (NINDS trial) was examined in the ECASS 3 trial. Results showed a modest but significant improvement in three month functional outcomes, with risk of symptomatic intracranial haemorrhage being similar to that in the 0–3-hour treatment trials. Though there was a short-term improvement in morbidity, overall mortality did not significantly change (also shown in 0–3-hour trials). It is important to note, however, that the ECASS 3 trial had more exclusion criteria compared to the NINDS trial, such as >80 years of age, NIHSS (National Institutes of Health Stroke Scale) >25, any anticoagulant use regardless of INR, and previous combination of stroke and diabetes.[4]

References

1. Hillis AE. Aphasia: progress in the last quarter of a century. *Neurology* 2007; **69**(2):200–13.
2. Crum RM et al. Population-based norms for the Mini-Mental State Examination by age and educational level. *JAMA* 1993; **269**(18):2386–91.
3. The National Institute of Neurological Disorders and Stroke rt-PA Stroke Study Group. Tissue plasminogen activator for acute ischemic stroke. *NEJM* 1995; **333**(24):1581–7.
4. Hacke W et al. Thrombolysis with alteplase 3 to 4.5 hours after acute ischemic stroke. *NEJM* 2008; **359**(13):1317–29.

Index